Illustrated Guide to Injectable Fillers

Basics | Indications | Uses

A CIP record for this book is available from the British Library

ISBN-13: 978-1-85097-251-8

QUINTESSENCE PUBLISHING

Quintessence Publishing Co, Ltd
Quintessence House
Grafton Road, New Malden, Surrey KT3 3AB
United Kingdom
www.quintpub.co.uk

Translated, revised and extended version (1. edition)

Important note:
As with every other science, medicine is subject to constant development. Research and clinical experience widen our knowledge base, particularly with regard to treatment modalities. If any dosages or methods of administration are mentioned in this book, the reader may have confidence that the authors, editors and publishers have taken great care to ensure that this information is in line with the latest knowledge available at the time of publication.

However, the publisher cannot give guarantees for any information regarding the filler choices, dosing instructions, and methods of administration. All users are requested to take great care to check the package insert leaflets of the products used and to consult the manufacturer/distributer, if necessary, to establish whether the recommendations or details of contraindications given therein differ in any way from the information provided in this book. This sort of check is particularly important with rare indications, treatment areas, or with minimally used or recently launched products. The use of any medication dose or method of administration takes place at the user's own risk. The authors and publisher appeal to all users to inform them if they spot any obvious inaccuracies.

Project management: Marie Bühler, Köln
Layout and typesetting: Gay & Sender, Bremen
Photos: Sixten Hofmann, Marburg; Stephan Ziehen, Hamburg; Marcus Karsten, Leipzig; Gerhard Sattler, Darmstadt
Editorial Chapter 4: Marcus Karsten, Leipzig
Graphics: Karl Wesker, David Kühn, Berlin
Production: Quintessenz Verlags-GmbH, Berlin
Printing: Drukarnia Dimograf, Bielsko-Biała/Poland

Printed in Poland

Illustrated Guide to Injectable Fillers

Basics | Indications | Uses

Gerhard Sattler

Uliana Gout

QUINTESSENCE PUBLISHING

London, Berlin, Chicago, Tokyo, Barcelona, Beijing, Istanbul, Milan, Moscow,
New Delhi, Paris, Prague, São Paulo, Seoul, Singapore and Warsaw

The Authors

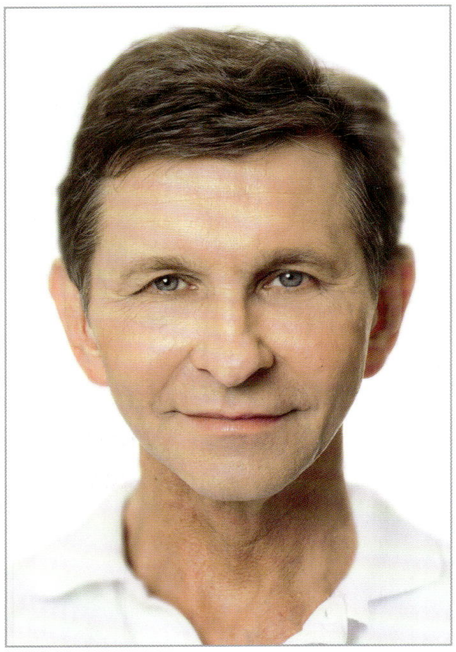

Dr Gerhard Sattler

is the President of the German Society of Aesthetic Surgery (Gesellschaft für Ästhetische Chirurgie Deutschland, GÄCD) and Executive Director of the International Society for Dermatologic Surgery, as well as being a member of numerous professional associations. He is also the Director of the Rosenpark Klinik, a leading aesthetic medicine and plastic surgery facility in Darmstadt, Germany.

Dr med Gerhard Sattler
Rosenpark Klinik
Heidelberger Landstraße 20
64297 Darmstadt
Germany

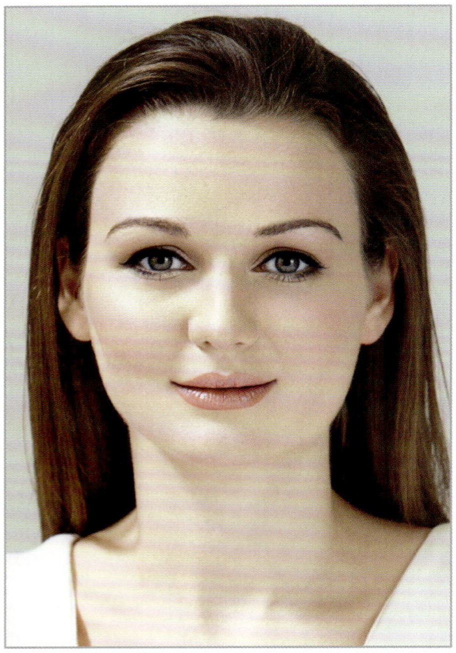

Dr Uliana Gout

is the Founder of London Aesthetic Medicine Services, London, offering clinical services as well as serving as an international training institution for non-surgical aesthetic medicine. Dr Gout is committed to developing the field of Aesthetic Medicine through evidence based medicine and is a regular speaker and educator on the international Aesthetic Medicine conference circuit, holding numerous advisory board, faculty and committee roles. Dr Gout is a Chairperson of the International Peeling Society and has also recently co-authored the *Illustrated Guide to Chemical Peels: Basics, Indications and Uses,* 2014, Quintessence Publishing Group.

London, United Kingdom
ug@london-aesthetic-medicine.com

Preface

We are proud to present to you the second edition of the *Illustrated Guide to Injectable Fillers*. To live up to the success of the first edition, this book is a combined knowledge base on classic augmentation techniques amassed during the initial period of volume augmentation, alongside the more recent innovative treatment approaches of the present.

We all appreciate the effects of ageing and the desire expressed by our patients to look fresh, youthful and healthy. This in turn has resulted in the demand to further understand how we as practitioners can satisfy our patients in a safe and effective manner. Importantly, today we see patients being drawn to non-surgical rejuvenation options. Minimally invasive procedures, which can be used to restore harmonious proportions while protecting the tissues, are currently at the focus of modern beauty-enhancing treatment concepts. Furthermore, patients are now seeking subtle, continuous natural improvements, rather than sudden dramatic changes. We believe this can only be met by a procedure that respects anatomy, individual beauty and treats the direct causes of the time-related signs of ageing.

This second edition therefore focuses on the latest understanding of facial attractiveness and its loss with time, the possibilities offered with the most up-to-date protective harmonising procedures, and the newer approaches with hyaluronic acid fillers to manage the causal elements of ageing.

The three key concepts of modern anti-ageing medicine, namely 'protection, restoration and proportionality' form the basis of volumetric rejuvenation with water-binding hyaluronic acid therapy. Today, with newly discovered anatomical findings and experience over the last decade or so with hyaluronic acid fillers, we now understand how to use fillers to correct the prime causes of the visible ageing symptoms, rather than just masking them superficially in the short term. Such restorative interventions have proven to give reproducible clinical outcomes.

This book explores in great detail the variety of injection techniques available using both needles and cannulas, and discusses the indications suited to each technique. Two novel techniques are introduced, namely vertical and horizontal mobilisation, aimed at treating the causes of the visible signs of ageing.

Vertical injections used needles in the supraperiosteal or supramucosal base at the site of the volume deficit within deep subcutaneous fat have proven to be a particularly revolutionary technique. The use of vertical filler depots can achieve a maximum lifting effect with the minimal volume of filler used without producing unnatural overcorrection or material accumulation. This technique directly targets the volume deficit and restores it immediately. Once these bases of volume deficit have been restored, the structures that have collapsed above due to atrophy below will rise up again on their own without having to inject more superficially. After all, over the years we have noted the limited benefits of superficial injections, which only mask the underlying defect for the short term, and are associated with impending disproportionate collapse of the filler shortly after the injection into the soft tissues below and thus requiring further injections. Furthermore, superficial injections are also commonly associated with excessive volumisation.

Horizontal tissue mobilising techniques using cannulas are also considered a breakthrough in modern volume augmentation. This form of filler application is not merely a way of distributing the filler evenly over larger areas, but more importantly, the motion of the cannula releases the fibrotic structures atraumatically, to achieve optimal harmonisation and ensures the filler works effectively in line with facial dynamics. In fact, in some cases we shall discuss how the mechanical effects of the cannula alone, without any filler injection can achieve significant clinical improvement. Furthermore, we shall discuss the longer-term effects of such mechanical stimulation, namely with regard to the activation of fibrinogenic neocollagen and neoelastin synthesis, and the resultant physiological regeneration of the tissues.

Another key improvement in this second edition is the focus on the key concepts and strategies to full-face rejuvenation, with the view of achieving overall harmony. A series of case studies document the before and after effects of the techniques outlined, to showcase to the reader the clinical outcomes achievable. Furthermore, extensive supporting anatomical drawings alongside the numerous videos have been created for the reader to allow them to visualise the injection techniques described. The video demonstrations can be easily accessed via the web link provided or by using the QR-code on a smartphone, and viewed while leafing through the book. In due course, a DVD containing the complete video collection will also become available as an accompaniment to the book. We hope this interactive method of teaching proves successful with our readers.

Our hope is that the extensive combination of written text, graphic illustrations, clinical photography and videos help the reader to learn the skills required and enable them to be applied directly.

We hope our readers enjoy this book and find it a useful tool to ensure our patients continue to receive the latest effective treatments. In these endeavours, we wish you much success and many happy patients!

Acknowledgements

I would like to thank many people, without whom the hard work needed to extend and improve the first edition of this book would not have been possible. Let me start with those who supported us with the first edition: thanks are owed to Mr Marcus Kasten (photographer; Leipzig University Hospital, Leipzig, Germany) for his editorial suggestions on the photographic case documentation series, to Mr Peter Lebovitz (Canfield Imaging Systems, Fairfield) for his valuable help in the 3D photo documentation section and to Sixten Hofman for producing the photographs.

Thanks also to Prof Friedrich Anderhuber MD (Institute of Anatomy, Medical University of Graz, Austria) and Dr Ulrike Pilsl MD (Institute of Anatomy, Medical University of Graz, Austria) for their support in preparing the anatomical drawings. Furthermore, my most profound thanks goes to the two illustrators, Karl Wesker and David Kühn (of the publishers KVM – Der Medizinverlag), who have now also brought this book to life with their magnificent drawings and graphics.

In addition, I wish to thank my whole family, especially my wife Sonja, as well as the entire team at the Rosenpark Clinic. Very special thanks must go to Ms Susanne Bernard, who actively supported this project at all times with her tireless commitment, and without whom the revision of this book would not have been possible.

Darmstadt, December 2015
Gerhard Sattler

Table of Contents

Abbreviations and Symbols

The following abbreviations are used in this book:

A./Aa.	Artery/Arteries
cm	centimetre
Lig./Ligg.	Ligament/Ligaments
M./Mm.	Muscle/Muscles
mg	milligram
ml	millilitre
mm	millimetre
N./Nn.	Nerve/Nerves
Proc.	Processus
R./Rr.	Ramus/Rami
ROOF	Retro-orbicularis oculi fat
SMAS	Superficial musculo-aponeurotic system
SOOF	Sub-orbicularis oculi fat
→	direction of motion

Abbreviations and symbols:

HAK	Horizontal Augmentation with a Cannula
SSRA	Skin Surface Regenerating Augmentation
MIAS	Minimally Invasive Augmentation Surgery
SAT	Superficial Augmentation Techniques
SHAC	Superficial Horizontal Augmentation with a Cannula
DHAC	Deep Horizontal Augmentation with a Cannula
TT	Tower Technique
VAT	Vertical Augmentation Techniques
VSDT	Vertical Supraperiosteal Depot Technique

	Injection point, insertion site
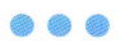	Point technique
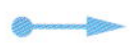	Linear technique, tunneling technique
	Vertical Supraperiosteal Depot Technique (VSDT)
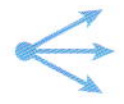	Horizontal Augmentation with a Cannula (HAC)
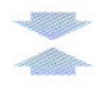	Compression technique
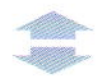	Stretching technique
	Injection volume, superficially (intradermally, subdermally) applied
	Injection volume, deeply (subcutaneously, supraperiosteally) applied
	Injection area (SHAC)
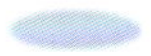	Injection area (DHAC)
	Windmill technique

1 The Skin

(Chapter written by U. Paasch)

1 The Skin

1.1 Structure and Function of the Skin

The skin is the largest organ in the human body. Its core function is to provide a protective barrier, by encasing all of the body's core structures. It is known as the **integument** *(integumentum commune)*.

In addition to being a purely mechanical barrier and providing UV protection, the skin also plays an important role in thermoregulation and water homeostasis. This structure also allows for direct communication with the outside world. For this reason, skin takes on many and varied functions involving the conduction of stimuli, which in turn inform us of the state of our surrounding environment. Furthermore, the skin performs a crucial role in preventing pathogens entering the body. In this context, it has evolved a variety of immunological activities. A diverse architecture of cellular and acellular components forms the basis of this complex range of functions.

With regard to the basic structure of this organ, the true upper skin or epidermis is of ectodermal origin, whereas the dermis (also known as corium) is of mesodermal origin. The basal membrane represents the link between these two structures, and is also known as the junction zone or interface. Below the dermis lies the subcutaneous tissue or subcutis, made up of adipose tissue.

Although the fundamental structure of skin is the same in all humans, there are significant differences in the epidermal architecture of the face between different genders and ethnicities. These are apparent in the form of differences in the size and number of pores, water content and elasticity (see image below).

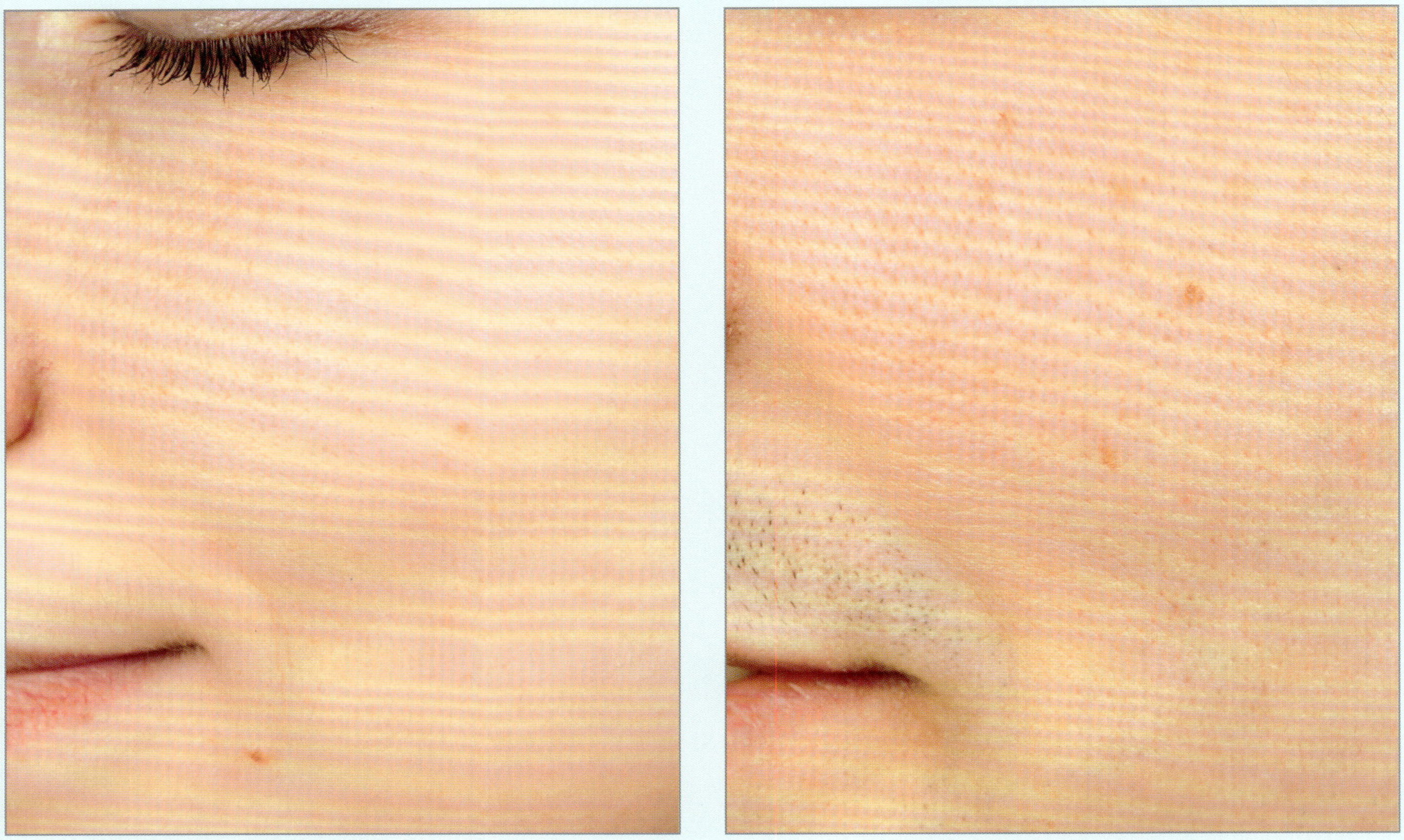

Fig. 1.1 Significant differences in the epidermal architecture of the skin of the face between different genders (female on the left, male on the right) and ethnicities. These are apparent in the form of differences in the size and number of pores, water content and elasticity.

1.1.1 The epidermis

The multi-layered epidermis is the outermost layer of the skin, and around 95 % of it is made up of keratinocytes. During their differentiation process, the keratinocytes migrate through all the layers of the epidermis until they reach the surface. Once there, having been transformed into corneocytes, they represent the skin's outermost boundary, the horny layer, and are eventually rejected. Accordingly, the various cells of the epidermis merely represent the various differentiation stages of a single cell type over a period of some 26–42 days, until they are rejected as dead skin cells.

The epidermis exerts its protective barrier function via its horny layer (stratum corneum). Nails, hair, sebaceous glands and sweat glands form its integral appendages.

Structure and function of the epidermis

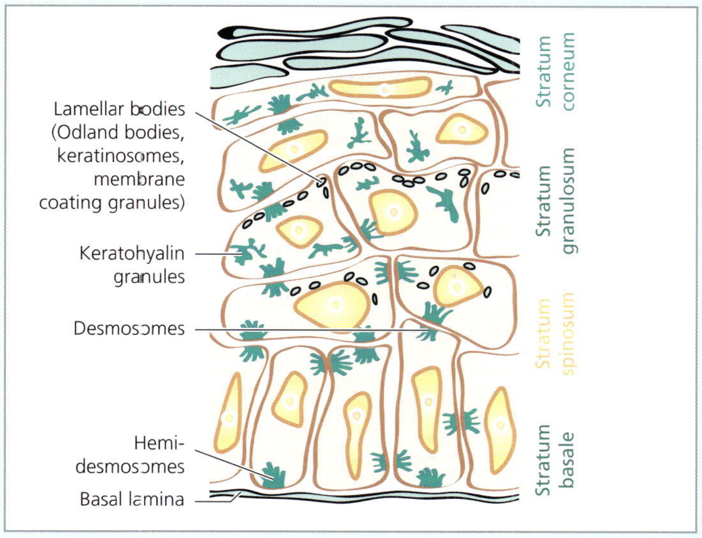

Fig. 1.2 Schematic structure of the skin. At the level of the stratum granulosum, the alignment of the keratinocytes changes into the regular, columnar structure of the horny layer through differentiation. With a diameter of c. 30 µm, the keratinocytes are among the largest cells of the human body. Adhesion organelles *(desmosomes, maculae adhaerentes)* and intermediate junctions *(zonulae adhaerentes)* mediate the bonding of the keratinocytes to each other and to the basal membrane (hemidesmosomes).

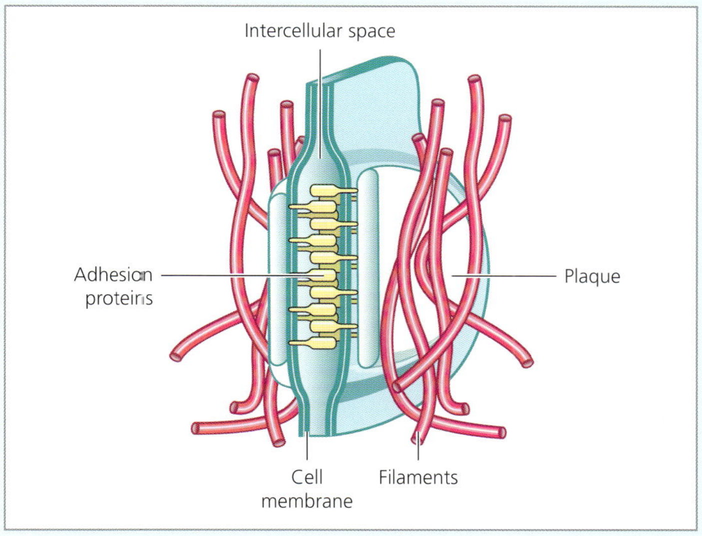

Fig. 1.3 Adhesion organelles mediate cell contact and cohesion. They are not static structures. Their constant generation and degeneration enables cell migration. The prickly appearance of the stratum spinosum is due to the fact that the cells shrink, but cannot detach themselves from the desmosomes. There are also communication channels, known as gap junctions.

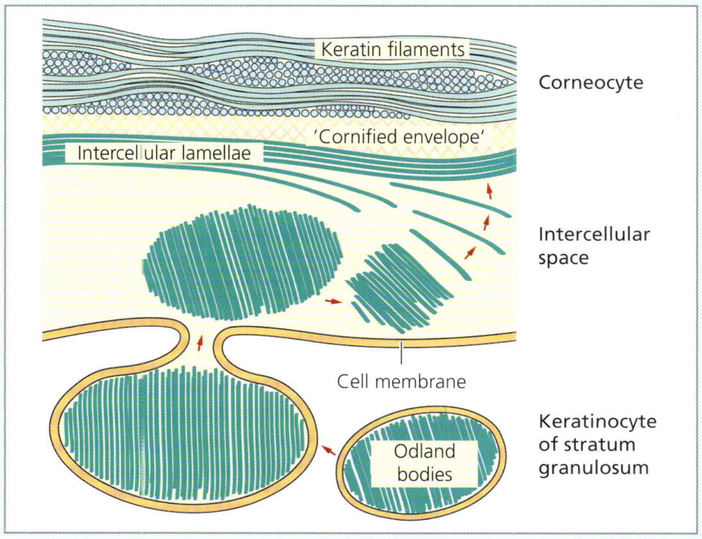

Fig. 1.4 Formation of lipid cement. The key differentiation stage of the keratinocytes occurs in the stratum granulosum. As the cell nucleus and organelles degenerate, what occurs is not just a morphological change into a hexagonal corneocyte. With dehydration, the cement-like lipid substance in the intercellular space and the cornified envelope is formed on the plasma membrane. The covalently bound envelope is juxtaposed onto this. Bound directly to the barrier lipid, this structure achieves considerable chemical resistance to alkalis, detergents or reducing substances, but not to proteolytic agents.

1

Structure and function of the epidermis

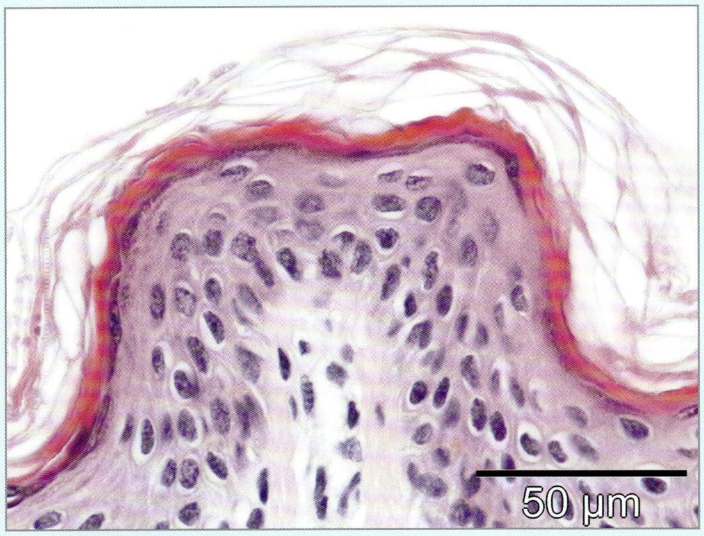

Fig. 1.5 Basket-weave orthokeratosis is characteristic of clinically smooth, non-flaky skin. The stratum lucidum can be seen immediately below this (HE 60×). The keratinocytes mature within 26–42 days, losing their cell nucleus. Two types of symbiotic dendrite cell are also found in the epidermis: the melanocytes in the basal layer and the Langerhans cells suprabasally.

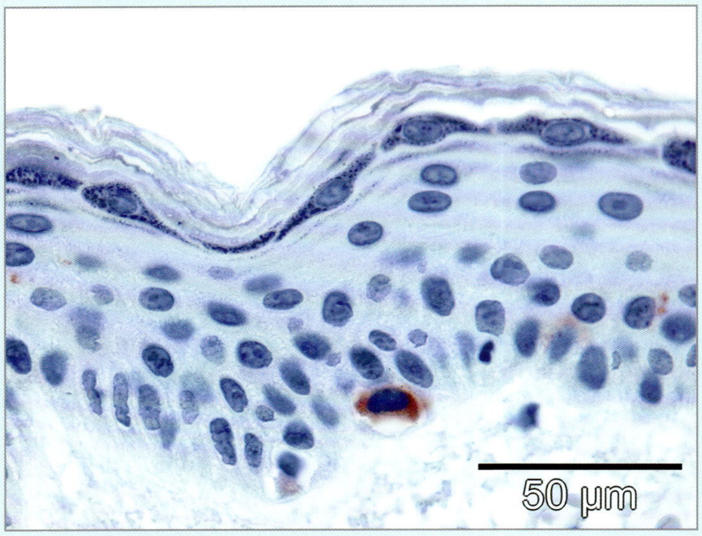

Fig. 1.6 Melanocytes are located between the basal keratinocytes in the epidermis (S100, 100×; melanocyte marked in red) and take on an important protective function by producing melanin and supplying it to the neighbouring keratinocytes. Each melanocyte makes contact with c. 30 keratinocytes.

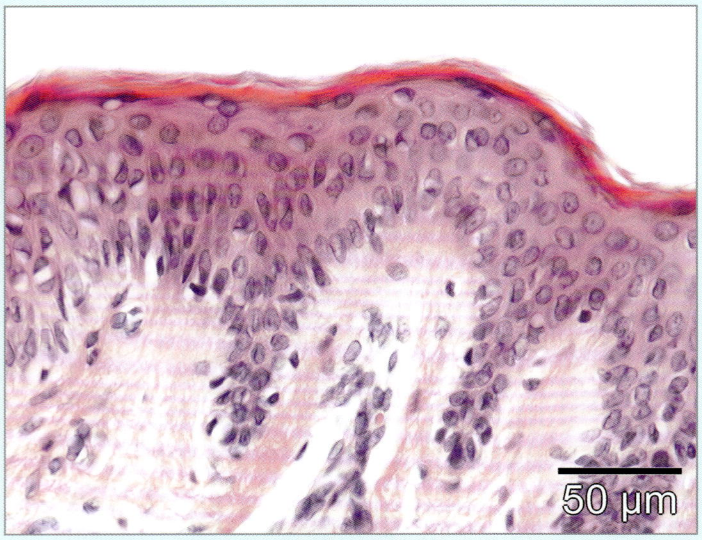

Fig. 1.7 Keratinocytes form four layers. The stratum basale forms the bottom layer of the epidermis and rests on the basal membrane. Above it is the stratum spinosum (prickle cell layer), followed by the stratum granulosum (granular layer). This is followed by a thin layer, the stratum lucidum, which shows strong eosinophilic staining. Lying uppermost is the stratum corneum (HE 60×).

Structure and function of the epidermis

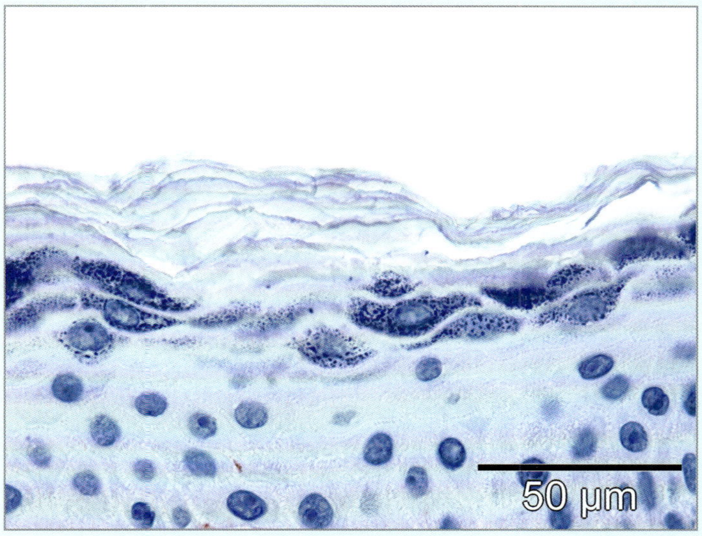

Fig. 1.8 Epidermal thickness (~0.1 mm) depends on its anatomical location and the mechanical stress on the skin. The granular cell layer (Hemalaun, 100×) in particular can vary in thickness, the granules being precursors of the keratin filaments, which make up the stratum corneum. The thickness of the skin without the subcutaneous fat varies regionally between 1.5 and 4.0 mm.

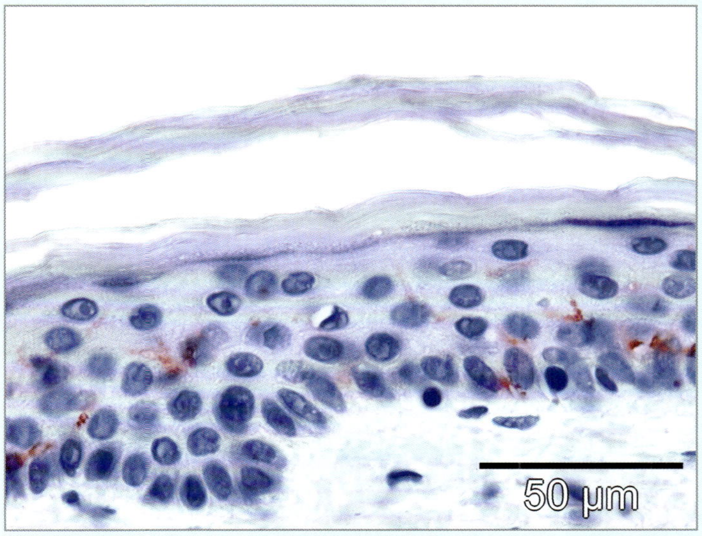

Fig. 1.9 Dendritic Langerhans cells can be found scattered in the suprabasal region of the epidermis (S100/Hemalaun, 100×). They occur in approximately the same numbers as the melanocytes and act as antigen-presenting cells. In addition, Merkel cells, which act as mechanoreceptors, can be found in considerably smaller numbers in the region of the hair follicles and the oral mucosa.

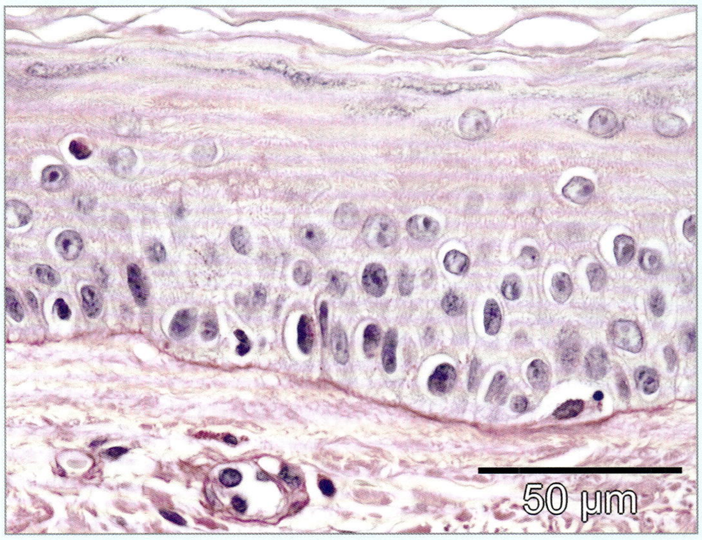

Fig. 1.10 A single row of cuboid cells fixed in place by hemidesmosomes rests on the basal membrane. The basal membrane shows up as PAS-positive (PAS 100×). Optimal interlocking between the two regions of the skin is ensured by the shape of the papillae. Regularly elongated rete ridges are found under normal physiological conditions. The upper squamous epithelium is made up of polygonal cells.

Structure and function of the epidermis

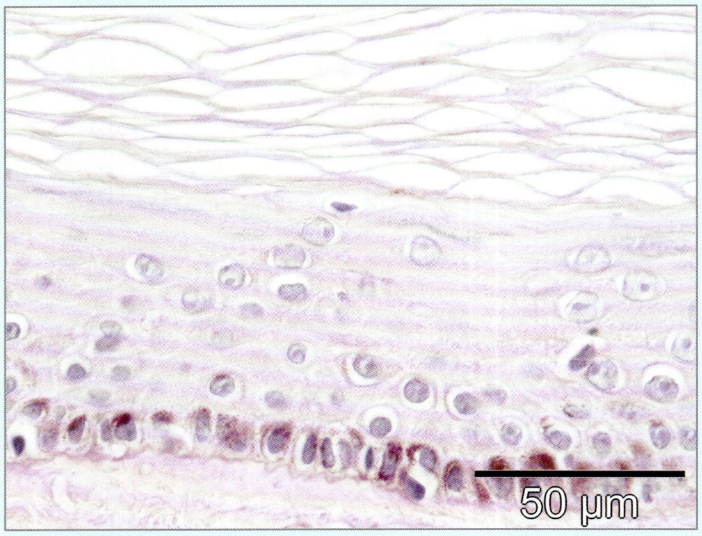

Fig. 1.11 Basal keratinocytes are pigmented in pale skin types. Melanin is only detectable in the upper epidermal layers in dark skin (PAS 100×).

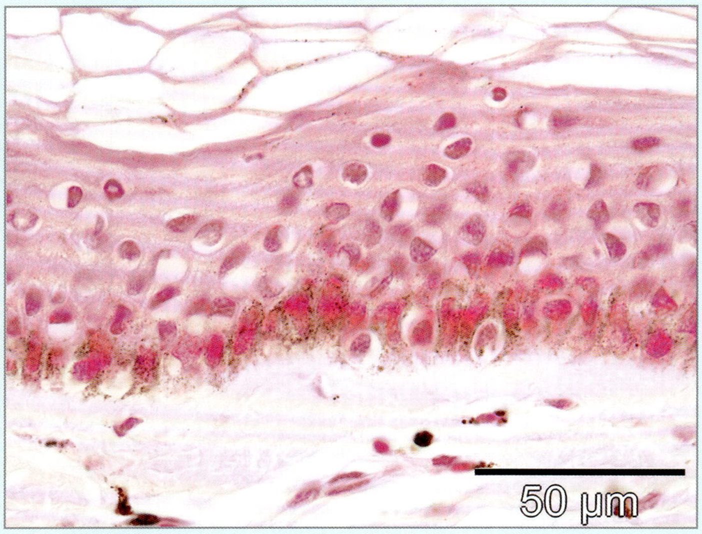

Fig. 1.12 Excess melanin 'leaks' or 'drips' downwards, especially following inflammation, and is stored by melanophages (Masson-Fontana 100×). Melanin located in the epidermis and dermis leads to visible pigmentary shifts.

1

1.1.2 The dermis

The dermis *(corium)* is a highly elastic, tear-resistant tissue, consisting mainly of fibrocytes, fibroblasts, collagen and elastin, all embedded into the extracellular matrix. The visible changes of skin ageing primarily affect this layer of the skin, which is also interspersed with nerves, blood vessels and lymphatic vessels. Appendages, also known as adnexal structures, are embedded in the dermis.

The dermis is known to vary somewhat in its constitution and levels activity according to skin type. Of interest, the dermis of black skin contains more fibres (which are also thicker), shows higher biosynthetic activity, has more vessels in the upper plexus as well as mixed apoeccrine sweat glands. Figure 1.13 shows the thick bundles of collagenous fibres in young skin. A fibroblast cell nucleus lies in the centre of the image (HE 100×; see Fig. 1.13).

Skin appendages

Skin appendages (adnexal organs) consist of hair roots, nails, sweat glands and sebaceous glands and are found deep in the dermis. Although they are located in the dermis, the skin appendages are of epidermal origin. A sebaceous gland consists of one or more lobes with a single duct, which releases the sebum along the hair follicle and onto the epidermis. The sebaceous glands vary in size, but this is not associated with hair thickness. In the face, they are particularly large in association with the vellus hairs. The periphery of the gland is made up of cuboid cells, which are eventually secreted into the central duct by holocrine secretion. Sebaceous glands are fully formed at birth.

Hair and fingernails

At any one time, approximately 84 % of the hairs on the head are in the anagen phase, 2 % in the catagen phase and 14 % in the telogen

Structure and function of the dermis

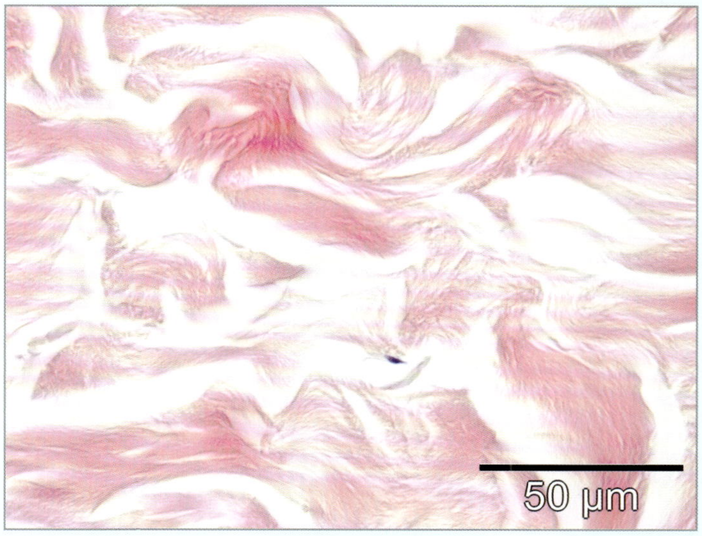

Fig. 1.13 The dermis is divided into the stratum papillare, which lies below the basal membrane, and above the underlying stratum reticulare. The papillary layer is made up of a fine network of collagenous fibres (type I and III) and elastic fibres in an ample matrix. In addition to the elastic fibres, the stratum reticulare consists of thick bundles of collagen type I fibres. The superficial and deep vascular plexuses, nerves, dermal cells and the matrix are also found here.

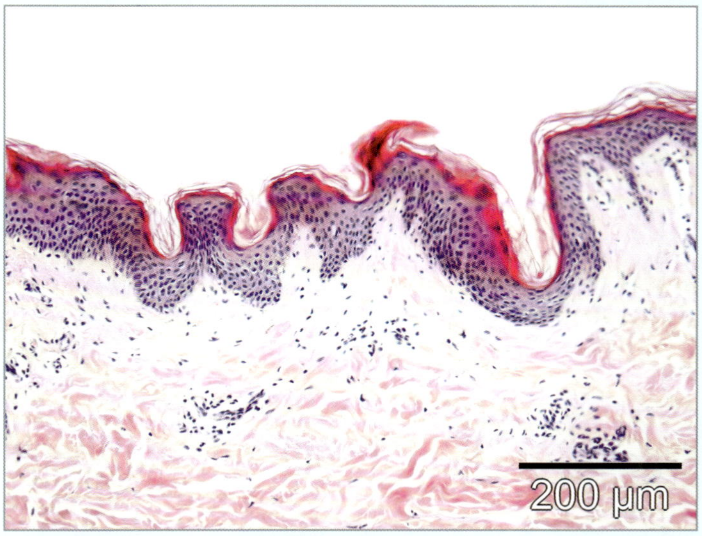

Fig. 1.14 Marked differences in connective tissue structure are apparent in the stratum reticulare and stratum papillare (HE 60×). Directly below the rete ridges, the fibres appear paler and thinner, with perpendicular alignment in places. Dermal fibroblasts produce the fibrils and the matrix. Histiocytes, mast cells and lymphocytes occur in small numbers.

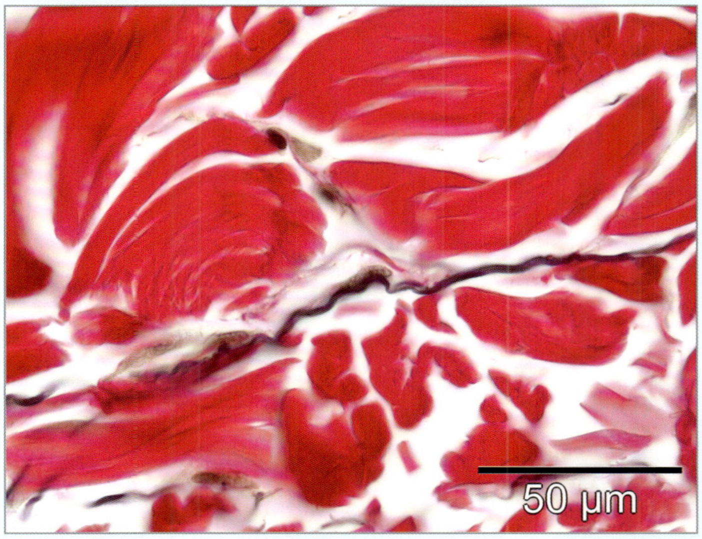

Fig. 1.15 Dermal tissue consists mainly of collagenous (red) and elastic (blackish-brown) fibres (Elastica van Giesson 100×). Collagen alone accounts for up to 70% of the dry weight. The interweaving fibrous architecture, together with the elastic fibres, gives the skin its elasticity. Between them is the matrix, consisting mainly of hyaluronic acid.

Structure and function of the dermis

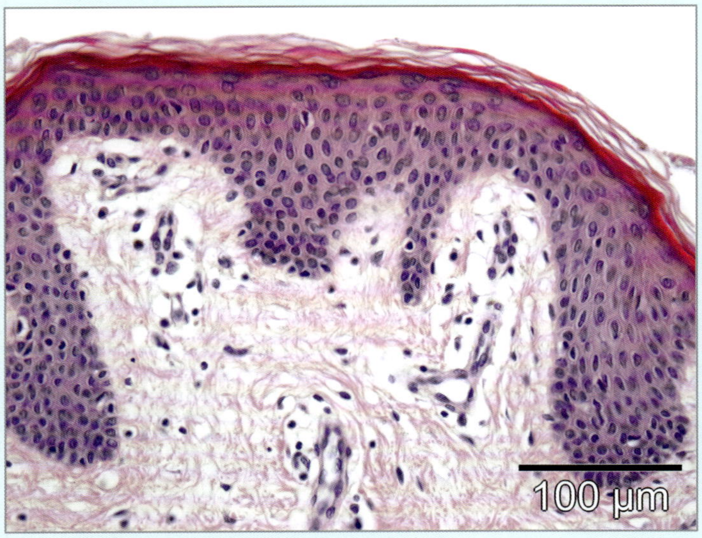

Fig. 1.16 Arterioles and venules can be found in the upper and lower vascular plexus of the skin. The superficially located sub-papillary plexus supplies the dermal papillae, the hair follicles and the eccrine glands (HE 40×).

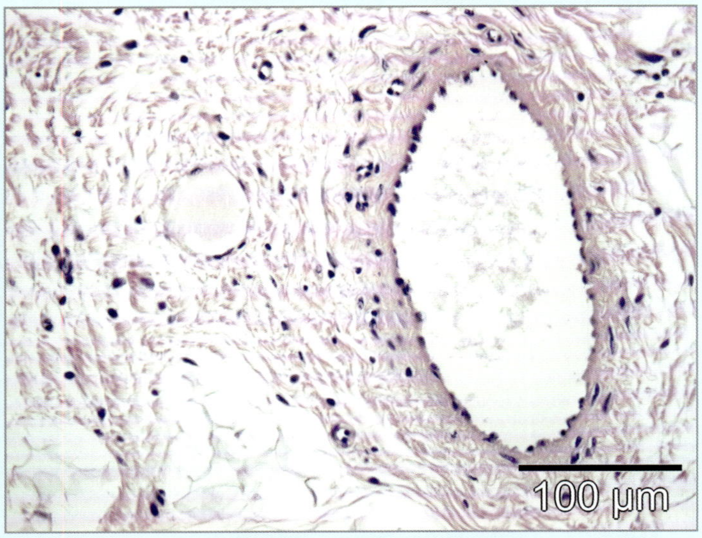

Fig. 1.17 The large arteries of the deep plexus ensure an optimal blood supply to the skin via the superficial plexus.

1

Skin appendages

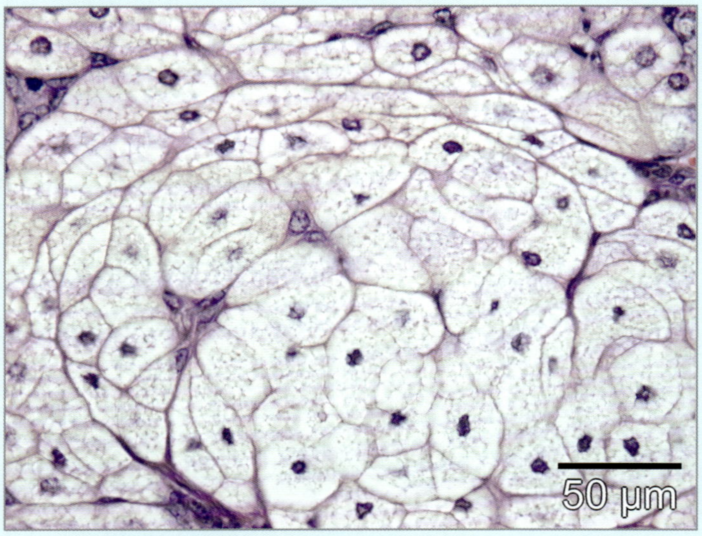

Fig. 1.18 Sebaceous glands (HE 60×) are important skin appendages, which develop from the epithelial buds of the hair follicles and therefore usually exist in association with hairs. They are thus found throughout the integument, with the exception of the palms of the hands and the soles of the feet. Sebaceous glands not associated with hair follicles occur around the areolae, the labia minora and the prepuce. The meibomian glands of the eyelids are modified sebaceous gland variants.

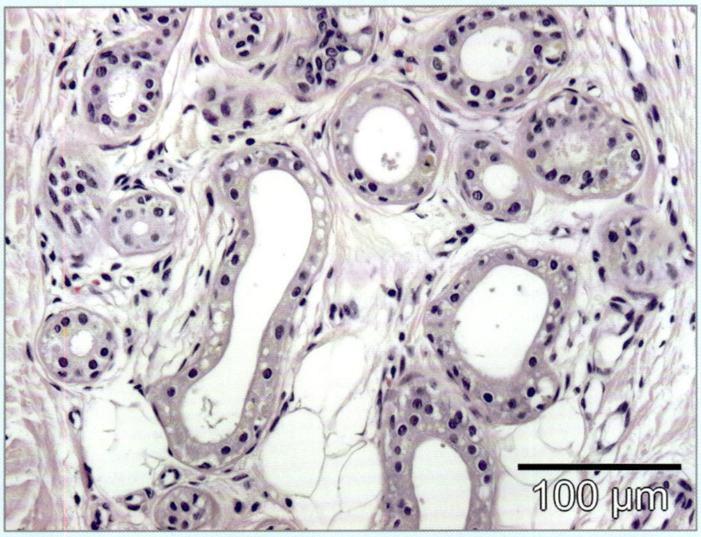

Fig. 1.19 Sweat glands occur in eccrine (sweat gland in the narrower sense) and apocrine (scent gland) from, and also in mixed form. Eccrine glands originate from the foetal epidermis and are therefore not associated with hair. They occur everywhere except on the mucous membranes and are responsible for thermoregulation. Apocrine glands originate from the follicular epithelium and are found predominantly in the axillae, on the areolae, the mons pubis, the labia minor, the prepuce, the scrotum and around the anus. They are in fact scent glands, and thus play an important role in the selection of sexual partners.

Hair and fingernails

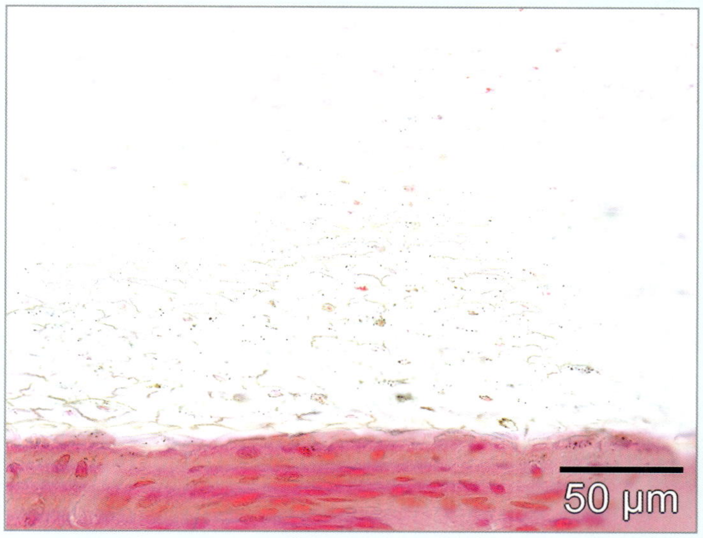

Fig. 1.20 Nails are appendages just like hair. The keratin of the nails becomes particularly hard and forms a nail plate which grows outwards from the nail bed. The nail is formed in the matrix (Masson-Fontana 60×).

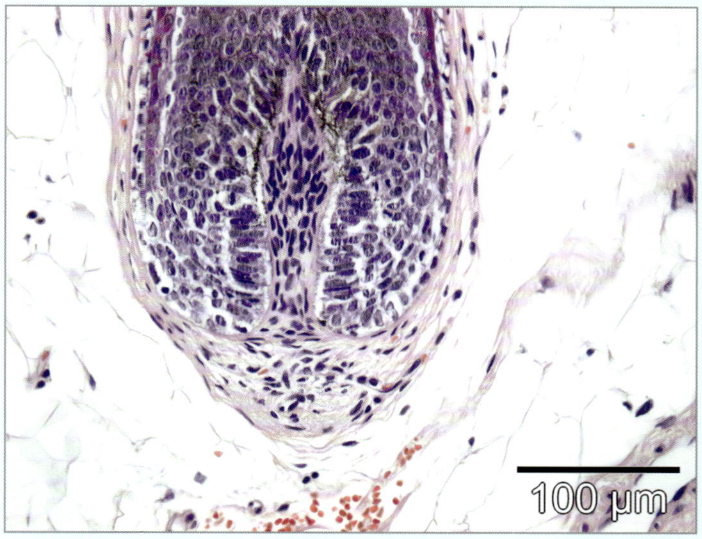

Fig. 1.21 The very fine vessels of the upper vascular plexus supply the hairs (HE 40×). The terminal hair papilla is of mesenchymal origin. It is located in the upper part of the subcutaneous tissue or in the deep dermis. The basophilic and often pigmented hair matrix surrounds the actual, centrally located papilla, whose stalk is fixed onto the underlying connective tissue bundle which surrounds the entire papilla. The suprabulbar zone begins immediately above the hair bulb.

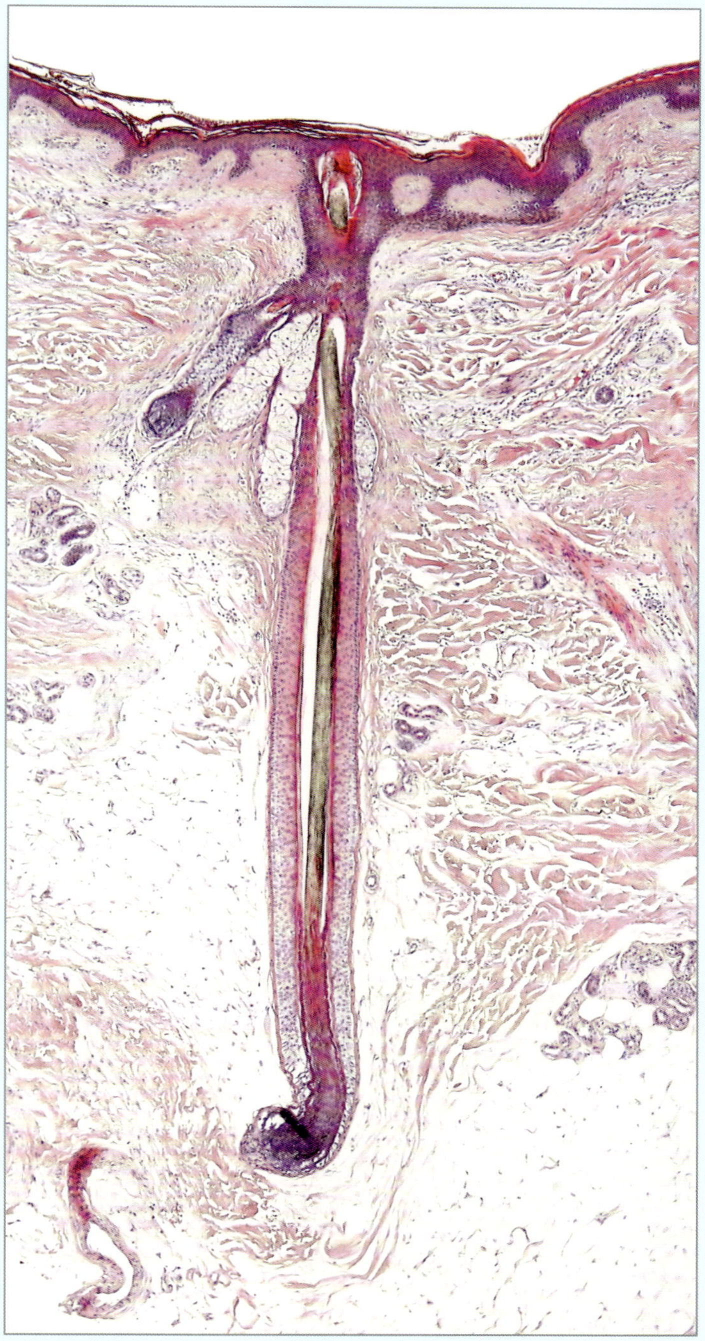

Fig. 1.22 Hair follicles originate from the basal keratinocytes. A hair is never found alone – the pilar unit always consists of a hair follicle, sebaceous gland and the erector pili muscle (HE 4×). The pilar unit is divided into three segments: infundibulum, isthmus and inferior segment. Hair growth follows a cycle consisting of growth (anagen phase, ~3 years), involution (catagen phase, 3 weeks) and the resting phase (telogen phase, ~3 months). Hair grows at an average rate of 0.4 mm per day.

Hair and fingernails

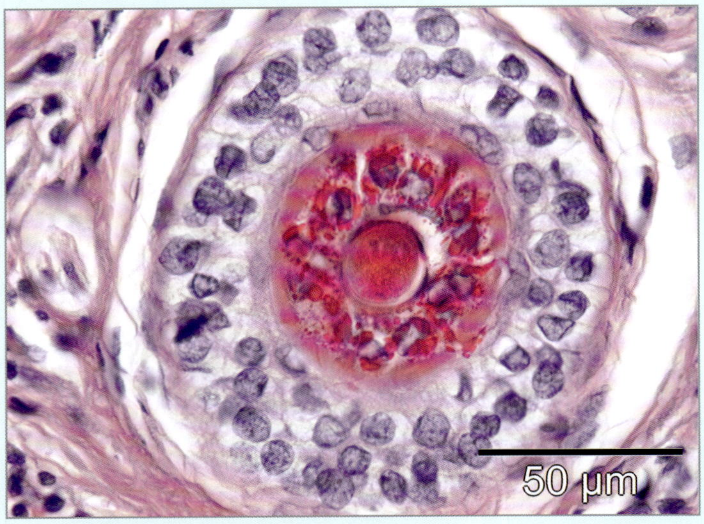

Fig. 1.23 Terminal hair in the anagen stage: transverse section through the suprabulbar region (HE 100×). Anagen, catagen and telogen hairs differ in structure and appearance. From the base upwards, anagen hairs are made up of the bulb, suprabulbar zone, isthmus and infundibulum.

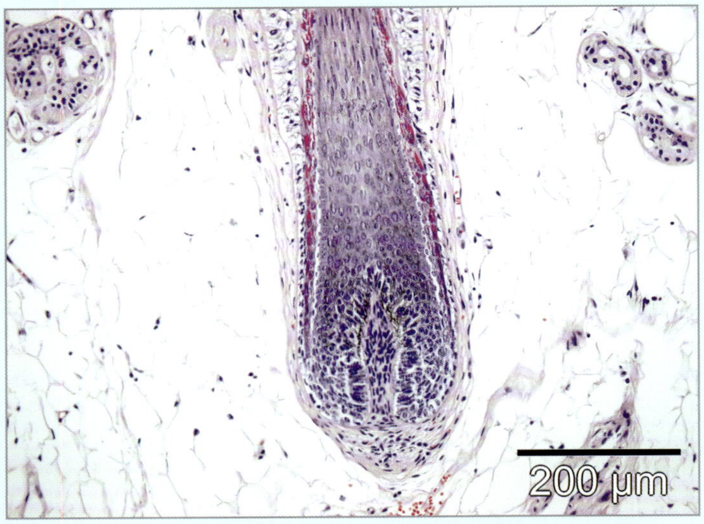

Fig. 1.24 The suprabulbar zone (HE 20×) above the papilla is made up of: the hair medulla, hair cortex, cuticle, inner root sheath (strong eosinophilic staining), outer root sheath (opaque cells), glassy membrane (eosinophilic staining) and the connective tissue sheath. The junction with the isthmus is marked by the insertion of the erector pili muscle. It ends at the opening of the sebaceous cell. The infundibulum lies above it.

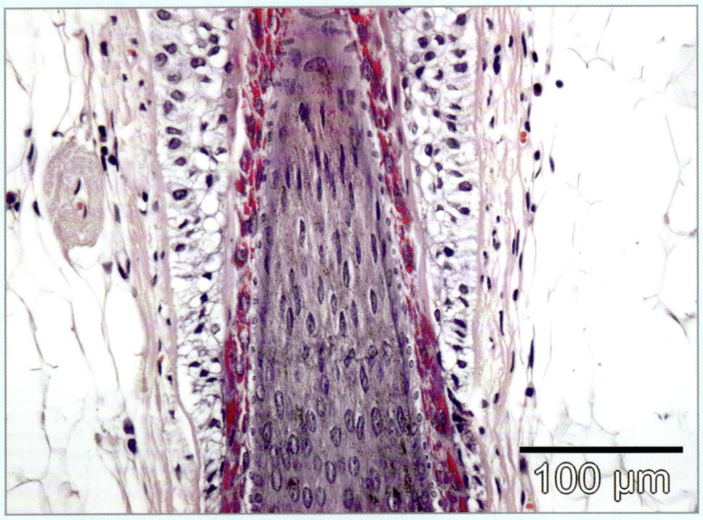

Fig. 1.25 Details of the suprabulbar zone (HE 40×) with the pigmented hair medulla, basophilic hair cortex, cuticle, inner root sheath (strong eosinophilic staining), outer root sheath (opaque cells with dark nuclei), glassy membrane (eosinophilic staining) and the connective tissue sheath located in the subcutaneous fat.

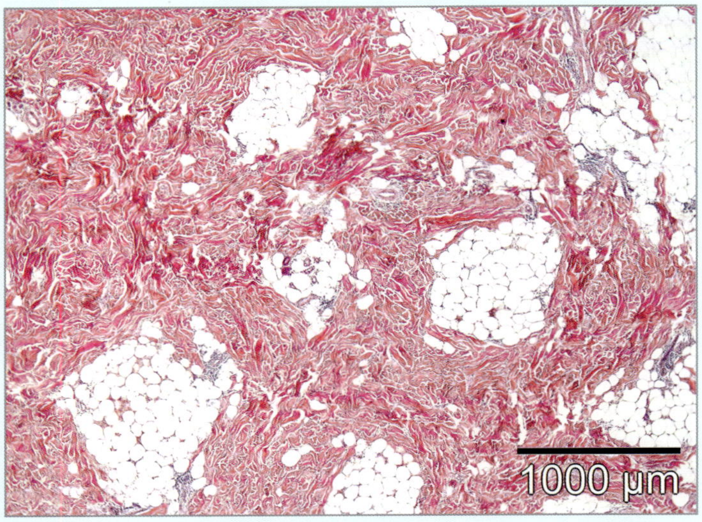

Fig. 1.26 Subcutis: the subcutaneous fat lies below the reticular dermis. In transverse section (HE 4×), one can see that, rather like the epidermis, it is anchored to the dermis by means of connective tissue septa.

phase. Most hair is pigmented. Hair colour is determined by the type of melanin granules present: erythromelanin in red hair, eumelanin in dark hair and phaeomelanin in blond hair. White hair is formed where there is a lack of melanin due to melanocyte inactivation following shedding. The appearance of grey hair occurs as a result of a mixture of pigmented and unpigmented terminal hairs.

1.1.3 The subcutaneous tissue

The subcutaneous tissue (subcutis, hypodermis, subcutaneous fat; see Fig. 1.26) is the deepest skin layer, varying in thickness from a few millimetres to several centimetres. Loose connective tissue divides the fat into clusters. The subcutaneous tissue is separated from the underlying tissues (e.g. muscles) by a fascia.

1.2 Skin Ageing

Ageing is a side effect of evolutionary imperfection. Human skin ages during the course of a lifetime. As the largest outer organ, it is directly exposed to all of the environmental influences throughout an individual's lifetime.

1.2.1 Introduction

Given the constant visibility of the skin in everyday life, its role is key in social interaction. The extent of skin ageing is determined by genetic (intrinsic) and exogenous (extrinsic) factors.

Skin ageing on the face

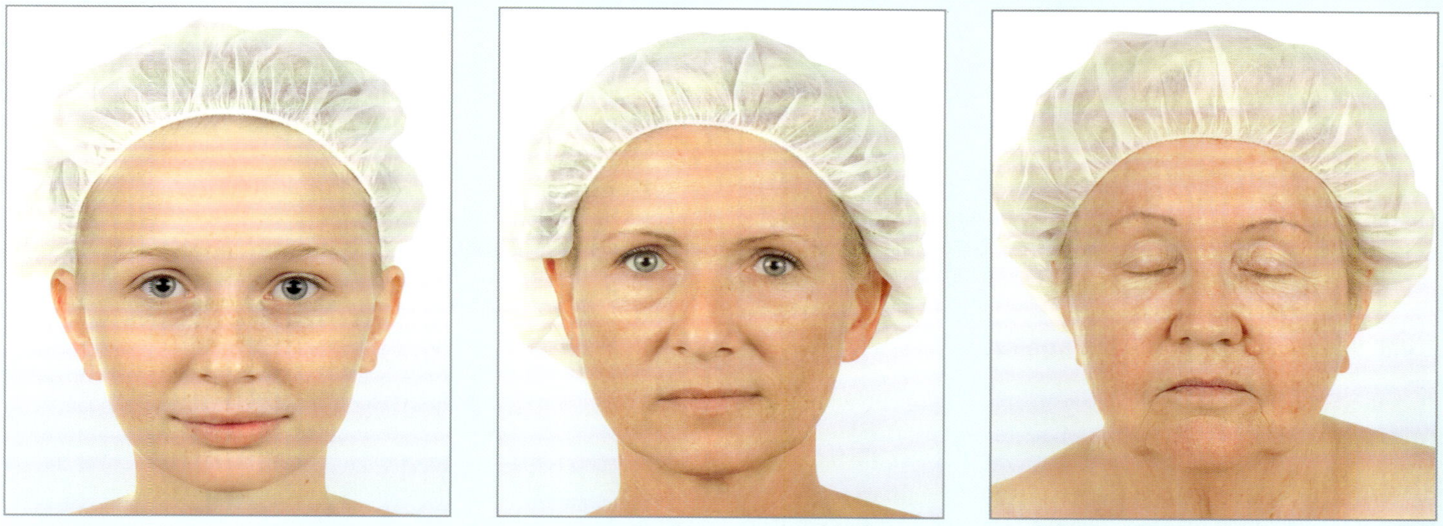

Fig. 1.27 Skin of the face – from right to left: grandmother, daughter and granddaughter.

Skin ageing on the hands and arms

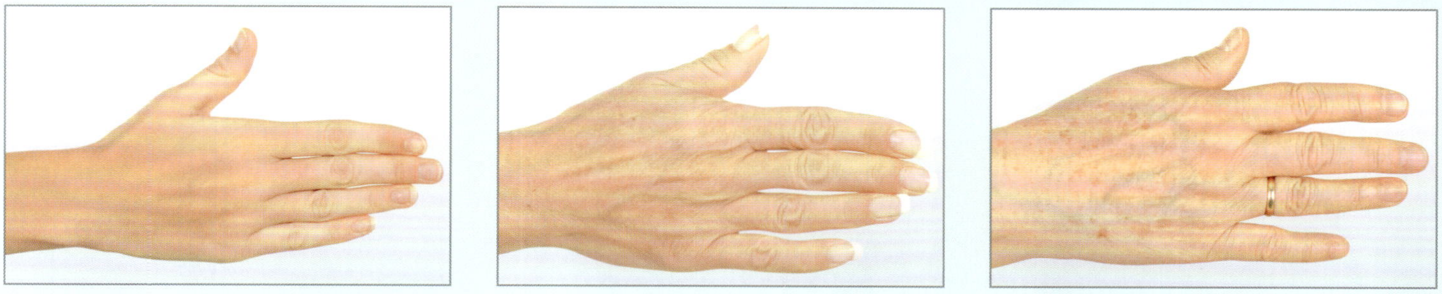

Fig. 1.28 Skin of the hand – from right to left: grandmother, daughter and granddaughter.

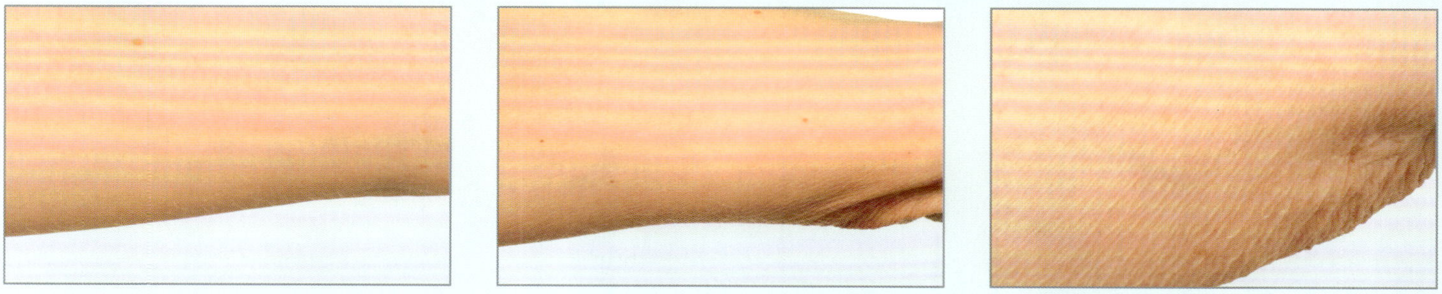

Fig. 1.29 Skin of the arm – from right to left: grandmother, daughter and granddaughter.

1.2.2 The appearance of ageing skin

As skin ages, it develops characteristic phenotypic features, such as dryness, lines and wrinkles, loss of elasticity, increased vulnerability, atrophy, pigmentary abnormalities, inflammation and an increase in neoplastic growth. Although UV-related ageing occurs independently of biological ageing and is characterised particularly by the loss of skin elasticity, the term *'senile elastosis'* was used for a long time, but has now been replaced by the term *'actinic elastosis'*.

Developments in microscopy have revealed the specific damage to elastic fibres resulting from UV radiation. In addition to causing the typical loss of elasticity, chronic UV exposure specifically triggers the development of cutaneous neoplasms. However, these can also be found on unexposed, intrinsically aged skin. The benign changes perceived as particularly unsightly throughout the world include senile lentigo (commonly known as age spots; see Fig. 1.31). Interestingly, it is only in Caucasians that wrinkling becomes apparent in middle age (see Fig. 1.30).

1.2.3 Specific aspects of skin ageing

Structural differences exist not only between different ethnic skin types and genders, but also with respect to extent of ageing. Under similar climatic conditions, Asian skin develops wrinkles a decade or so later compared to Central European skin. In contrast, ageing in Europeans tends to have a linear course, whereas Asians rapidly and dramatically begin to show the features of ageing between the ages of 40 and 50 years. The damaging effect of UV-B light is also accurately identifiable within the Asian population.

Furthermore, in European skin it is the presence of wrinkles which is perceived as unattractive, while in dark skin, pigmentary changes play a more significant role in perception of attractiveness. It is noted that the number of melanocytes decreases by 8–20 % per decade of life. Interestingly, it is only in persons of Oriental origin that the risk of hyperpigmentation does not increase with increasing body mass index. Chronic UV exposure very clearly leads to the typical lesions on white skin, but actinic damage can also develop on dark skin given sufficient exposure.

Dark skin is also characterised by low trans-epidermal water loss, a lower pH, greater elasticity, higher electric capacity and also a higher density of *Propionibacterium acnes*.

Appendages: hairs, sweat glands, scent glands and sebaceous glands

The appendages age similarly to the skin itself. However, intrinsic and extrinsic processes have different effects. The reduction in sebaceous and sweat glands seen with age leads to the typical presentation of senile xerosis with itching *(senile pruritus)*. Hair becomes white and thin, and hair loss occurs. The subcutaneous fat looses its thickness and strength.

In contrast, the extrinsic UV effects on the appendages manifest as Favre–Racouchot syndrome. As with acne, these lesions are found with comedones at the pilosebaceous orifices.

The sebaceous glands appear dilated when viewed under the microscope. In contrast, sebaceous gland hyperplasia refers to the clinically visible hypertrophy of the sebaceous glands, which develops particularly on the forehead in the form of small umbilicated papules, as a consequence of chronic UV exposure.

1.2.4 Extrinsic and intrinsic skin ageing

Characteristic features of the ageing face include not only the degeneration of the subcutaneous fat in the midface, but also the

Appearance of ageing skin

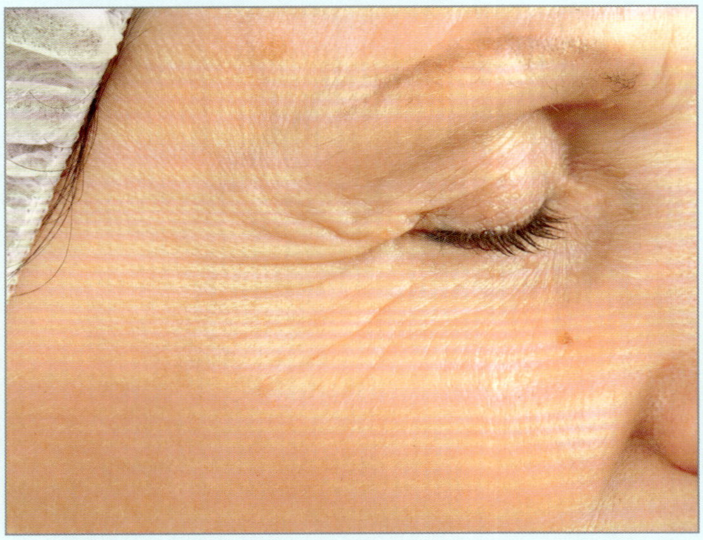

Fig. 1.30 Crow's feet.

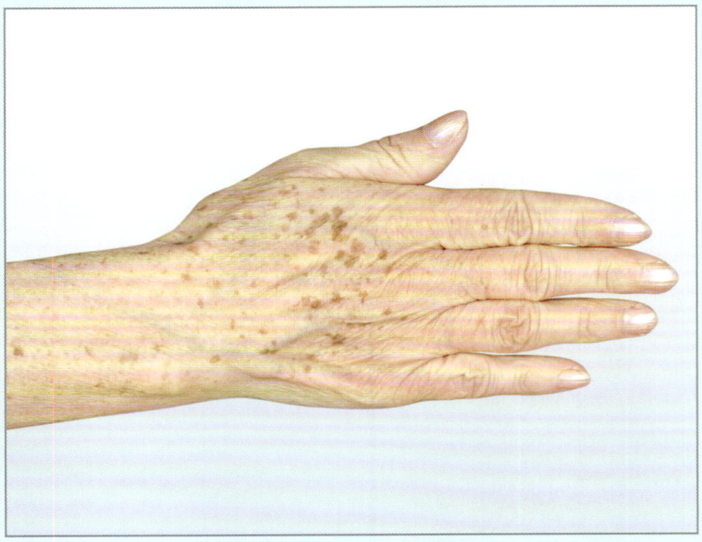

Fig. 1.31 Senile lentigines.

typical signs of intrinsic and extrinsic skin ageing, i.e. loss of elasticity and wrinkling. However, the consequences of extrinsic and intrinsic skin ageing differ considerably.

Extrinsic skin ageing

In lighter skin types, the clinical appearance of extrinsically aged skin tends to be one of atrophy, whereas zones of thickening predominate in darker skin types. Deep lines are seen (see Fig. 1.32), including ones which influence facial expression (see Fig. 1.33–1.35, 1.37), solar elastosis (see Fig. 1.36), pigmentary abnormalities (see Fig. 1.38, 1.39, 1.40), teleangiectasias (see Fig. 1.41), ecchymoses (see Fig. 1.43) and areas of inflammation (see Fig. 1.42). In addition, hair follicles, sweat glands and sebaceous glands decrease in number.

Triggering factors

Key factors that contribute to extrinsic ageing include UV exposure, smoking, ionising radiation, excessive alcohol intake, malnutrition or a poor diet, and emotional stress alongside many others. However, ultraviolet light alone contributes up to 80% to the overall damage, making it the most important exogenous trigger of skin ageing, particularly in lighter skin types.

Short-wave UV-B light (290–320 nm) is largely absorbed by the epidermis. Even below the erythema threshold, it activates transcription factors, which leads to the increased production of enzymes that contribute towards the breakdown of the extracellular matrix (matrix metalloproteinases, MMPs). Keratinocytes and the symbiotic den-

Extrinsic skin ageing

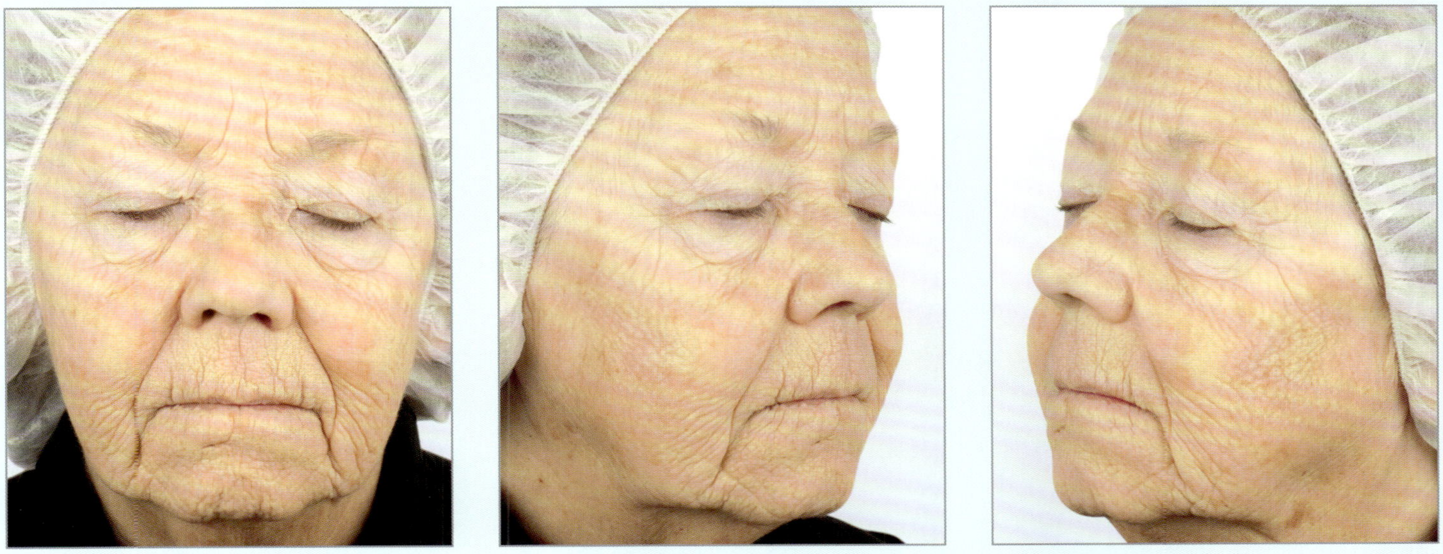

Fig. 1.32 Deep facial lines.

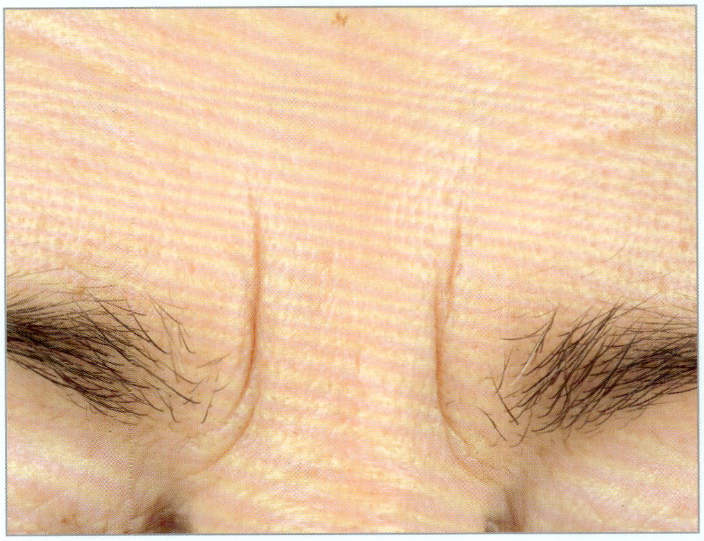

Fig. 1.33 Glabellar lines.

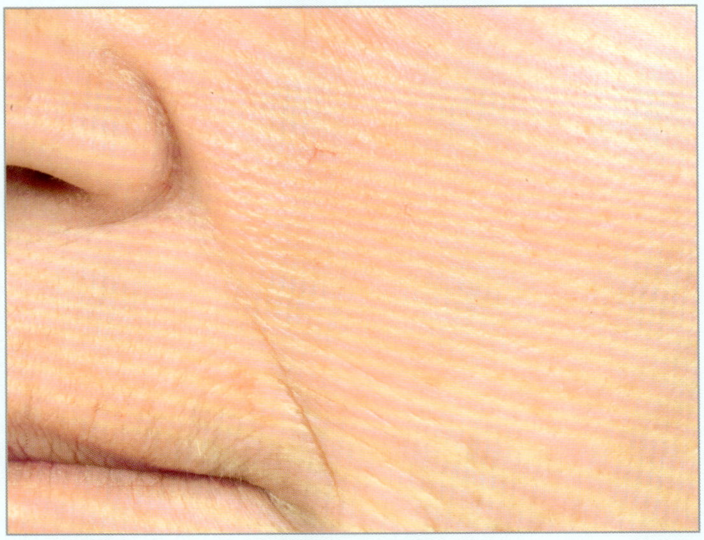

Fig. 1.34 Nasolabial lines.

1

Extrinsic skin ageing

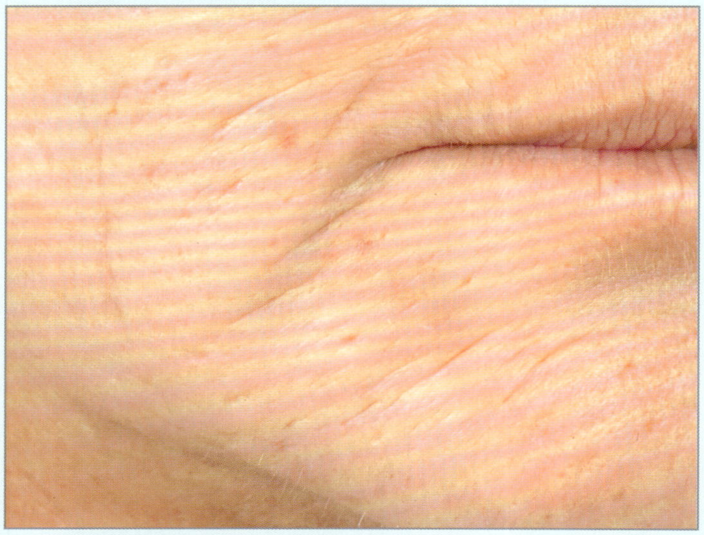

Fig. 1.35 Melomental folds (marionette lines).

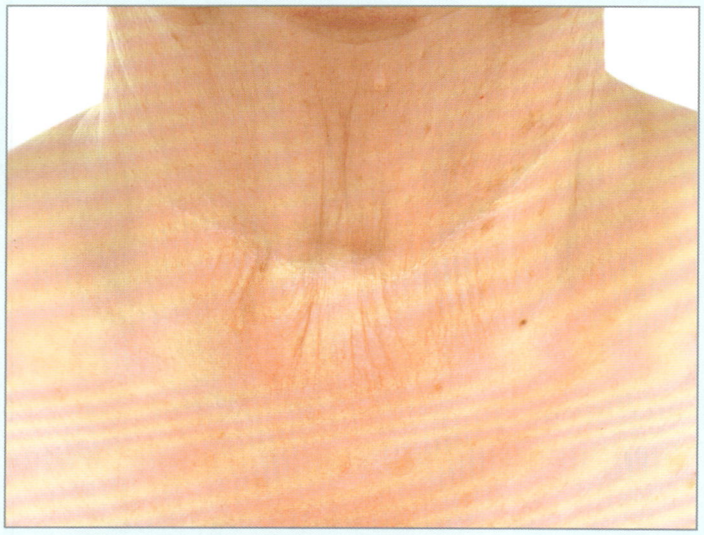

Fig. 1.36 Solar elastosis on the neck.

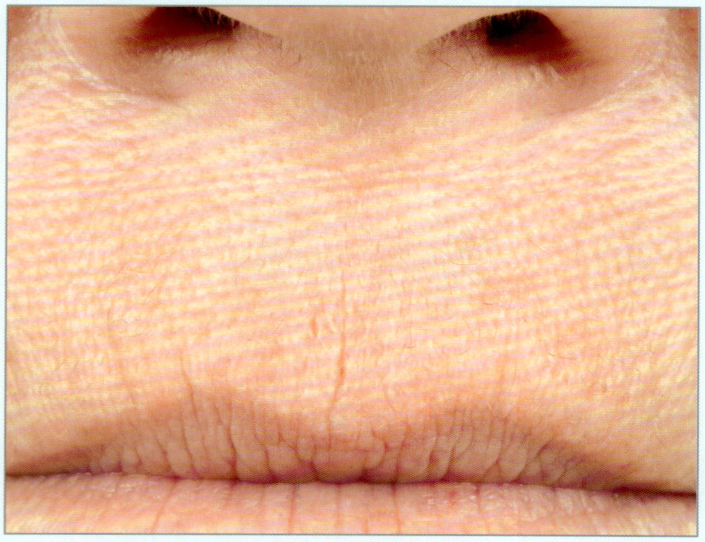

Fig. 1.37 Radial lip lines.

Extrinsic skin ageing

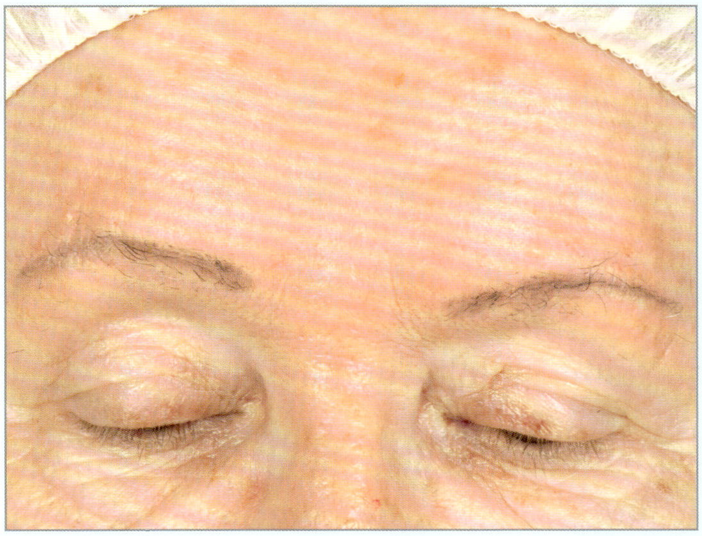

Fig. 1.38 Pigmentation abnormality on the face.

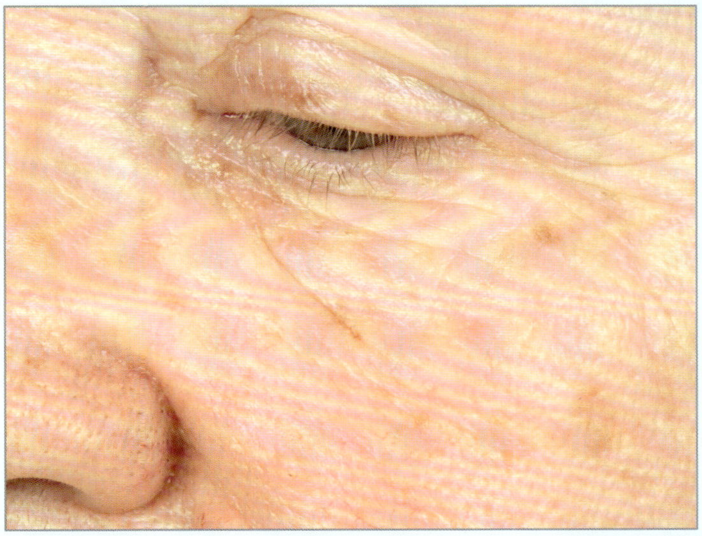

Fig. 1.39 Pigmentation abnormality on the face.

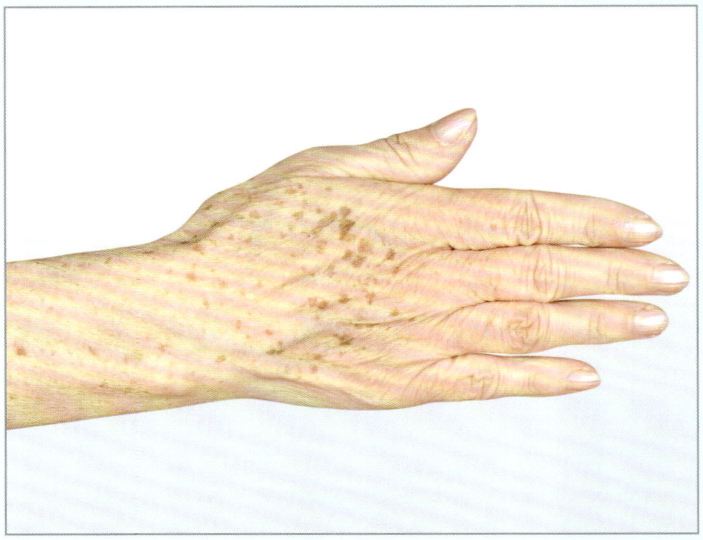

Fig. 1.40 Pigmentary abnormality on the dorsal aspect of the hand.

Extrinsic skin ageing

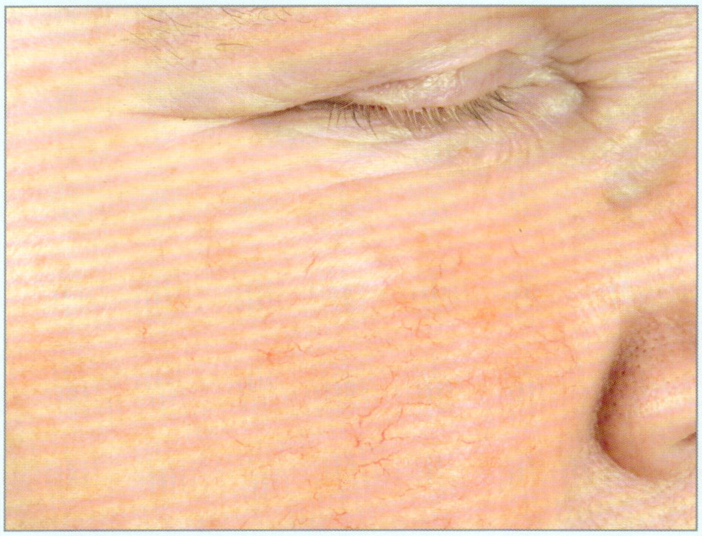

Fig. 1.41 Teleangiectasias.

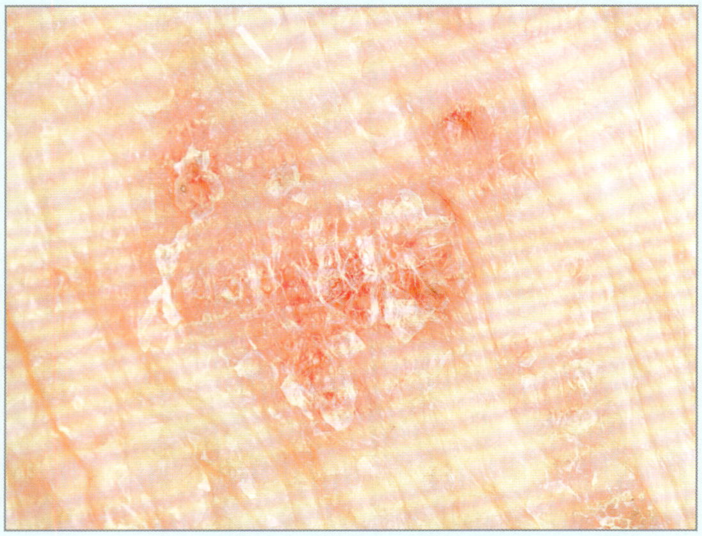

Fig. 1.42 Inflamed aged skin.

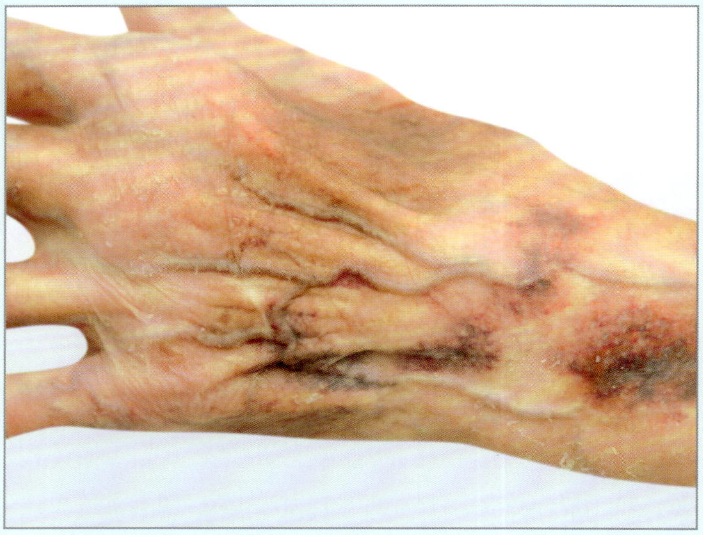

Fig. 1.43 Ecchymoses.

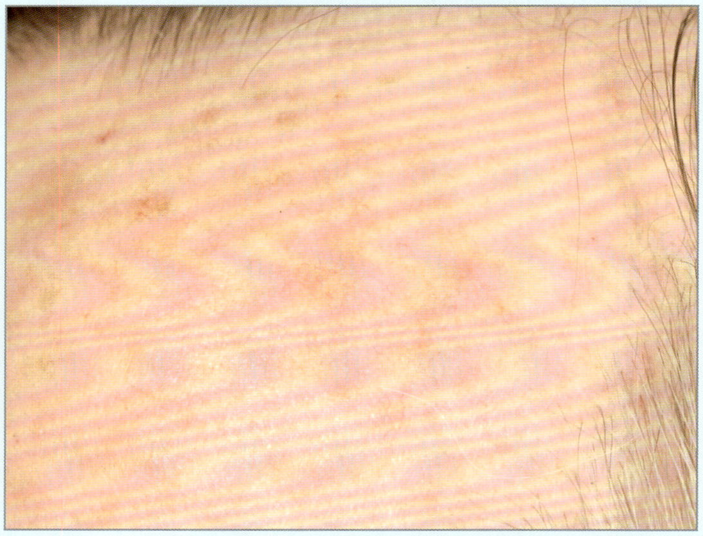

Fig. 1.44 Actinic keratoses.

dritic cells are damaged as a result. Covalently bound thymidine dimers, known as UV fingerprints, appear following sun exposure. Microscopically detectable sunburn cells occur 8–12 hours following the effects of UV light. The skin's ability to repair itself decreases with increasing age, resulting in accumulation of mutations.

UV-A light (320–400 nm) penetrates the epidermis and the upper layers of the dermis with damaging effects. Although it is a thousand times less harmful, it still contributes considerably to skin wrinkling.

Importantly, it is worth noting that even long-wave infrared light (720–1,000 nm) has an ageing effect on the skin.

Causes

There is a general consensus that UV light is a key catalyst of skin ageing, even if the exact molecular mechanisms of this process have not yet been fully elucidated. Furthermore, there is an increase in the quantity and activity of the enzymes that break down collagen (matrix metalloproteinases, MMPs), which is coupled with inhibition of new collagen synthesis. Reactive oxygen species, which themselves directly lead to DNA strand fractures in the cells, are formed at the same time. The chronic overload of the body's own detoxification mechanisms caused by this cumulative oxidative stress leads to protracted ageing. A key role in this process is played by the interaction of fibroblasts and the fibre network, which exerts a strong pull on them.

Extrinsic skin ageing

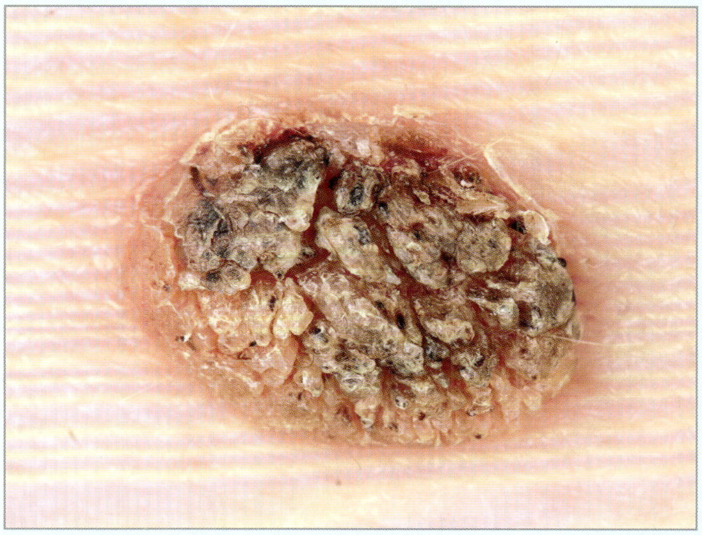

Fig. 1.45 Seborrheic keratosis.

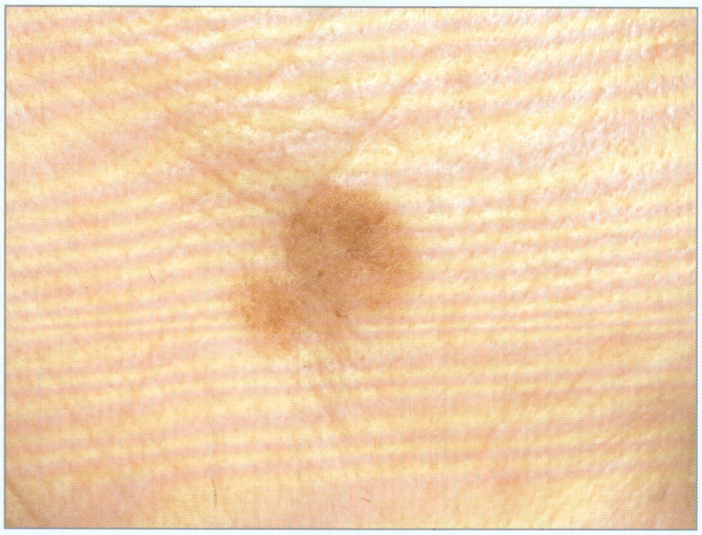

Fig. 1.46 Solar lentigo.

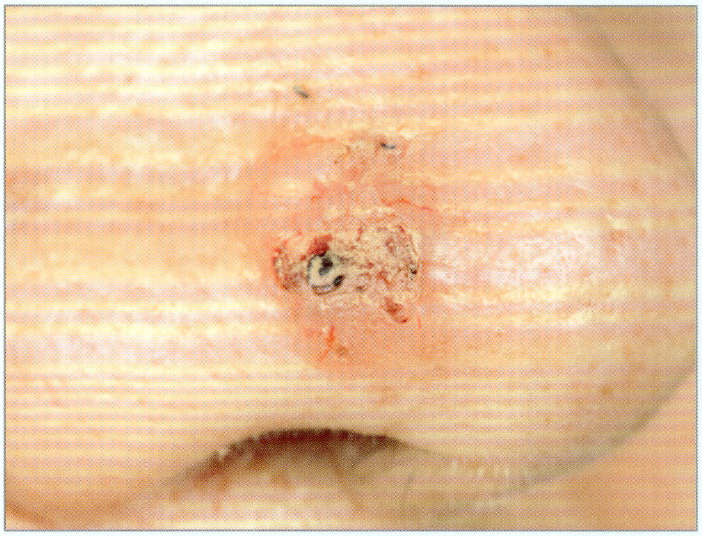

Fig. 1.47 Basal cell carcinoma.

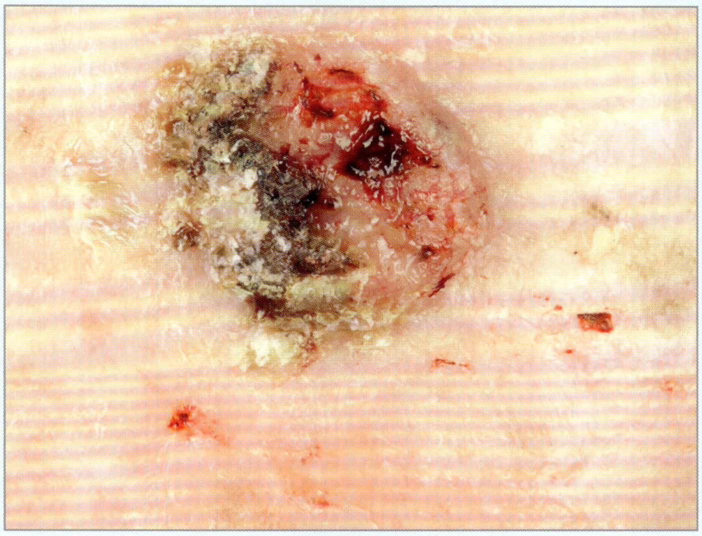

Fig. 1.48 Squamous cell carcinoma.

With increasing fragmentation of this fibre network, the fibroblasts lose their function in direct correlation with the decrease in the pull exerted on them. This gives rise to interesting interventional approaches, some of which have already been introduced into therapy and are being intensively researched.

Neoplasms occur more frequently with ageing: these include actinic and seborrheic keratoses (see Fig. 1.44, 1.45), solar lentigines (see Fig. 1.46), malignant tumours, particularly non-melanoma skin cancer, as well as melanomas.

At the microscopic level, orthokeratosis with a basket-weave pattern characterises clinically smooth, non-flaky skin, which remains pre-

Caution

Non-melanoma skin cancer

Non-melanoma skin cancer refers to all malignant tumours which do not originate from the skin's pigment cells, and thus comprise the very common tumour entities of basal cell carcinomas (BCCs) (see Fig. 1.47) and squamous cell carcinomas (SCCs), (see Fig. 1.48). Melanomas on the other hand, are malignant tumours of the pigmented cells and are associated with a high mortality.

Extrinsic skin ageing

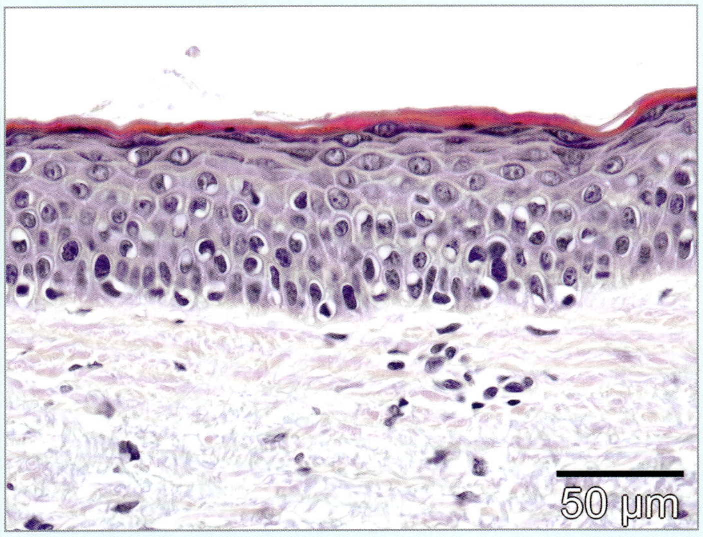

Fig. 1.49 Atrophic effacement of the rete ridge. Loss of normal alignment of keratinocytes; histological image.

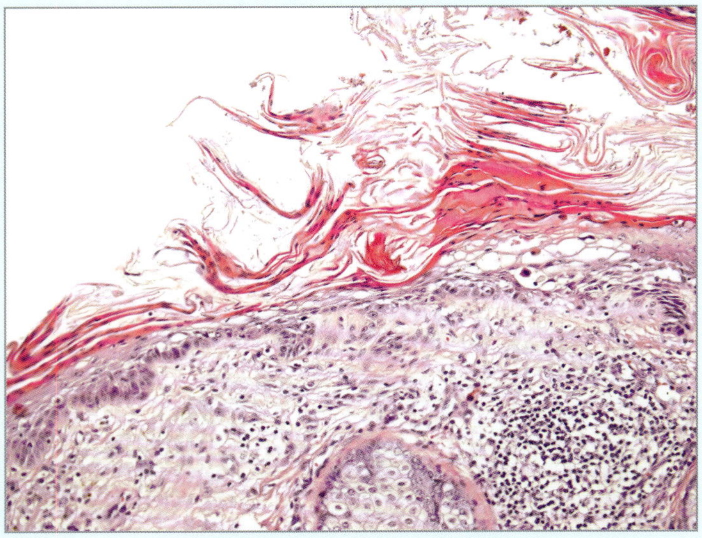

Fig. 1.50 Actinic keratosis; histological image.

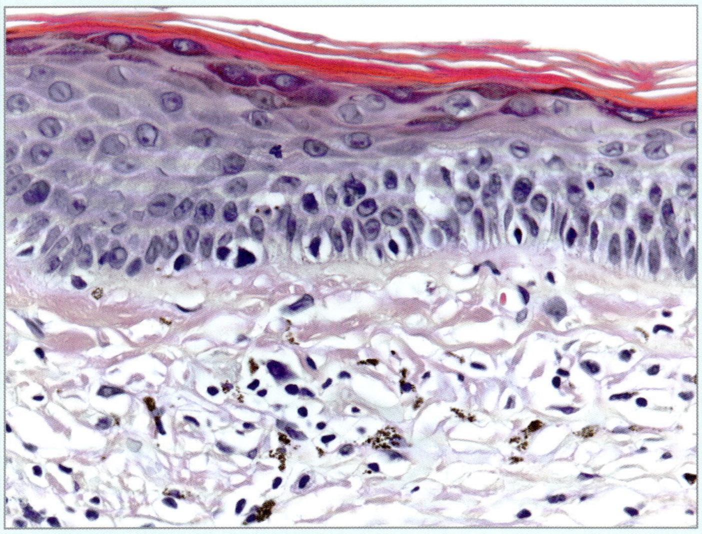

Fig. 1.51 Pigment leakage and melanophages; histological image.

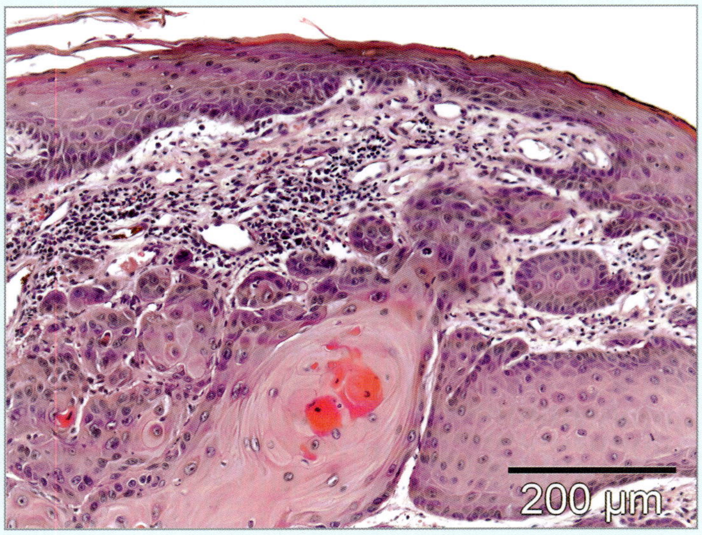

Fig. 1.52 Squamous cell carcinoma; histological image.

served with age if effective skincare is maintained. However, the rete ridges often become effaced (see Fig. 1.49). Failure to compensate for the changes typical of age with effective skincare results in a skin surface that is rough to the touch due to flaking, presenting histologically as loss of the basket-weave orthokeratosis, later followed by para(hyper)keratosis, associated with compacting, vesticulations and protein inclusions in the stratum corneum. Variable thickening of the stratum lucidum is typical.

The actinic damage to the keratinocytes leads to cytomorphological changes, which are evident as a loss of normal cell polarity in the basal cell layer (see Fig. 1.50).

Langerhans cells are also noted to decrease in number and functional activity, which explains the reduced immunological capacity of the integument in old age.

Atypical mitotic figures and apoptotic keratinocytes can also be found. The density of the melanocytes and Langerhans cells decreases, and in turn they begin to show more irregular distribution and activation. Maculate pigmentation abnormalities develop, with 'pigment leakage' into the dermis and subsequent storage of pigment in melanophages (see Fig. 1.51).

This leads to squamous cell carcinomas with strands and nests of tumour cells proliferating into the underlying tissue, variably dif-

Extrinsic skin ageing

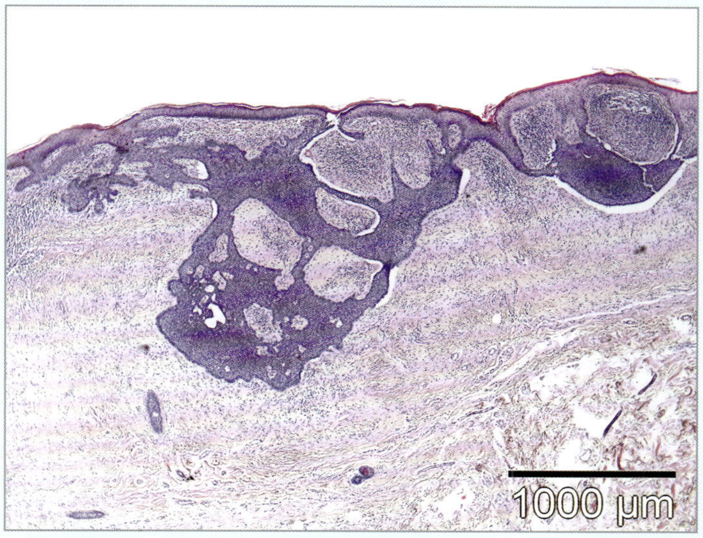

Fig. 1.53 Basal cell carcinoma; histological image.

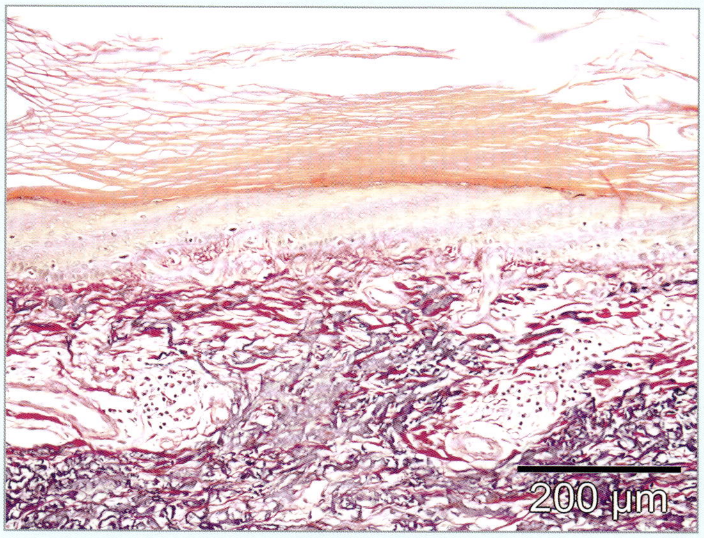

Fig. 1.54 Elastosis; histological elastic Van Giesson stain.

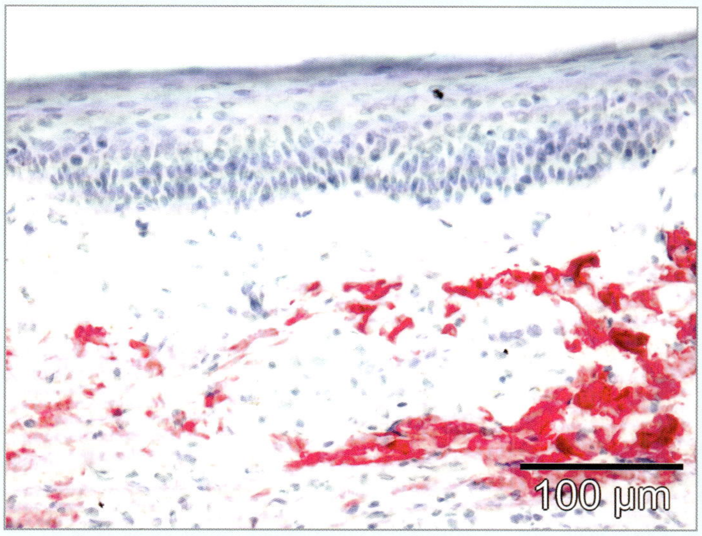

Fig. 1.55 Elastosis; immunohistological anti-elastin staining.

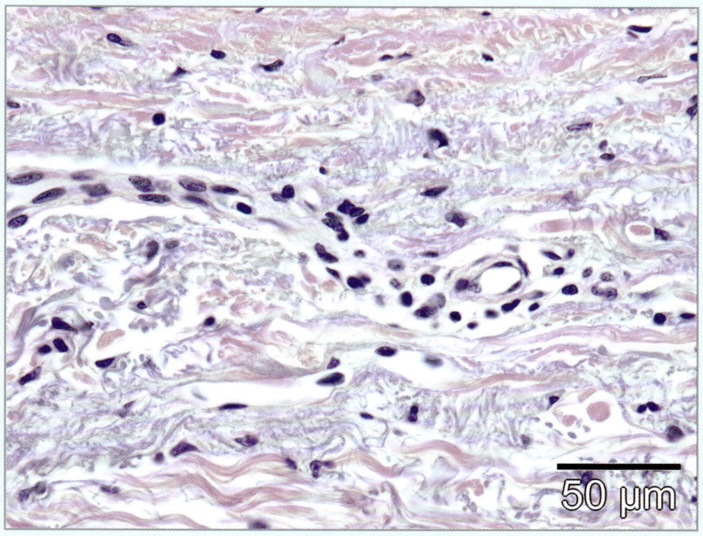

Fig. 1.56 Elastosis; histological HE stain. Amorphous fibres.

ferentiated squamous epithelial cell elements with an increased mitosis rate, atypical mitotic figures, as well as cornification of individual cells and cell groups (see Fig. 1.52). In BCCs, the findings include nests of cell elements with basaloid differentiation forming a typical peripheral palisade, retraction artefacts away from the adjacent connective tissue, and an increased mitosis rate (see Fig. 1.53).

In pronounced extrinsic skin ageing, atypical melanocytes are found not only in the basal layer, but also above it. If such cells occur in nests, the lesion is diagnosed as a malignant lentigo. This is classified as an in situ variant of lentigo maligna melanoma.

A high level of clinical expertise is needed to distinguish malignant neoplasms reliably from benign age-related changes. If there is any doubt, a definitive diagnostic process must always precede any aesthetic interventions.

Changes in the dermis

The extracellular matrix is made up of collagenous and elastic fibres which ensure the structural integrity of the dermis. Ageing of the connective tissue leads to non-elastic, loose skin via the induction of matrix metalloproteinases (MMPs). The number and density of elastic fibres decreases, with amorphous masses of elastolytic material found as the key sign of exogenous, UV-triggered skin ageing. The shortening, thinning and number of the elastic fibres is a significant determinant of wrinkle depth (see Fig. 1.54, 1.55). Furthermore, water is increasingly found in unbound form, since glycosaminoglycans are bound into elastotic material. Histologically, this is characterised by the appearance of the typical blue colour in the polygonal polymorphic fibres, which are no longer clearly identifiable as a network (see Fig. 1.56).

Directly below the basal membrane is a junction zone consisting of a narrow band of dense collagen fibrils laid parallel to the surface, as an expression of microscarring. The classical histological methods do not show up the changes in the elastic fibres. Special stains reveal the thickened, coarse elastic fibres, which have aggregated into clumps (see Fig. 1.55). Perivascular infiltrates are also found around the frequently dilated vessels, as an expression of chronic inflammation. This impaired vascular function manifests in the form of red blood cell extravasation (see Fig. 1.56).

Intrinsic skin ageing

Chronological or intrinsic skin ageing proceeds uniformly across the entire organ and affects all of its functions. Clinically, the skin becomes thin and parchment-like, with very fine wrinkles. Thinning of 10–50% can be seen between the third and eighth decades of life, accompanied by marked hypocellularity. There is a particularly pronounced decrease in the thickness of the stratum granulosum, even though reports to the contrary exist. Pigmentation becomes uniformly silvery. The skin appears loose due to the reduction in the subcutaneous fat pads. Nevertheless, the easily lifted skin folds spring back quickly and almost completely, as the collagenous and elastic fibres do not undergo dramatic changes. Apart from genetic predisposition, another factor that contributes towards intrinsic skin ageing is the decline in sex steroids. Consequently, there is a potential for skin ageing to be influenced through exogenous hormone replacement. In fact, transdermal testosterone replacement therapy has now become firmly established. Nevertheless, it does have its drawbacks, as the topical application of testosterone has negative effects on the epidermal barrier.

All these changes make the skin susceptible to minor trauma, leading to frequent sugillations. This leads to senile purpura.

A number of additional changes are noted, including:

- wounds healing slows down
- benign skin tumours develop, e.g. seborrheic keratoses (see Fig. 1.57). Nevi, on the other hand, decrease from the third decade of life, and any new ones formed subsequently tend to be a sign of malignant disease
- reduction in sebaceous and sweat glands also leads to typical senile xerosis with itching *(pruritus senilis)*
- hairs turn white and reduce in number
- the thickness and strength of the subcutaneous fat decreases.

1

Intrinsic skin ageing

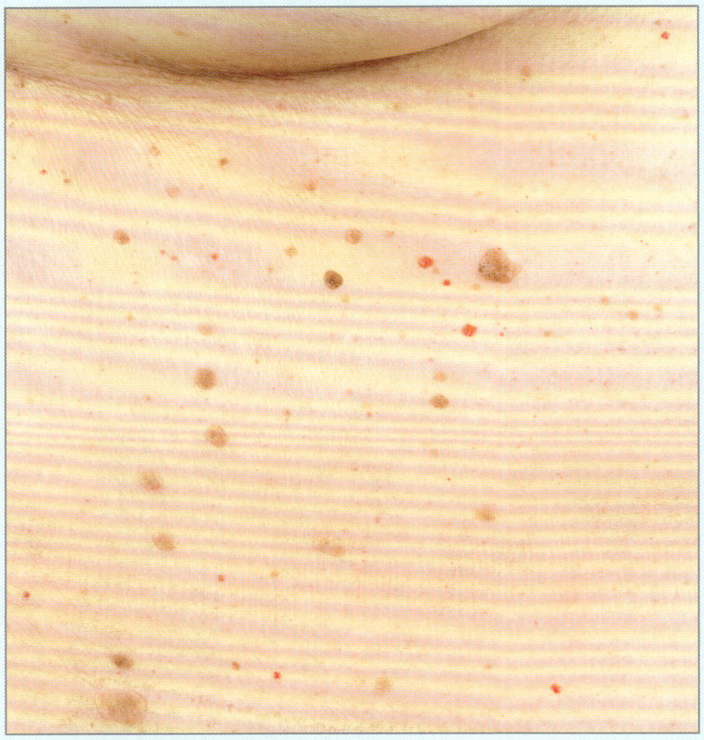

Fig. 1.57 Seborrheic keratoses, clinical view; identifiable by the dirty-brown pigmentation.

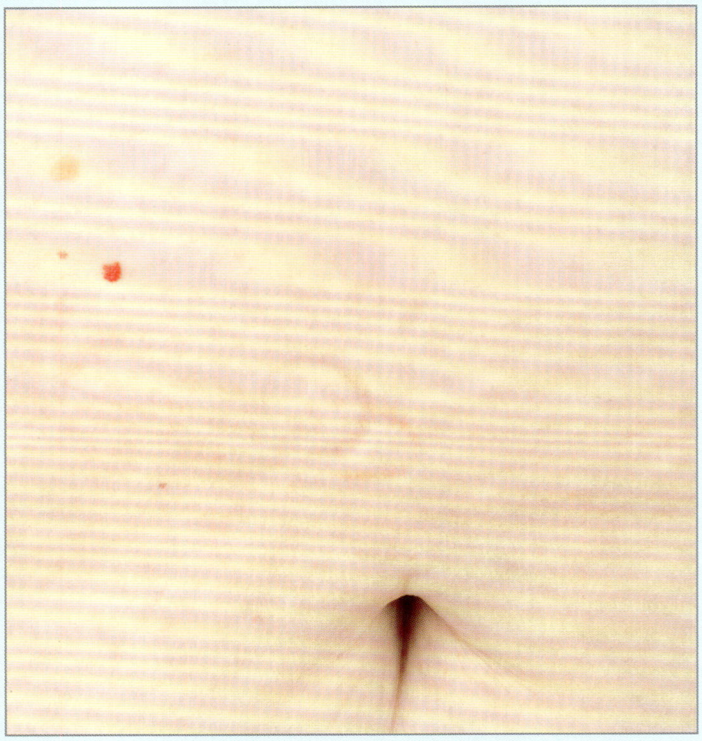

Fig. 1.58 Senile haemangioma on intrinsically aged skin.

Clinical appearance of intrinsically aged skin		
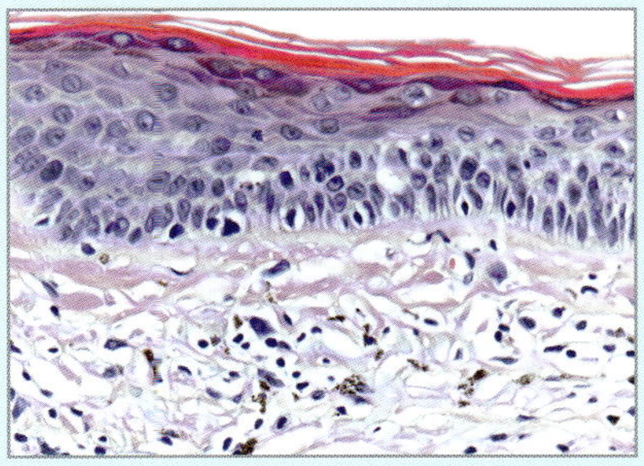	**Epidermis/dermis**	**Thin, rough, non-elastic, transparent skin with fine lines** • Decreasing barrier function • Reduced integumental reactivity • Increased vulnerability
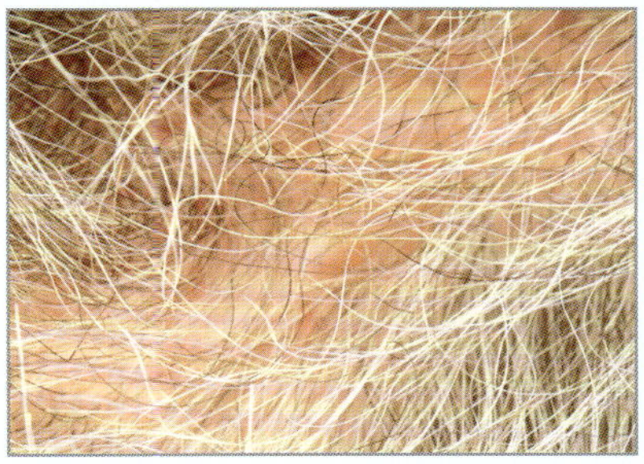	**Hair pigmentation**	**Loss of hair pigmentation** • Appearance: grey hair • Pigment shifts on hairless skin
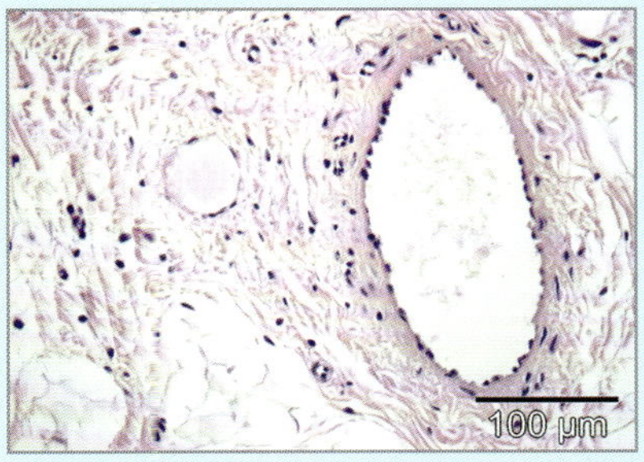	**Blood vessels**	**Regression, involution and disorganisation of the vascular plexuses** • Impaired thermoregulatory function • Sugillations, ecchymoses, purpura • Haemangiomas
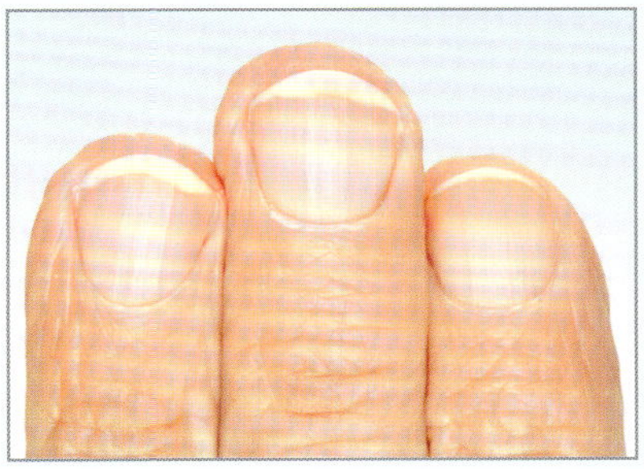	**Appendages**	**Regression, involution and disorganisation of the appendages** • Reduction in sebum and sweat production – sebostasis, pruritus – impaired thermoregulatory function • Loss of hair pigmentation, reduction in hair number; proliferation of vellus hairs • Thinning of the nail plate, roughness of the nail surface, formation of ridges • Reduction in nervous stimulability
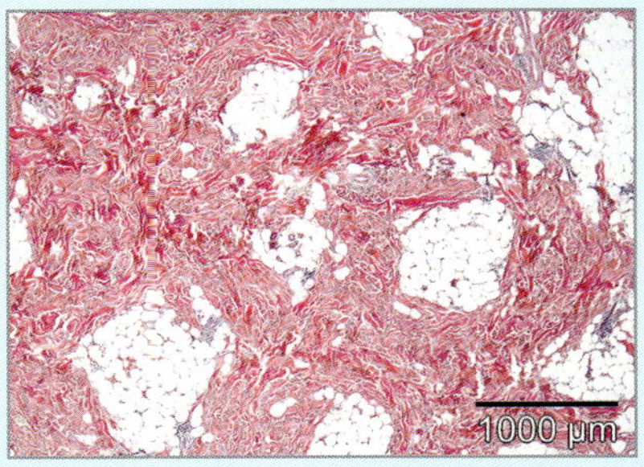	**Subcutaneous tissue**	**Regression, involution and disorganisation of the subcutaneous tissue** • Reduction in fatty tissue • Osteoporosis of the underlying bone layers leads to sagging skin folds (e.g. jowling)

Tab. 1.1 Clinical appearance of intrinsically aged skin.

Clinical appearance of skin subjected to chronic UV damage		
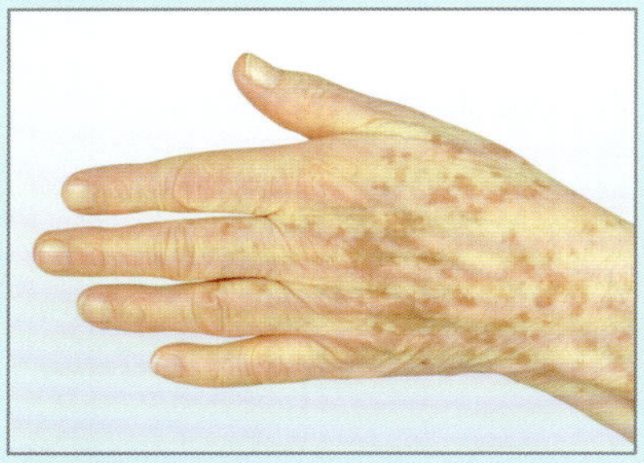	**Pigmentation**	• Lentigines • Guttate hypomelanosis • Irregular hyperpigmentation
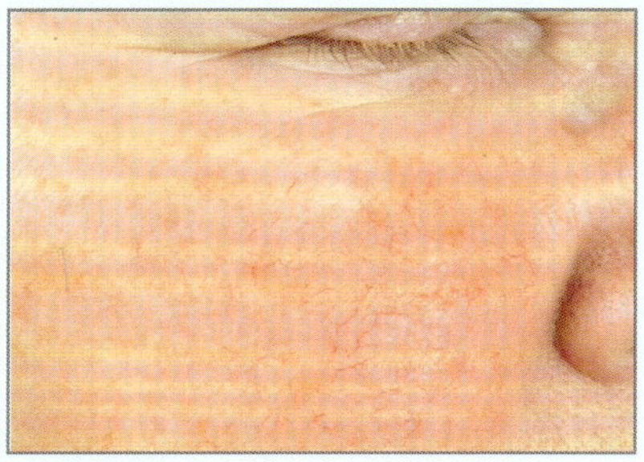	**Blood vessels**	• Telangiectasias • Ecchymoses • Haemangiomas
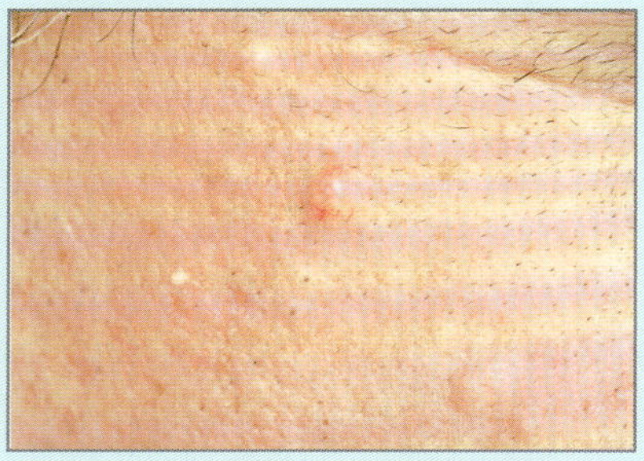	**Appendages**	• Sebaceous gland hyperplasia • Favre–Racouchot syndrome
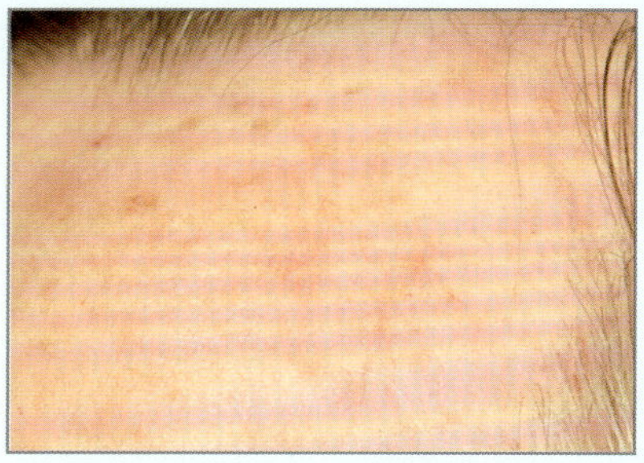	**Neoplasms**	• Actinic keratosis lesions • Basal cell carcinoma • Squamous cell carcinoma • Malignant melanoma
	**Epidermis/dermis**	• Scars • Actinic granuloma

Tab. 1.2 Clinical appearance of skin subjected to chronic UV damage.

1

2 Facial Anatomy and Ageing

2 Facial Anatomy and Ageing

The face has always been the primary focus of beauty-enhancing efforts in aesthetic dermatology and surgery. Driven by attempts to optimise these procedures, our understanding of the facial anatomy and of the mechanisms of facial ageing is constantly expanding.

The knowledge gained over the past two decades or so has provided some particularly significant insights. Importantly, there has been a paradigm shift from a two-dimensional to a three-dimensional approach to viewing and understanding the face. In particular, the crucial role of the subcutaneous fat pads in providing soft tissue volume, and of skin atrophy caused by a decrease in blood flow in the facial ageing process have become increasingly better understood. The new strategy of attributing the structural changes of ageing to deficits that are likely to be influenced by minimally invasive treatments laid the foundation for a groundbreaking approach to the treatment of facial ageing.

Whereas potentially destructive surgical techniques were mainly used in the 1990s, anti-ageing medicine has increasingly focused on restorative techniques since the turn of the millennium. These new techniques should enable us to finally start treating the root causes, and not just the symptoms of the loss of attractiveness due to the process of ageing.

Minimally invasive soft tissue augmentation with filler agents with high water-binding capacity has pioneered the way in this wave of innovation. The clinical results obtained over more than two decades of experience with this treatment show that facial proportions can be naturally restored and harmonised by compensating the volume and fluid losses within the soft tissues. Importantly, this treatment approach does not damage the key anatomical structures, and in fact activates physiological regenerative processes. Since its inception, this treatment method has been dynamically refined and revolutionised based on new clinical, scientific and technological achievements. Today, deep soft tissue augmentation techniques are available that enable causal and proportional treatments to harmonise the structural effects of ageing in the entire face (Fig. 2.1).

The clinical and anatomical information presented in the following pages is of paramount importance, as it enables the aesthetic practitioner to independently perform the treatment concepts described in this book.

2.1 The Face and Attractiveness

The face, with its characteristic features, plays a crucial role in society, particularly in distinguishing people and especially in social interactions. The face conveys a continuous flow of personal information. This occurs both consciously (i.e. when engaging in verbal and non-verbal communication) and subconsciously. Certain facial features reveal a plethora of information about one's age, mood and stress levels, state of relaxation, alongside physical and mental state. As an observer we subconsciously form opinions about people's personality, whether they are likeable or not, and whether attractive or not within that initial glance. No other part of the body plays as significant a role in emotional and social processing.

The consequences of the ageing process are not as visible in any other part of the body as soon or as obviously as in the face, which is continuously exposed to the external environment. For these reasons, it is not surprising that it has always been the primary focus of the beauty, skincare and cosmetic industry. As such, clinical interventions to counteract the visible signs of ageing on a deeper level, which cannot be accessed by the application of daily skin care and decorative cosmetic products, are becoming increasingly popular. The desire to achieve beautification and rejuvenation is inherent in society worldwide and no longer accessible to just the ranks of the 'rich and famous' anymore.

2.1.1 Criteria for facial attractiveness

How are beauty and attractiveness defined? This has not proved to be an easy question to answer. Beauty ideals are subject to constant change given they ultimately stem from specific historical, socio-cultural and individual contexts. Therefore, it is not possible to establish a *de facto* global definition of 'the epitome of beauty'.

Attractiveness is also a very subjective value. According to the etymological origin of the word (from Latin *tractum* 'to draw, pull' and *ad* = 'to'), it is based on a property that can be universally assessed and compared. An attractive person exerts a 'force of attraction' upon others. This attractive force may therefore be due to the person's physical appearance, personality traits, and material or social status.

Thus, attractiveness consists of more than just specific attributes of external beauty. Research has shown that physical appearance has a tremendous impact on an individual's social and personal relationships. Studies by Dr Martin Gründl and his team at the University of Regensburg (Braun et al, 2001) have shown that independent observers subconsciously associate positive character traits such as success, likeability, creativity and intelligence with 'attractive' faces, and predominantly negative character traits with less attractive faces. This has highlighted a positive correlation between physical attractiveness and social acceptance. Social acceptance, in turn, is closely associated with personal self-esteem. This implies that it is generally easier for attractive people to develop their potential and achieve their professional and personal goals compared to less attractive people. Attractiveness is therefore considered a desirable trait at all stages of life.

In a study titled 'Beautycheck', Braun et al (2001) conducted a series of experiments designed to obtain empirical answers to fundamental questions regarding the perception of attractiveness in contemporary Western culture (Tab. 2.1). Original male and female faces and 'morphed' prototype faces generated by facial averaging were rated for attractiveness and compared (Fig. 2.2). In this manner, the study identified attractiveness criteria of the male and female face by pairwise comparison of prototypes of attractive versus unattractive faces. Below are the criteria associated with an attractive male and female face as highlighted by the study.

2.1.2 Characteristics of age-related loss of attractiveness

Regardless of how attractive one was in their youth, an age-related loss of physical attractiveness inevitably occurs over the course of time. A loss of facial volume and proportions can generally be observed in different parts of the face over time. A gradual loss of the

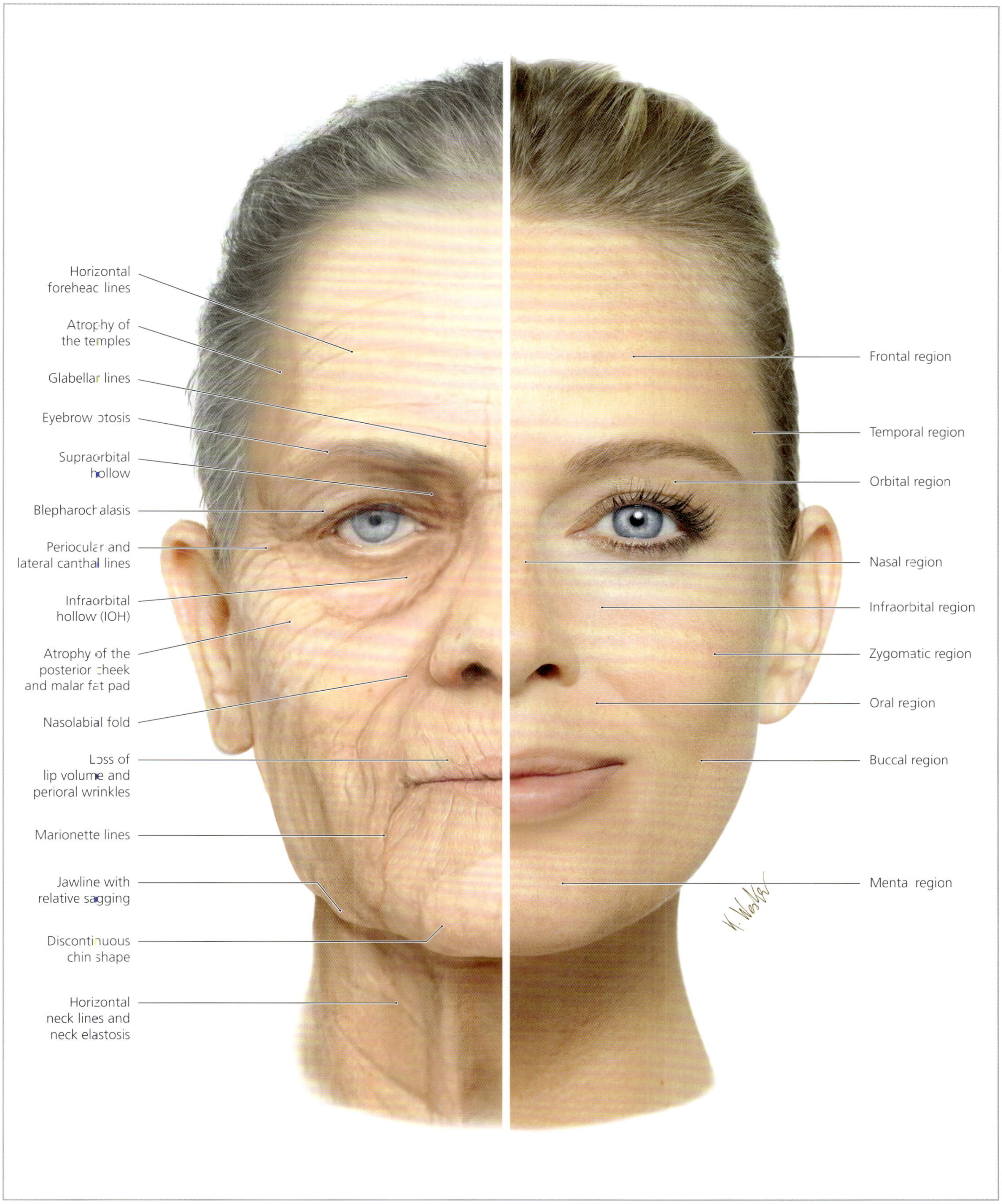

Fig. 2.1 Clinical characteristics of the ageing face.

Attractive versus unattractive faces

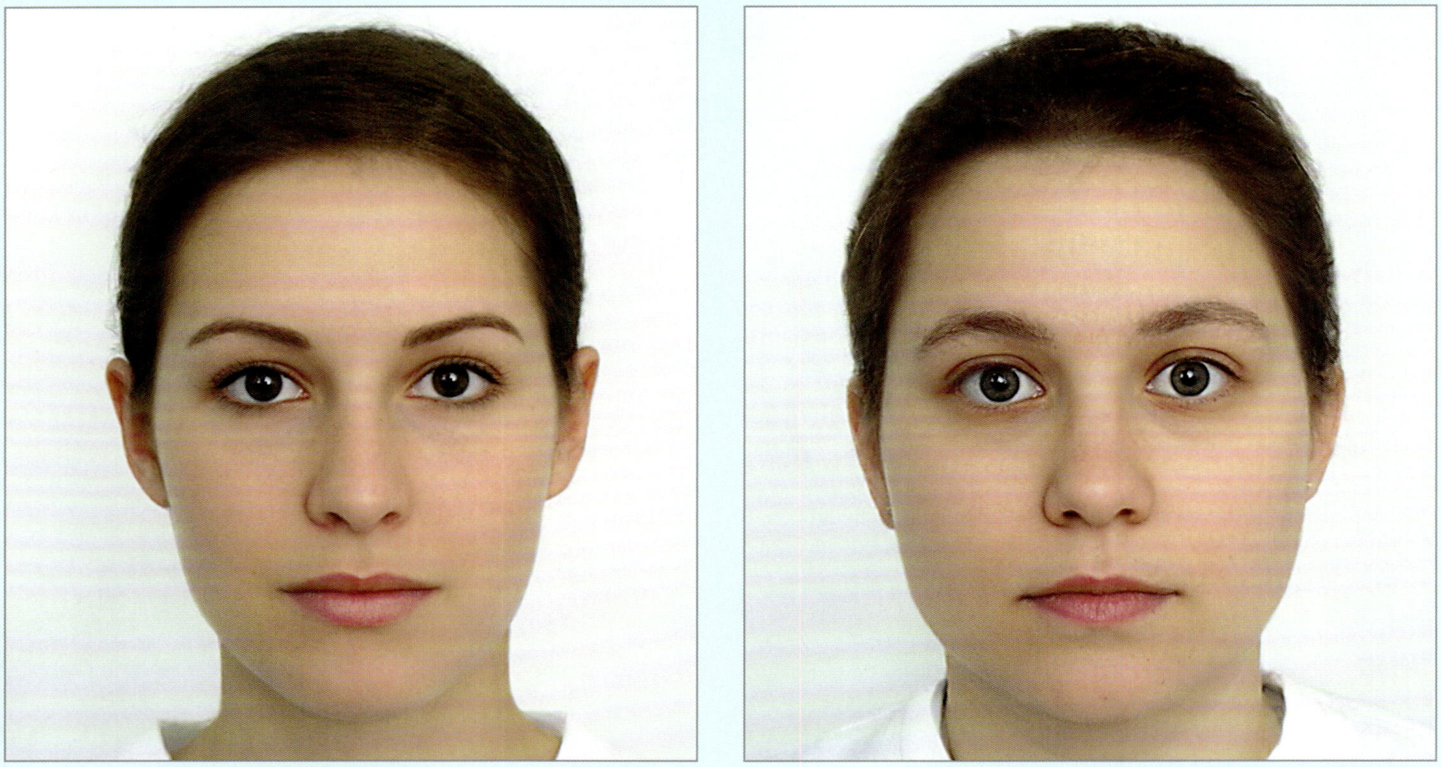

Fig. 2.2 Morphed prototype of the attractive (left) versus the unattractive (right) female face. Prototype faces were artificially generated from mathematical averages of original photographs of several different faces that had previously been evaluated and rated for levels of attractiveness. The main characteristics that distinguish attractive faces from unattractive faces were then identified by directly comparing different face pairs. A homogeneous skin surface and a childlike appearance were identified as the main criteria of facial attractiveness. Average proportions and facial symmetry proved to be marginal attractiveness criteria.

Characteristic features of an attractive female face	Characteristic features of an attractive male face
• Clear skin • Sun-tanned skin • Narrow face (and neck) • Limited fatty tissues • Well-kept, full lips • Dark, thin eyebrows • Smaller distance between the tarsus and the eyelid fold • Fuller, longer and darker eyelashes • No dark circles under the eyes (due to volume loss) • High cheekbones • Narrower nose • Midface volume greater than chin volume	• Clear skin • Sun-tanned skin • No receding hairline • Narrow face (and neck) • Broader upper half of the face • Dark, thin eyebrows and dark eyelashes • High cheekbones • Full lips and symmetrical mouth • Prominent lower jaw and chin

Tab. 2.1 Characteristic features of attractive male and female faces (from Braun et al, 2001).

underlying soft tissue occurs in the upper midface region in conjunction with the downward migration and redistribution of the superficial buccal fat. Consequently, the upside-down triangle associated with a youthful face associated with most volume in the midface gradually inverts and becomes associated with a heavier lower third of the face. In addition, the increased loosening of the attachment between the skin and the soft tissue base results in the formation of skin folds.

Facial features begin to gradually lose the delicate characteristics of youth. At the same time, structures that disturb facial proportions start to emerge and become ever more prominent.

Clinical course of facial ageing

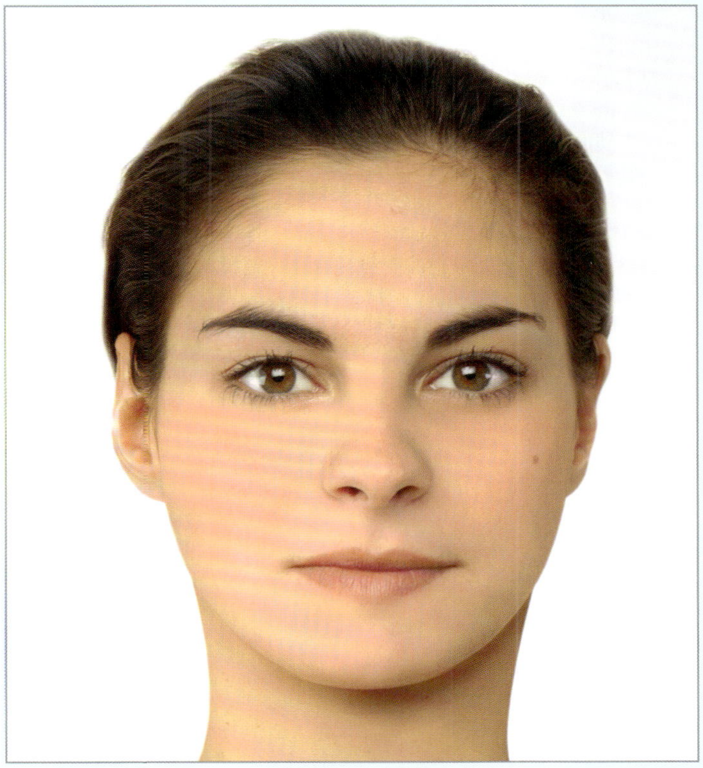

Fig. 2.3 Face at the age of 15 years.

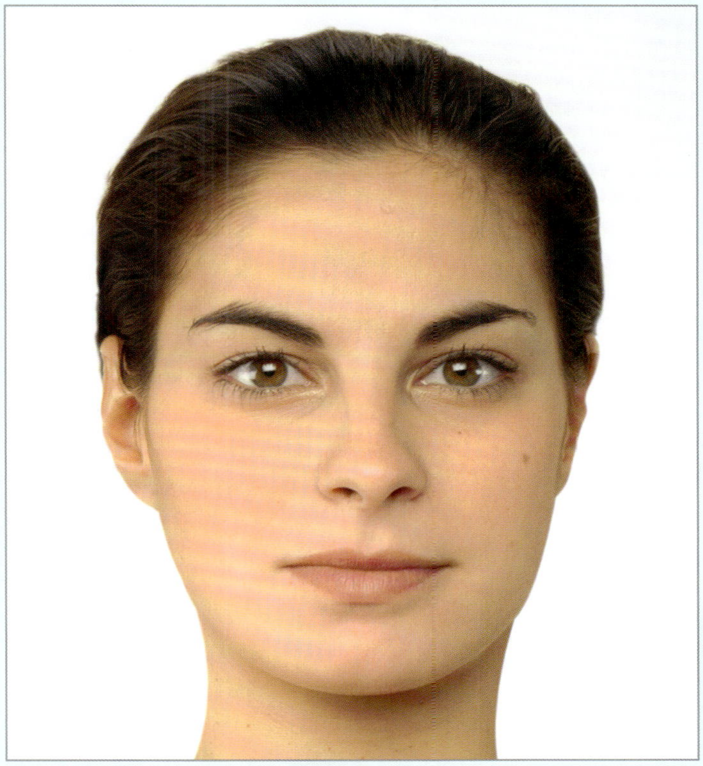

Fig. 2.4 Face at the age of 25 years.

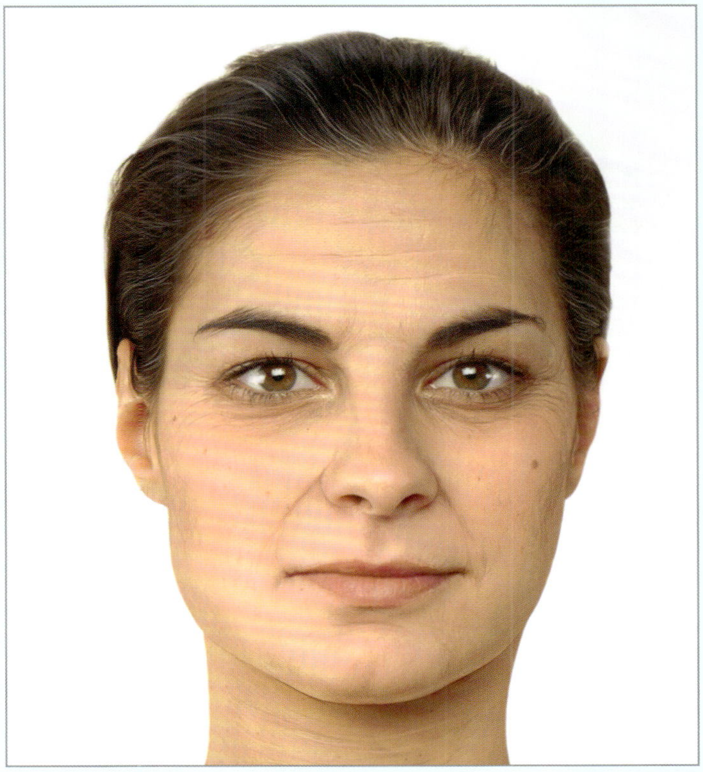

Fig. 2.5 Face at the age of 45 years.

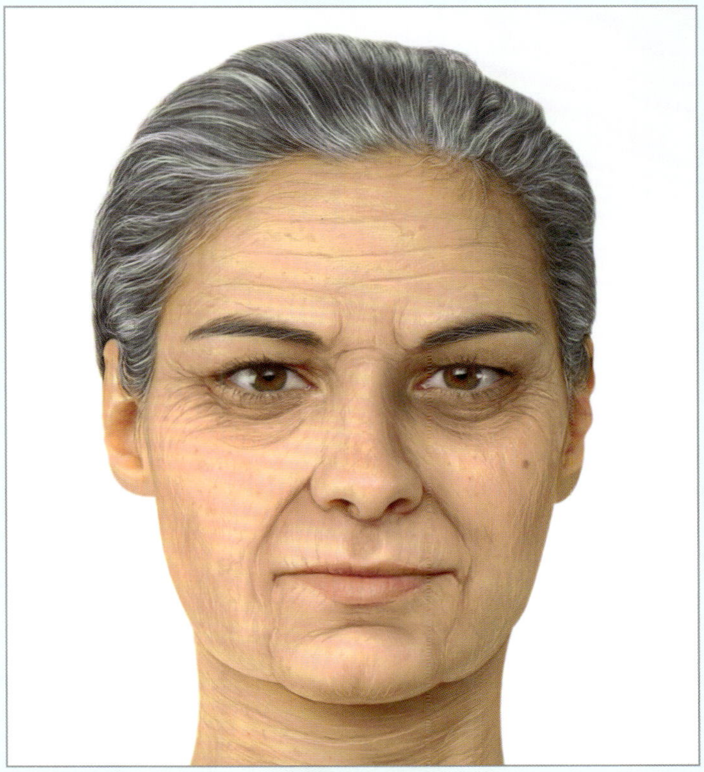

Fig. 2.6 Face at the age of 65 years.

Direct comparison of the chronological changes in the faces of different individuals clearly shows that the visible characteristics are different but comparable. Each individual face ages at its own speed and with an individual extent of changes in regional structures. However, there are certain basic characteristics that are common to all aged faces, and include:

- Inversion of the youthful upside-down triangle of the face
- Irregular skin surface (creases, rough patches, wrinkles)
- Skin discolouration (dark circles, superficial capillaries, pigmentary disorders)
- Loss of proportion of the skin envelope (loss of subcutaneous fat, downward sagging of the soft tissues)
- Glabellar lines
- Sagging of the eyebrows (ptosis)
- Sunken eyes (supraorbital hollowness)
- Wrinkles around the eyes
- Infraorbital hollowness (dark circles under the eyes, tear trough deformity)
- Fat atrophy in the upper cheek region (malar fat pad)
- Deep nasolabial folds
- Wrinkles around the mouth
- Loss of lip volume and perioral wrinkles
- Drooping corners of the mouth and jowls (marionette lines)
- Wrinkle below the lips (sublabial fold)
- Irregular chin contour and 'sagging'

The occurrence of common inter-individual characteristics of ageing suggests that their mechanism of development is based on a system of which the causality can be explained and influenced by aesthetic treatments to a certain extent. The anatomical relationships described below are fundamental to this understanding of ageing.

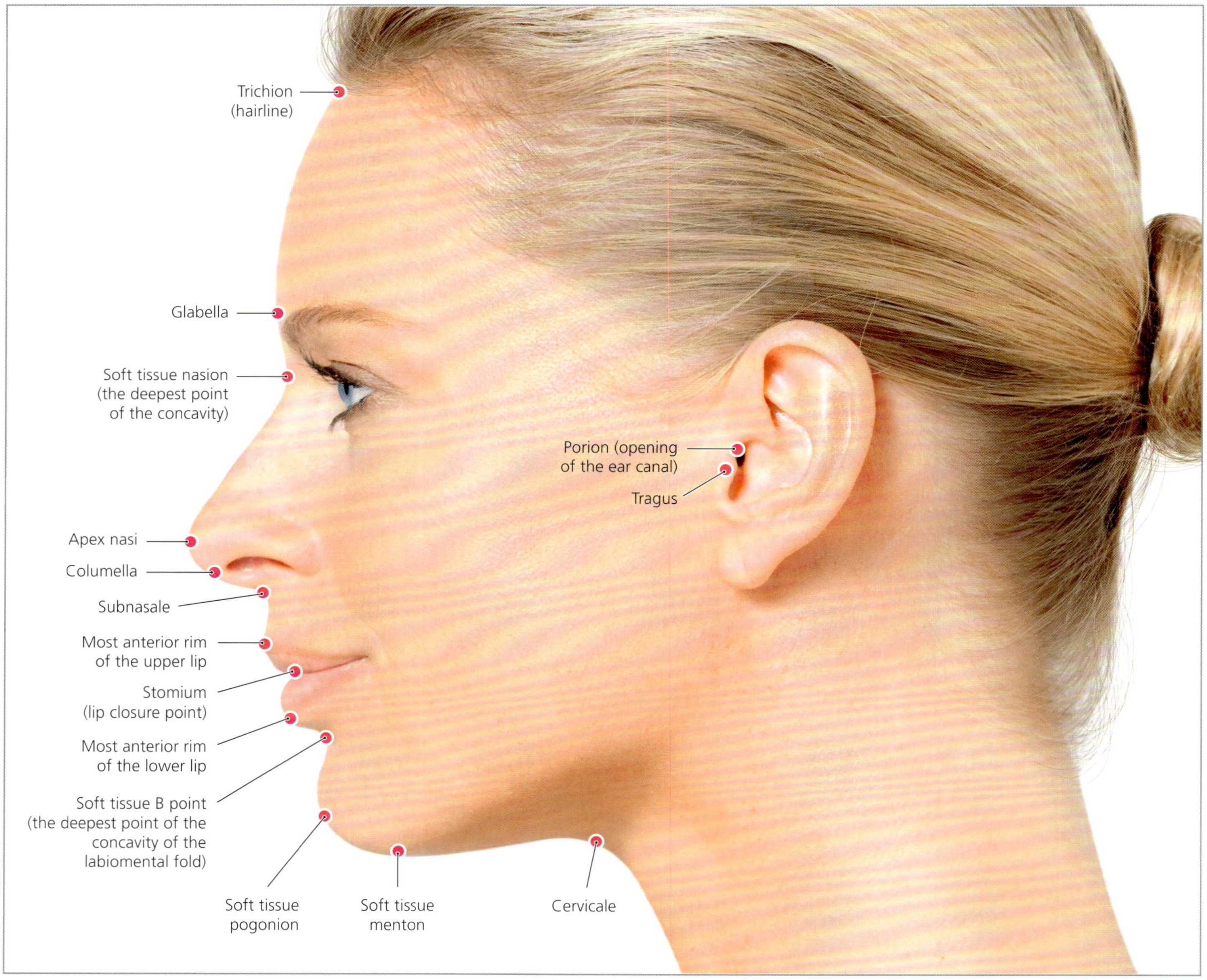

Fig. 2.7 Landmarks that may be used for facial measurements (lateral view).

2.2 Anatomical Structures of the Face

Every face is constructed of an anatomical blueprint that is common to all humans yet characteristic in each individual, making each person unique. The human face is comprised of the following basic anatomical structures:

- Bones
- Muscles
- Retaining ligaments
- Subcutaneous fat and connective tissue
- Neurovascular and lymphatic tissue
- Skin

A network of nerves, blood vessels and lymph vessels permeate the tissue complex to innervate the individual tissue compartments and to ensure the flow of nutrients and fluids. The anatomical tissues of the face are not static, but rather a dynamic tissue complex subject to the dynamics of muscle activity in different parts of the face.

There are several ways to obtain standardised measurements of facial structures and proportions and to assess them from an aesthetic viewpoint (Fig. 2.7). Knowledge of theoretically 'ideal' facial proportions is certainly important when planning measures to enhance facial attractiveness (Fig. 2.8). However, these 'ideals' should not be used alone, but rather in conjunction with the patient consultation, whereby their subjective concerns and ideas are also taken into account. Furthermore, differences between male and female faces, as well as those between different ethnic backgrounds and age groups should also be considered.

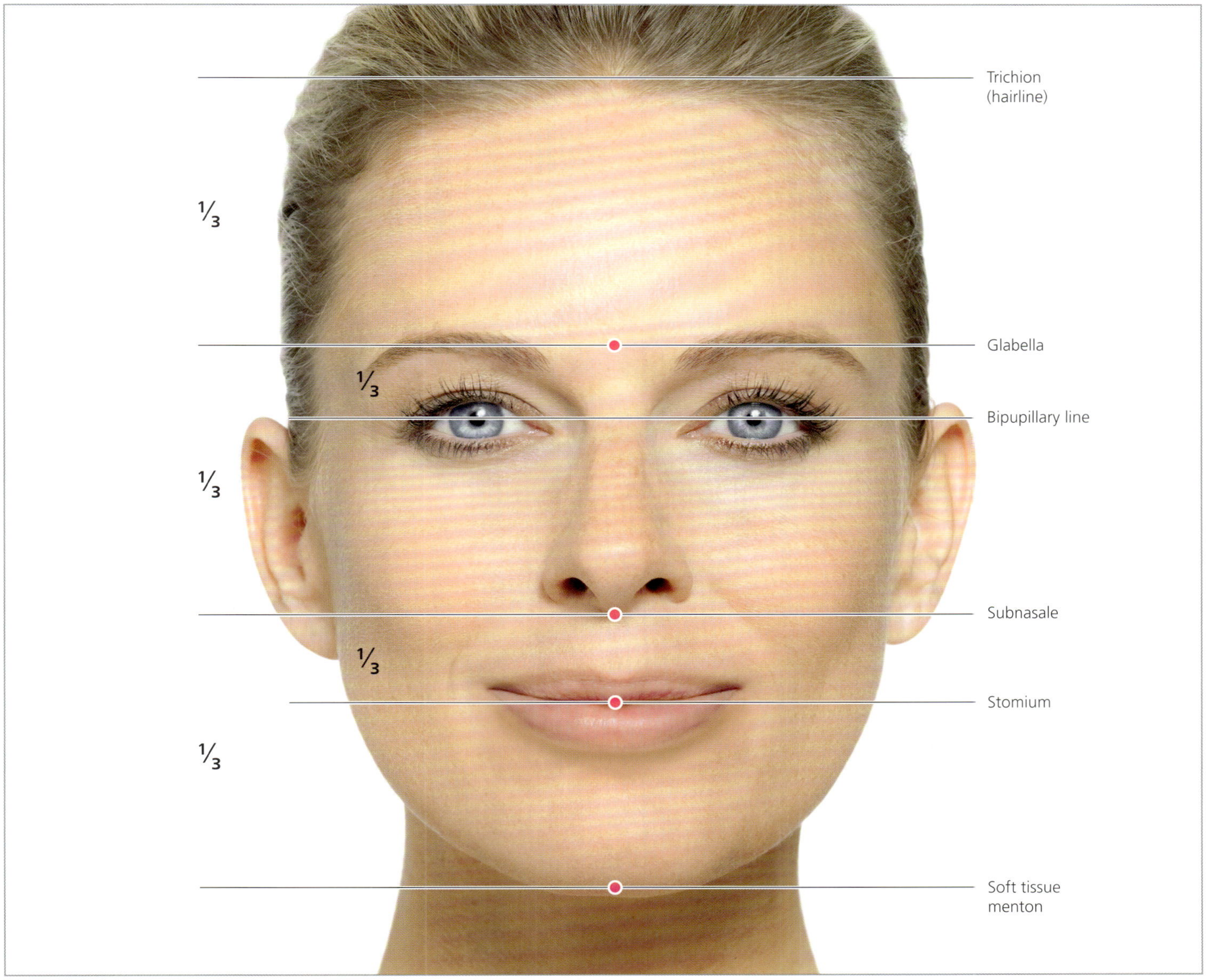

Fig. 2.8 'Ideal' facial proportions.

2

2.2.1 Facial skeleton

The skull forms the bony platform of the face. The skull provides attachment sites for the facial muscles and ligaments (Figs 2.9 and 2.10). Some of these attachment sites are raised areas (e.g. the masseteric tuberosity), while others are simply indentations (e.g. the temporal fossa).

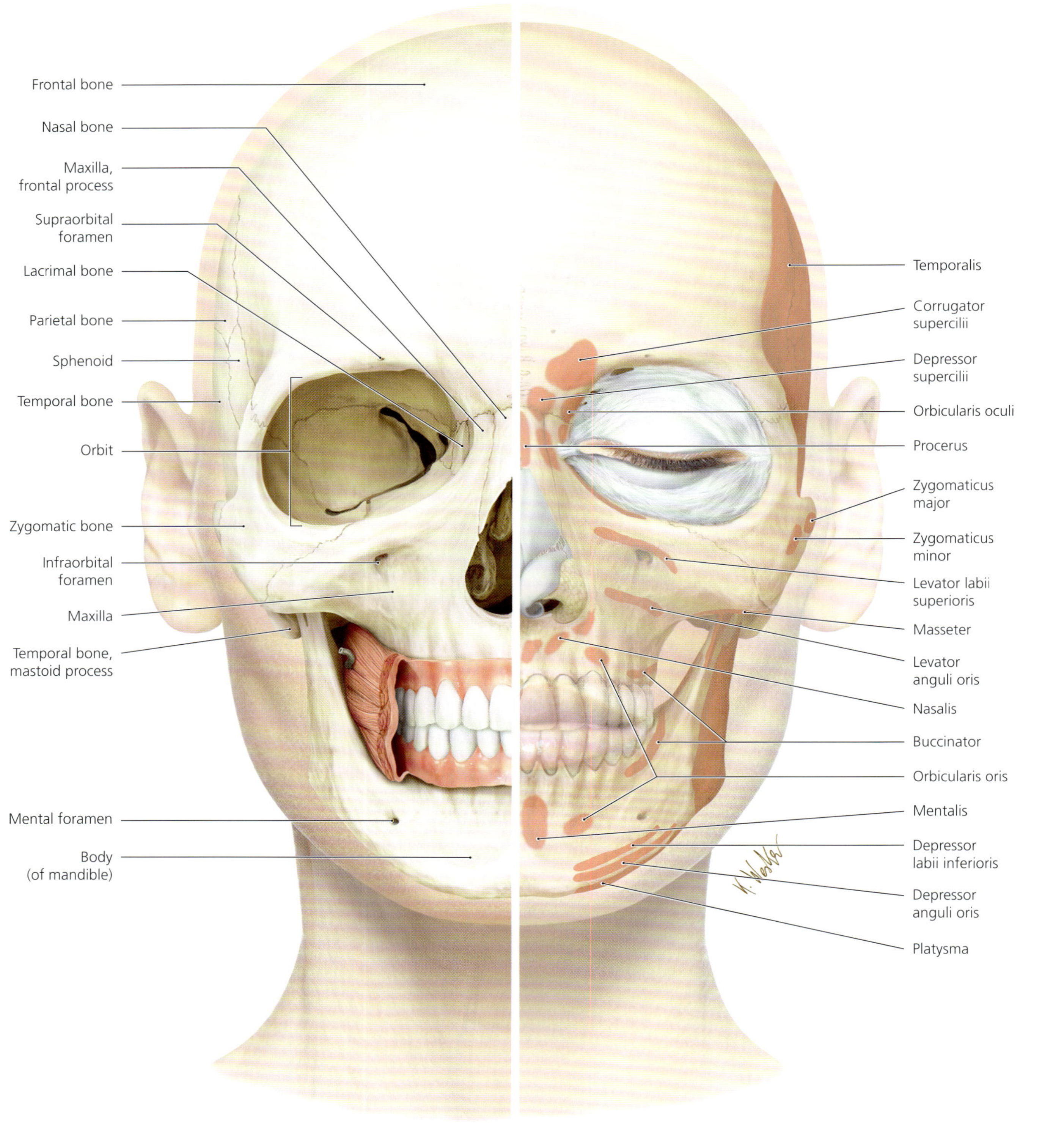

Fig. 2.9 The facial skeleton (right side of the face) and muscle attachment sites projected onto it (left side of the face).

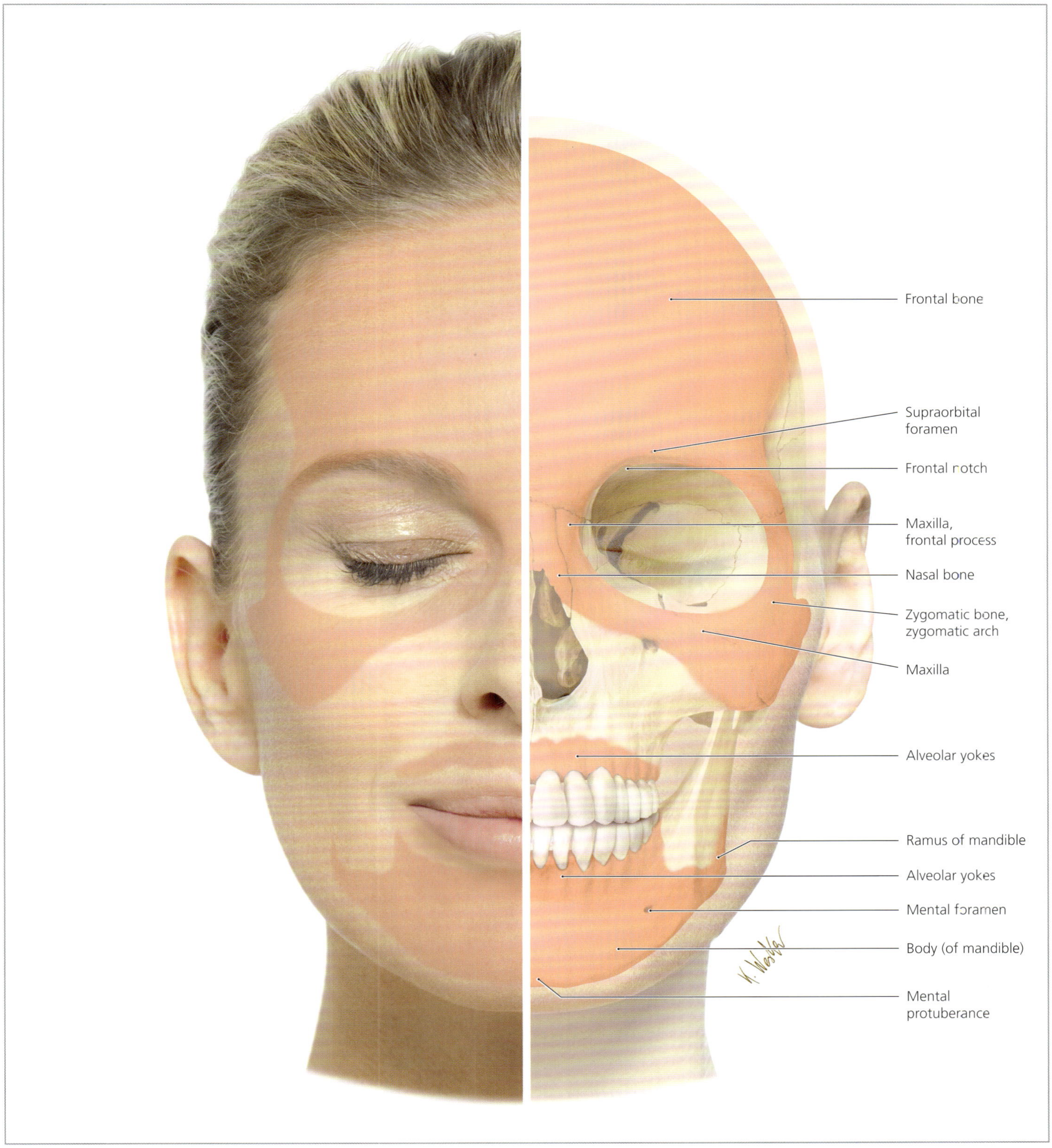

Fig. 2.10 Schematic representation of the palpable parts of the facial skeleton (red). Right: clinical appearance. Left: anatomical view.

2.2.2 Muscles of the face

The face consists of a total of 30 different muscles that are functionally divided into four paired muscles of mastication and 22 muscles of facial expression. According to Amar, the muscles of facial expression can be further subdivided according to their plane of depth (Amar R. E., Fox D. M. [2011]). Three muscle planes are thus distinguished: superficial, middle and deep (Fig. 2.11). As dynamic co-players in the soft tissue complex, the muscles of the face play an extremely important role in the mechanisms of facial ageing.

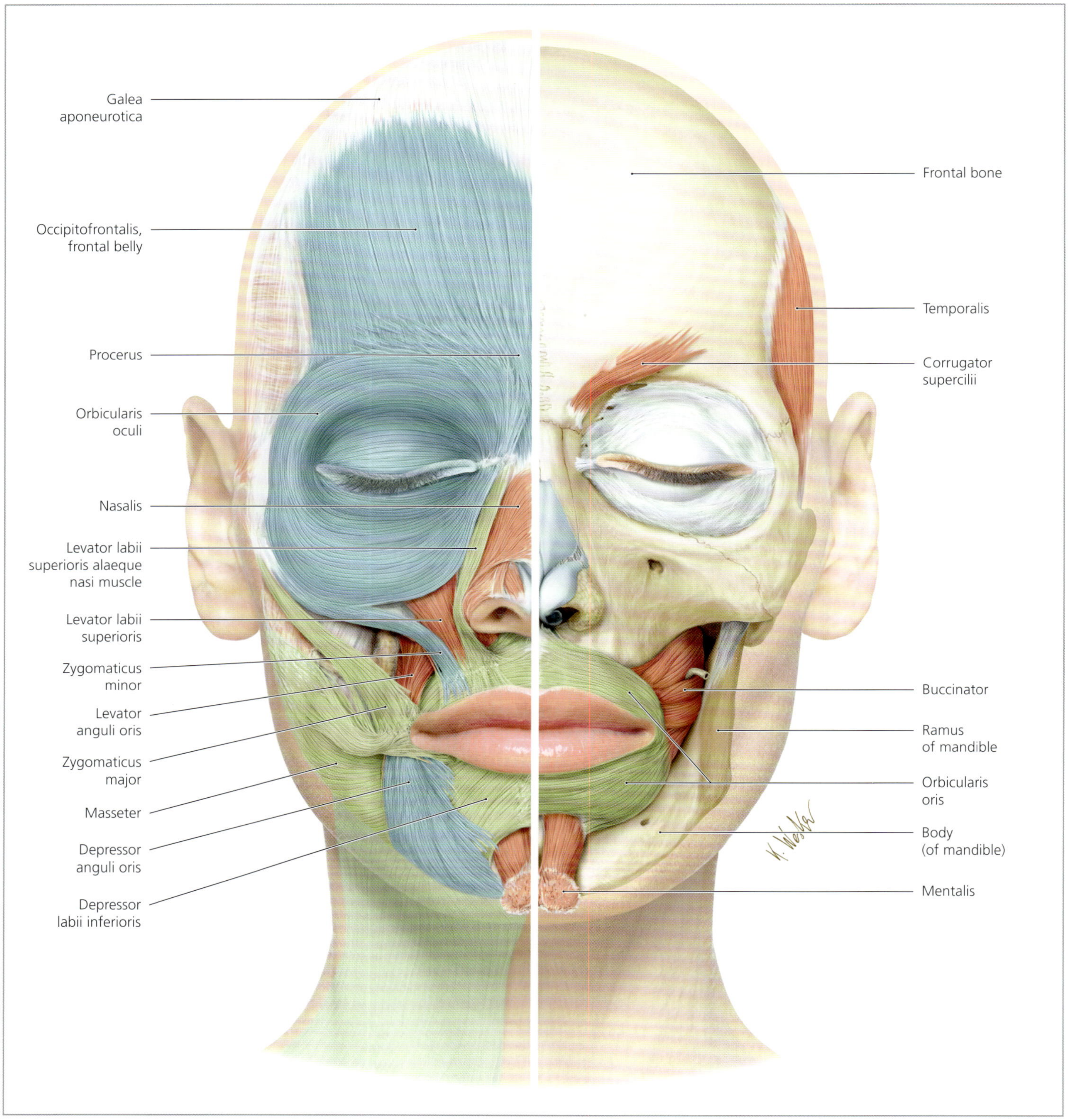

Fig. 2.11 Schematic representation of the facial muscles in three planes according to Amar: superficial (green), middle (blue) and deep (red).

2.2.3 Muscles of facial expression

The muscles of facial expression are mostly superficial muscles that lie just under the skin. Hence, they are also referred to as the 'skin muscles'. Dynamic wrinkles form due to the contraction of these muscles during the expression of emotions (Fig. 2.12). With age, these muscles tend to become hypertrophic, resulting in the development of persistently visible wrinkles that are involuntary and undesirable.

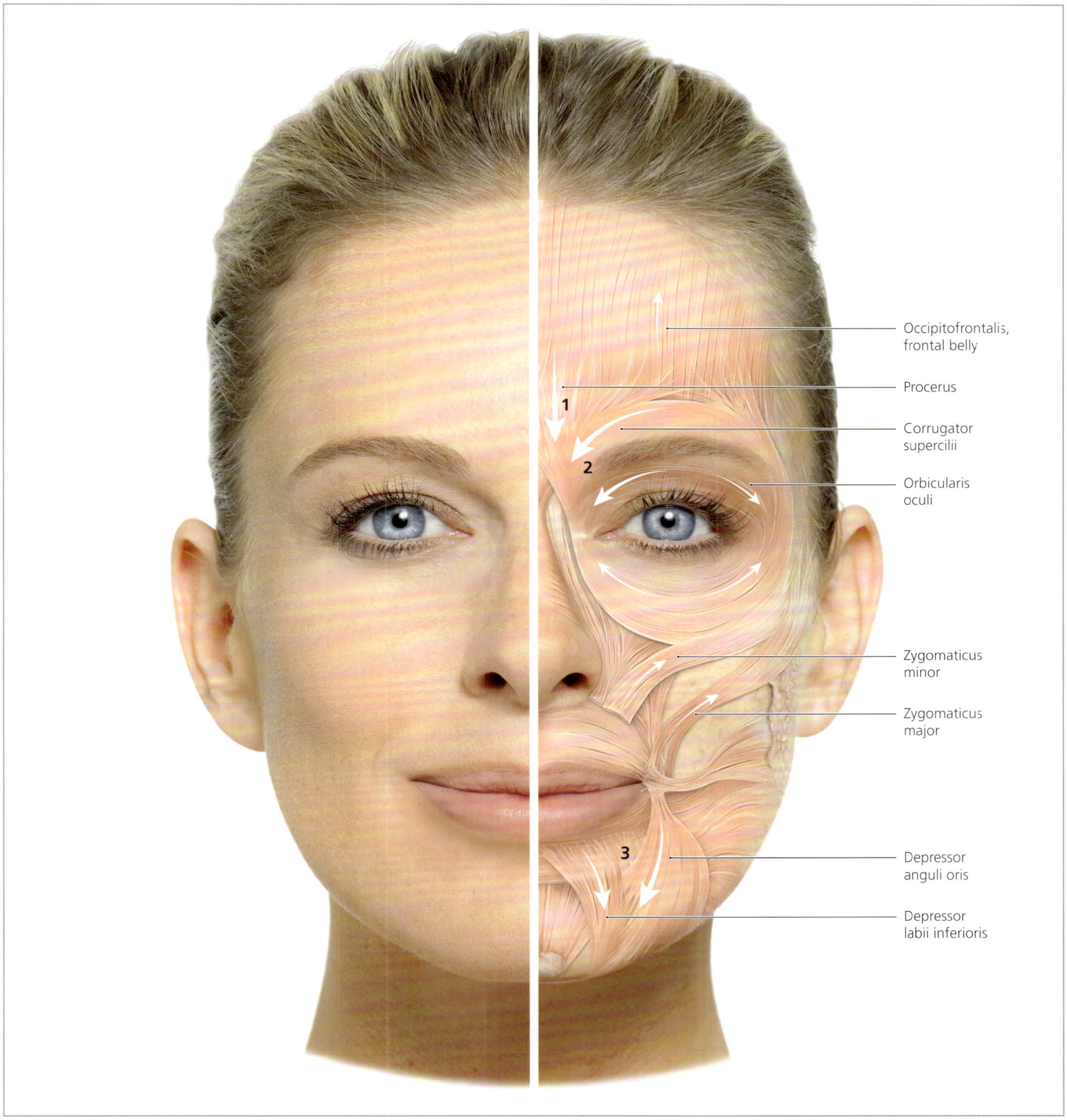

Fig. 2.12 Overview of the muscles of facial expression and schematic representation of the contraction forces (arrows) involved in the facial expression of emotion. An increase in depressor muscle activity (1, 2, 3) and a decrease in elevator muscle activity generally occurs with age.

A gradual shift in the balance of power between the facial elevator and depressor muscles also occurs, which contributes to the development of the age-related changes seen in the face. An increase in the depressor muscle activity and a decrease in the elevator muscle activity generally occur with age.

2.2.4 Subcutaneous fat and connective tissue

The subcutaneous fat embedded in the connective tissue of the face acts as a 'volumising agent' in the facial soft tissue complex. It provides a mechanical and physiological support cushion for the skin and the underlying structures. It not only functions as a 'shock absorber' that protects the face from external injury but it also ensures a continuous supply of essential fluids and nutrients to the facial tissue complex.

Two main fat compartments can be distinguished in the face: a continuous superficial fat compartment located superior to the superficial fascia of the superficial musculo-aponeurotic system (SMAS), and a discontinuous deep fat compartment located inferior to the SMAS.

The superficial fat compartment is a coherent system of small, highly septate fat lobules with a honeycomb-like appearance. Morphologically, it resembles fish skin whereby the skin attaches to the SMAS. This provides the skin with a layer of biomechanical support. In facial areas with a well-defined superficial fat compartment, the skin surface is more homogeneous and the facial features softer. In a youthful face the superficial fat layer is well-defined, particularly in facial areas in and around the cheeks, the nasolabial folds, the glabella, and the jaw–chin region, as well as in front of the neck above the platysma (Fig. 2.13). However, there is little superficial fat in the area

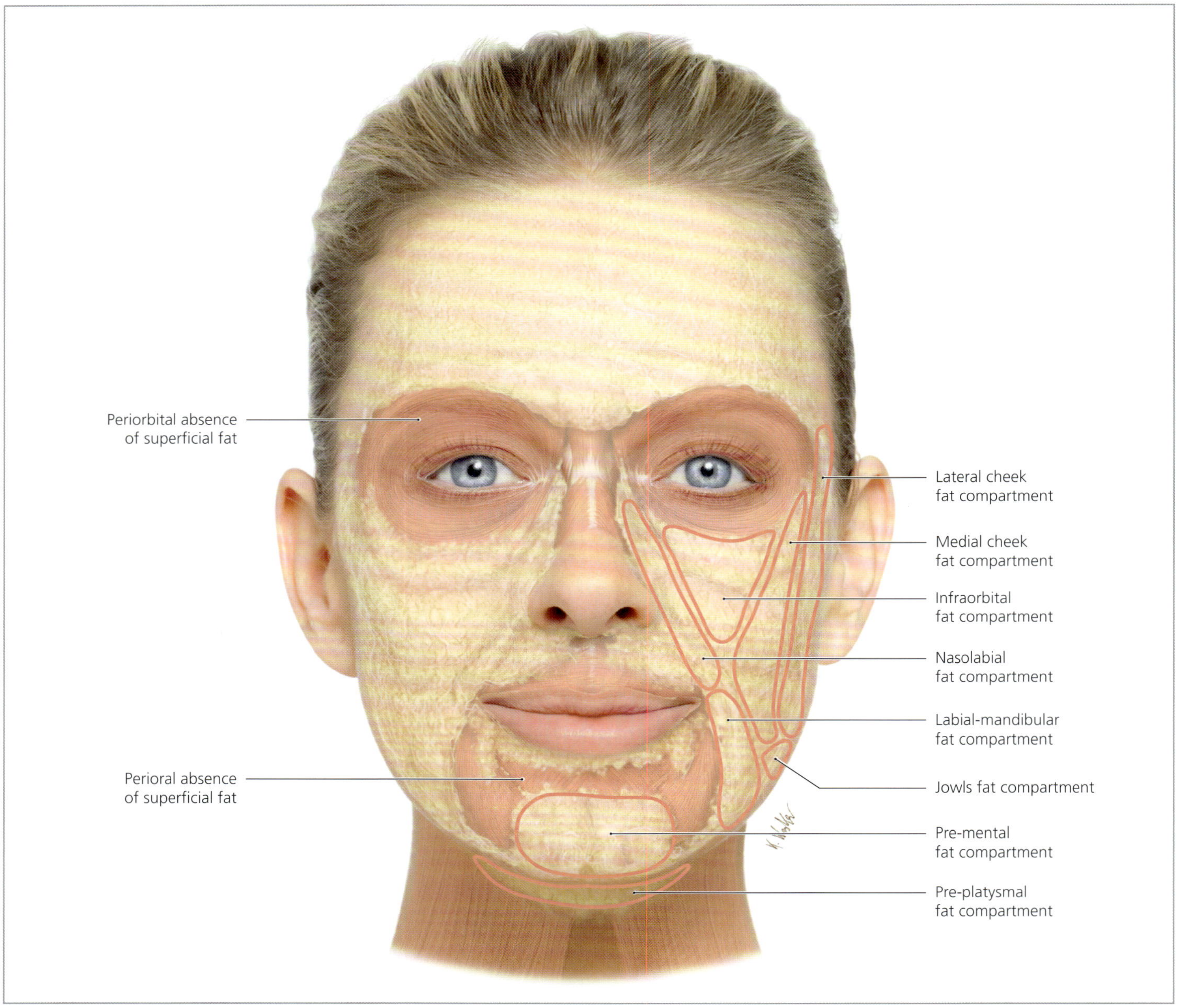

Fig. 2.13 Superficial fat distribution in the face.

of the temples and the forehead, and almost none in the periorbital and perioral region.

The deep fat layer lies inferior to the SMAS. In contrast to the superficial fat, it has a discontinuous structure composed of separate, individual fat bodies that resemble lipomas. These fat pads are larger and contain hardly any septae. The deep fat not only serves as padding for the structures embedded within it, but also functions as an energy store and an endocrine organ. In a youthful face, the deep fat pad provides a base of support and volume to the other facial soft tissues, and increases skin tone in the entire facial tissue complex in an augmentative manner. Atrophy and loss of volume of the deep fat in the natural ageing process is the main initiator of development of the externally visible signs of ageing. Moreover, the trophic conditions of the deep fat layer determine the quality of the blood supply and fluid balance in the peripheral tissue layers (Fig. 2.14).

Deep fat compartments of the face:

- Sub-orbicularis oculi fat (SOOF); inferior to the *orbicularis oculi* muscle (periorbicular)
- Retro-orbicularis oculi fat (ROOF); superior to the *orbicularis oculi* muscle (periorbicular)
- Buccal fat pad (Bichat's fat pad)
- Malar fat pad (in the zygomatic muscle region)
- Temporal fat pad
- Glabellar fat pad
- Submental fat compartment (chin fat)

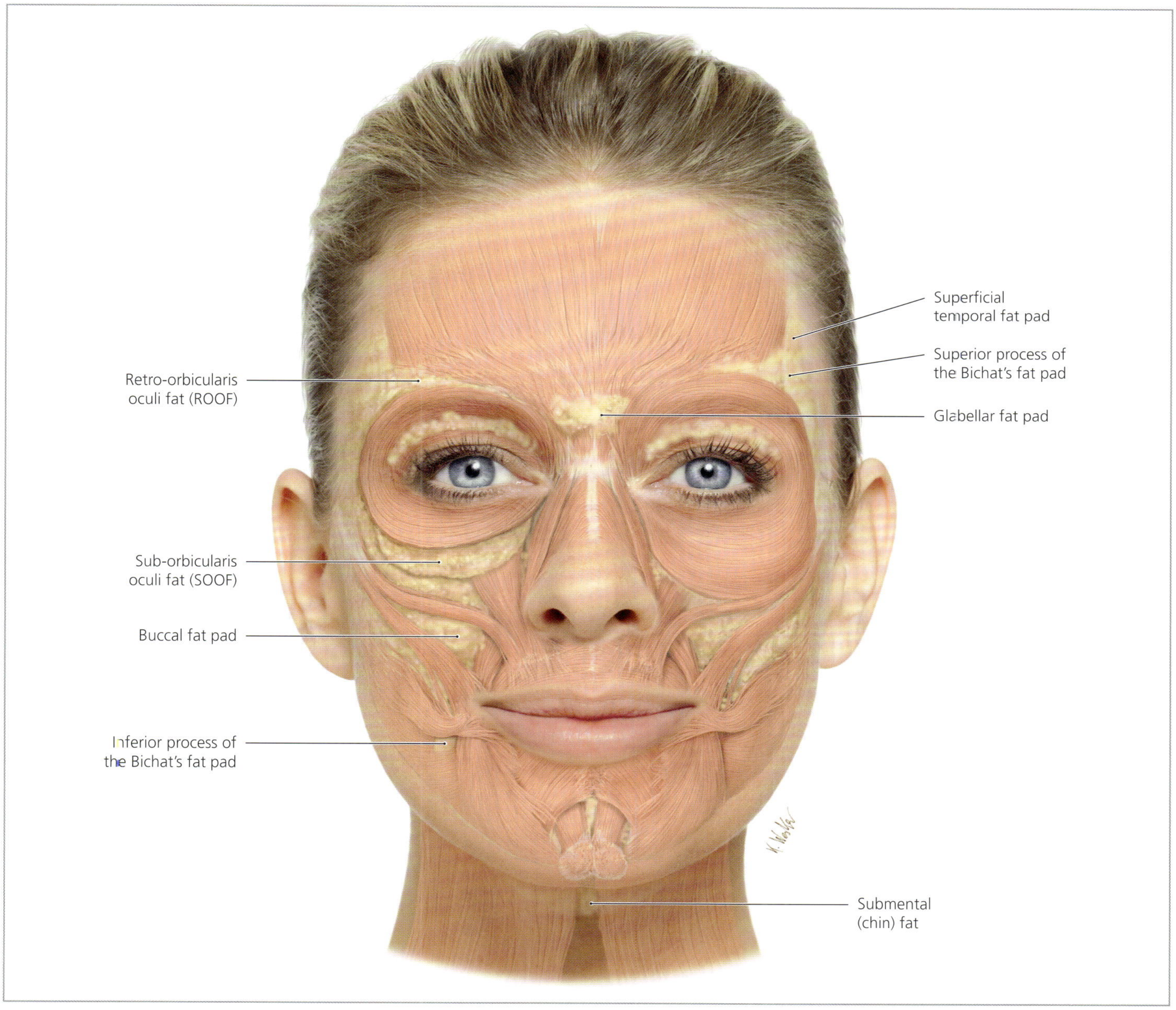

Fig. 2.14 Deep fat compartments of the face.

2.2.5 Retaining ligaments

Bands of fibrous connective tissue attach the skin to the underlying soft tissues and the skeletal structures. These fibrous bands are interchangeably referred to as the 'retaining ligaments' and 'skin ligaments' *(ligamentae retinacula cutis)*. Retaining ligaments that attach the skin to the bone are classified as 'true' retaining ligaments (Fig. 2.15), and those that attach the skin to the muscle fascia or to the superficial musculo-aponeurotic system are referred to as 'false' retaining ligaments.

True retaining ligaments are dense fibrous bands that function to provide facial integrity and compartmentalisation. When an injury occurs in one area of the face, the retaining ligaments form a diffu-

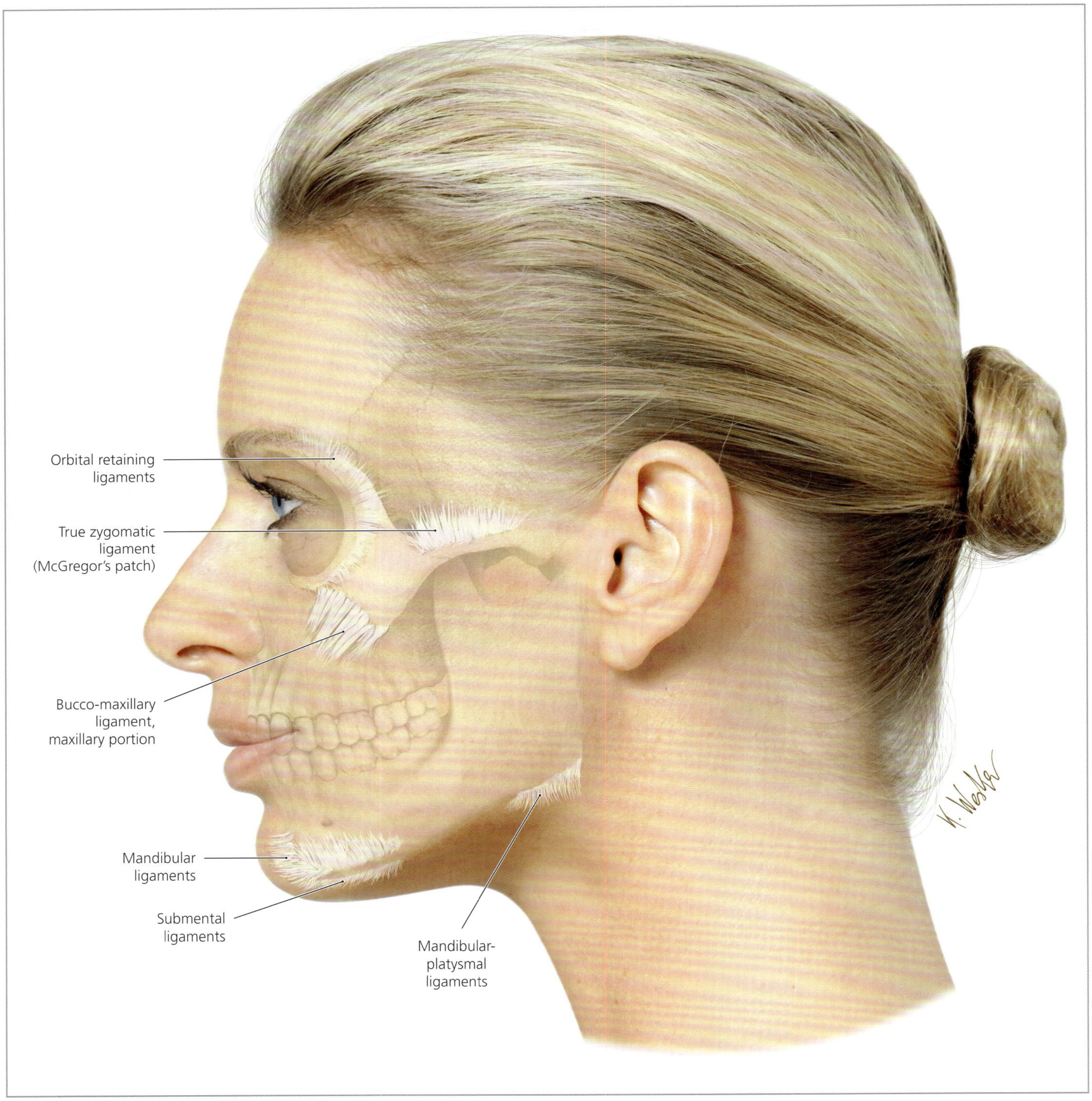

Fig. 2.15 True retaining ligaments.

sion barrier that prevents the redistribution of tissue fluids to other areas of the face. Thus the true retaining ligaments can be described as the 'pillars of the face'.

False retaining ligaments, on the other hand, tend to be longer and less dense (Fig. 2.16). They resemble a picket fence with spaces between the pickets and, thus, do not constitute a diffusion barrier. False retaining ligaments serve to stabilise the overall facial soft tissue complex by virtue of their attachment to the skin. Accordingly, they are responsible for the natural compartmentalisation of the facial skin surface, and for the tensile forces acting on it. In the initial stages of ageing, atrophy and weakening of these attachment elements results in the downward migration of the facial skin and the underlying soft tissues.

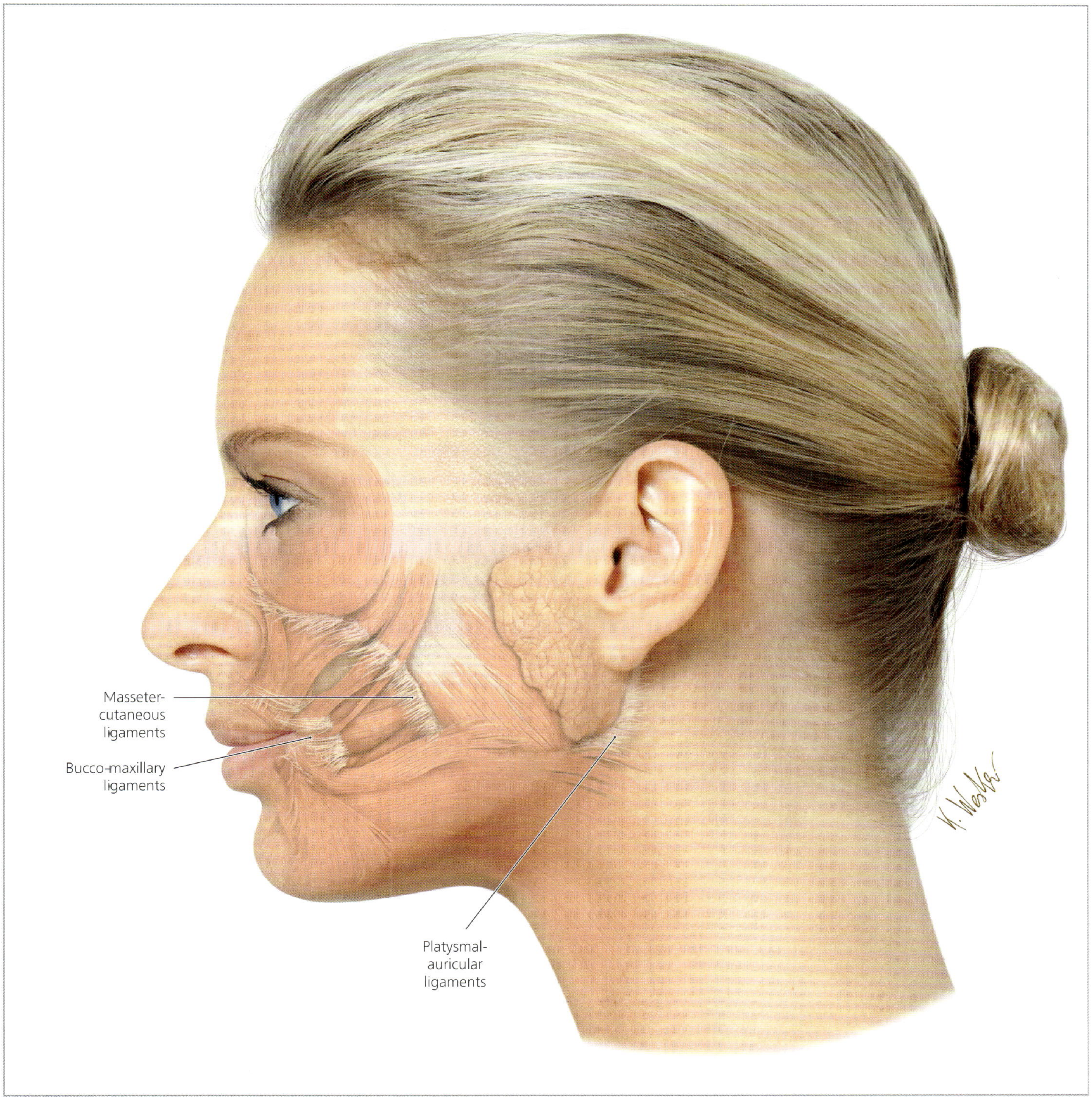

Fig. 2.16 False retaining ligaments.

2.2.6 Areolar planes

In order for individual tissue compartments to glide past one another or over the underlying periosteum, there exists a small space between these structures. Small areolar tissue compartments exist between the fascia, the connective tissue structures that surround other soft tissues (e.g. between a deep fat pad and the periosteum) (Fig. 2.17). Such structures are known as areolar or gliding planes.

Major areolar planes are found in the following parts of the face (Fig. 2.18):

1. Temporal (between the temporal and temporoparietal fascia)
2. Forehead (between the galea aponeurotica and the periosteum)
3. Midface (between the superficial SMAS and the parotidomasseteric fascia)
4. Neck (between the platysma and superficial cervical fascia).

These areolar zones can be considered as the sites where the downward migration of the facial soft tissue begins in the ageing process.

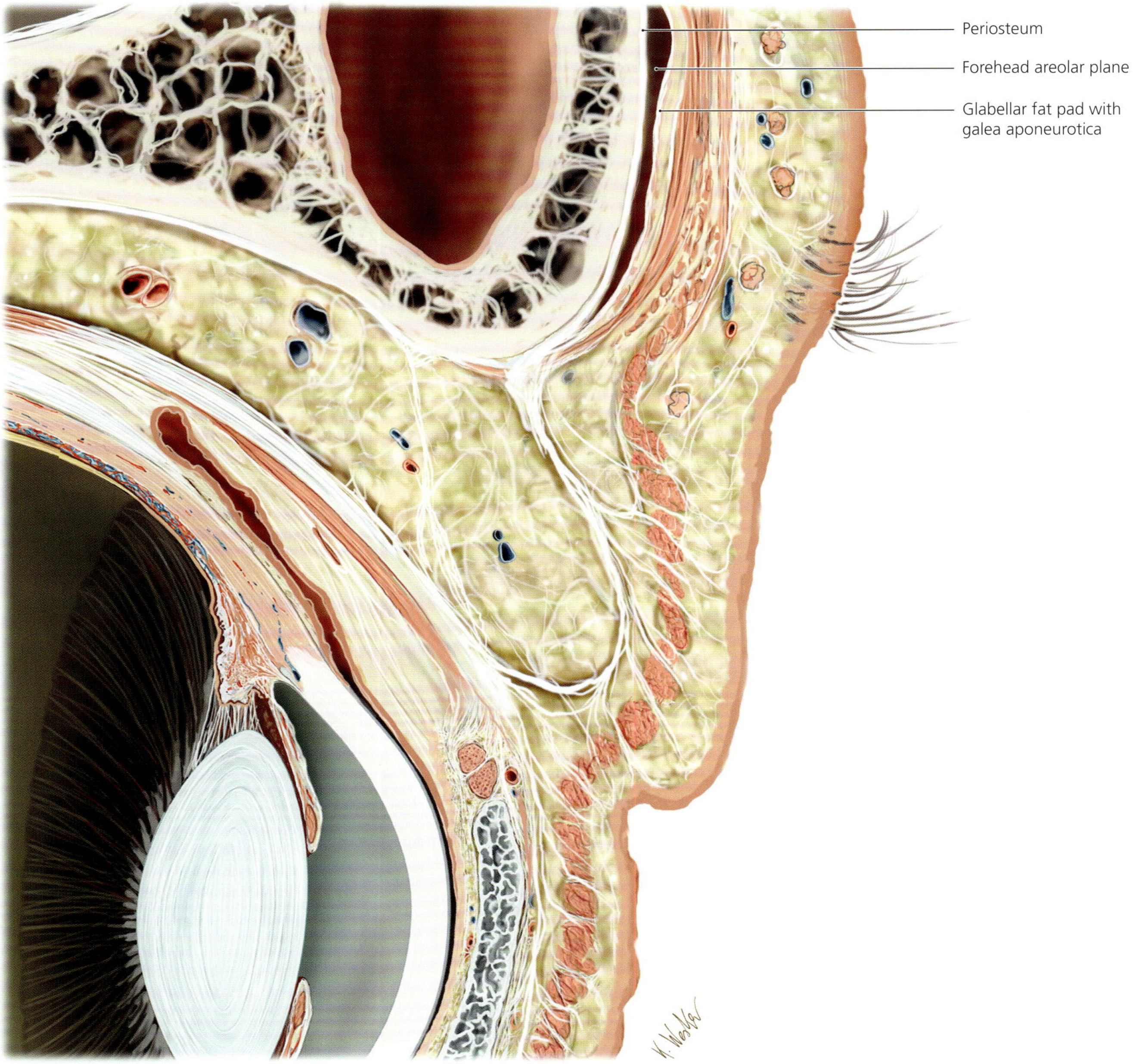

Fig. 2.17 Cross-section of the supraperioral region showing the forehead areolar plane.

2

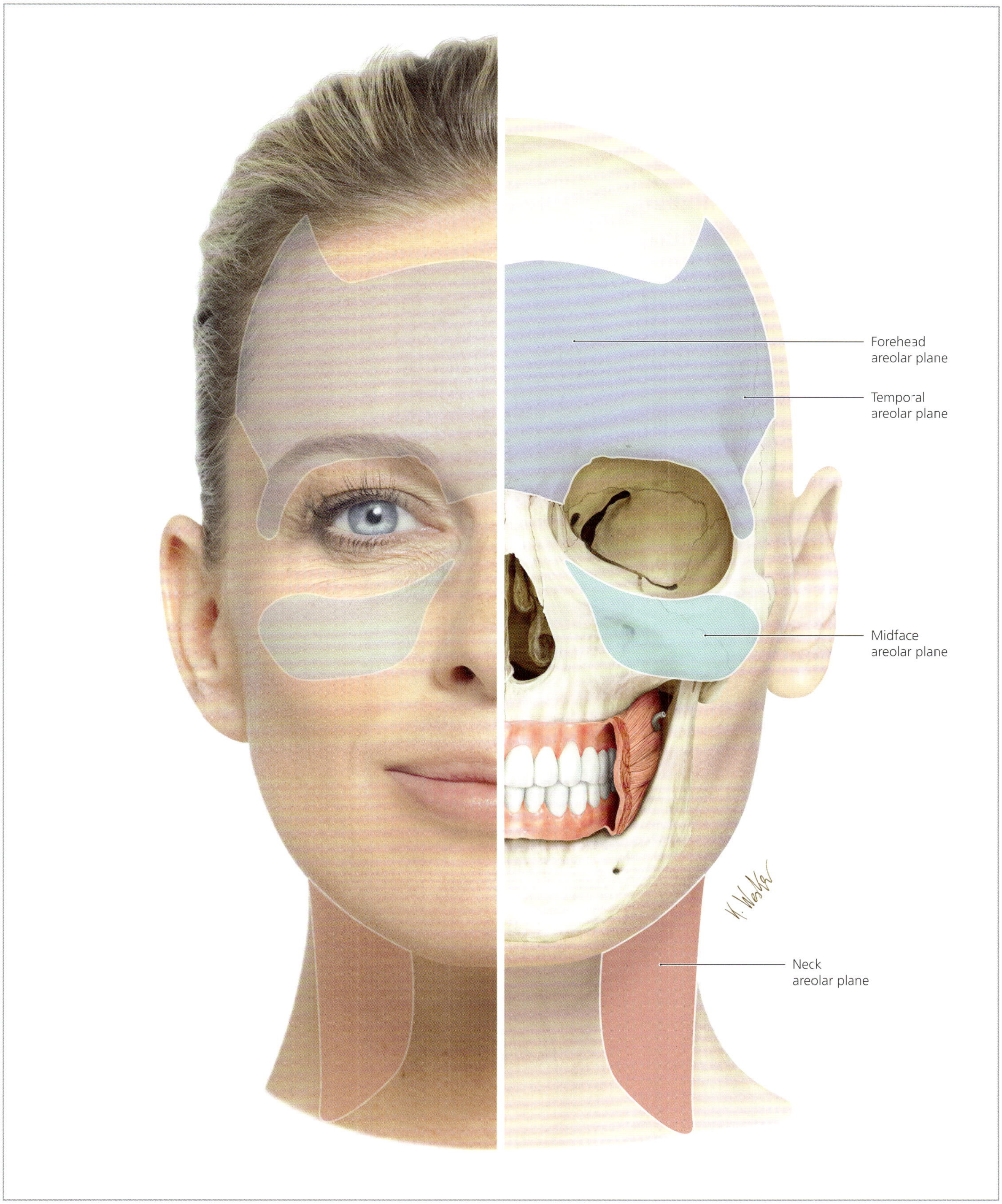

Fig. 2.18 Areolar planes of the face, projected onto the skin surface (right) and cranial skeleton (left).

2.2.7 Blood supply

A complex vascular network is at work to continuously transport blood alongside a steady supply of nutrients to the subcutaneous soft tissues. The peripheral skin layers however receive blood from fine capillary vessels. Because the epidermis receives its nutrients by diffusion alone, an adequate supply of blood and fluids to the skin and subcutaneous tissues is therefore imperative for a healthy and even complexion.

When performing any treatment resulting in microtrauma to the face, a thorough knowledge of the whereabouts of the major blood vessels is crucial, especially for the avoidance of complications relating to intravascular injection (Fig. 2.19).

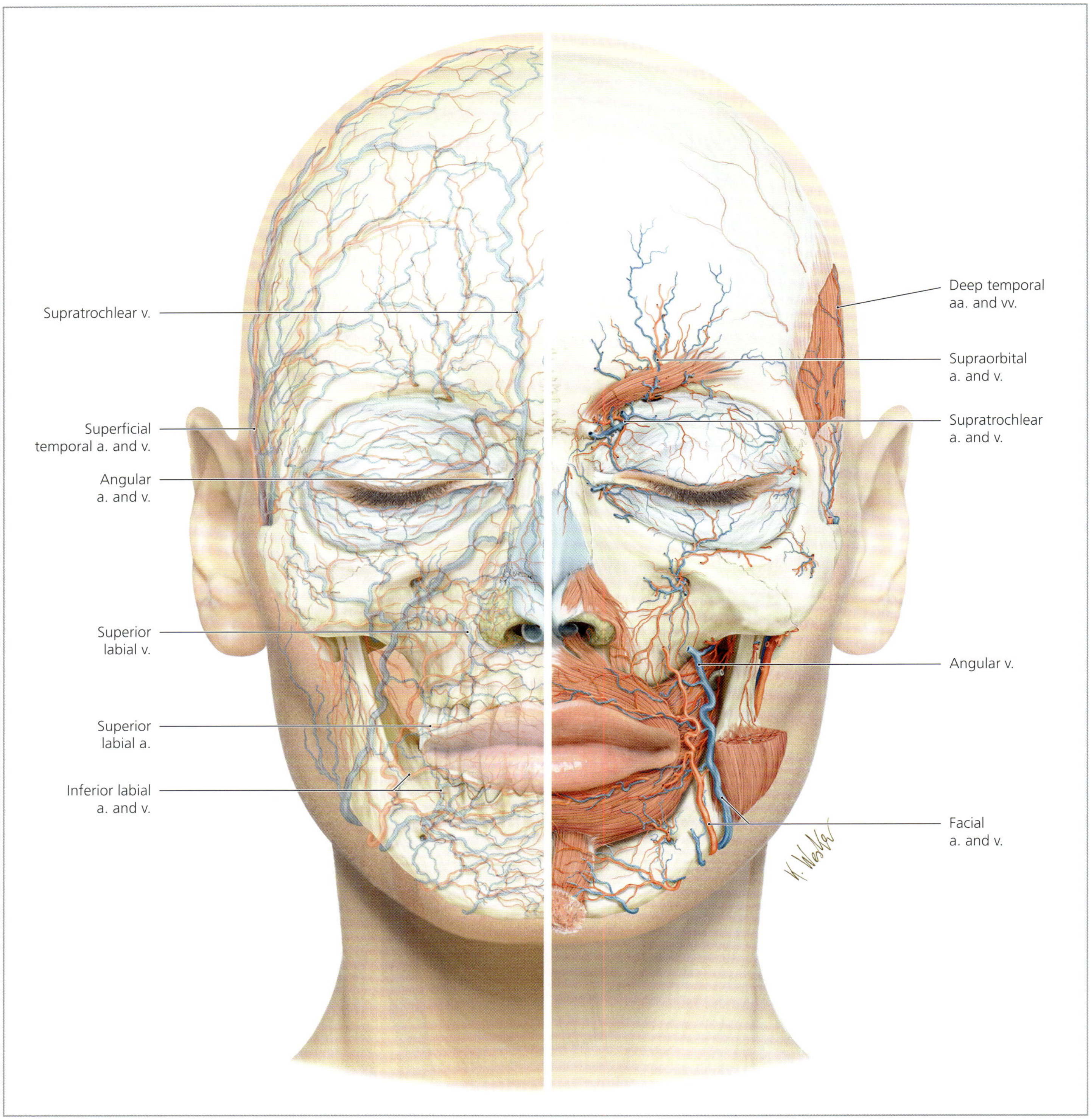

Fig. 2.19 Blood vessels of the face, projected onto the facial skeleton (right side), and the position of the deep arteries and veins of the face relative to the deep muscles (left side) (a. = artery, aa. arteries, v. = vein, vv. veins).

Because of the biological support function of the subcutaneous fat, an adequate blood supply to the subcutaneous fat is of critical importance for the maintenance of the fluid balance (volume) and the trophic condition of the overall soft tissue complex of the face (Fig. 2.20). In the young face, the subcutaneous soft tissues are well supplied with blood; however, a decrease in blood supply occurs at a relatively early age, and is accelerated by factors such as smoking. This results in two initial features of ageing, namely:

1. Facial volume loss due to atrophy
2. Deterioration in the supply of fluid, oxygen and nutrients to the skin.

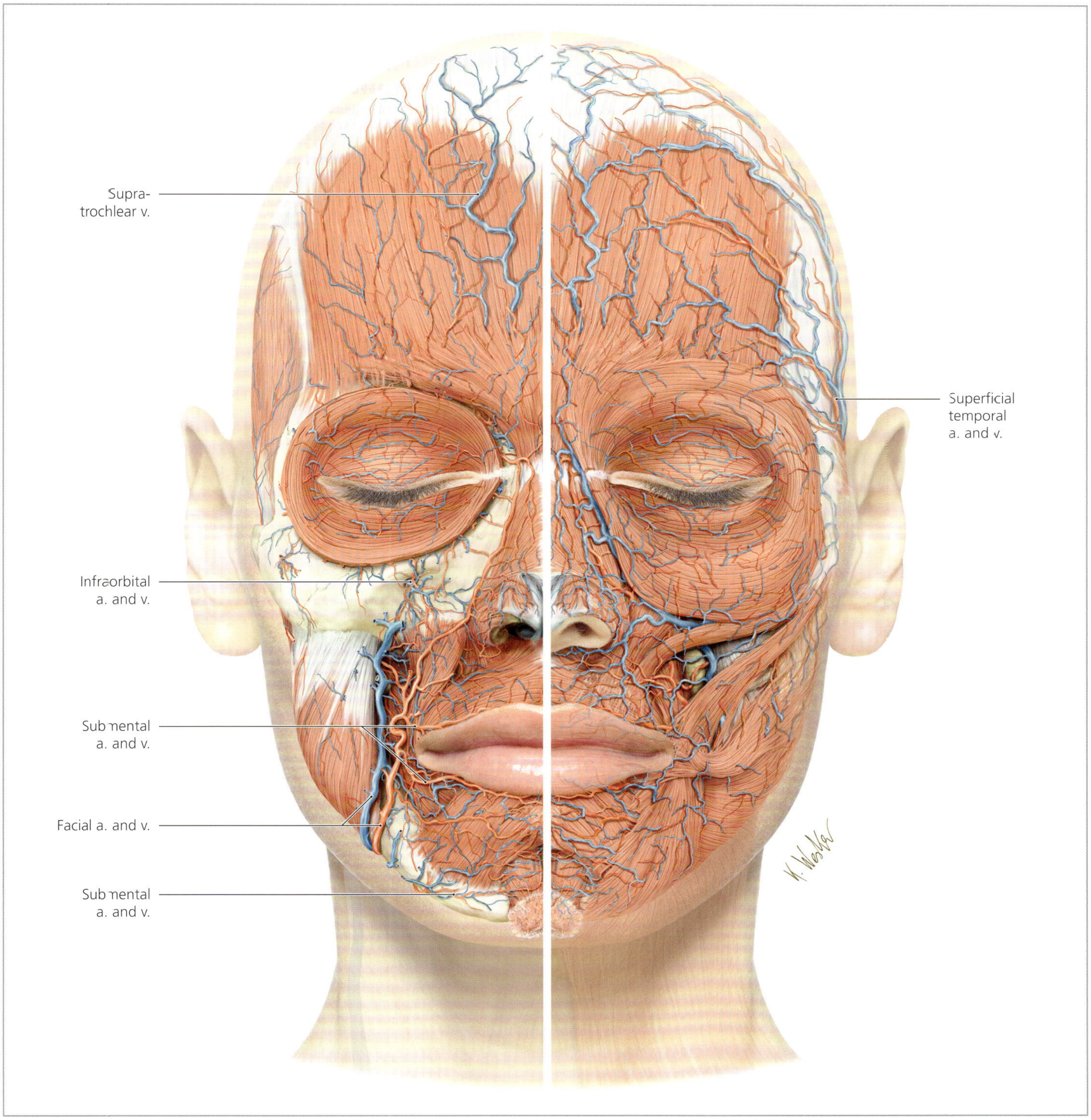

Fig. 2.20 Position of the facial arteries and veins relative to that of the moderately deep (right side) and superficial muscles (left side) (a. = artery, v. = vein).

2.2.8 Innervation

Innervation of the face arises mainly from the divisions of two major nerves: the trigeminal and the facial nerve.

The trigeminal nerve (cranial nerve V) is responsible for the sensory innervation of the face. Divisions of the trigeminal nerve include the ophthalmic nerve (V_1), the maxillary nerve (V_2), and the mandibular nerve (V_3). The ophthalmic nerve (V_1) exits the orbit via the supraorbital foramen and fissure, supplying sensation to the upper part of the face. The maxillary nerve (V_2) arises from the infraorbital foramen and innervates the midface. The mandibular nerve (V_3) innervates the mandibular and temporal regions (Fig. 2.21).

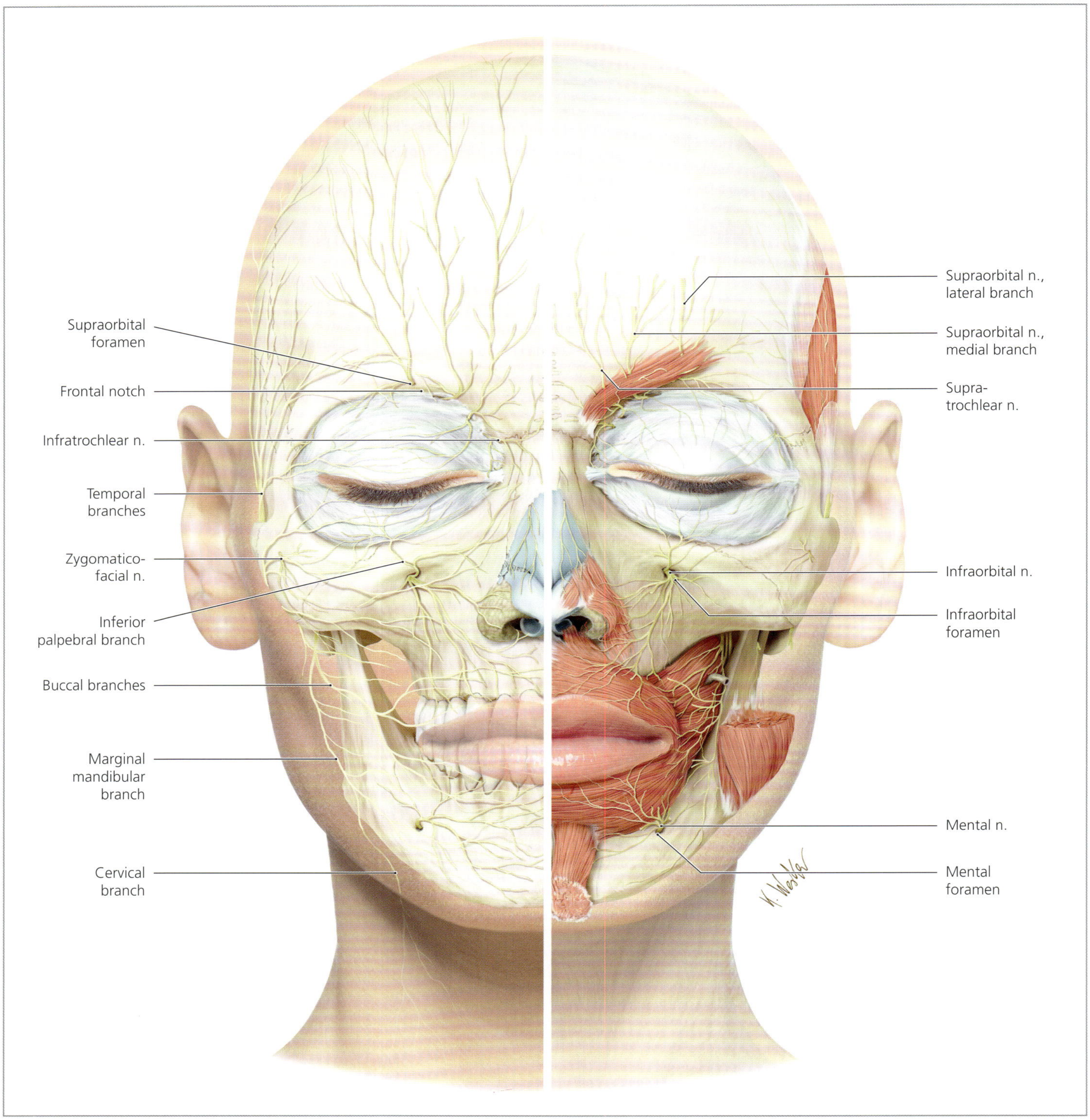

Fig. 2.21 Overview of the nerves of the face (right side of the face), and position of the deep facial nerves relative to the deep muscles (left side of the face) (n. = nerve).

The facial nerve (cranial nerve VII) innervates the muscles of facial expression. Within the parotid gland, it divides into five major branches, including the temporal, zygomatic, buccal, marginal mandibular and cervical. They run superficial to a number of muscles (Fig. 2.22).

The temporal branch of the facial nerve supplies the temporal, frontal and palpebral muscles. The zygomatic branch of the facial nerve innervates the muscles of the zygomatic region and lower eyelid; the buccal branches of the facial nerve extend to the muscles of the cheeks and the periorbital region. Meanwhile, the marginal mandibular branch of the facial nerve innervates the muscles of the chin region, and the cervical branch of the facial nerve supplies the platysma.

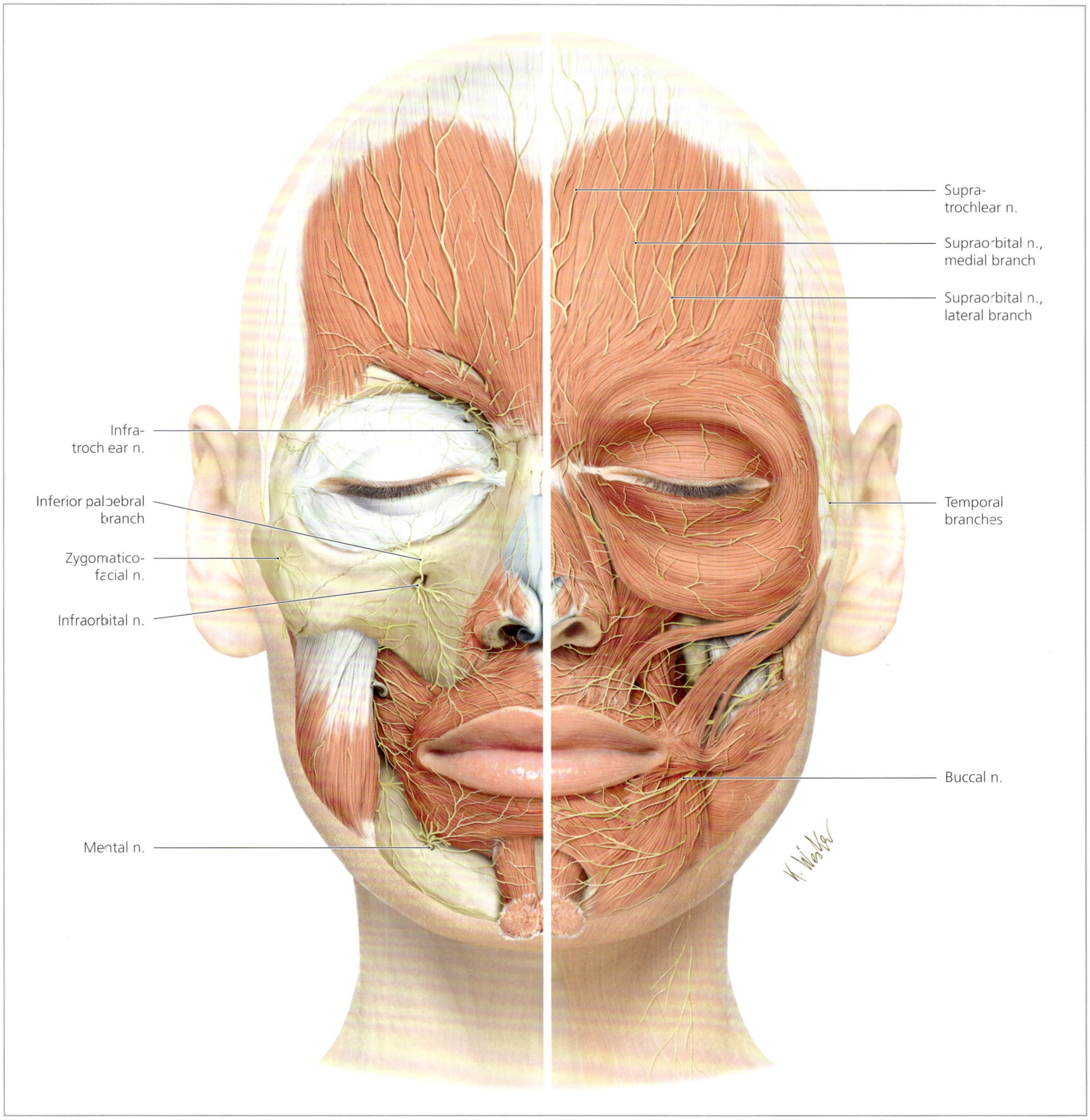

Fig. 2.22 Position of the facial nerves relative to the moderately deep (right side of the face) and superficial muscles (left side of the face) (n. = nerve).

2.3 Mechanisms of Facial Ageing and Their Clinical Consequences

Due to the complex interplay of intrinsic as well as extrinsic factors, age-related changes in the facial structures gradually arise over the course of time. Initially they occur at an anatomical level below the skin surface, and eventually become clinically apparent on the skin surface. Certain parts of the face are particularly susceptible to these changes. The first clinical signs of ageing manifest at sites on the skin surface with little superficial fat. For sites where superficial fat is absent, alongside facial atrophy due to deep fat loss, the clinical signs of ageing become apparent at a particularly early age. Sites of fat loss around the eyes and mouth are therefore considered to be facial ageing 'hot spots' (Fig. 2.23).

The face is comprised of different regional units or compartments. Therefore, the facial ageing process can be understood as a series of spatially isolated events, which are proportionally related to each other.

When attempting to develop causal therapeutic strategies, it is critical to consider the mechanisms of ageing:

- within the individual tissue compartments
- their regional interplay with adjacent structures
- in the global context of the face as a whole.

In order to restore a youthful, the proportional facial structure, it is important to consider not only the position of structural changes of ageing in the three-dimensional context of the face, but also the dynamic changes in the facial structures in the context of facial expressions.

2.3.1 Age-related changes in facial tissues

Changes in the skin

The skin is subject to intrinsic and extrinsic ageing processes, as described in the previous section. In summary, cumulative UV damage results in a gradual loss of collagen and a decrease in skin elasticity over time. Metabolism is impaired and cell division rates slow due to the biological degradation mechanisms, enhanced by the decrease in blood supply and the atrophy-related general deterioration of the trophic condition of the tissues. This results in impairment of the regeneration capacity, barrier function and immune function of the skin. The main clinical signs and consequences of skin ageing are increasing dryness and inhomogeneity of the skin surface, accompanied by an increased susceptibility to injury and infection.

At the same time, the relative surface area of the skin envelope increases due to the progressive soft tissue atrophy, and the stabilising tension produced by the retaining ligaments decreases. Skin laxity is not only caused by a loss of elasticity, but also by the loosening of the attachment of the skin to the other soft tissues and underlying structures. The consequences are gravity-induced sagging of the skin, skin folds and wrinkles.

Changes in the subcutaneous fat

Although all facial skin ages at a uniform rate, the visible signs of ageing tend to be more or less concentrated in some areas more than others. This highlights that changes in the skin surface alone cannot be the sole factor responsible for the occurrence of the clinical signs of ageing.

Therapeutic implications – blood supply

A decrease in the blood supply and subcutaneous tissue atrophy result in the deterioration of the trophic condition of the skin, the related decrease in the relative moisture content of the stratum corneum, the degradation of dermal collagen, and water loss. These are some of the main causes of the visible signs of skin ageing. The dermis and the subcutaneous fat can be resaturated with fluids via the injection of water-binding filler substances, such as hyaluronic acid. This can compensate for the deficits and restore the vitality and barrier function of the skin by natural means. Clinically, this results in a more homogeneous, more elastic and smoother skin surface with a 'fresher' complexion. Therefore, superficial hyaluronic acid injections are useful for skin rejuvenation in the treatment and prevention of premature skin ageing.

Topographical comparisons at the sites of subcutaneous fat distribution versus those of the clinical signs of ageing (see Fig. 2.23) show that the appearance of the structural changes of ageing are associated with the distribution and condition of the subcutaneous fat deposits. The periorbital and perioral regions are the starting points for the loss of the subcutaneous fat in the clinical ageing process. Since the skin in these areas lacks a biomechanical support layer, the surface is particularly susceptible to the visible effects of anatomical degeneration. Importantly, the externally visible signs, including wrinkles, skin laxity and the loss of a homogeneous skin surface, should not be regarded as the causes of age-related changes in the facial appearance. The causes of these visible changes most likely occur at deeper tissue levels that are not clinically visible.

Recent anatomical findings suggest that deep fat atrophy is significantly affected by age-related decrease in blood flow (Anderhuber, 2012 and personal communication). Hence, vascular degeneration is considered the main initiator of the development of the structural changes of ageing. Importantly, blood flow to the supraperiosteal fat pads deteriorates at a relatively early age, and is furthermore accelerated by factors such as smoking (Anderhuber, 2012 and personal communication). Therefore, a decrease in the supply of fluids, oxygen and nutrients, as well as shrinkage of the deep fat stores occurs in young adulthood in some cases. The gradual loss of volume and physiological blood supply from the underlying subcutaneous tissue results in the decrease of skin tone and fluid levels in the entire facial tissue complex.

Furthermore, the retaining ligaments slacken and lose their ability to provide adequate support to the skin and other soft tissues. The facial skin envelope begins to sag, and downward migration of the underlying soft tissues occurs via the areolar planes. The condition of the skin surface deteriorates due to the diminishing support from below.

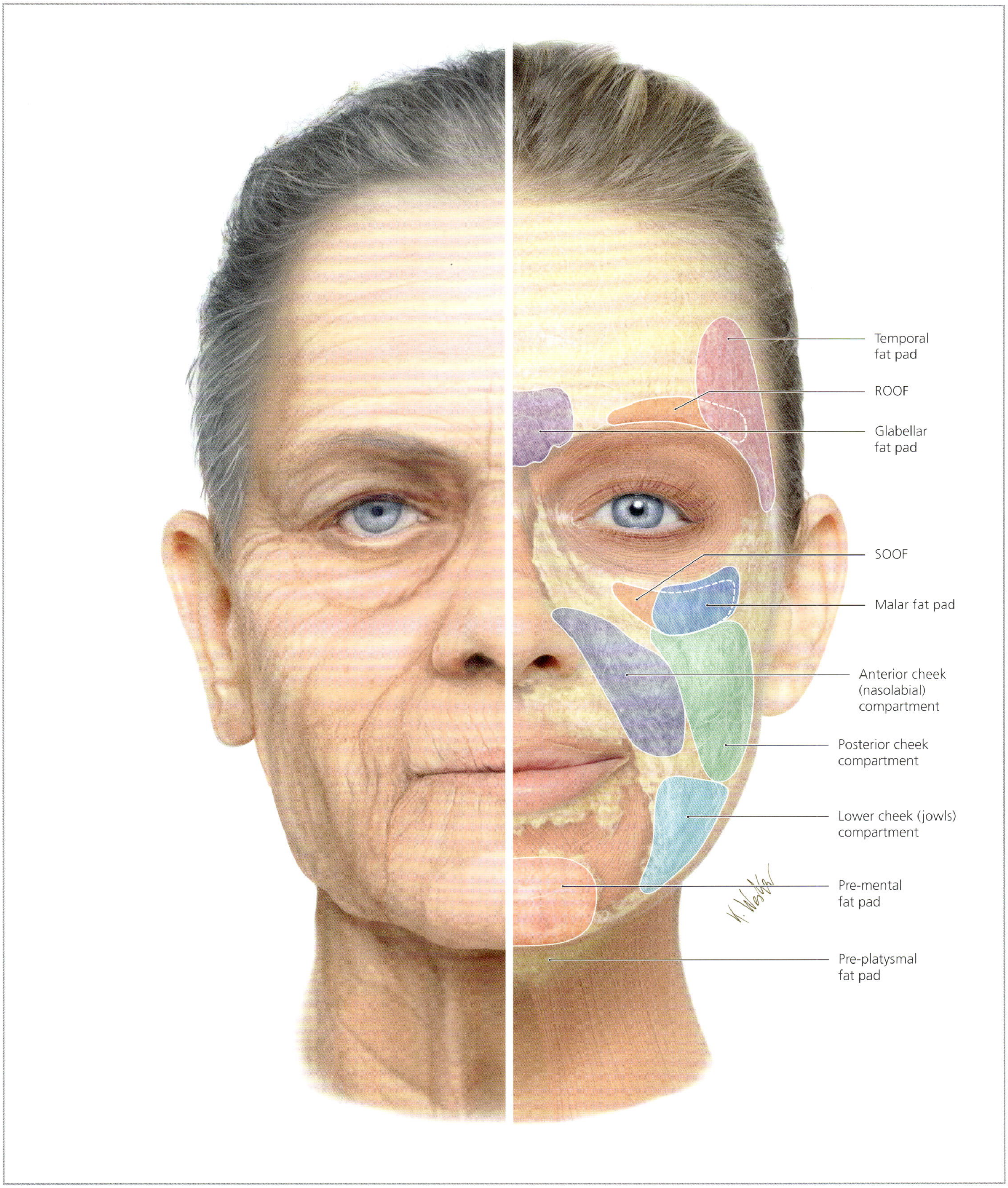

Fig. 2.23 Split view of the clinical signs of ageing and subcutaneous fat distribution of the face. It is apparent at first glance that there is a correlation between them. At sites where superficial fat is absent, alongside facial atrophy due to deep fat loss, the clinical signs of ageing become apparent at a particularly early age. Sites of fat loss around the eyes and mouth are therefore considered to be facial ageing 'hot spots'.

In view of the multifactorial causes of these blood flow-related processes, it is understandable why the clinical signs of ageing occur at a point in time where the effects of purely chronological changes (e.g. within the bone) are not yet expected. This also explains why there are inter-individual differences in the severity and time of occurrence of the individual structural changes.

Therapeutic implications – subcutaneous fat

The subcutaneous fat plays a key role in the initial process of facial ageing. Atrophy of the supraperiosteal fat pad and the associated loss of elasticity of the tissue complex are considered to be the main causes of the occurrence of the clinical signs of facial ageing. As observed after injecting hyaluronic acid filler into the deep subcutaneous tissues, these visible structural changes in the face can be treated directly by compensatory volume and fluid replacement. This treatment strategy achieves results superior to previous approaches aimed at either superficial masking or surgical resection of the structural changes in the face. Contrary to the original theory of facial ageing, the clinical signs of ageing can be attributed to soft tissue deficits, which can be effectively treated with minimally invasive, tissue-sparing restorative procedures. Such anti-ageing treatments and preventative techniques, including soft tissue augmentation using filler agent with a high water-binding capacity, are the forerunners of modern anti-ageing medicine of the 21st century.

Changes in the retaining ligaments

For a long time, the role of the facial retaining ligaments was virtually ignored when considering possible clinical-anatomical correlations with ageing. Today we know that the skin ligaments are primarily responsible for the three-dimensional compartmentalisation of the skin surface, and that they play a leading role in the development of most of the structural changes of facial ageing.

The facial retaining ligaments produce tension between the skin and other tissues, thus tightening the overall tissue complex and stabilising its three-dimensional structure. The loss of the underlying soft tissue volume associated with ageing results in a general decrease in tension. Particularly the false retaining ligaments, which are less stable, slacken at a relatively early age and increasingly lose their ability to sufficiently augment the stability of the skin, muscle and fatty tissues. This triggers and/or promotes the gravity-induced downward migration of the skin and soft tissues, resulting in the disproportionate redistribution of the tissues and the development of skin folds.

The buccal part ('false ligament') of the buccal–maxillary retaining ligament is considered the weakest of the retaining ligaments. Its rapid weakening leads to the early sagging of soft tissues in the anterior cheek region, resulting in the characteristic formation of the nasolabial folds – one of the initial signs of ageing.

True retaining ligaments are column-like connectors that attach skin to bone. If an atrophy-related decrease in the underlying soft tissue base occurs, visible indentations in the skin surface appear at the ligament attachment sites. This contributes to the development of the visible signs of ageing, such as eye bags and malar fat pads in the cheekbone area (buccal–maxillary retaining ligament), nasolabial folds in the midface region, marionette lines in the lower third of the face, and changes in the jaw–chin line. In some cases, the significant atrophic situation and fluid deficit also leads to accelerated degeneration (fibrosis) of the retaining ligaments in connection with an increasing loss of elasticity (Fig. 2.24).

Therapeutic implications – tensile forces

The tensile forces exerted by the retaining ligaments are also determined by conditions in the subcutaneous fat. Age-related atrophy and loss of the underlying tissue volume leads to the impairment of the overall skin tone, which promotes the downward migration of the destabilised soft tissues via the areolar planes. This results in the early appearance of prominent structural changes of ageing, such as ptosis and nasolabial folds.

Furthermore, the centralised tension forces from the true retaining ligaments lead to indentations in the skin surface over the atrophied areas. Depression of the surface below the original level at ligament attachment sites is thus a more likely explanation for some oedema-like visible signs of ageing (e.g. sagging cheeks) rather than bulging due to fat prolapse. The fibrotic adhesion of ligaments to their atrophied attachment sites may increase the severity of these manifestations.

By injecting water-binding hyaluronic acid fillers to compensate for the loss of the deep subcutaneous tissue volume, the slackened retaining ligaments can be tightened, and the overall soft tissue complex can be lifted. This is extremely important when treating problems such as the infraorbital hollow.

Anatomical release of the possibly fibrotic retaining ligaments attached to the dehydrated underlying tissues with subsequent filler injections at the attachment sites may further reduce the tension on the skin and smooth out the deep indentations (i.e. nasolabial folds and marionette lines) harmoniously and without static overprojection.

Retaining ligaments

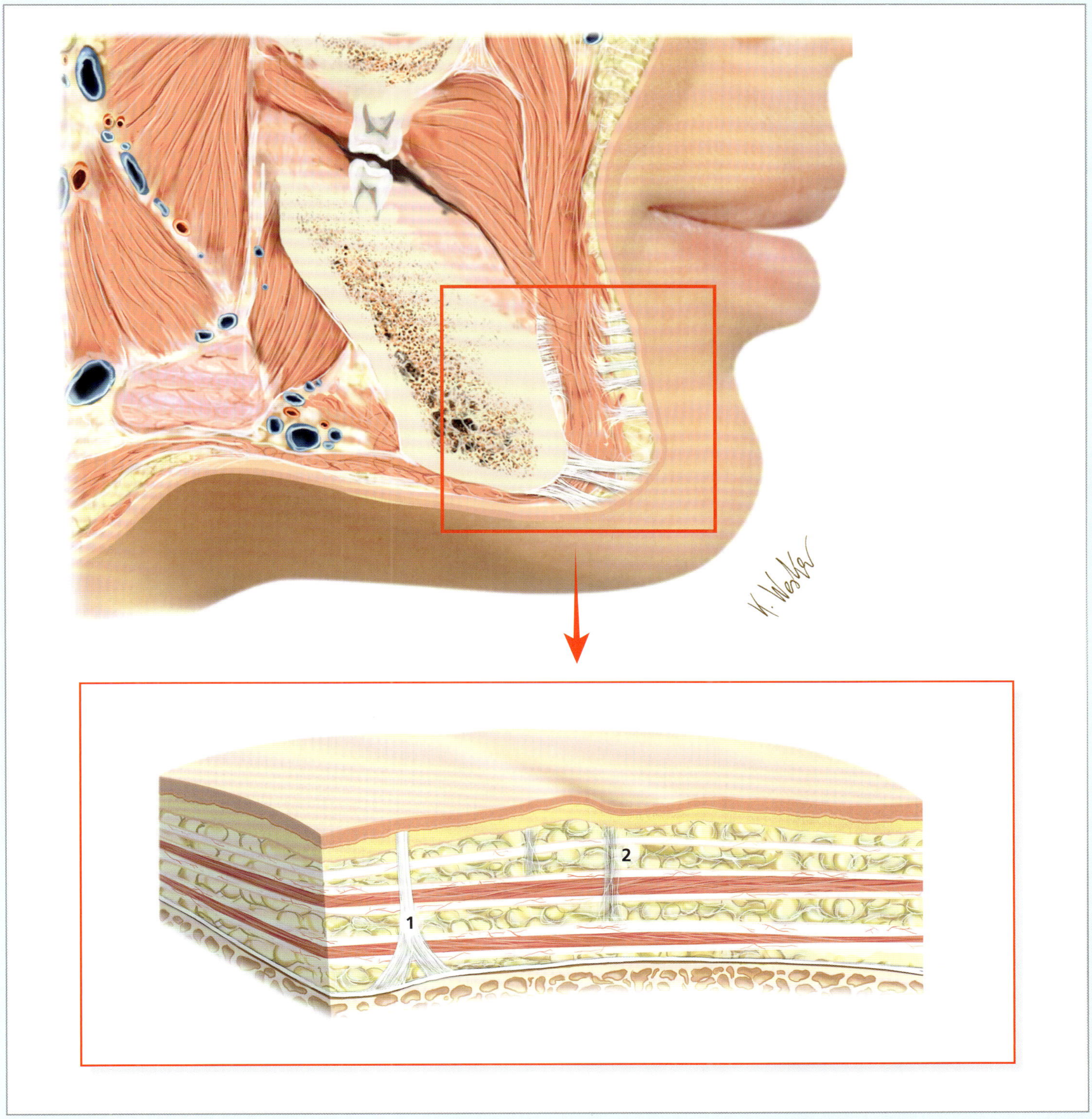

Fig. 2.24 Schematic representation of the true **(1)** and false **(2)** retaining ligaments and their role in compartmentalisation of the face. True retaining ligaments act as solid columns, whereas false retaining ligaments form a permeable elastic barrier between the skin and other parts of the tissue complex. Laxity of the retaining ligaments occurs due to atrophy and loss of the underlying subcutaneous tissue volume, resulting in destabilisation and gravity-induced sagging of the skin and soft tissues. Continuous tension on the skin at the attachment sites of true retaining ligaments results in visible indentations on the skin surface. Both of these clinical signs of ageing can be successfully treated by deep-tissue volume augmentation with agents such as hyaluronic acid fillers.

Role of the muscles of facial expression

A loss of muscle mass generally occurs in the ageing process. The muscles of facial expression exhibit characteristic features in this context. An increase in average muscle tone can be observed whereas the bellies of these muscles get lengthened following age-related softening of the connective tissues together with enduring functional stress. Consequently, the extent of muscle activity decreases, although the muscles are generally in a state of continuous tension. As a result, wrinkles and lines that can be voluntarily produced in areas of facial expression remain visible, even when the face is relaxed.

A gradual shift in the balance of power between the depressor and elevator muscles (agonists and antagonists) also occurs with age. Muscle activity increases in the depressor muscles (e.g. the corrugators and depressor anguli oris muscles), and decreases in the elevator muscles (e.g. the frontalis and levator angulis oris muscles). With age this imbalance provokes the appearance of an increasingly negative, upset and unfriendly facial expression, and contributes to the development of the characteristic signs of ageing, such as sagging of the eyebrows (eyebrow ptosis) and drooping of the corners of the mouth.

Therapeutic implications – wrinkle smoothing

As the facial expression muscles become hypertrophic with age, lines and creases that once occurred only in dynamic states become persistent. Glabellar frown lines are the most prominent example. When planning the aesthetic correction of wrinkles, the clinician must first determine whether the wrinkles are being induced dynamically (by muscle activity) or statically (due to atrophy). If induced by muscle activity, dose-dependent botulinum toxin type-A administration is always the first treatment of choice. Thereafter, if still necessary the wrinkle-smoothing effect can be further optimised by adjuvant hyaluronic acid filler injections. Ideally, facial harmonisation therapy is a combination of fillers for volume augmentation and botulinum toxin type-A for muscle relaxation.

Changes in the facial skeleton

The facial skeleton also undergoes gradual, age-related changes, which contribute to the development of the visible signs of ageing. In very advanced age, a significant loss of the bone mass in the facial skeleton can be observed, especially within the orbital region. This can promote the downward migration of the fat compartments and the skin above these regions. For decades, this hypothesis has been used to explain the development of the visible signs of ageing. However we would like to propose further thoughts and ideas on this hypothesis and perhaps refute that skeletal changes is the key influencing factor responsible for the initial visible signs of ageing. Rather, the authors would like to propose that the initial signs of ageing arise from changes in the conditions within the soft tissues, namely relating to the blood supply, connective tissue elements, alongside the activity of the muscles and the ligaments etc. As an example, we have previously discussed the significant impact that vascular degeneration has on the atrophy of the deeper fat pads. Similarly, the cumulative stress on the skeletal structures arising from the constant muscular and ligamentous activity should also be considered in this context. Hence, the onset and the development of facial ageing is a complex process.

Therapeutic implications – ageing causes

Clinically, the facial ageing process can be understood as the result of multifactorial transformation mechanisms in a three-dimensional tissue complex comprised of the skin, muscles, subcutaneous fat, connective tissue and the skeleton. In terms of clinical significance, specific causes and events certainly play an important role at different stages of life. Whereas soft tissue atrophy resulting from a decreased blood supply is now thought to be the primary initial factor, chronologically progressive deformation of the skeleton was believed to be the main cause of ageing until only a few years ago. Today, it is believed that skeletal deformation plays a minor role in the initial stages of ageing, and does not have clinically relevant effects until a much later stage in the ageing process.

2.3.2 Regional changes

Ageing in the periorbital region

The periorbital region is one of the main 'hot spots' for the development of the initial signs of facial ageing. This is largely due to the absence of a superficial fat layer to cushion the area. Atrophy- and muscle-related changes in the deeper tissues therefore have immediately visible effects (Fig. 2.25).

Changes in the supraorbital region involving gradual atrophy of the retro-orbicularis oculi fat pad can trigger the gradual descent of the eyebrow fat pad (ROOF) in the frontal areolar plane. Clinically, this manifests as sagging of the eyebrows (ptosis) in combination with skin folds and hollowing in the upper lid region ('sunken eyes', supraorbital hollows). The decreased activity of the brow elevator muscles *(frontalis muscles),* increased activity of the forehead depressor muscles, and the gradual loss of skin elasticity associated with ageing, can all aggravate these processes.

Changes in the infraorbital region involving atrophy of the sub-orbicularis oculi fat occur, starting at the medial part ('tail') of the SOOF. The resulting absence of a superficial fat pad leads to the appearance of a visible 'hole' in the infraorbital region *(infraorbital hollow, IOH).* This leads to the appearance of a tear trough deformity (medially), as well as to a prominence of the lower eyelid furrow (laterally). The overall impression, depending on the individual position of the superficial fat, is that of periorbital 'dark circles'. The orbital retaining ligaments, which separate the infraorbital fat 'bald spot' from the part of the cheek padded with superficial fat, extend along the orbital rim. This further emphasises the infraorbital margin.

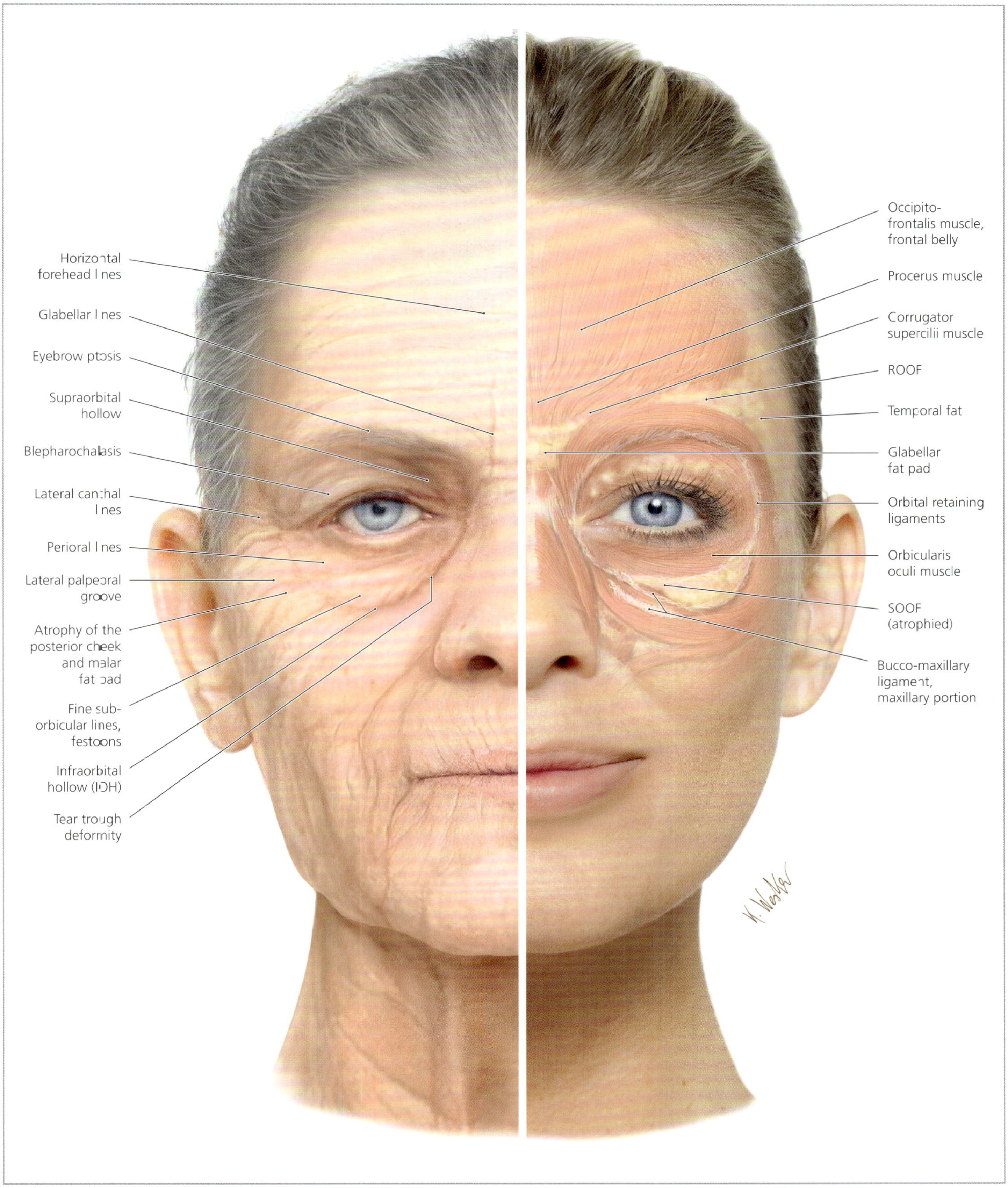

Fig. 2.25 Split view of the clinical signs of ageing and anatomical structures in the periorbital region.

2

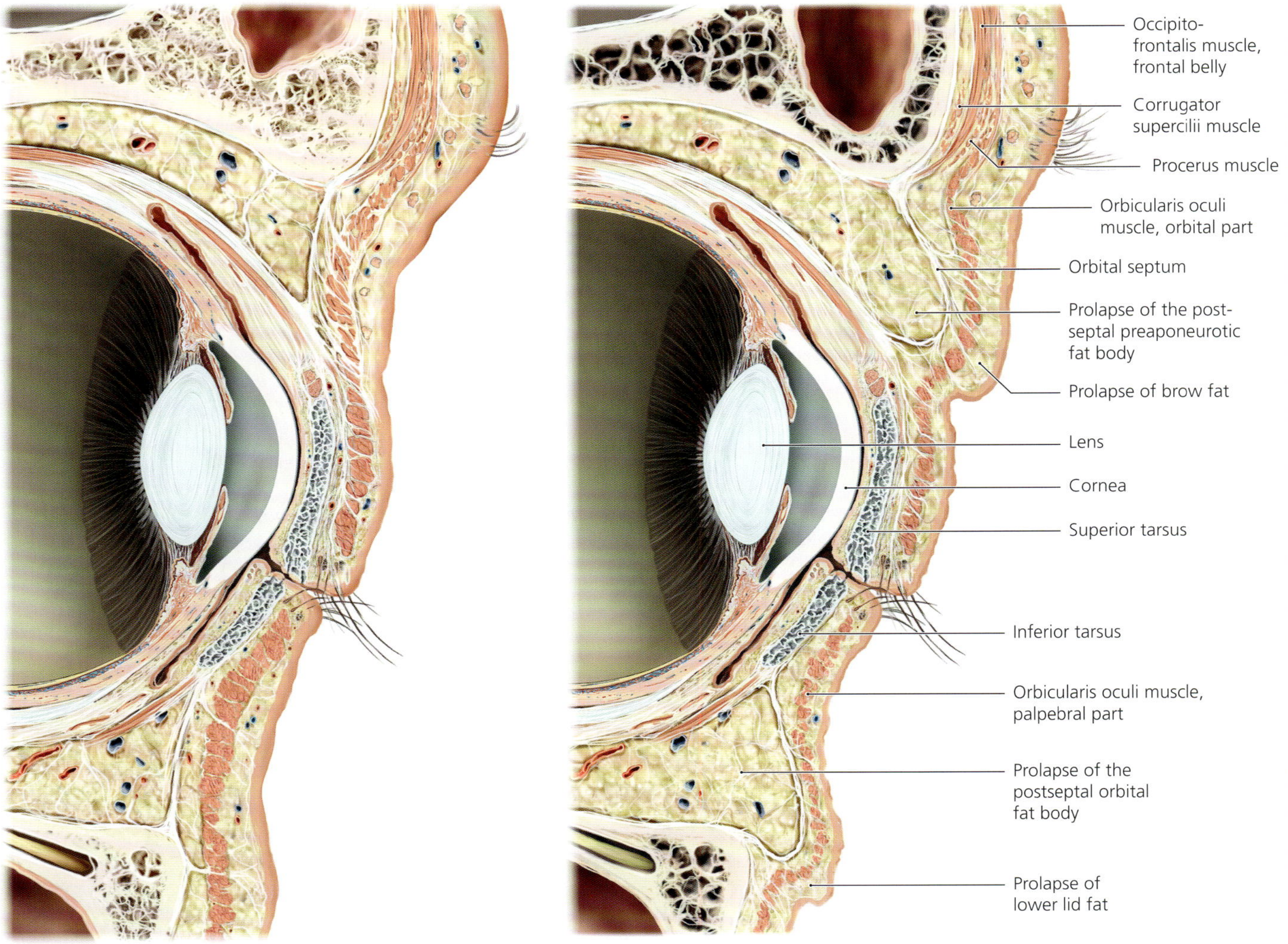

Fig. 2.26 Sagittal section through the periorbital region of a young face (left) and an older face (right) based on the 'old theory' of facial ageing. Supra- and infraorbital prolapse of the intraorbital fat occurs as a consequence of ageing. The orbicularis oculi muscle volume decreases and the ligaments and skin slacken, resulting in sagging (ptosis) of the tissues. Previously, this was mainly attributed to very gradual bone loss in the orbital region, degenerative loss of elasticity of the skin and connective tissue septa, and the consequent sliding and prolapse of the various structures. Today, atrophy and loss of the underlying tissues and a loss of tension from the ligaments are believed to be the primary causes of age-related sagging of the skin and soft tissues in this area. Tension on the skin at the attachment sites of the true retaining ligaments results in the visible indentations on the skin surface, making the fat pads more prominent. The recent clinical findings of one of this book's authors (Sattler) suggest that bags under the eyes are most likely caused by the lymphatic congestion over the buccal–maxillary retaining ligaments, and that the prolapse of intraorbital fat plays a subordinate role.

A loss of muscle volume also occurs in conjunction with an increase in orbicularis oculi muscle tone, resulting in an atrophy-related decrease in skin tone. This, in turn, leads to the appearance of fine wrinkles around the lower eyelid and outer corners of the eye, which can be aggravated by the progressive loss of skin elasticity.

'Eye bags' may also appear in advanced age. Previously, this was thought to be due to the prolapse of the inner orbital fat. However, the clinical results obtained by treating the periorbital region with botulinum toxin type-A suggest that the appearance of the bags under the eyes is more likely caused by lymphatic congestion in the infraorbital compartment above the orbital and/or buccal–maxillary retaining ligament. Like the impaired tissue drainage observed when someone has a bad cold or after botulinum toxin type-A chemodenervation in the periorbital region, infraorbital lymph fluid accumulates above the segmented ligament, resulting in the appearance of the 'bags' (Fig. 2.26).

Ageing in the perioral region

The perioral region is another 'hot spot' for the development of the visible signs of ageing (Fig. 2.27). It can be described as a superficial fat 'bald spot'. Because an underlying cushion of supporting fat is

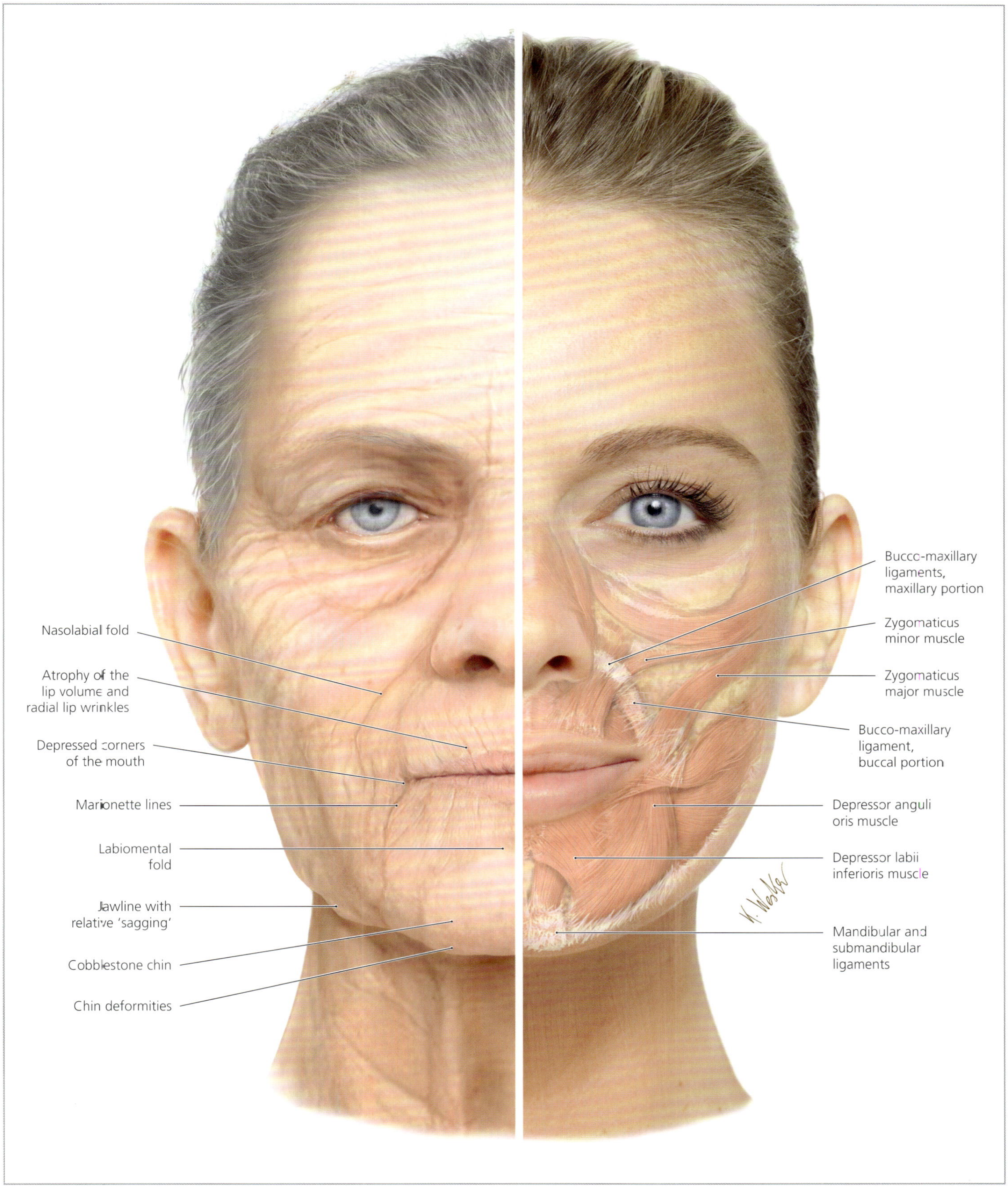

Fig. 2.27 Split view of the clinical signs of ageing and the anatomical structures in the perioral region.

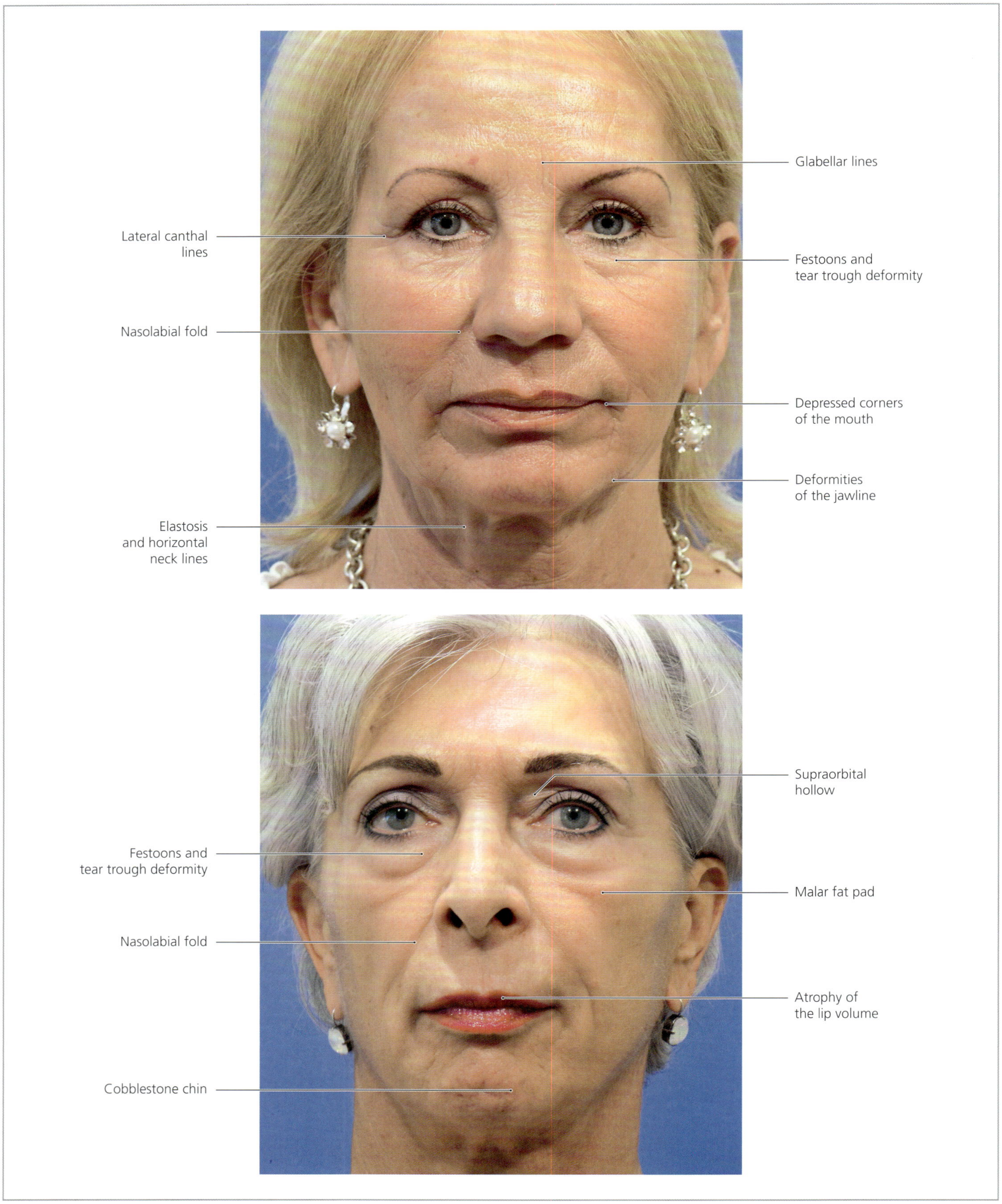

Fig. 2.28 Clinical appearance of the visible signs of ageing.

absent, visible signs of ageing appear around the mouth at a relatively early age.

The maxillary (true ligament) part of the buccal–maxillary retaining ligament plays a role in the development of a fold at the nasolabial junction to the fat pad of the cheek, which becomes more and more prominent with age. Nasolabial fold development is aggravated by gradual ptosis of the upper cheek fat due to a lack of sufficient tension from the buccal (false ligament) part of the buccal–maxillary retaining ligament, which tends to slacken at an early age.

With age, the volume of the muscle that encircles the mouth (orbicularis oris muscle) decreases, while the tone of the muscle increases. This in conjunction with the progressive loss of lip volume results in the appearance of fine radial lines around the upper and lower lip. The 'balance of power' between the depressor anguli oris muscle and the antagonist levator anguli oris muscles progressively tilts in favour of the depressor muscle, dragging the corners of the mouth further downward. The junction between the fat accumulating in the lower cheek and the perioral fat 'bald spot' becomes increasingly prominent and extends into the chin region. In this area, the depressor *labii inferioris* muscle attaches directly to the mucosa. This leads to further deepening of these so-called marionette lines (Fig. 2.28).

Further regional changes

With regard to the upper third of the face, in the forehead region, horizontal forehead lines and glabellar lines appear and become increasingly prominent due to the combined effects of the subcutaneous volume loss, muscle hypertrophy, slight bone loss and gravity. In the temple region, a loss of fat and muscle volume leads to the visible bulging of blood vessels at the temples.

With regard to the midface, as the upper cheek fat gradually descends with age, the 'inverted triangular shape' of the youthful face slowly rotates and acquires a triangular shape. In the cheekbone area, the malar fat pads may become visible due to the atrophy-related redistribution of fat and laxity of the true retaining ligaments.

Depending on the original cartilage condition, age-related enlargement of the nose and ears may occur as cartilage growth in the tip of the nose, nostril and ears continues with age.

In lower third of the face, the chin region is affected by the laxity of numerous ligaments, which in turn contributes to the development of prominent age-related changes in facial contours. Furthermore, weakening of the mental ligaments is involved in the development of a 'cobblestone' chin. Laxity of the atrophied mandibular and mandibular–platysmal ligaments, in conjunction with volume loss and destabilisation of the underlying soft tissues, contributes to sagging of the cheeks.

In the cervical region, the loss of the deep fat and slackening of the retaining ligaments leads to the development of horizontal lines on the neck and progressive loosening of the skin envelope. Furthermore, the vertical lines (platysmal banding) on the neck are formed by an overactive platysma muscle.

2.4 Summary and Treatment Implications

According to the old school of thought, facial ageing was primarily conceived as gravity-induced sagging of the facial tissues, progressive bone resorption, and decreased tissue elasticity of the skin envelope. This view implied that the visible signs of ageing could only be treated symptomatically, and certainly not by minimally invasive means.

Today it is known that the processes responsible for facial ageing are much more complex than previously believed, yet more responsive to minimally invasive treatments than was previously assumed. These multidimensional processes unfold in a multi-layered tissue complex comprising of skin, subcutaneous fat, connective tissues, muscles, and bone.

Facial volume loss and decreasing soft tissue quality are two key factors involved in the initial ageing process. Both occur due to the decreased blood flow and the consequent loss of the subcutaneous fat pads, which have the physiologically important function of supporting the facial tissue complex. The externally visible changes in the tissue structures, including the increasing wrinkling and folding of the skin, can be explained as secondary consequences of atrophy-related destabilisation of the soft tissues in association with decreased elasticity.

Aesthetic treatment strategies based on the old theory of facial ageing were designed to eliminate the external symptoms, but not the underlying subcutaneous causes of the externally visible signs of ageing. Surgical treatments such as facelifts were performed in an attempt to harmonise the external proportions of the face at a deeper level. Unsightly tissues were simply cut off, resulting in concomitant irreversible destruction of the healthy tissues. Moreover, this strategy failed to address the actual causes of facial ageing, involving deep tissue defects that can only be addressed at the subclinical stage.

The advent of soft tissue augmentation procedures using water-binding fillers brought about a paradigm shift in the treatment of facial ageing. The results of clinical experience and clinical studies by the authors have shown that soft tissue volume augmentation with hyaluronic acid fillers extensively improves the visible signs of ageing, with natural results (see Ch. 8, p. 231). Initially, clinicians tried to mask deficits mainly by superficial intradermal injection techniques. However, augmentation treatments in the deep subcutaneous structures achieved the final breakthrough. Maximal effect and facial harmony can now be achieved with minimal material consumption and maximal protection of the natural facial structures.

Regarding the secondary tissue-regenerating effects of hyaluronic acid fillers due to an improved supply of fluids, recent evidence supports the importance of this treatment as a causal therapeutic approach to counteracting the ageing process at the physiological and anatomical level.

The following treatment goals can now be achieved with hyaluronic acid fillers, using a combination of traditional superficial injection techniques and the newer vertical and horizontal atraumatic injection techniques:

- Volume augmentation to compensate for atrophy-related volume loss in the subfascial fatty tissues
- Remodelling of facial contours
- Horizontal tissue mobilisation and homogenisation (using atraumatic cannulas)
- Superficial repair of the deficits not related to atrophy
- Rehydration and revitalisation of the skin surface
- Restoration of ligament tensile strength (re-stabilisation and natural augmentation of the soft tissues)
- Bio-regeneration and saturation of the target tissues with fluids
- Induction of fibrogenetic tissue regeneration via atraumatic microlesions (triggering neocollagenesis and neo-elastin synthesis)

Due to the broad spectrum of filler applications and clinical outcomes, the authors prefer to call the newer, holistic approach to treatment with hyaluronic acid fillers 'Minimally Invasive Augmentation Surgery' (MIAC). This book focuses on the principles and applications of this treatment approach, while taking both traditional and innovative approaches into account.

3 Injectable Fillers

3 Injectable Fillers

3.1 Introduction

To date, numerous injectable agents have been utilised for skin augmentation. Several hundreds of different filler agents with plumping and tissue-saturating effects are currently available on the international market. Product choice depends on several factors, namely the indication, area to be treated, desired clinical effect and the intended mode of administration. This chapter shall discuss the different types of fillers available and their properties, based on some of the key features outlined below:

I Degradability
1. Absorbable (degradable)
2. Delayed absorption (slowly degradable, semi-permanent)
3. Permanent (non-degradable)

II Bio-identical/non-bio-identical

III Injection depth
1. Dermal
2. Subdermal/subcutaneous
3. Submuscular/supraperiosteal

IV Filler origin
1. Heterogeneous (animal or fermentative)
2. Allogeneic
3. Autologous (obtained from the patient)
4. Synthetic

A number of criteria are required to be met when considering the introduction of filler agents into the international market. Ideally, a facial filler should have all of the following properties:
- Non-infectious
- Non-pyrogenic
- Biocompatible
- Easy to inject
- Associated with minimal discomfort and pain upon injection and thereafter
- Remaining at the injection site post-treatment (no migration)
- Longevity (the filling effect is as long-lasting as possible)
- Natural look and feel post-treatment
- Cost-effective

Furthermore, filler agents have to satisfy the various indications requested by the patients and clinicians. They range from the treatment of lines and wrinkles of varying depth, to the deeper contouring and volumising of larger areas of the face including the chin and cheeks, augmentation of the lips, and pan-facial augmentation of the face (e.g. in HIV-associated lipodystrophy).

A number of filler agents have been utilised over the years, with changing patient and practitioner requirements driving innovation. The very first filling agents recorded dates back to 1893, with the injection of autologous fat by Gustav Neuber (Neuber, 1892) Paraffin was introduced soon after in the years 1900 to 1935, but was eventually declared an unsuitable filler. Liquid silicone, first produced and used for breast-implants by Dow Corning Corporation in 1962, was also soon deemed an inappropriate filler agent. More recently, the industry has seen the use of bovine collagen in 1981 and more recently hyaluronic acid has pioneered the way internationally, being first introduced into the market in 1997. Today, more than 150 new injectable filler products of varying composition exist within the international arena.

Many would argue, however, that even among the large choice of fillers available today, the 'ideal filler' yet remains to be discovered, and each agent's advantages and disadvantages need to be carefully weighed up on a case-by-case basis. Today, it has proved challenging to find a filler agent that will fulfil all of the above criteria. For example, degradable fillers have proved popular for their lower complication rates post-treatment and hence better tolerance, however, on the other hand, they have to be re-injected often (every 4–12 months, depending on the agent used), which is a disadvantage for patients seeking treatment longevity. Conversely, semi-permanent and permanent fillers have shown to offer longer-lasting clinical effects, but this has been offset by a higher rate of complications, which have proved very challenging or impossible to remedy.

The licensing of the filler products in the USA is subject to the Food and Drug Administration's (FDA) assessment of the filler properties with regard to their efficacy and safety profiles. In Europe, each country's appropriate authority is responsible for regulating this.

The use of injectable fillers is limited to licensed, insured and trained medical practitioners, who have demonstrated precise knowledge of the filler agent and injection techniques, and also of the corresponding anatomy of the treatment areas. It is up to the practitioner to select the correct filler product and volume required based on the patient's needs, desired treatment outcome, planned injection site, injection technique and depth of injection.

Below is a list compiled by the authors outlining some of the key considerations with regard to absolute and relative contraindications to injectable fillers.

3.1.1 Absolute contraindications

- Acute or chronic skin conditions in the area to be treated
- Active infection or inflammation at the injection site (e.g. labial herpes, cold sore, or acne)
- Allergy to any of the filler constituents
- Pregnancy and breastfeeding (or actively planning to be during the period of time the filler is in situ)
- Injection into blood vessels, bones, tendons, ligaments, or muscles
- Existing autoimmune systemic reactions

3.1.2 Relative contraindications

- Immunosuppressed patient
- Children and adolescents below the age of 18 years (only in exceptional cases)
- Predisposition to keloid and hypertrophic scarring
- Use of non-steroidal anti-inflammatory drugs (NSAIDs)
- Connective tissue disorders (applies for superficial injections of stabilising fillers only)
- Thin, atrophied skin
- Anticoagulant medication (life-saving anticoagulant medications should not be stopped for the treatment, and it is advisable to

check the status of clotting, e.g. INR levels before treatment. However, non-life-saving anticoagulant medications can be discontinued in good time pre-treatment and restarted after if necessary)
- Clotting disorders
- Existing autoimmune disease (decision to be made on a case-by-case basis, special monitoring needed)
- Granulomatous inflammation
- Recent dermabrasion, laser treatment or chemical peeling (i.e. when skin has not fully healed)
- Caution in patients with diseases caused by Streptococci (recurrent tonsillitis/sore throat, acute rheumatic arthritis); no injection in case of cardiac involvement
- Caution when injecting areas previously treated with another filler

3.1.3 Potential side effects

Side effects are broadly divided into immediate-onset and delayed-onset. They may be related to numerous factors, namely the administered product itself, the injection tool used, the injection technique used, as well as the conditions immediately pre- and post-treatment (e.g. disinfection of the treatment area). Immediate post-treatment short-lived erythema, oedema and bruising are to be expected, and hence patients should be pre-warned of these in advance of the treatment. Delayed onset complications can present as late as many years post-treatment (e.g. due to immunological reactions to the product used, and may present with foreign body granulomas). This sort of complication has been associated primarily with permanent fillers.

To minimise the occurrence of preventable side effects, only specially trained medical practitioners should administer filler injections. Detailed knowledge of the filler agents, indications, anatomical considerations, injection techniques and depths of injection is fundamental in the avoidance of side effects. Furthermore, successful treatments require meticulous and careful patient selection, history taking and examination pre-treatment. In addition, it is essential that patients receive informed consent, whereby they are fully informed and educated on all the treatment options available and are able to weigh up the pros and cons of the treatments proposed when making a final decision, as well as to the full treatment process (see section 5.6, p. 92).

A large body of published evidence exists on the subject of side effects associated with injectable fillers, which the reader is encouraged to review on a regular basis to keep up-to-date.

3.1.4 Complications

Frequent complications
- Haematomas
- Pain
- A feeling of tension

Rare complications

Acute
- Allergic/anaphylactic reactions (these tend to be more frequent with agents containing a local anaesthetic than with agents not containing one)
- Hypo- or hypersensitivity at the injection site
- Inflammatory reactions (erythema, oedema), sometimes with itching and tenderness
- Ischaemia (caused by intravascular injection or compression)
- Abscesses, sometimes with fistulation
- Blistering

Subacute
- Non-specific flu-like symptoms (fever, headache, muscle aches, malaise, nausea, dizziness, joint and nerve pains)
- Nodules (nodules occurring during the injection are usually caused by uneven distribution of the introduced material and are not tender or inflamed, whereas inflamed, erythematous nodules are caused by an infection or a tissue reaction)
- Foreign body granulomas: ranging from subclinical (only histologically detectable) to inflammatory, livid, disfiguring changes in the form of nodules, cords or more widespread, disc-like lesions
- Infection (bacterial, viral, fungal). Recurrence of herpes in the perioral region (appropriate drug treatment is required)

Chronic
- Unintentional over- or undercorrection, failure to achieve the desired effect
- Migration/dislocation of the filler (primarily with permanent fillers in gel form or as a result of mechanical pressure)
- Skin colour changes at the injection site, pigmentation abnormalities
- Keloid and hypertrophic scarring
- Lipoatrophy
- Scarring, necrosis (particularly in the glabellar region; it is therefore advisable to respect anatomy and be aware of the high risk zones, chose appropriate filler agents and injection techniques to avoid vascular compromise)
- Thrombosis (with highly viscous fillers)
- Indurations/scabs
- Necrosis
- Blindness (following intravascular injection and necrosis)
- Reactivation of existing autoimmune systemic reactions

> **Caution**
>
> **Biopsy and bacterial culture is always required in the event of symptoms including fever, leukocytosis and exhaustion.**

3.2 Filler Types

This section summarises the different types of filler agents used to date. Because of the emphasis on historical completeness, some of the filler agents included in the list below may not be relevant in current clinical practice.

Types of filler agents used:
- Absorbable/biodegradable (temporary)
  - Hyaluronic acid (HA)
  - Collagen
  - Autologous fat

3

- Delayed absorption (long-lasting, slowly degradable, semi-permanent)
  - Poly-l-lactic acid (PLLA) microspheres
  - Calcium hydroxylapatite (CaHA) microspheres
- Non-absorbable/non-biodegradable (permanent)
  - Polyacrylamide
  - Polymethylmethacrylate (PMMA) microspheres

In recent years hyaluronic acid (HA) has become the most widely used biodegradable filler worldwide. Consequently, this book focuses mainly on augmentation procedures using HA fillers.

3.2.1 Absorbable/biodegradable (temporary) fillers

Hyaluronic acid (HA) fillers

Hyaluronic acid (new nomenclature: hyaluronan, abbreviated: HA) is a clear, viscous liquid and a natural component of skin, bones, cartilage and connective tissue. It is a glucosaminoglycan, composed of N-acetylglucosamine and glucuronic acid molecules, and is formed on the cell surface by HA synthases. It is broken down enzymatically by hyaluronidases (Fig. 3.1).

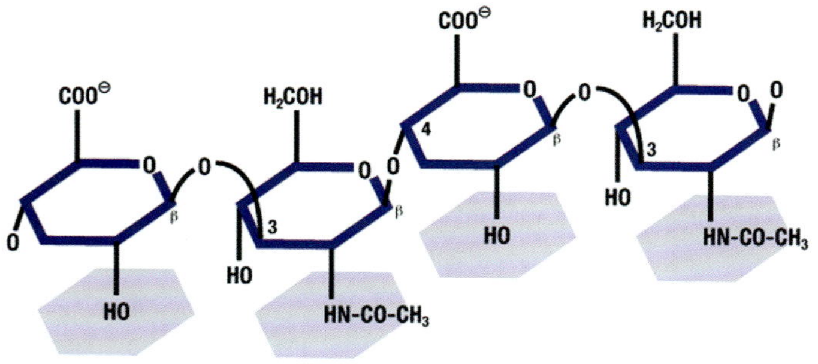

Fig. 3.1 Two disaccharide repeating units of hyaluronic acid.

The most important property of HA is its high water-binding (hydrophilic) capacity. This gives the skin its moisture, elasticity and resilience. However, the skin's hyaluronic acid content decreases with time due to various physiological and environmental effects, among them being the natural ageing process alongside UV exposure. The skin loses moisture and becomes less elastic, resulting in visible lines and wrinkles.

Degradable hyaluronic acid fillers have been successfully used since 1996 to correct these skin changes. Post-therapeutic investigations of the skin using scientific analysis instruments (e.g. cutometer, corneometer) after injections of hyaluronic acid fillers have shown that these treatments achieve a significant and persisting enhancement in the skin's moisture content and elasticity.

The sources of the hyaluronic acid used in fillers are either bacteria (i.e. produced by non-pathogenic bacterial fermentation) or avian in origin (i.e. derived from rooster combs). In both cases, thorough sterilisation is a key factor in avoiding unwanted side effects and complications. Avian hyaluronic acid is subjected to sterile filtration and then autoclaved. The molecule obtained by bacterial fermentation is also sterilised by filtration, and some manufacturers also autoclave it and additionally test for endotoxins and viruses.

A clear distinction should be made between native, non-cross-linked and cross-linked hyaluronic acid. Whereas the native form stimulates the anabolic metabolism of the fibroblasts, the cross-linked form is used for volume replacement due to its insolubility in water. 1,8-diepoxyoctane (DEO), divinyl sulphone (DVS) or 1,4-butanediol-diglycidyl ether (BDDE) are used as cross-linking agents for this purpose. DEO-cross-linked products are more resistant to enzymatic breakdown, as the agent produces double cross-linking via an ether and an ester bond. It should also be highlighted that cross-linking agents used in filler manufacturing are also associated with allergic reactions, and hence practitioners should be aware of this when performing filler injections.

The essential properties of HA fillers during and after injection are determined by the content of the cross-linked HA and the method of cross-linking used (i.e. bioengineering technology). The effects of cross-linking include:

- The **water-binding capacity** of the filler increases with the degree of cross-linking
- The **duration of effect** of the filler increases with the degree of cross-linking due to slowing of the degradation process
- The **elasticity and viscosity** of the filler is influenced by cross-linking
- The **viscosity** ('stiffness') of the filler increases with the degree of cross-linking, but is also dependent on the type of cross-linking technology used.
  - **High-viscosity hyaluronic acid** results in increased tissue resistance, making the substance harder to inject. Although it has a rather large projection effect, it cannot be modelled well post-injection. High-viscosity hyaluronic acid fillers are suitable for supraperiosteal applications
  - **Medium-viscosity hyaluronic acid** has a certain projection effect but still has good modelling properties and is relatively easy to inject. It is used for medium and deep injections
  - **Low-viscosity hyaluronic acid** is soft and easy to inject. Due to the good horizontal propagation of the filler, it creates smooth transitions between areas; accordingly, it has a minor projection effect. Low-viscosity hyaluronic acid fillers are used for superficial injections.

The manufacturers of hyaluronic acid fillers have developed different cross-linking technologies, designed to give their fillers specific clinical characteristics. One such innovation is the biphasic HA gel: after cross-linking, the gel is broken into small particles and mixed with water or non-cross-linked HA to make the filler suitable for injection with a very thin needle. In general, it is accepted that:

1. The smaller the particles, the more biodegradable the material and, thus, the shorter the duration of the filling effect
2. Fillers with small particles and low viscosity have greater horizontal spread and are mainly used for superficial injections
3. Fillers with larger particles have higher viscosity and are mainly used for medium to deep injections.

Hyaluronic acid is considered the 'all-round', 'all-purpose' filler on the global market today. It is applicable to all parts of the body and has a wide range of applications. Importantly is has a low side effect profile, and allows for effective and reproducible treatment outcomes.

Importantly, a key advantage of hyaluronic acid is that any potential unwanted aggregation or nodules that it might cause can be dissolved by injecting hyaluronidase (e.g. brand name Hylase®) into the affected area; this is a major safety benefit over other injectable fillers.

A recently proven additional benefit of HA fillers is their secondary tissue-regenerating effect. Due to its strong hydrophilic properties, HA injection not only results in temporary compensation for the volume loss, but also in biological improvement by supplying the tissues with additional fluids. This is why HA treatment results in continuous clinical improvement over time, even in patients who do not receive further treatments (see Ch. 8, p. 231). Furthermore, recent data by Wang et al, 2007 has highlighted that HA fillers also stimulate long-term collagen production, which is an important consideration and opens up further discussions for the future.

Caution

In addition to the side effects and contraindications that apply to all injectable fillers, the incompatibility of hyaluronic acid with quaternary ammonium salts needs particular mention. Disinfectants such as benzalkonium chloride and instruments treated with them must on no account come into contact with hyaluronic acid fillers, as this would cause hyaluronic acid to precipitate out.

Collagen fillers

In recent years collagen fillers have received less interest, due to the development of longer-acting and better tolerated fillers, namely hyaluronic acid.

Historically, bovine collagen was one of the first collagen fillers introduced back in 1981 for the treatment of lines and wrinkles. At one point it was considered an economical and well-established filler; however today it is rarely used due to the associated high allergenic risk. Since then, a variety of collagen fillers have been introduced from a number of sources: xenologous (bovine); homologous/allogeneic (human, but not the patient's own); or autologous (the patient's own). Human collagen has better immunologic compatibility and has shown promising results in the initial studies; however further research is necessary to evaluate its full potential.

Accurate knowledge of their short- and long-term effects has been amassed due to the many years of use worldwide. However, the duration of the filling effect is only limited to a few months in general, as degradation of the collagen by the body's own collagenases begins directly after the injection. Furthermore, collagen fillers need to be stored in a refrigerator and injected with overcorrection. Their side effects and contraindications correspond to those of all injectable fillers.

Overall, however, the newer hyaluronic acid fillers have succeeded collagen fillers with their more attractive safety and efficacy profile.

Autologous fat

Until recently, autologous fat grafting used to be a popular treatment option for advanced atrophy-related volume loss of the face, but has now been largely replaced by new hyaluronic acid-based fillers developed specifically for this purpose.

One of this book's authors, G. Sattler, views autologous fat as a useful filler agent particularly in the treatment of the infraorbital hollow, in comparison to the effects achieved with hyaluronic acid fillers for this indication. However, the author also believes that the overall results obtained with autologous fat are generally less predictable. Because of the lower water-binding properties of autologous fat, swelling tends to be less severe but the desired fluid replenishing and tissue-regenerating effects such as those associated with hyaluronic acid fillers are lacking here. Therefore, the author generally prefers the use of hyaluronic acid fillers for deep injection with tissue volumising effect over autologous fat.

3.2.2 Delayed absorption fillers (long-lasting, slowly degradable, semi-permanent)

Semi-permanent (long-lasting), absorbable fillers contain slowly degrading polymer microspheres dissolved in a resorbable fluid. While the fluid is broken down with time, new endogenous connective tissue forms around the microspheres.

The diameter of the particles determines the effect of the filler. They should be between 30 and 100 µm in diameter. Particles that are too small (< 10 µm) are either phagocytosed by macrophages or are at risk of flooding into the capillaries (< 30 µm). If, on the other hand, they are too big (> 100 µm), the filler cannot be injected adequately.

Two kinds of commonly used long-lasting fillers are currently employed:

- Calcium hydroxylapatite (CaHA, e.g. Radiesse®, produced by Merz)
- Poly-l-lactic acid (PLLA, e.g. Sculptra®, produced by Sanofi-Aventis)

Their side effects and contraindications correspond to those of all injectable fillers. A particular point of note is that any overcorrection may persist for longer periods and is more difficult to remedy. Both fillers require specific preparation, and specific post-treatment care should be taken with PLLA with regard to massage.

3.2.3 Non-absorbable/non-biodegradable fillers (permanent)

Due to the associated risk of permanent, irreversible side effects, the authors do not generally advise the use of permanent fillers. However, they are mentioned here for the purposes of completeness.

The contraindications and potential side effects associated with non-absorbable fillers correspond to those of all injectable fillers. Furthermore, it is worth noting that these fillers tend to become very protuberant with the associated age-related atrophy of the skin and subcutaneous tissue with time.

It is generally accepted that when using permanent fillers, one should not attempt to achieve full correction in one session, as there is a risk of permanent overcorrection. Instead, the defects should be refilled gradually over several sessions.

Examples of permanent filler agents include.

- Polyacrylamide (e.g. Aquamid©)
- Polymethyl methacrylate microspheres (PMMA, e.g. Artefill®)
- Acrylic hydrogel fragments

3.3 'Filler Navigator'

A summary of the different (mainly hyaluronic acid-based) commercial fillers, called the 'Filler Navigator', is presented in the following pages. The authors have attempted to compile a representative selection of the available products that they recommend, based on their own reproducible treatment results.

In general, the available fillers can be classified in terms of the following features:
- Concentration and degree of cross-linking of hyaluronic acid (determines the viscosity and elasticity of the gel)
- Specific filler properties post-injection (e.g. lifting/projection effect, modelling capacity, biodegradability)
- Depth of desired injection (injection plane)
- Lumen diameter of the needle or cannula used to inject the filler

The fillers presented below are classified into groups according to their intended depth of injection and indication (Filler Navigator classification). The following chapters will make reference to this classification when discussing special applications or loco-regional treatments. We hope this classification proves useful in distinguishing the fillers available based on their intended indication, plane of placement and injection technique.

Filler Navigator classification

1 Superficial injection (intradermal augmentation)

2 Medium injection (subdermal augmentation)

3 Deep injection (subcutaneous augmentation)

4 Ultra-deep injection (supraperiosteal augmentation)

A Special indication: skin surface regeneration and mesotherapy (skin boosters)

B Special indication: lips – perioral complex and tear trough

Important note

The product information provided in this book was derived from the manufacturers' product descriptions and was verified by the manufacturers in 2015. It is quite possible that the manufacturers may have placed new fillers on the market or removed some of those listed in this book in the interval between the date of verification and the date of publication. Therefore, we make no claim of completeness for the data presented on the following pages. For current and additional information, please refer to the websites of the filler manufacturers.

The classification of fillers into the individual indication groups below has been provided solely as a navigation aid. The individual decision regarding the selection of a particular product depends on clinical findings and product-specific compatibility (indication/contraindication).

Further information on the indications, contraindications and interactions may be found in the fillers advice sheets, provided by the manufacturers and should be regarded as the primary and up-to-date source of advice.

1 Fillers for superficial injections (p. 62)

Depth of injection: intradermal

Indications:
- Fine modulation (camouflage) of various very superficial deficits
- Relining of the skin and homogenisation of the skin surface
- Improvement of skin texture (revitalisation and rehydration)
- Fine facial wrinkles

Filler properties:
- ⇩ Degree of cross-linking
- ⇩ Viscosity and/or particle size
- ⇧ Horizontal distribution of the filler
- ⇩ Projection effect
- ⇩ Duration of effect (due to the biochemical properties of the fillers)

Injection tool:
- 30 G needle

2 Fillers for medium injections (p. 63)

Depth of injection: subdermal, superficial subcutis

Indications:
- Decorative correction and concealment (camouflage) of volume deficits
- Remodelling of the skin surface relief
- Relining of the skin and homogenisation of the skin surface
- Improvement of skin texture
- Scars
- Lips
- Fine wrinkles not due to volume loss
- Hands

Filler properties:
- ⇩/⇦ Degree of cross-linking
- ⇩ Viscosity and/or particle size
- ⇦ Horizontal distribution of the filler
- ⇩/⇦ Projection effect
- ⇩ Duration of effect (due to the biochemical properties of the fillers)

Injection tool:
- 27 G needle or cannula

3 Fillers for deep injections (p. 66)

Depth of injection: subcutaneous, supramucosal

Indications:
- Remodelling of the facial contours
- Volume augmentation to compensate for loss of the subfascial fat
- Widespread tissue mobilisation and relining with a blunt cannula
- Focused volume projection of wrinkles over non-bony areas
- Soft tissue stabilisation
- Forehead
- Temples
- Eyebrows
- Sunken eyes (supraorbital hollow)
- Cheeks
- Nasolabial folds
- Lips (including lip atrophy)
- Marionette lines
- Neck volumisation
- Scars

Filler properties
- ⇦/⇧ Degree of cross-linking
- ⇦ Viscosity and/or particle size
- ⇦ Horizontal distribution of the filler
- ⇦/⇧ Projection effect
- ⇦ Duration of effect

Injection tool:
- 25–28 G needle
- 22–25 G cannula

4 Fillers for ultra-deep injections (p. 67)

Depth of injection: supraperiosteal

Indications:
- Remodelling of the facial contours
- Compensation for volume loss in the supraperiosteal fat plane
- Greatest possible lifting/projection effect with minimum filler consumption
- Tightening of the retaining ligaments
- Focused volume projection of wrinkles over bony areas
- Static tissue stabilisation
- Forehead wrinkles
- Infraorbital hollows
- Rhinoplasty
- Nasolabial fold (proximal part)
- Chin volumisation
- Jawline recontouring (sagging)
- Scars

Filler properties
- ⇧ Degree of cross-linking
- ⇧ Viscosity and/or particle size
- ⇩ Horizontal distribution of material
- ⇧ Projection effect
- ⇧ Duration of effect (due to the biochemical properties of the filler)

Injection tool:
- 25–27 G needle

A Special indications: skin surface regeneration and mesotherapy (skin boosters) (p. 69)

Depth of injection: intradermal, subdermal (mesotherapy: subcutaneous, supraperiosteal)

Indications:
- Rehydration and revitalisation of the skin surface
- Prevention and treatment of wrinkles
- Harmonisation of the skin appearance
- Refreshing the overall complexion

Filler properties:
- ⇩ Degree of cross-linking
- ⇩ Viscosity and/or particle size
- ⇧ Horizontal distribution of material
- ⇩ Projection effect
- ⇩ Duration of effect (due to the biochemical properties of the fillers)

Injection tool:
- 30–32 G needle
- 25–27 G cannula

B Special indications: lips – perioral complex and tear trough (p. 70)

Depth of injection: intradermal, subdermal, subcutaneous/supramucosal

Indications:
- Lip volumisation
- Lip contouring
- Lip surface regeneration

Filler properties:
- Dependent on the indication and/or depth of injection

Injection tool:
- 30–32 G needle
- 25–27G cannula (depending on the indication and filler used)

The here given **'durations of effect'** refer to the relative duration until the next injection is required due to the biochemical properties of the filler. The comparison between different products is made based on general practical aspects following the authors' experiences. An absolute comparison is not possible since this duration depends on skin type, indication, application site and injected volume among others.

1	Fillers for superficial injections						
	Product name	**Manu-facturer**	**Indications**	**Injection depth(s)**	**Amount of hyaluronic acid and cross-linking**	**Injection tool**	**Material properties**	**Website**
	BELOTERO® Soft Lidocaine	Merz Aesthetics	Correction of fine lines, e.g. crow's feet, perioral lines, fine forehead lines	Injection into the superficial dermis at approx. 10 degrees	Cross-linked sodium hyaluronate: 20 mg/ml; lidocaine hydrocholoride: 3.0 mg/ml; cross-linking: +	30 G needle	Combination of low-viscosity and high cohesivity that enables to integrate smoothly the superficial dermis for optimal fine line treatment	www.belotero.com
	BELOTERO® Hydro	Merz Aesthetics	Skin hydration, e.g. face, neck, décolletage, back of hands	Injection into the superficial dermis or the dermo-epidermal junction	Sodium hyaluronate: 18 mg; glycerol: 21 mg/ml; cross-linking: none	30 G needle	Unique and patented combination of non-cross-linked HA and glycerol for synergistic effect in skin elasticity, tone and radiance restoration	
	Hyal® ACP	Merz Aesthetics	Skin hydration, e.g. face, neck, décolletage, back of hands	Injection into the superficial dermis or the dermo-epidermal junction	Auto-cross-linked hyaluronate 20 mg/ml	30 G needle	Unique and patented auto-cross-linked HA for long-lasting biorevitalising of the skin, improvement of skin elasticity, tone and radiance restoration	www.hyal-acp.de
	Juvéderm® ULTRA®2	Allergan	Filling any medium-sized depressions of the skin via mid-dermis injection, as well as for lip definition	Mid-dermis injections and injections in the mucous membrane of the lips	24 g/ml cross-linked HA (HYLACROSS™ technology)	30 G1/2″ needle (filler is presented in a graduated, pre-filled, disposable 0.55 ml syringe)	Sterile, pyrogen-free, physiological gel, with 0.3% lidocaine	www.juvederm.eu
	Juvéderm® VOLBELLA®	Allergan	Treatment of any fine lines and medium-sized skin depressions due to conditions such as premature ageing. Enhancement and pouting of the lips to correct structural defects such as asymmetry, contour deformities, volume loss	Superficial or mid-dermis injection or lips mucosa injection	15 mg/ml cross-linked HA (VYCROSS™ technology)	30 G1/2″ needle (filler is presented in a graduated, pre-filled, disposable 1 ml syringe)	Sterile, pyrogen-free physiological gel, with 0.3% lidocaine; good distribution	
	Juvéderm® HYDRATE™	Allergan	Improving skin hydration and elasticity	Multi-injection into the dermal epidermal junction and into the superficial dermis	13.5 mg/ml non-cross-linked HA	Graduated pre-filled syringe for single use	Sterile apyrogenic, physiological solution of hyaluronic acid containing 0.9% mannitol	
	Emervel® Touch	Galderma	Superficial lines, e.g. perioral lines, periorbital lines	Superficial dermis	20 mg/ml low cross-linked HA (Optimal Balance™ technology)	30 G 1/2″ UTWN microcannula 30 G, 25 mm UTWN	Very soft gel with small particle size and moderate lifting capacity	www.emervel.com

1 Fillers for superficial injections

Product name	Manu-facturer	Indications	Injection depth(s)	Amount of hyaluronic acid and cross-linking	Injection tool	Material properties	Website
TEOSYAL® First Lines	Teoxane	Correction of fine lines and wrinkles in thin skin – crow's feet	Superficial dermis	20 mg/ml cross-linked HA	30 G 1/2 needle	Easy to inject, well tolerated, with lidocaine	www.teoxane.com
TEOSYAL® RHA1	Teoxane	Treatment of superficial and fine wrinkles on the face (forehead lines, perioral area, crow's feet), neck and neckline	Superficial to mid-dermis	15 mg/ml mix of non-cross-linked and cross-linked HA (preserved network technology)	30 G 1/2 needle	Easy to inject, high stretch value, good integration of the product into the dermis, with lido-caine. Gel composed of longer HA chains, specially designed to respect face dyna-mism	

2 Fillers for medium injections

Product name	Manu-facturer	Indications	Injection depth(s)	Amount of hyaluronic acid and cross-linking	Injection tool	Material properties	Website
BELO-TERO® Balance Lidocaine	Merz Aesthetics	Correction of moderate lines, e.g. moderate perioral wrinkles, lip contour-ing, philtrum	Injection into the superficial to mid-dermis at approx. 15 degrees	Cross-linked sodium hyaluro-nate: 22.5 mg/ml; lidocaine hydro-choloride: 3.0 mg/ml; cross-linking: ++	27 G needle, 30 G needle	Combination of low-viscosity and high cohesive cross-linked HA for outstanding dermal integration to treat any lines or moder-ate wrinkles	www.belotero.com
Juvéderm® ULTRA®3	Allergan	Filling mid and/or deep depressions of the skin via mid and/or deep dermis injection; lip definition and enhancement	Mid and deep dermis	24 mg/ml cross-linked HA (HYLACROSS™ technology)	27 G 1/2" needle (filler is presented in a graduat-ed, pre-filled, disposable 1 ml syringe)	Sterile, pyrogen-free physiological gel with 0.3% lidocaine	www.juvederm.eu
Juvéderm® ULTRA®4	Allergan	Filling any deep depressions of the skin via deep dermis injection; lip enhancement; cheekbone augmen-tation	Deep dermis injection and injections in the mucous membrane of the lips	24 mg/ml cross-linked HA (HYLACROSS™ technology)	27 G 1/2" needle (filler is presented in a graduated, pre-filled, disposable 1 ml syringe)	Sterile, pyrogen-free physiological gel with 0.3% lidocaine	
Juvéderm® ULTRA SMILE®	Allergan	Filling mid and/or deep depressions of the skin via mid and/or deep dermis injection; lip definition and enhancement	Mid and deep dermis	24 mg/ml cross-linked HA (HYLACROSS™ technology)	30 G 1/2" needle (filler is presented in a graduated, pre-filled, disposable 0.55 ml syringe)	Sterile, pyrogen-free physiological gel with 0.3% lidocaine	

2 Fillers for medium injections

Product name	Manu-facturer	Indications	Injection depth(s)	Amount of hyaluronic acid and cross-linking	Injection tool	Material properties	Website
Juvéderm® VOLBELLA®	Allergan	Treatment of any fine lines and medium-sized skin depressions due to conditions such as premature ageing. Enhancement and pouting of the lips to correct structural defects such as asymmetry, contour deformities, volume loss	Superficial or mid-dermis injection or lips mucosa injection	15 mg/ml cross-linked HA (VYCROSS™ technology)	30 G 1/2″ needle (filler is presented in a graduated, pre-filled, disposable 1 ml syringe)	Sterile, pyrogen-free physiological gel with 0.3 % lidocaine; good distribution	www.juvederm.eu
Juvéderm® VOLIFT®	Allergan	Treatment of any deep skin depressions due to conditions such as premature ageing. Face contouring and volume restoration to correct facial structural defects such as asymmetry, contour deformities, volume loss in the lips, cheeks, chin, lower face	Deep dermis or lips mucosa injection	17.5 mg/ml cross-linked HA (VYCROSS™ technology)	30 G 1/2″ needle (filler is presented in a graduated, pre-filled, disposable 1 ml syringe)	Sterile, pyrogen-free physiological gel with 0.3 % lidocaine; good distribution	
Juvéderm® VOLIFT® Retouch	Allergan	Treatment of any deep skin depressions due to conditions such as premature ageing. Face contouring and volume restoration to correct facial structural defects such as asymmetry, contour deformities, volume loss in the lips, cheeks, chin, lower face	Deep dermis or lips mucosa injection	17.5 mg/ml cross-linked HA (VYCROSS™ technology)	30 G1/2″ needle (filler is presented in a graduated, pre-filled, disposable 0.55 ml syringe)	Sterile, pyrogen-free physiological gel with 0.3 % lidocaine; good distribution	
Emervel® Classic	Galderma	Nasolabial folds, marionette lines	Mid-dermis	20 mg/ml moderately cross-linked HA (Optimal Balance™ technology)	30 G 1/2″ UTWN icrocannula 27 G, 38 mm UTWN	Soft gel with small particle size and moderate lifting capacity, with 0.3 % lidocaine	www.emervel.com
Emervel® Lips	Galderma	Lip volume, lip contour	Vermilion lip, submucosal tissue	20 mg/ml highly cross-linked HA (Optimal Balance™ technology)	30 G 1/2″ UTWN Microcannula 27 G, 38 mm UTWN	Moderately soft gel with small particle size and moderate lifting capacity, with 0.3 % lidocaine	

2	Fillers for medium injections						
Product name	**Manu-facturer**	**Indications**	**Injection depth(s)**	**Amount of hyaluronic acid and cross-linking**	**Injection tool**	**Material properties**	**Website**
Restylane®	Galderma	Moderate wrinkles, e.g. nasolabial folds, marionette lines	Mid-dermis	20 mg/ml stabilised HA (NASHA technology)	29 G 1/2" TWN; Pix'L™-Microcannula 27 G, 40 mm; Pix'L+™-Microcannula 28 G, 40 mm	Firm gel with medium particle size and moderate lifting capacity, with or without 0.3% lidocaine	www.restylane.com
Restylane® Perlane	Galderma	Midface and cheeks, deep wrinkles, e.g. nasolabial folds, marionette lines	Deep dermis or surface of subcutis	20 mg/ml stabilised HA (NASHA Technology)	29 G 1/2" TWN; Pix'L™-Microcannula 25 G, 40 mm; Pix'L™-Microcannula 23 G, 50 mm; Pix'L+™-Microcannula 25 G, 40 mm	Firm gel with big particle size with high lifting capacity, with or without 0.3% lidocaine	
Restylane® Lip Volume	Galderma	Lip volume, lip contour	Submucosal tissue	20 mg/ml stabilised HA (NASHA Technology)	29 G 1/2" TWN; Pix'L™-Microcannula 27 G, 40 mm; Pix'L™-Microcannula 25 G, 40 mm	Firm gel with medium particle size with moderate to high lifting capacity, with 0.3% lidocaine	
TEOSYAL® Global Action	Teoxane	Filling of moderately pronounced wrinkles	Mid-dermis	25 mg/ml cross-linked HA	30 G 1/2 needle	Moderate viscosity, with lidocaine	www.teoxane.com
TEOSYAL® Touch up	Teoxane	Ideal for touch up as complement of a first TEOSYAL® injection	Mid-dermis	25 mg/ml cross-linked HA	30 G 1/2 needle	Moderate viscosity, without lidocaine	
TEOSYAL® RHA1	Teoxane	Treatment of superficial and fine wrinkles on the face (forehead lines, perioral area, crow's feet)	Superficial to mid-dermis	15 mg/ml mix of non-cross-linked and cross-linked HA (preserved network technology)	30 G 1/2 needle	Easy to inject, high stretch value, good integration of the product into the dermis, with lido-caine. Gel composed of longer HA, specially designed to respect face dyna-mism	
TEOSYAL® RHA2	Teoxane	Treatment of moderate wrinkles, in particular fore-head lines, perioral area, crow's feet, glabella, accordion lines and nasolabial folds	Mid-dermis	23 mg/ml cross-linked HA (preserved network technology)	30 G 1/2 needle	Easy to inject, high stretch value (less than RHA1), high integration of the product into the dermis, with lido-caine. Gel composed of longer HA chains, specially designed to respect face dyna-mism	

3 Fillers for deep injections

Product name	Manu-facturer	Indications	Injection depth(s)	Amount of hyaluronic acid and cross-linking	Injection tool	Material properties	Website
BELO-TERO® Intense Lidocaine	Merz Aesthetics	Correction of deeper lines, e.g. severe nasolabial fold, lip volume, oral commis-sures, marionette folds	Injection into the mid and deep dermis at approx 30 degrees	Cross-linked sodium hyaluronate: 25.5 mg/ml; lidocaine hydro-choloride: 3.0 mg/ml; cross-linking: +++	27 G needle	Outstanding elasticity for excellent tissue support to treat any severe winkles or folds	www.belotero.com
Radiesse®	Merz Aesthetics	Radiesse® is a medical device, indicated for plastic and reconstruc-tive surgery, including deep dermal and subdermal soft tissue augmentation of the facial area. Excessive volume deficits that occur due to HIV-asso-ciated facial lipoatro-phy or age-related volume loss of the hands. *Please note:* All information based on CE-certification	Deep dermis or subder-mally near the subcuta-neous structure at 30–45 degrees, depends on physician's preferred practice and injection depth respectively	Radiesse® is a sterile, latex-free, non-pyrogenic, semi-solid, com-pletely bio-degrad-able, cohesive injectable filler. Radiesse® principal components are: • 30 % calcium hydroxylapatite (CaHA) micro-spheres (25–45 μm) • 70 % sodium carboxyl methyl-cellulose (CMC) resorbable aque-ous gel carrier	27 G 1/2 needle; 28 G 3/4; 25 G 1 needle	Excellent lifting and contouring effects with long-term collagen stimulation	www.radiesse.com
Juvéderm® ULTRA®4	Allergan	Filling any deep depressions of the skin via deep dermis injection; lip enhancement; cheekbone augmenta-tion	Deep dermis injection and injections in the mucous membrane of the lips	24 mg/ml cross-linked HA (HYLACROSS™ technology)	27 G 1/2″ needle (filler is presented in a graduated, pre-filled, disposable 1 ml syringe)	Sterile, pyrogen-free physiological gel with 0.3 % lidocaine	www.juvederm.eu
Juvéderm® VOLUMA®	Allergan	Restore volume of the face	Subcutane-ous, upper-periostea, or into the deep dermis	20 mg/ml cross-linked HA (VYCROSS™ technology)	27 G 1/2″ needle (filler is presented in a graduated, pre-filled, disposable 1 ml syringe)	Sterile, pyrogen-free physiological gel with 0.3 % lidocaine available; low distribution because of strong cohesion	
Juvéderm® VOLIFT®	Allergan	Treatment of any deep skin depressions due to conditions such as premature ageing; face contouring and volume restoration to correct facial structural defects such as asymmetry, contour deformities, volume loss in the lips, cheeks, chin, lower face	Deep dermis or lips mucosa injection	17.5 mg/ml cross-linked HA (VYCROSS™ technology)	30 G 1/2″ needle (filler is presented in a graduated, pre-filled, disposable 1 ml syringe)	Sterile, pyrogen-free physiological gel with 0.3 % lido-caine; good distribution	

3 Fillers for deep injections

Product name	Manu-facturer	Indications	Injection depth(s)	Amount of hyaluronic acid and cross-linking	Injection tool	Material properties	Website
Juvéderm® VOLIFT® Retouch	Allergan	Treatment of any deep skin depressions due to conditions such as premature ageing. Face contouring and volume restoration to correct facial structural defects such as asymmetry, contour deformities, volume loss in the lips, cheeks, chin, lower face	Deep dermis or lips mucosa injection	17.5 mg/ml cross-linked HA (VYCROSS™ technology)	30 G 1/2″ needle (filler is presented in a graduated, pre-filled, disposable 0.55 ml syringe)	Sterile, pyrogen-free physiological gel with 0.3 % lidocaine; good distribution	www.juvederm.eu
Emervel® Deep	Galderma	Midface and cheeks, deep wrinkles, e.g. nasolabialfolds, marionette lines	Deep dermis	20 mg/ml very highly cross-linked HA (Optimal Balance™ technology)	27 G 1/2″ UTWN Microcannula 27 G, 38 mm UTWN	Moderately firm gel with medium particle size and high lifting capacity, with 0.3 % lidocaine	www.emervel.com
Restylane® Perlane	Galderma	Midface and cheeks, deep wrinkles, e.g. nasolabial folds, marionette lines	Deep dermis or surface of subcutis	20 mg/ml stabilised HA (NASHA Technology)	29 G 1/2″ TWN; Pix'L™-Microcannula 25 G, 40 mm; Pix'L™-Microcannula 23 G, 50 mm; Pix'L+™-Microcannula 25 G, 40 mm	Firm gel with big particle size with high lifting capacity, with or without 0.3 % lidocaine	www.restylane.com
TEOSYAL® Deep Lines	Teoxane	Filling of highly pronounced wrinkles	Deep dermis	25 mg/ml cross-linked HA	27 G 1/2 needle	Moderate viscosity, with lidocaine	www.teoxane.com
TEOSYAL® RHA3	Teoxane	Treatment of deep wrinkles in particular nasolabial fold, glabella, accordion lines, marionettes lines, perioral area, crow's feet and temples	Deep dermis	23 mg/ml cross-linked HA (preserved network technology)	27 G 1/2 needle	Easy to inject, moderate stretch value associated with high strength value, high integration of the product into the dermis, with lidocaine. Gel composed of longer HA chains, specially designed to respect face dynamism	

4 Fillers for ultra-deep injections

Product name	Manu-facturer	Indications	Injection depth(s)	Amount of hyaluronic acid and cross-linking	Injection tool	Material properties	Website
BELO-TERO® Volume Lidocaine	Merz Aesthetics	Restoration of facial volumes e.g. cheeks, temples, facial volume loss	Injection into deep dermis, subcutaneously or in the upper periostea	Cross-linked sodium hyaluronate: 26 mg/ml; lidocaine hydrocholoride: 3.0 mg/ml; cross-linking: ++++	30 G + 27 G needle; 27 G cannula	Unique combination of elasticity and plasticity that provides high projecting capacity with possibility to model the implant for natural outcomes	www.belotero.com

4 Fillers for ultra-deep injections

Product name	Manu-facturer	Indications	Injection depth(s)	Amount of hyaluronic acid and cross-linking	Injection tool	Material properties	Website
Radiesse®	Merz Aesthetics	Radiesse® is a medical device, indicated for plastic and reconstructive surgery, including deep dermal and subdermal soft tissue augmentation of the facial area. *Please note:* All information based on CE-certification	Injection into the deep dermis or subdermally near the subcutaneous structure at 30–45 degrees	Radiesse® is a sterile, latex-free, non-pyrogenic, cohesive injectable filler. Radiesse® principal components are: • 30 % calcium hydroxylapatite (CaHA) microspheres (25–45 µm) • 70 % sodium carboxyl methylcellulose (CMC) resorbable aqueous gel carrier	27 G 1/2; 28 G 3/4; 25 G 1 needle	Radiesse® combines excellent lifting and rejuvenating properties with a very natural look and feel. Treating the key areas of the face with Radiesse® can lead to excellent lifting and contouring effects. Re-volumising key areas (most commonly cheeks, jawline, and chin) can result in a synergistic effect which restores the harmony of upper, mid and lower face. Moreover, Radiesse® may be used to correct excessive volume deficits that occur due to HIV-associated facial lipoatrophy or age-related volume loss of the hands	www.radiesse.com
Juvéderm® VOLUMA®	Allergan	Restore volume of the face	Subcutaneous, upper-periostea, or into the deep dermis	20 mg/ml cross-linked HA (VYCROSS™ technology)	27 G 1/2″ needle (filler is presented in a graduated, pre-filled, disposable 1 ml syringe)	Sterile, pyrogen-free physiological gel with 0.3 % lidocaine available; low distribution because of strong cohesion	www.juvederm.eu
Juvéderm® ULTRA®4	Allergan	Filling any deep depressions of the skin via deep dermis injection; lip enhancement; cheekbone augmentation	Deep dermis injection and injections in the mucous membrane of the lips	24 mg/ml cross-linked HA (HYLACROSS™ technology)	27 G 1/2″ needle (filler is presented in a graduated, pre-filled, disposable 1 ml syringe)	Sterile, pyrogen-free physiological gel with 0.3 % lidocaine	
Juvéderm® VOLIFT®	Allergan	Treatment of any deep skin depressions due to conditions such as premature ageing. Face contouring and volume restoration to correct facial structural defects such as asymmetry, contour deformities, volume loss in the lips, cheeks, chin, lower face	Deep dermis or lips mucosa injection	17.5 mg/ml cross-linked HA (VYCROSS™ technology)	30 G 1/2″ needle (filler is presented in a graduated, pre-filled, disposable 1 ml syringe)	Sterile, pyrogen-free physiological gel with 0.3 % lidocaine; good distribution	
Juvéderm® VOLIFT® Retouch	Allergan	Treatment of any deep skin depressions due to conditions such as premature ageing. Face contouring and volume restoration to correct facial structural defects such as asymmetry, contour deformities, volume loss in the lips, cheeks, chin, lower face	Deep dermis or lips mucosa injection	17.5 mg/ml cross-linked HA (VYCROSS™ technology)	30 G 1/2″ needle (filler is presented in a graduated, pre-filled, disposable 0.55 ml syringe)	Sterile, pyrogen-free physiological gel with 0.3 % lidocaine; good distribution	

4 Fillers for ultra-deep injections

Product name	Manu-facturer	Indications	Injection depth(s)	Amount of hyaluronic acid and cross-linking	Injection tool	Material properties	Website
Emervel® Volume	Galderma	Volume for facial contours, e.g. cheek-bones, cheeks, chin, jawline	Supra-periosteally or subcuta-neously	20 mg/ml highly cross-linked HA (Optimal Balance™ technology)	For 1 ml syringes: 27 G 1/2" UTWN; Microcannula 27 G, 38 mm UTWN. For 2 ml syringes: 23 G 1" UTWN; Microcannula 22 G, 50 mm UTWN	Moderately soft gel with big particle size and very high lifting capacity, with 0.3% lidocaine	www.emervel.com
Restylane® SubQ	Galderma	Volume for facial contours, e.g. cheek-bones, cheeks, chin, jawline	Supra-periosteally or subcuta-neous fatty tissue	20 mg/ml stabilised HA (NASHA Technology)	Sharp needle 21 G 1" Pix'L™-Microcannula 21 G, 60 mm Blunt cannula 16–21 G	Very firm gel with bigger particle size and very high lifting capacity, with or with-out 0.3% lidocaine	www.restylane.com
TEOSYAL® Ultimate	Teoxane	Volume recovery for wide areas (face oval, cheeks, temples)	Subcutane-ous or pre-periosteum	22 mg/ml cross-linked HA	23 G 1 (3 ml syringe), 27 G 1/2 (1 ml syringe)	High volumising capacities in large areas, with lidocaine	www.teoxane.com
TEOSYAL® Ultra Deep	Teoxane	Volume creation for targeted areas (cheekbones, chin) and correction of deep wrinkles in thick skin	Subcutane-ous or pre-periosteum	25 mg/ml cross-linked HA	25 G 1 needle	High projection abilities, with lidocaine	
TEOSYAL® RHA4	Teoxane	Volume creation in extended areas (chin, cheeks, mandibular area, temples), filling deep wrinkles (mari-onette lines, nasolabial fold)	Subcutane-ous or pre-periosteum	23 mg/ml cross-linked HA (preserved network technology)	27 G 1/2 needle	Easy to inject, moderate stretch value associated with high strength value, high integration of the product into the dermis, with lido-caine. Gel composed of longer HA chains, specially designed to respect face dyna-mism	

A Special indications: skin surface regeneration and mesotherapy (skin boosters)

Product name	Manu-facturer	Indications	Injection depth(s)	Amount of hyaluronic acid and cross-linking	Injection tool	Material properties	Website
Hyal® ACP	Merz Aesthetics	Skin hydration, e.g. face, neck, décolle-tage, back of hands	Injection into the superficial dermis or the dermo-epidermal junction	Auto-cross-linked hyaluronate 20 mg/ml	30 G needle	Unique and patented auto-cross-linked HA for long-lasting biorevitalising of the skin, improvement of skin elasticity, tone and radiance restoration	www.hyal-acp.de

A Special indications: skin surface regeneration and mesotherapy (skin boosters)

Product name	Manu-facturer	Indications	Injection depth(s)	Amount of hyaluronic acid and cross-linking	Injection tool	Material properties	Website
Juvéderm® HYDRATE™	Allergan	Improving skin hydration and elasticity	Multi-injection into the dermal epidermal junction and into the superficial dermis	13.5 mg/ml non-cross-linked HA (VYCROSS™ technology)	Graduated pre-filled syringe for single use	Sterile apyrogenic, physiological solution of hyaluronic acid containing 0.9% mannitol	www.juvederm.eu
Restylane® Skinboosters™ Vital Light	Galderma	Rejuvenation and skin quality improvement of face, neck, hands and décolletage for young or delicate skin	Mid-dermis	12 mg/ml stabilised HA (NASHA Technology)	29 G TWN Smart Click System; 30 G Pixl™ cannula; 29 G TWN injector	Soft gel with small particle size, with or without 0.3% lidocaine	www.restylane.com
Restylane® Skinboosters™ Vital	Galderma	Rejuvenation and skin quality improvement of face, neck, hands and décolletage; also for mature and photodamaged skin	Mid to deep dermis	20 mg/ml stabilised HA (NASHA Technology)	29 G TWN Smart Click System; 30 G Pixl™ cannula; 29 G TWN injector	Soft gel with slightly bigger particle size (compared to Vital Light), with or without 0.3% lidocaine	
Emervel® Touch	Galderma	Perioral lines, periorbital lines	Superficial dermis	20 mg/ml low cross-linked HA (Optimal Balance™ technology)	30 G 1/2" UTWN; Microcannula 30 G, 25 mm UTWN	Very soft gel with small particle size and moderate lifting capacity	www.emervel.com
TEOSYAL® Meso	Teoxane	Revitalisation and hydration of the face	Superficial dermis	15 mg/ml non-cross-linked HA	30 G 1/2 needle	Light gel, ideal for mesotherapy	www.teoxane.com
TEOSYAL® Redensity I	Teoxane	Hydration and rejuvenation of the face, neck and décolletage	Superficial to mid-dermis	15 mg/ml non-cross-linked HA + patented Dermo-Restructuring Complex (8 amino acid + 3 antioxidants + zinc, copper + vitamin B6)	30 G 1/2 needle	Skin rejuvenation – well tolerated, with lidocaine	

B Special indications: lips – perioral complex and tear trough

Product name	Manu-facturer	Indications	Injection depth(s)	Amount of hyaluronic acid and cross-linking	Injection tool	Material properties	Website
BELOTERO® Balance Lidocaine	Merz Aesthetics	Correction of moderate lines, e.g. moderate perioral wrinkles, lip contouring, philtrum	Injection into the superficial to mid-dermis at approx. 15 degrees	Cross-linked sodium hyaluronate: 22.5 mg/ml; lidocaine hydrocholoride: 3.0 mg/ml; cross-linking: ++	27 G needle	Outstanding tissue integration for optimal treatment of the lips contours	www.belotero.com
BELOTERO® Intense Lidocaine	Merz Aesthetics	Correction of deeper lines, e.g. severe nasolabial fold, lip volume, oral commissures, marionette folds	Injection into lips mucosa	Cross-linked sodium hyaluronate: 25.5 mg/ml; lidocaine hydrocholoride: 3.0 mg/ml; cross-linking: +++; Phosphate buffer pH 7 q.s.: 1 ml	27 G needle	Outstanding elasticity for excellent tissue support to project the lips	

B Special indications: lips – perioral complex and tear trough

Product name	Manu-facturer	Indications	Injection depth(s)	Amount of hyaluronic acid and cross-linking	Injection tool	Material properties	Website
Juvéderm® VOLBELLA®	Allergan	Treatment of any fine lines and medium-sized skin depressions due to conditions such as premature ageing. Enhancement and pouting of the lips to correct structural defects such as asymmetry, contour deformities, volume loss	Superficial or mid-dermis injection or lips mucosa injection	15 mg/ml cross-linked HA (VYCROSS™ technology)	30 G 1/2" needle (filler is presented in a graduated, pre-filled, disposable 1 ml syringe)	Sterile, pyrogen-free physiological gel with 0.3% lido-caine; good distribution	www.juvederm.eu
Juvéderm® ULTRA®3	Allergan	Filling mid and/or deep depressions of the skin via mid and/or deep dermis injection. Lip definition and enhancement	Mid and deep dermis	24 mg/ml cross-linked HA (HYLACROSS™ technology)	27 G 1/2" needle (filler is presented in a graduated, pre-filled, disposable 1 ml syringe)	Sterile, pyrogen-free physiological gel with 0.3% lidocaine	
Juvéderm® ULTRA SMILE®	Allergan	Filling mid and/or deep depressions of the skin via mid and/or deep dermis injection. Lip definition and enhancement	Mid and deep dermis	24 mg/ml cross-linked HA (HYLACROSS™ technology)	30 G 1/2" needle (filler is presented in a graduat-ed, pre-filled, disposable 0.55 ml syringe)	Sterile, pyrogen-free physiological gel with 0.3% lidocaine	
Juvéderm® VOLIFT®	Allergan	Treatment of any deep skin depressions due to conditions such as premature ageing. Face contouring and volume restoration to correct facial structural defects such as asymmetry, contour deformities, volume loss in the lips, cheeks, chin, lower face	Deep dermis or lips mucosa injection	17.5 mg/ml cross-linked HA (VYCROSS™ technology)	30 G 1/2" needle (filler is presented in a graduat-ed, pre-filled, disposable 1 ml syringe)	Sterile, pyrogen-free physiological gel with 0.3% lido-caine; good distribution	
Juvéderm® VOLIFT® Retouch	Allergan	Treatment of any deep skin depressions due to conditions such as premature ageing. Face contouring and volume restoration to correct facial structural defects such as asymmetry, contour deformities, volume loss in the lips, cheeks, chin, lower face	Deep dermis or lips mucosa injection	17.5 mg/ml cross-linked HA (VYCROSS™ technology)	30 G 1/2" needle (filler is presented in a graduat-ed, pre-filled, disposable 0.55 ml syringe)	Sterile, pyrogen-free physiological gel with 0.3% lido-caine; good distribution	
Emervel® Classic	Galderma	Nasolabial folds, marionette lines	Mid-dermis	20 mg/ml moderately cross-linked HA (Optimal Balance™ technology)	30 G 1/2" UTWN Microcannula 27 G, 38 mm UTWN	Soft gel with small particle size and moderate lifting capacity, with 0.3% lidocaine	www.emervel.com
Emervel® Lips	Galderma	Lip volume, lip contour	Vermilion lip, submucosal tissue	20 mg/ml highly cross-linked HA (Optimal Balance™ technology)	30 G 1/2" UTWN Microcannula 27 G, 38 mm UTWN	Moderately soft gel with small particle size and moderate lifting capacity, with 0.3% lidocaine	

B Special indications: lips – perioral complex and tear trough

Product name	Manu-facturer	Indications	Injection depth(s)	Amount of hyaluronic acid and cross-linking	Injection tool	Material properties	Website
Restylane® Lip Volume	Galderma	Lip volume, lip contour	Submucosal tissue	20 mg/ml stabilised HA (NASHA Technology)	29 G 1/2" TWN; Pix'L™-Microcannula 27 G, 40 mm; Pix'L™-Microcannula 25 G, 40 mm	Firm gel with medium particle size with moderate to high lifting capacity, with 0.3% lidocaine	www.restylane.com
TEOSYAL® Kiss	Teoxane	Harmonisation of the lip contour and volume	Labial mucosa	25 mg/ml cross-linked HA	27 G 1/2 needle	Moderate viscosity, with lidocaine	www.teoxane.com
TEOSYAL® Global Action	Teoxane	Filling of moderately pronounced wrinkles	Mid-dermis	25 mg/ml cross-linked HA	30 G 1/2 needle	Moderate viscosity, with lidocaine	
TEOSYAL® Redensity II	Teoxane	Correction of the eye circle, tear trough, palpebromalar groove, minimal palpebral or malar bags	Supraperi-osteal, deep sub-orbicular	15 mg/ml mix of non-cross-linked and cross-linked HA + Dermo-Restructuring Complex	30 G 1/2 needle	Specific product for tear trough correction, well tolerated, with lidocaine	
TEOSYAL® RHA1	Teoxane	Treatment of superficial and fine wrinkles on the face (forehead lines, perioral area, crow's feet)	Superficial to mid-dermis	15 mg/ml mix of non-cross-linked and cross-linked HA (preserved network technology)	30 G 1/2 needle	Easy to inject, high stretch value, good integration of the product into the dermis, with lidocaine. Gel composed of longer HA, specially designed to respect face dynamism	
TEOSYAL® RHA2	Teoxane	Treatment of moderate wrinkles, in particular forehead lines, perioral area, crow's feet, glabella, accordion lines and nasolabial folds	Mid-dermis	23 mg/ml cross-linked HA (preserved network technology)	30 G 1/2 needle	Easy to inject, high stretch value (less than RHA1), high integration of the product into the dermis, with lidocaine. Gel composed of longer HA chains, specially designed to respect face dynamism	
TEOSYAL® RHA3	Teoxane	Treatment of deep wrinkles in particular nasolabial fold, glabella, accordion lines, marionettes lines, perioral area, crow's feet and temples	Deep dermis	23 mg/ml cross-linked HA (preserved network technology)	27 G 1/2 needle	Easy to inject, moderate stretch value associated with high strength value, high integration of the product into the dermis, with lidocaine. Gel composed of longer HA chains, specially designed to respect face dynamism	

4 Medical Photography

4 Medical Photography

One of the key convincing and objective ways of demonstrating the efficacy of the increasing number of non-invasive treatments is through medical photography. For this reason, professional, standardised medical photographs charting the course of the treatment play a key role in the medical aesthetic practice today. Photographic documentation of a treatment not only provides a communication medium in the consultation, but also promotes patient loyalty during the more prolonged treatments. Furthermore, follow-up images are part of a clinic's quality management procedure and, last but not least, provide a safeguard in the event of a dispute.

This chapter provides an overview of the basics of photographic documentation in the medical practice, and in addition focuses on the advantages and practical applications of 3D photography in aesthetic medicine.

4.1 General Requirements for Medical Photography

Digital photography has long since superseded conventional analogue photography. Professional photographic documentation should fulfil the following requirements:

- Ease of use, allowing the picture-taking process to be delegated
- Cost-effectiveness
- Standardisation of the baseline and follow-up shots for optimum comparability
- Analysis of the images
- Patient-referenced archiving and analysis
- Report-writing
- Suitability for use in publications

4.2 Photographic Documentation

4.2.1 Room

It is advisable to take medical photographs in a dedicated room or, at least, in a separate area without direct sunlight.

4.2.2 Background

The background must be free of extraneous objects that distract the eye from the subject, such as books, plants or other people. Furthermore, the patient being photographed should not simply be placed in the middle of the room: this makes the image background impossible to control or reproduce for subsequent photographs. The optimal way is to set up a fixed documentation spot within the practice premises, with a uniform, neutral background, e.g. back of the door, wall or room divider. Furthermore, photographs of the head, arms, legs and feet, for example, can be taken against the neutral surface colour of an examination couch. This ensures that no extraneous, distracting objects are visible in the background.

The ideal background is homogeneous and in a single, neutral colour. Colours that are too bright and glaring or too dark are best avoided. Standard grey is ideal when assessing skin changes. The background should be reproducible throughout the documentation period.

> **Practice tip**
>
> Homogeneous backgrounds of single colour hues such as cream, white or grey, make a suitable background.

4.2.3 Lighting

Every light source has different colour temperatures, with differing effects on colour reproduction. Artificial light sources pose particular problems, since mixtures of different light sources do not provide good follow-up documentation due to the colour variations involved.

Mixed light situations (i.e. daylight, various fluorescent lamps or other artificial light sources) almost always occur in the practice setting, which makes it more difficult to reproduce the true colours of the subject and/or require time-consuming processing with associated poorer quality. Mixed light situations can be avoided by using a bright, artificial light source for the shots. The use of a dedicated flash unit is the optimal solution. This allows reproducible results to be achieved regardless of the natural light source and also, in most cases, regardless of any existing ambient lighting. Exposure times suitable for excluding ambient light can be achieved with shorter shutter speeds from 1/125 s.

Lighting with a **flash** offers a few advantages, provided that the ground rules are followed (Figs 4.1 and 4.2). There are two variants: direct and indirect flash. For a direct flash, the adjustable reflector is directed at the subject. In the indirect technique, the reflector is directed onto a large white surface, e.g. the ceiling or the wall of the room. The flash bounces off this surface, lighting the subject indirectly.

4.2.4 Taking the photographs

The following section describes the basic practical features of photographic documentation. The sample shots shown here were taken with a digital reflex camera. It is generally accepted that this is the most suitable documentation tool in a medical aesthetics context.

Posture and pose

For optimum results the patient should be instructed to keep still during the photography, while holding the chosen pose. A series of images are advised to capture a variety of expressions (e.g. in static repose, dynamic repose: smiling, frowning, etc) and from a variety of perspectives (e.g. from the front, 45 degree lateral, full lateral, view from above, view from below). From the operator's perspective, a tripod is ideal to ensure quality images, otherwise the photographer can chose to hold the camera with the elbows pressed tightly against the body for maximum control.

Handling

Ensure that any measuring instruments and sensors are not covered with the hand or any other objects. They are there to ensure that the automatic lighting and focus functions work correctly.
The lenses and viewfinder should be cleaned regularly with appropriate cleaning agents. However, the sensor must not be cleaned or

Effects of different light sources on the subject

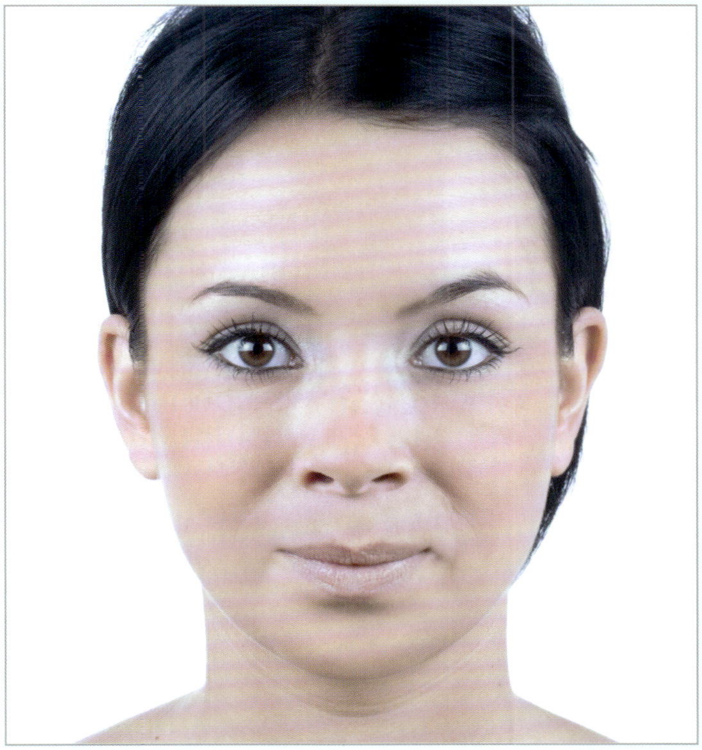

Fig. 4.1 Light source: flash, set manually to cold light → colour is falsified.

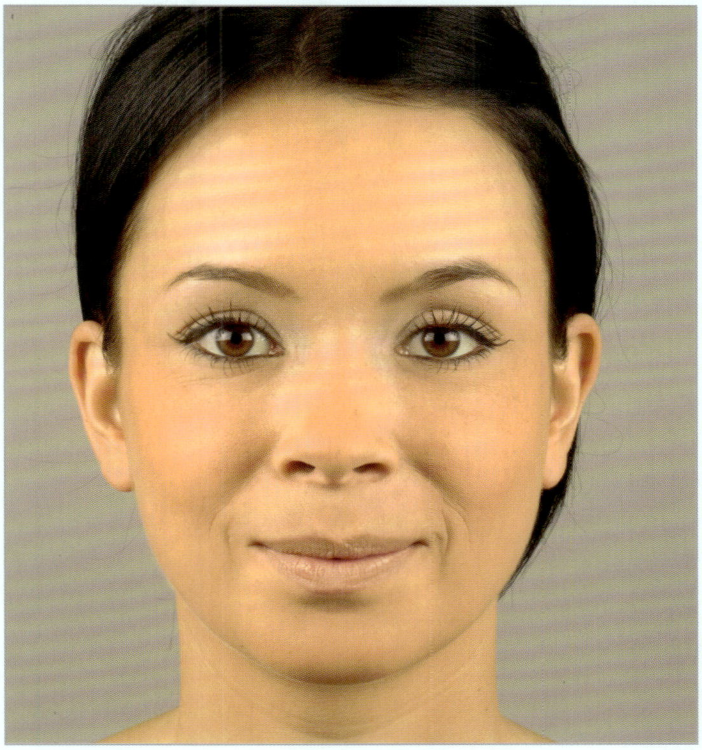

Fig. 4.2 Light source: flash, set manually to incandescent flash → colour is falsified.

touched. In essence, a defective sensor surface equals complete damage to a digital reflex camera.

Reference image, baseline shot

The first or baseline photograph of a documentation series should be taken very carefully and conscientiously, as it represents the reference image (Fig. 4.3). All the images taken at follow-up will thereafter be compared with this reference image (Figs 4.4 and 4.5).

Detail shots

Prior to taking detail photographs/shots, it is best to focus in on the desired location gradually. If some time has passed since the last photographic session, it can often be difficult to recall which area was last photographed. Where this is the case, a general view helps to find the correct location for subsequent shots.

Treatment course documentation

The reference image must always be used when documenting a patient's treatment course. This photograph shows the selected distance, angle, light setting, and location. These criteria are sufficient for most treatment course documentation series. Higher-cost complete solutions (camera, tripod, light) are available for the purpose of conducting studies. With these, photographs can always be taken under the same conditions.

Distance from the shot area

A certain distance needs to be maintained from the area being photographed, as the shot can otherwise become distorted or out of focus. Every focal length has its advantages and disadvantages in this respect. For example, shots taken with a wide-angle lens of less than 50 mm produce undesirable distortions (rather like viewing someone through a spy-hole), which are not appropriate for documentation purposes. It is better to zoom in on the subject from a slightly greater distance. On the other hand, one should also avoid zooming in too far, as this can cause blurring.

Camera angle

The camera should always be held parallel to the subject, since standard cameras can only produce a sharply focused image in a plane parallel to the image sensor or the camera. A partially blurred image is produced if the camera is tipped or tilted relative to the imaging plane.

Lighting

Assessing light through the camera display alone provides some guidance, at best. An image that is too dark on the display indicates that there is too little light, whereas a very bright display indicates too much light. Different cameras (even those of the same type) can have different displays, and thus react differently to variations in lighting. The following parameters must be taken into account with regard to lighting:

Treatment course documentation: using the reference image as a guide

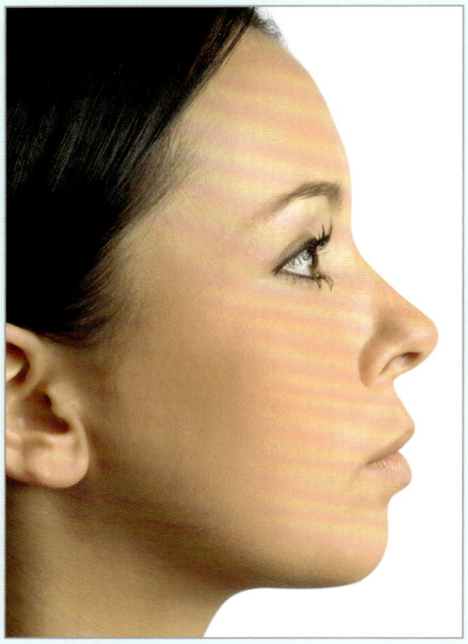
Fig. 4.3 Reference image.

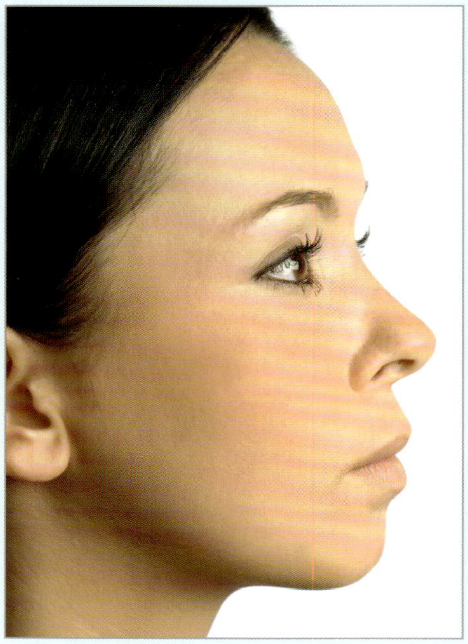
Fig. 4.4 Follow-up image 1.

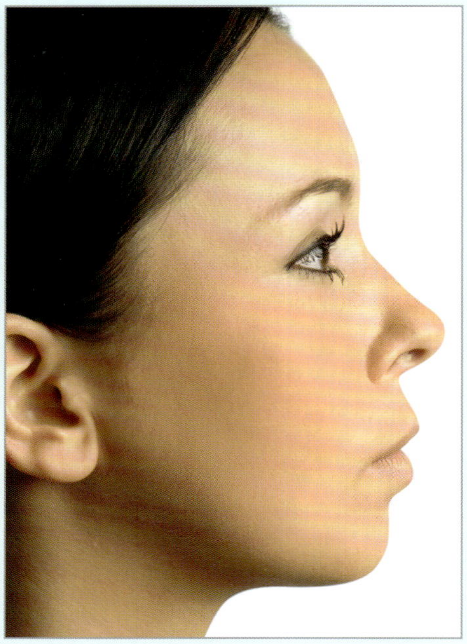
Fig. 4.5 Follow-up image 2.

- ISO speed
- Lens aperture
- Flash unit performance

The following settings are recommended: ISO speed over a range of 200–800; maximum possible lens aperture; an exposure time which fades out most of the ambient light when a flash is used, but which should never be longer than 1/50 s.

Uncertainties regarding correct lighting can be avoided by using a histogram. A histogram is a graphic representation of the brightness distribution within a photograph and provides a much better way of controlling this variable than the camera's own display. The two ends represent dark (left) and bright (right) areas in the image. However, a balanced, correctly lit photograph requires medium values in addition to the shadows and highlights. Depending on the camera model, the histogram can be displayed before or while taking the shot, or it can be integrated into the playback mode after the shot has been taken.

Clinical measurements

The simplest way of making measurements in the image is with the use of a ruler. If any features need to be documented with a 'yardstick', a good option, for hygienic and practical purposes, is to use disposable rulers. These are usually 10 cm long and 2 cm wide, self-adhesive and can easily be written on with a ballpoint pen.

4.2.5 Camera types

A choice of three camera types are available: compact (point-and-shoot); reflex; and bridge cameras.

Compact cameras are all-round machines. They are small, easy to use, have an integrated flash and are suitable for simple documentation work.

The standard is a digital **reflex camera** with all its add-on options including lenses, flash, dermatoscope attachment and lens filters. If configured correctly, the digital reflex camera delivers the highest optical performance.

The final option is the **bridge camera**. These combine the advantages of the digital reflex and point-and-shoot cameras in compact form.

Which of these three variants is selected depends on the user's individual requirements (see Tab. 4.1). In general, the selected camera should be suitable for its specialised use in medical documentation.

Practice tip

The camera should be tested prior to purchase. To do this, take long-distance and close-up shots of some skin areas against single-colour backgrounds. If the results are not reproducible, the camera's inbuilt features are not suitable for this purpose. Before using a new camera, users should take time to familiarise themselves with its technical features and mode of operation.

Digital compact camera	Digital reflex camera	Bridge camera
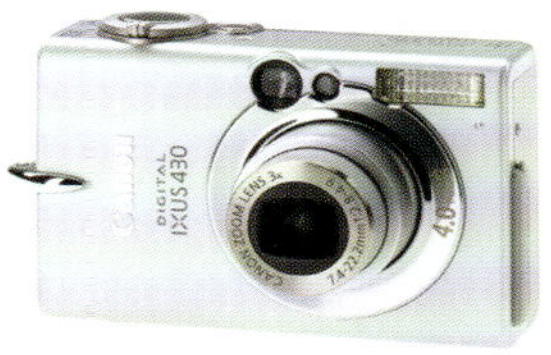	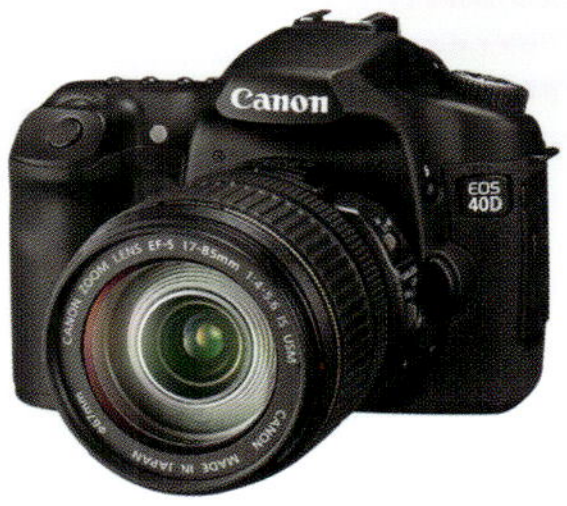	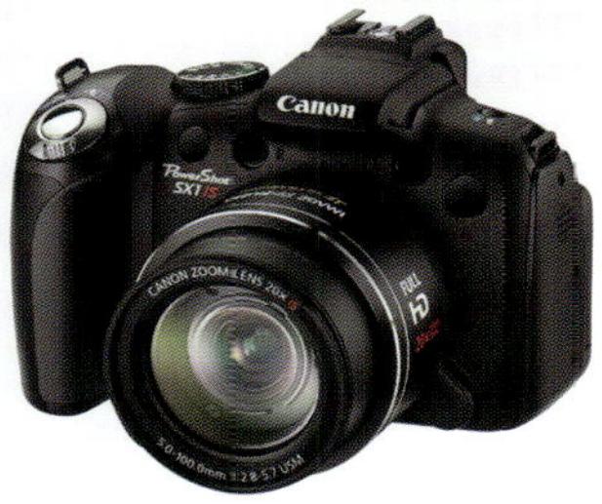
	Advantages	
+ Easy to use	+ Wide range of accessories on offer	+ Small and compact
+ Pre-programmed image modes	+ Simple manual operation	+ Can be operated manually
+ Economical to buy	+ High optical performance	
+ Small and compact	+ Lenses can be changed	
	+ Special attachments (e.g. dermatoscope)	
	Disadvantages	
– Few accessories	– Unwieldy	– Accessories expensive, few available
– Limited applications	– Basic knowledge of photography required to operate	– Lenses cannot be changed
– Manual operation complicated/few options		– Basic knowledge of photography required to operate
– No indirect flash		

Tab. 4.1 Camera types compared.

4.3 Three-dimensional (3D) Photography

3D photography has been used in medicine for more than 20 years. However, historically the required technical skills and associated high costs meant that routine use within medical premises was challenging and inappropriate.

Today, the development of high-performance graphics cards for the consumer sector, alongside compact cameras with high resolution, quick processors and cutting-edge software, have enabled the real-time synthesis (rendering) of two-dimensional images into complex three-dimensional forms. This means that compact systems for use in medical practices are now available. The following section presents practice-related information on the use of 3D photography in aesthetic medicine.

The aesthetic medicine sector was virtually predestined for the use of 3D imaging. 3D imaging enables a substantial dialogue to be conducted with the patient. Starting with a baseline image, which represents the present state, various interventions can then be simulated in real time. Conversely, the patient can be shown what effects a desired modification will have on their appearance.

In business management terms, the use of 3D imaging as part of the practitioner–patient communication process represents a substantial competitive advantage. For the patient, the before/after simulation provides further information and support when making the decision to go ahead with the treatment. Ultimately, the 3D view allows the clinical result of the treatment to be viewed and experienced in more tangible terms. Furthermore, it also makes it easier for the practitioner to explain the benefits of the various combined treatment options, e.g. the combination of injectable fillers with botulinum toxin type-A.

Caution

It is essential that the practitioner thoroughly explains to the patient that the simulation is only a helpful exercise and the final treatment results cannot be fully guaranteed to resemble the image(s) shown.

4.3.1 Overview of the 3D systems

3D systems consist of various components. The exact configuration depends on the purpose for which they are used and on the manufacturer's technology.

Detailed reproduction of the face requires the highest degree of resolution and the most precise lighting. The system's user-friendly technology is a key consideration. The corresponding software should ideally be easily understood, logical, and intuitive to use (Fig. 4.6).

Cameras

The cameras in 3D imaging systems have a number of purposes. Firstly, their positioning defines the spatial geometry of an object; secondly, they also record all the surface details on the skin with regard to colour and structure.

A software package then computes the digital images taken by the cameras into virtual 3D models.

Lighting

The lighting in 3D systems needs to be precisely adjusted in order to reproduce contours and surface details. A xenon flash with a pulse of a few milliseconds' duration is the preferred option. These short illumination periods ensure that the subject's movements do not impair the final image. In addition, the high intensity of the xenon light enables the photographs to be taken under normal indoor light conditions.

Positioning

Both the cameras and the light sources need to be positioned to ensure the correct angle and the correct distance from the subject at all times. Systems used for photography of the face and neck are usually fixed. The subject is then placed into the optimum position for photography with the aid of appropriate devices. Systems used to take pictures of the body need to be height-adjustable to cater for different-sized patients.

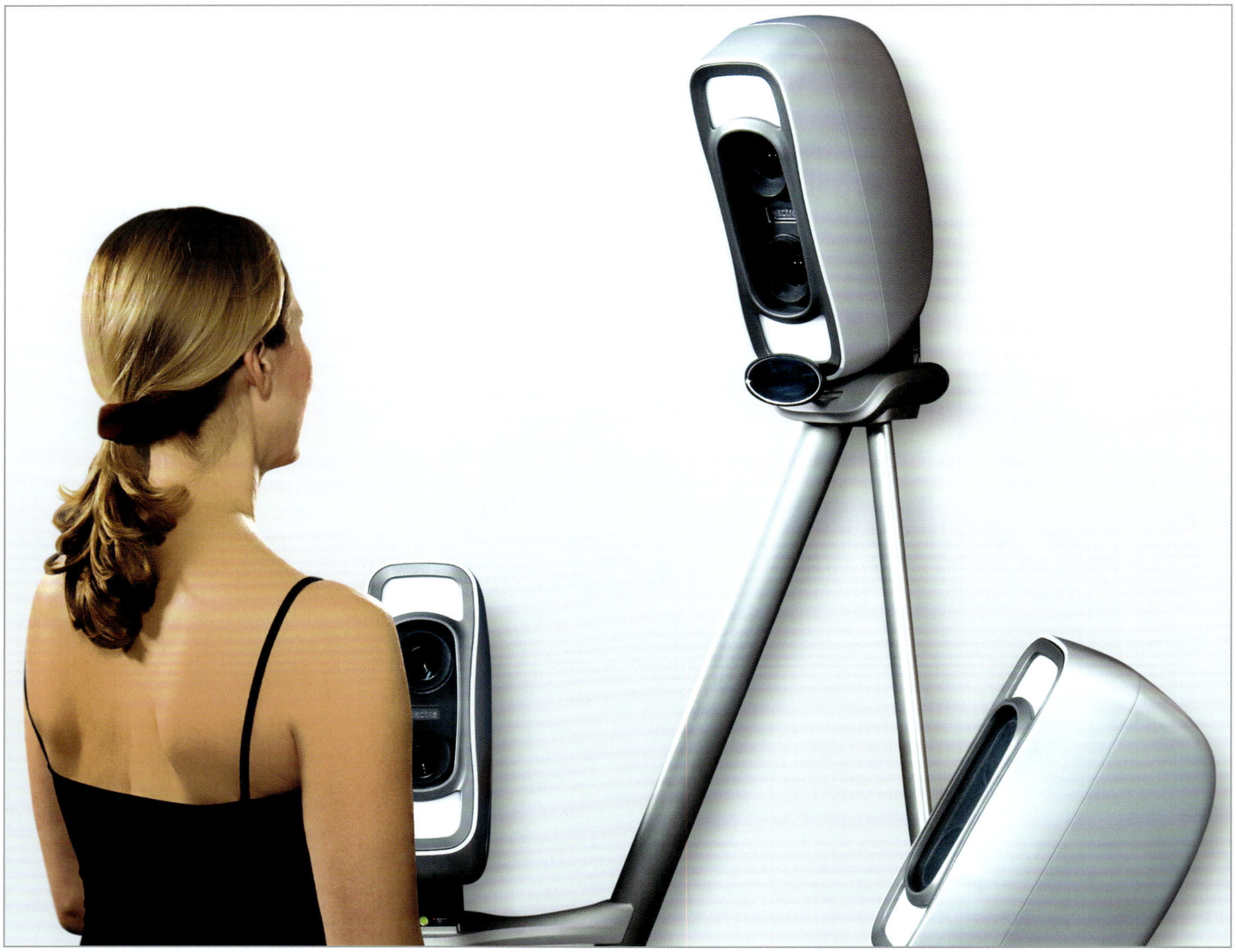

Fig. 4.6 The VECTRA M3 system (Canfield Imaging Systems) is one example of a camera that delivers high-resolution 3D models of the face and upper body.

Computer systems

Most systems are based on a commercially available, high-performance PC with large storage capacities. An equally high-performance graphics card will be needed due to the high volume of data that has to be processed and transformed into 3D models. In most cases, the computer is integrated into a local area network, to allow access to the images during the consultation and to make regular data back-up easier. An internet connection is important to enable remote diagnosis and other services.

Software

A suitable software package contains a number of modules. From the user's point of view, the following functions should be available:

1. Taking photographs and storing the images thereafter: in simple terms, the software allows the practitioner to generate a 3D image of the subject. Once the user is satisfied with the result, they can store the image locally or on the server.
2. Image analysis: software modules allow lines, surfaces and volumes to be measured and analysed. This ensures that the results of the clinical procedures can be visualised and compared with one another at different points in time. In the example shown here, the software has calculated the volume required for an augmentation treatment in the midface using fillers (Fig. 4.7).

4.3.2 Practical applications

Documenting the baseline status

The baseline status, i.e. the reference image, is the cornerstone of the consultation process. The first step involves the generation of the reference photograph, which reproduces the actual status at the time of the consultation. This reference photograph forms the basis for all the simulations that may be carried out later. Furthermore, this image serves as a reference against which to compare the subsequent results of the treatment. The reference photograph should therefore be taken with great care, to ensure that the baseline status clearly represents the patient's current physical state. The authors advocate taking baseline images in a static and also dynamic repose (i.e. with no expression alongside several expressions, e.g. smiling).

The following basic requirements must be met when taking the reference photograph:

- The patient's skin should be dry, clean and free of all cosmetic products.
- If the face is the focus of the treatment, it should not be obscured by hair.
- A strong light source, e.g. direct sunlight, should be avoided.
- The patient should be in a comfortable position when being photographed, to minimise movement before or while the image is being taken.
- If the face is being photographed, the patient should adopt a relaxed and neutral facial expression. Clinical images of dynamic expressions, e.g. smiling, frowning, pouting, etc are also advantageous for the baseline images, and care should be taken to ensure the facial expression is natural and reproducible as much as possible. Images taken in dynamic motion are useful to assess and evaluate how fillers have integrated with the natural tissues and how they exert their enhancing effects.

Volume measurement and simulation

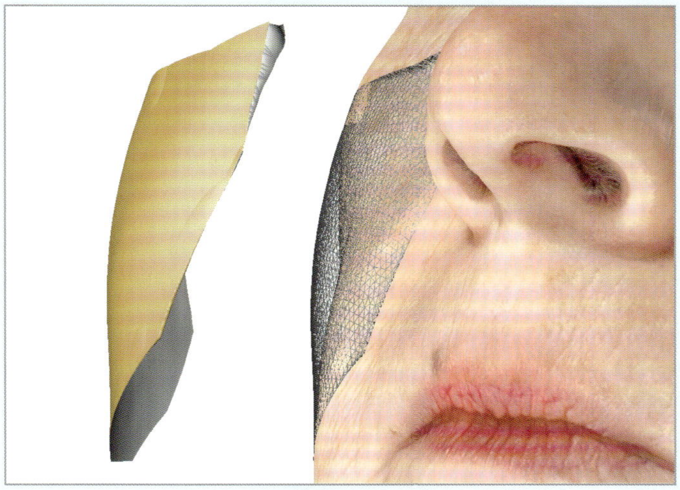

Fig. 4.7 Volume measurement for a midface augmentation treatment with fillers.

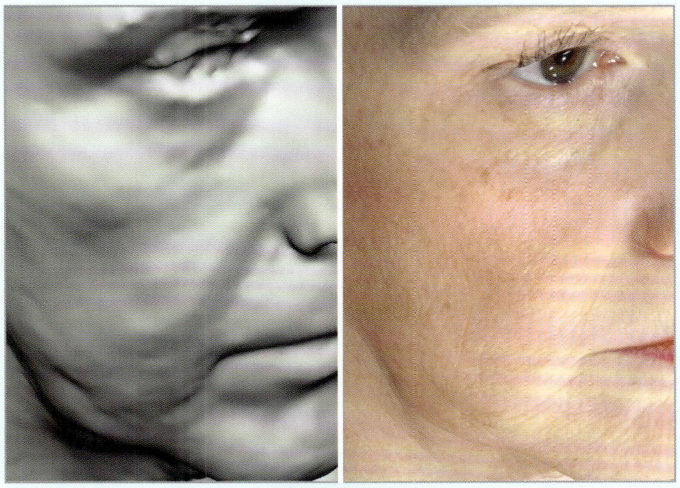

Fig. 4.8 Removing skin colour and the superficial structures results in an excellent representation of the contours of the face.

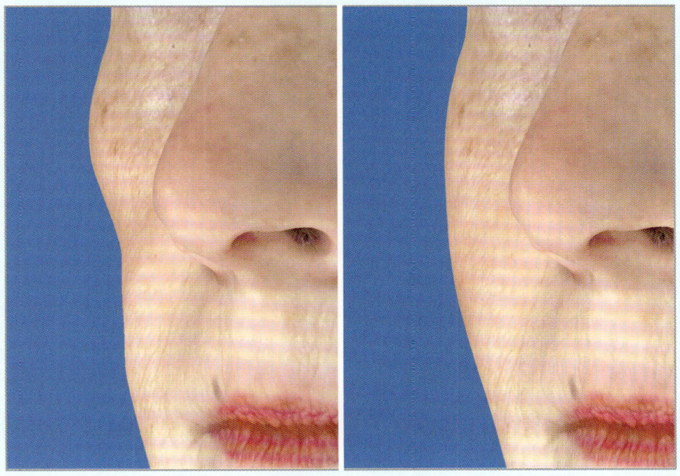

Fig. 4.9 Simulation of a midface augmentation treatment with fillers.

Evaluation

The evaluation of the baseline image forms the basis for assessing the efficacy of a treatment. Furthermore, this baseline image can be used to determine which treatment options are worth considering. Specific software can be used to remove the skin colour, showing the surface of the skin in shades of grey (Fig. 4.8). This image modification allows much better visualisation of the surface contours and highlights uneven areas.

Generating simulations

The greatest value of 3D visualisation lies in the simulation of the results of a planned modification. This gives the patient a chance to look at the effects of a potential treatment result with the aid of spatial imaging, from all the sides and points of view (Fig. 4.9).

Experience has shown that patients are far more likely to agree to the proposed procedure if 3D visualisation is used as part of the aesthetic consultation. In addition, it gives the practitioner the option of demonstrating the advantages of additional combined treatment modalities, which could improve the results of the treatment. The option of demonstrating any features that cannot be corrected, and explaining why, is also just as important. Ultimately, a consultation based on a 3D visualisation or 3D simulation results in a well-informed and satisfied patient.

4.3.3 Examples of potential uses

Lip augmentation

Patients who want to have fuller lips can benefit from lip volume augmentation with fillers. By using an appropriate software tool, the practitioner can simulate the change in size of the upper or lower lip in accordance with the patient's wishes. The figures show both the baseline image and the simulation of the fuller lips (see Fig. 2.23, p. 45).

Volume therapy with fillers

In older patients, volume replacement is particularly effective at producing a more youthful and healthy appearance. In this case, the practitioner needs to define the specific areas of the face where additional volume will be required. To do this, they can use a specific software tool to simulate the desired effect (Fig. 4.10).

The baseline and the simulation image(s) can also be shown in a single 3D image, with the added volume shown as a semi-transparent overlay (Fig. 4.11). This is particularly useful if subtle differences are difficult to detect in a side-by-side comparison. It is even possible to calculate the difference in volume (i.e. the volume of filler required for the treatment) between the reference and the simulation image (Fig. 4.12).

4

Visualising differences in volume

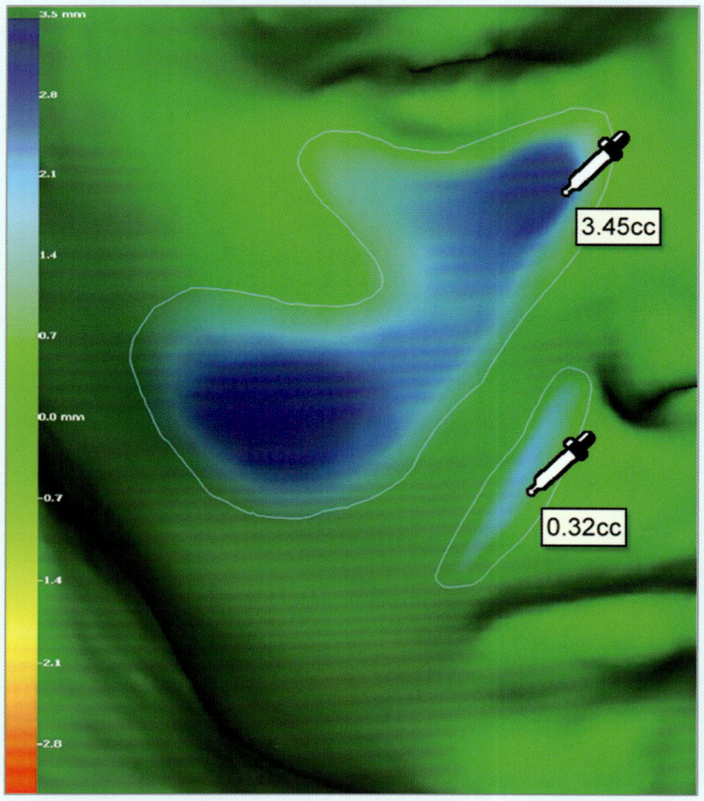

Fig. 4.10 Colour profiles identify and visualise volume differences in the areas to be treated.

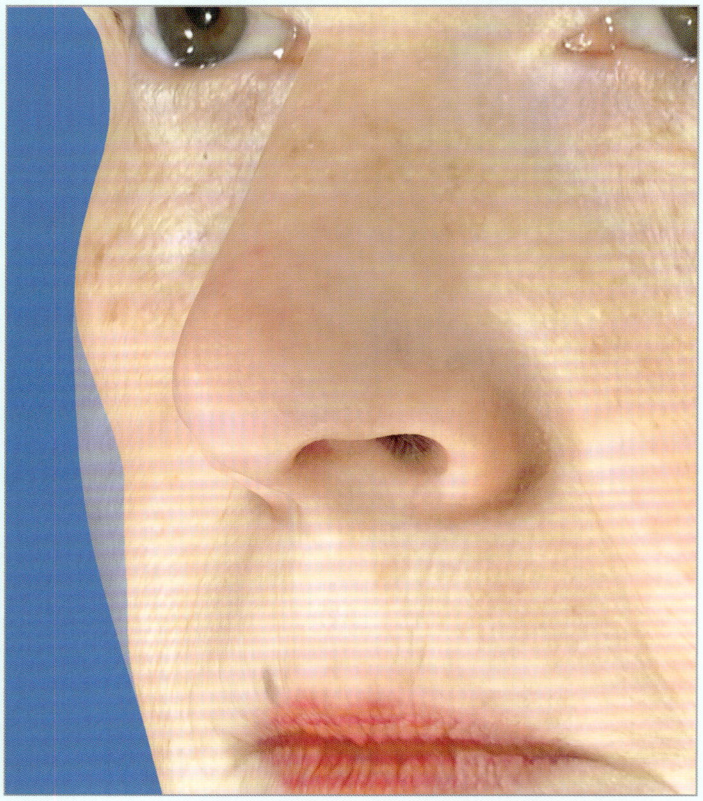

Fig. 4.11 A semi-transparent overlay shows up subtle differences.

Simulated lip augmentation

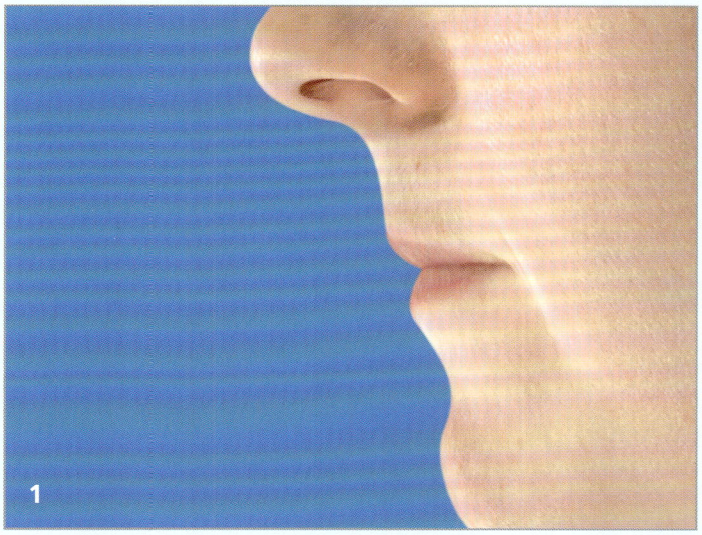

Fig. 4.12
1 Prior to the treatment.

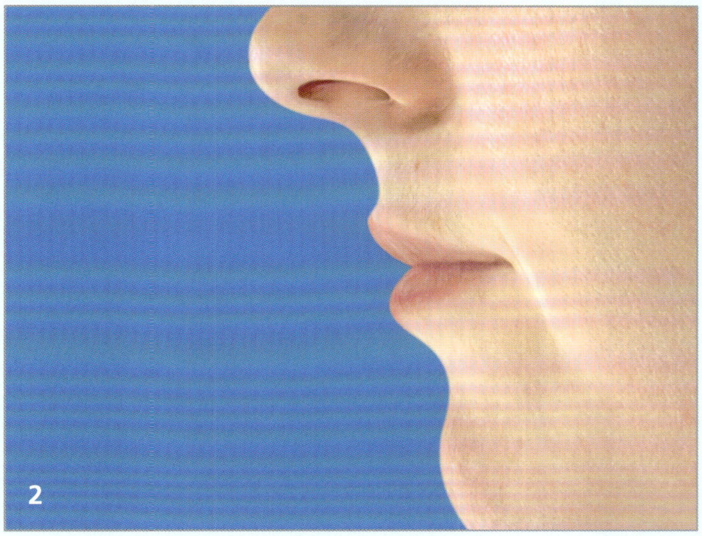

2 Simulated result.

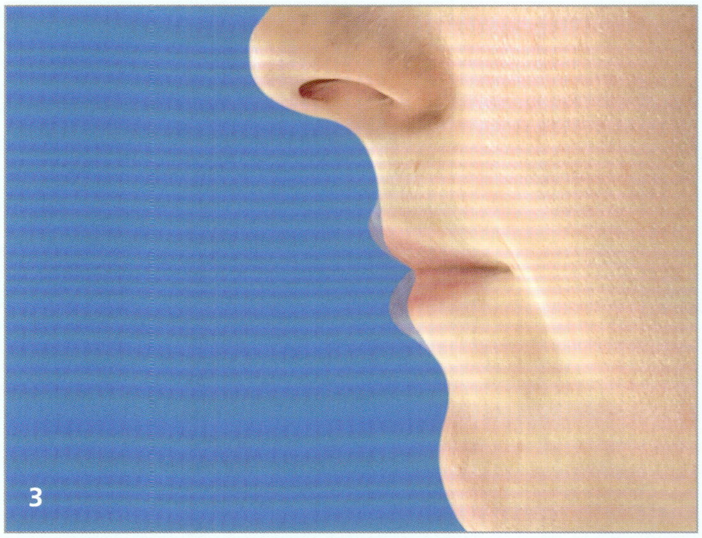

3 Before and after simulation for comparison.

Treating lines with fillers and botulinum toxin type-A

The reduction of wrinkles and lines with the aid of fillers, for example in the glabellar region, can be simulated using what is known as a 'smoothing' tool (see Fig. 4.13). This software tool can be used to select the lines to be treated and fill them to the desired extent. The smoothing tool can be used in a similar way to show a simulation of the line reduction treatment on other areas (e.g. the forehead). Since the 3D effect in this form of simulation is not as pronounced, the patient can be given the option of looking at the result from various viewpoints.

Simulated reduction of lines

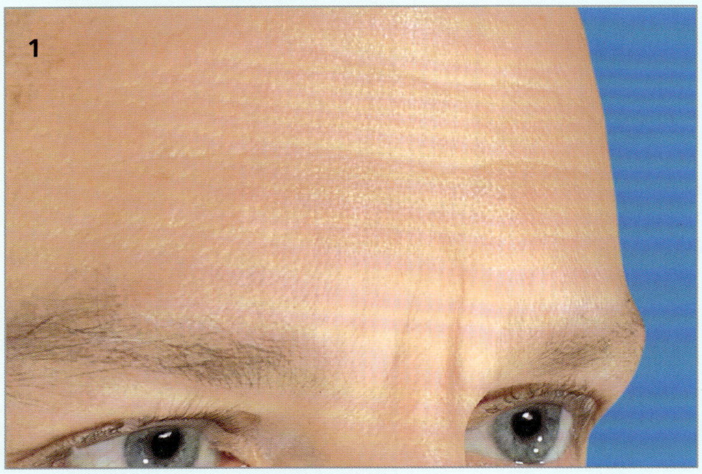

Fig. 4.13
1 Prior to the treatment.

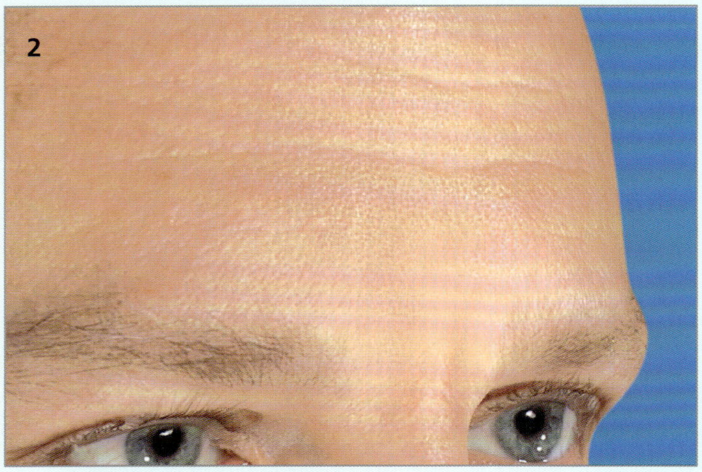

2 Simulated augmentation of the glabellar lines.

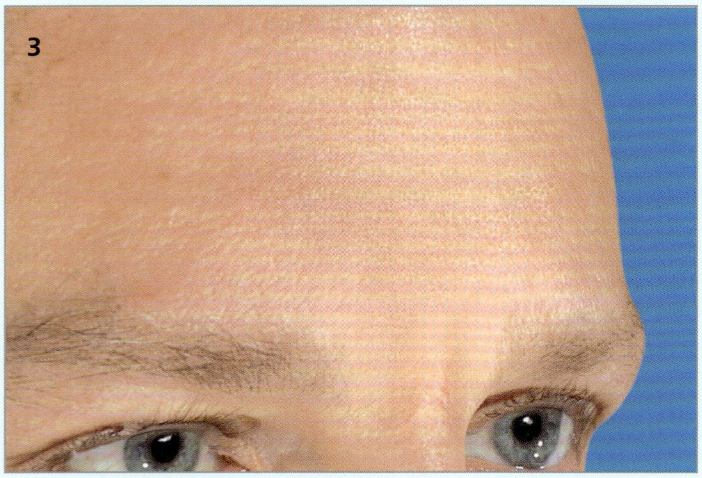

3 Simulated treatment of the forehead with botulinum toxin type-A.

4

5 Consultation

5 Consultation

5.1 Basics

An aesthetic consultation differentiates itself from a classic medical consultation in the sense that most patients present seeking to enhance or change a feature in their appearance, rather than seeking a diagnosis or treatment for a physical health problem. Furthermore, most patients present with very high expectations of the results. It is therefore essential not only to understand the subjective patient's impressions of their aesthetic needs and problems, but also to simultaneously evaluate the situation objectively. The consultation process should cover the following points:

- Understand the patient's desires in explicit, accurate terms
- Understand the timeline for improvement being sought
- Examination of the area that treatment is being sought for (assessing the extent of the ageing processes involved and/or rejuvenation being sought)
- Record the baseline findings in a clear and concise manner, alongside medical photography (see section 4.2)
- Perform a psychological examination
- Discuss the treatment options available, while educating the patient on their pros and cons, as well as discussing the financial implications

The practitioner's main aim is therefore to assess the patient's request and gauge how feasible and easy it is to satisfy their needs in a safe, natural and cost-effective manner. This requires a thorough consultation followed by an appropriate examination, coupled with a detailed and educational discussion with the patient. Documentation is a key element in recording the above findings and discussion points, and serves as an essential reference guide with the baseline findings for any future treatments.

Checklist: discussions and information provision

1. Given that many of the procedures offered within the aesthetic arena are not necessary for medical purposes, are elective and mostly off-label, it is essential that each patient receives adequate information both in written and verbal format to allow them to understand their treatment options, risks and benefits, and long-term strategy options alongside the associated financial implications.
2. The initial consultation cannot be rushed and plenty of time should be set aside to allow the patient to ask questions and hold a thorough discussion. Importantly, adequate information should be provided with regard to the possibility of complications and adverse events to ensure patients receive informed consent.
3. The discussion regarding treatment costs needs to be had during the initial consultation and as part of informed consent. Patients should have access to all treatment costs to allow them to make their final decisions.
4. Clear and thorough written documentation of the initial consultation proceedings, price discussions, examination findings, consent and the treatment process should be completed and filed for future purposes. Furthermore, any additional photographic documentation should be made with the patient's consent, and should the practitioner wish to use any of the images for future teaching or marketing purposes this should be clearly discussed, agreed and signed by the patient in the photographic consent paperwork.
5. **Most importantly,** as practitioners we need to respect that patients may need adequate time to decide on whether to go ahead with the proposed treatment, and hence allow the patient to take the relevant information away with them to consider further, prior to committing to a treatment.

5.2 Clarifying Expectations

Gauging the patient's expectations of the consultation itself, as well as any future treatments, is one of the most important aspects during the first consultation. Importantly, this is a crucial point for the practitioner to assess how realistic and feasible the requests are, and to advise the patient about these.

Often, one is faced with two typical scenarios: firstly, the patient being very precise and specific about a particular feature they point out; and secondly, the patient being generally dissatisfied with their overall appearance and not being specific enough. The former is certainly easier to manage, whereas the latter may be an outright indication that the patient may not ever be satisfied with the treatment given there may be other factors affecting how they perceive themselves, which in turn may need to be addressed first and foremost.

The use of a mirror is essential during this part of the consultation, alongside asking the patient to point directly to the feature, or features, they wish to discuss further. At times, however, the practitioner may be drawn to a feature or an area that the patient does not seem to mention, and yet one that the practitioner feels requires addressing. For instance, a patient may enquire about the management of mild perioral lines and seem oblivious to the large, hairy mole on the upper lip, which may be far more unsightly and noticeable. This requires careful management, and perhaps can be pre-empted by the practitioner offering the patient an objective assessment of their face if they should wish. If the response is positive or neutral, it is then more likely that the patient will not take offence at the observations noted, in the hope that they will be open to guidance and advice from an objective perspective. After all, patients only see themselves in a two-dimensional perspective, whereas those around them see them in a three-dimensional perspective. Overall, it is our duty to offer an objective global assessment of the patient as part of a thorough consultation, and it is equally assumed that patients should seek an honest and objective assessment to aid them in their decision-making.

Certain features that imply dissatisfaction, anger and tiredness are worth noting to the patient, namely the glabellar furrows, downturned corners of the mouth, hollow eyes, etc. After all, these features if left untreated will continue to project a certain emotion regardless, even if other areas have been well rejuvenated. Often, these features lie within the central facial triangle (demarcated by the

5

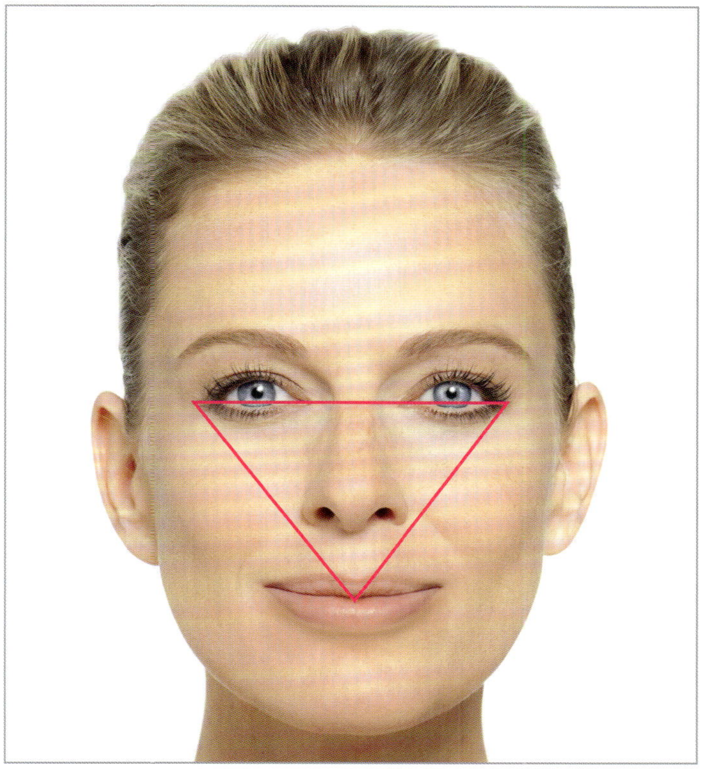

Fig. 5.1 The central facial triangle according to Yarbus (1967).

eyes and the mouth) and given they are the areas most commonly viewed by the observer, they need to perhaps be addressed at an early stage (Fig. 5.1). However, of course, this needs to be balanced with the patient's views and demands.

Interestingly, treatment expectations and requests are different when comparing male and female patients. Male patients usually seek a more focused, detailed, structured and shorter consultation. Female patients usually wish to explore their options further and are happy to discuss for longer. However, it is important to assess each patient as an individual, and gauge cautiously what their requirements are.

Overall, the consultation should offer a platform for the practitioner to build a rapport with the patient, manage their expectations and to educate them on the importance of achieving a natural, well-balanced and harmonious treatment outcome. It is also essential to point out treatments that may simply not be appropriate for a particular age group, e.g. a female in her 70s requesting full lips amidst a face that is heavily photodamaged, presenting with marked tissue laxity and loss of subcutaneous tissues. Respecting the human form and ensuring that our treatments do not result in unsightly discrepancies is an essential element of our work.

Checklist to clarify the patient's wishes

- What exactly does the patient wish to change?
- What is the motivation behind the desire for the treatment?
- What are the expectations of the treatments?
- Can the potential risks be accepted?
- How high is the patient's level of self-esteem and confidence?
- What are the patient's levels of anxiety?
- What is the patient's attitude to the practitioner and the clinic staff?
- How compliant will the patient be with the post-treatment advice?

5.3 History Taking and Examination

An accurate history taking and examination allows the practitioner and patient to understand what treatment options are feasible and reduce the occurrence of complications.

Ultimately this process needs to further elucidate the patient's level of expectations and highlight any concerns. Should the practitioner then feel the patient's expectations are somewhat unrealistic, this would be the time that a thorough discussion should be had to see if the patient could accept a more realistic treatment outcome, or whether the practitioner should discourage or even refuse to perform the treatment completely.

Following the history taking and examination, the patient should be offered time to think about the proposed treatment strategy before having the treatment.

5.3.1 History taking

During the history taking, the practitioner needs to clarify not only the patient's medical and medication history, but also discuss their aesthetic treatment history and aesthetic concerns. The later discussion should elucidate both surgical and non-surgical procedures, when they took place, what products/agents/devices were involved, the perceived clinical outcomes and whether any adverse reactions or complications were noted. It is particularly significant to understand the specifics of the surgical interventions carried out, in order to recognise any areas where the anatomy may be altered, as this will in turn bear implications on further treatments alongside the potentially heightened risks involved.

If patients cannot remember or simply do not know what procedures/treatments they had, it is advisable to ask them to liaise with their previous practitioners to gather the relevant information. Certainly, any complications after previous treatments performed elsewhere should be noted by the practitioner or by the patient. It is advisable not to rush into further treatments but to consider the risks involved and how to best remedy the situation, even though the patient may insist on this not being a problem for them. The balance of risk versus benefit should always underpin the evaluation of the consultation and the examination process.

The psychological assessment will take part during the history taking as well as the examination, and forms an essential part of the consultation. Should any concerns arise, it is important to discuss them further to understand if patients are able to consent and, furthermore, if the treatment should be carried out at all.

Below is an overview list of some key questions worth clarifying:
- Past aesthetic treatments (both surgical and non-surgical, perceived outcomes, adverse reactions and complications).
- Pregnancy, breast feeding, or planning to become pregnant in the near future.
- Illnesses or diseases (active, in remission or past). In particular, it is important to screen for autoimmune conditions, which can potentiate rejection of foreign agents, e.g. fillers. Diabetes mellitus, vascular disorders, kidney disease, liver disease, autoimmune and malignant disorders can affect the treatment success, introduce risks of complications and affect the healing process. Vitamin and mineral deficiencies, e.g. vitamin C, vitamin A and zinc may also affect wound healing. Blood-borne infections are also worth noting, e.g. HIV, hepatitis B or C. Clotting disorders are also important to screen for due to the associated risks with injection treatments. Hormonal disorders can also affect the treatment plan and outcome. Psychiatric conditions (body dysmorphic syndrome, depression, psychosis, etc) need to be thoroughly understood to evaluate the suitability of the aesthetic procedure.
- Skin conditions (active, in remission or past). Pre-cancerous/cancerous lesions, acne lesions, rosacea, pigmentary conditions, e.g. hyper or hypopigmentation, hypertrophic and keloid scarring are particularly important to note.
- Medications (both regular and occasional). Non-steroidal anti-inflammatory agents, corticosteroids, anticoagulants, chemotherapy agents, immunosuppressants, colchicine, penicillamine, herbal remedies, etc are worth screening for due to the increased risk of delayed healing, increased bruising and possible rejection reactions.
- Allergies or anaphylactic reactions. Particular focus on reactions to anaesthetic agents, sedative agents, filler agents and their additive constituents, animal proteins, disinfectants, antibiotics, etc should be discussed. Caution should be taken however: a negative history does not rule out future allergic reactions.
- History of herpes simplex (cold sores).
- Smoking status. This may affect the rate of healing.
- Use of sunbeds and sun exposure (past and present).
- Dietary habits.
- Levels of stress and work-life balance.
- Hormonal balance.
- Alcohol consumption.

5.3.2 Examination – visual assessment

The examination process involves both a visual assessment alongside a manual examination/palpation. The initial visual assessment entails observing the patient while they behave naturally, taking note of the skin quality, volume of the soft tissues, bony proportions, and symmetry alongside how the tissues move with facial expressions. Examination should ideally be conducted not just from the front but also from a three-quarter view and the full lateral.

It is important to also assess the adjacent body parts, as well as the most visible body areas, e.g. décolleté, neck and hands, to ensure a harmonious global body rejuvenation approach.

The visual assessment entails analysis of:
- Fitzpatrick skin type (see Tab. 5.1)

Fitzpatrick skin classification

Skin type	Geographical areas of frequent occurrence	Sunburn potential	Tanning potential	Potentially suitable peels
I	Ireland	High	Never	Superficial to deep
II	Northern Europe	High	Rarely	Superficial to deep
III a	Southern Europe	Moderate to slight	Frequently	Superficial to deep
III b	East Asia	Given to slight	Frequently	Superficial to deep
IV	South America	Slight	Always	Superficial to medium[1]
V	Asia	None	Always	Superficial to medium[1]
VI	Africa	None	Always	Superficial to medium[1]

Tab. 5.1 Assessment of skin pigmentation and sensitivity to sunlight according to Fitzpatrick (Fitzpatrick, 1988).

1 Deep chemical peels can be performed on Fitzpatrick skin types IV to VI, but they have a greater risk of significant pigmentary changes. The authors therefore recommend such cases to be treated only by very experienced practitioners.

Glogau type	Age in years	Characteristics
I	28–35	• Small wrinkles appearing when face is in motion
II	35–50	• Wrinkles appearing when face is in motion • First signs of dyspigmentation • Incipient elastosis
III	50–60	• Persistent wrinkles in areas of facial mobility • Frequent pigmentation abnormalities • Elastosis dependent on posture • Teleangiectasias
IV	> 60	• Persistent wrinkles in mobile and non-mobile facial areas • Yellowish-grey skin colour • Solar lentigines • Teleangiectasias • Regions of actinic keratosis with and without transition into invasive growths are possible • Pronounced elastosis

Tab. 5.2 Classification of actinic damage/photoageing; adapted from Glogau (1996).

- The adapted version of Glogau classification of photoageing (see Tab. 5.2)
- Wrinkle types (see below)
- Activity of the sweat glands as a marker of the skin's overall activity
- Skin condition and surface findings (i.e. naevi, pigmentation abnormalities and teleangiectasies, and skin efflorescences)

This is used to evaluate the levels of photoageing/actinic damage (Glogau, 1996). Whereas the qualitative changes are clear, the age classification needs to be adjusted according to the genetic and geographical context of the patient (Tab. 5.2).

Skin condition and surface findings

Skin colour can change with certain underlying disorders and therefore should be analysed before treatment:

- Reddening can be a sign of high blood pressure, focal inflammation, alcohol misuse or localised/generalised skin disorder (e.g. rosacea).
- Bluish skin discolouration, due to a decreased haemoglobin or oxygen level in the blood, may be seen in lung disorders such as bronchial asthma.
- Yellowish discolouration may be caused by liver disease or due to the use of certain food supplements, such as carotenoids.
- Brown-yellow pigmented spots may occur in increased numbers during pregnancy and with liver disease.

The condition of the skin is affected by a variety of external factors (i.e. type of skincare used, extent of photodamage, stress levels, hormone balance, etc):

- In many cases, dry skin is the result of overintensive skincare use alongside photodamage. However, it can also be a sign of a disease including hypothyroidism, in which the skin of the face in particular appears thickened and rough.
- Autonomic reactions, such as may occur with anxiety or nervousness, can lead to increased skin moisture.
- Acne commonly develops on greasy skin, particularly during times of hormonal change (e.g. puberty, treatment with hormonal agents).
- Efflorescences may be an indication of inflammatory skin disorders, potentially representing a contraindication to injection treatment in the affected area (see below).
- A predisposition to acne or scarring should be taken into account when determining which treatment is proposed, to ensure that it has a positive effect on these conditions.

Skin efflorescences

Efflorescences may by a sign of inflammatory skin disorders, potentially representing a contraindication to treatments involving injections in the affected area. The individual types of efflorescence are explained in the images below.

5

Efflorescences

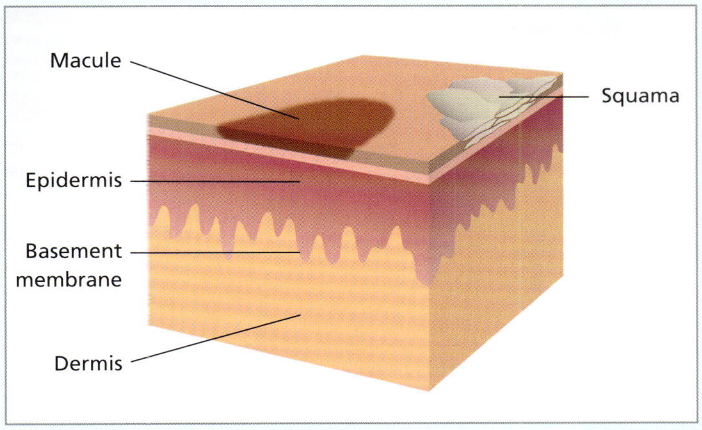

Fig. 5.2
Macule: A macule is a circumscribed area of skin discolouration, which is smaller than 5 mm in diameter and is not accompanied by elevation, hardening or scaling. If the change is larger than 5 mm, it is sometimes referred to as a patch.

Squama: A scale is referred to as a squama. It consists of flat corneal cells, which have become detached from the stratum corneum (horny layer).

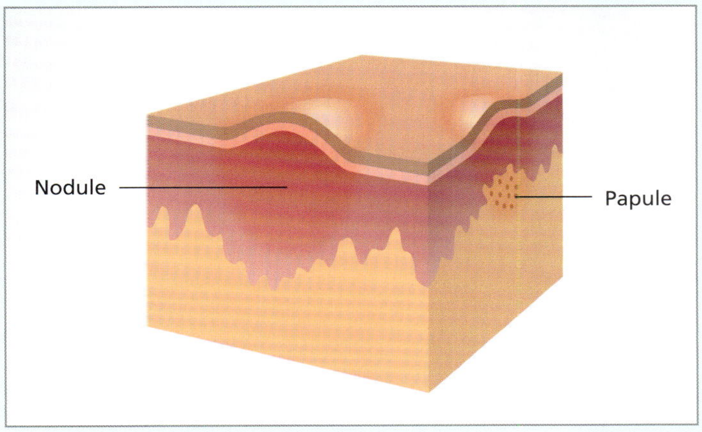

Fig. 5.3
Papule: A papule is a circumscribed skin elevation that is smaller than 5 mm. If it is larger than 5 mm, it is referred to as a nodule.

Efflorescences

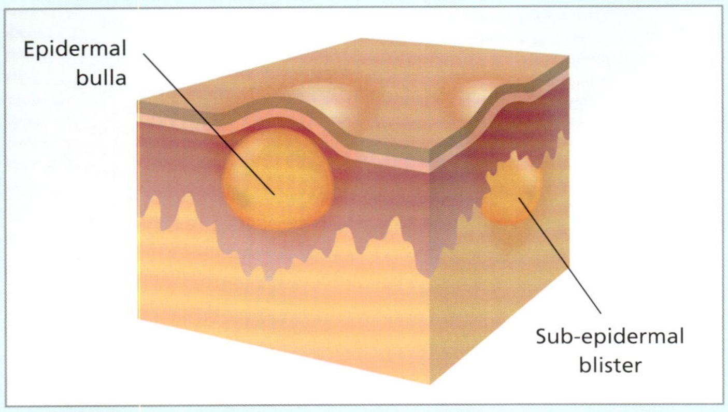

Fig. 5.4
Bulla (blister): A hollow space filled with fluid is referred to as a bulla. If the efflorescence is smaller than 5 mm, it is more likely to be referred to as a vesicle or a small blister.

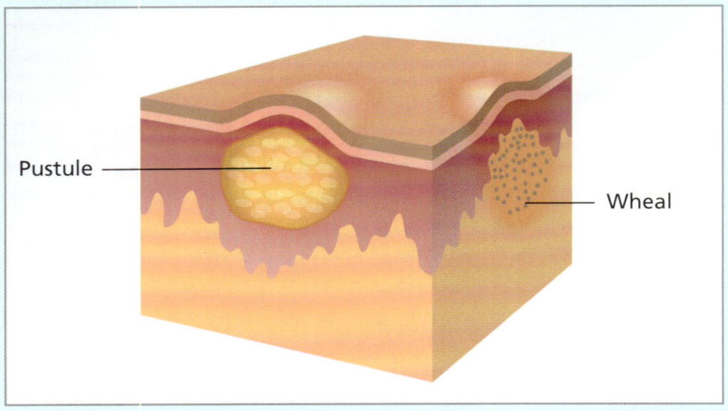

Fig. 5.5
Pustule: A pustule is a hollow space filled with pus.

Wheal (urtica): A wheal is a transient, raised, itchy, usually pink swelling, formed as a result of oedema in the dermis.

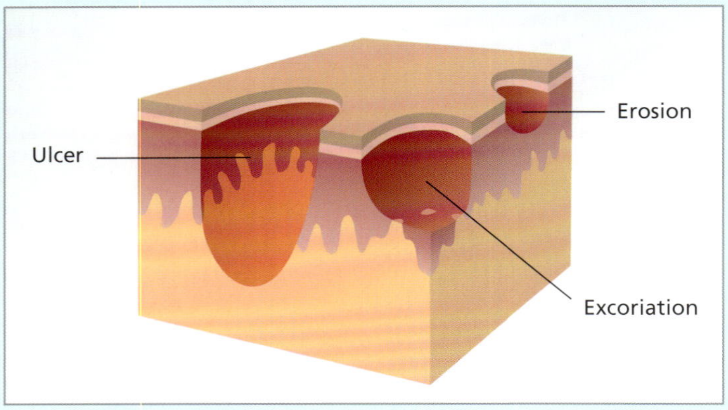

Fig. 5.6
Erosion: An erosion is defined as the loss of the epithelium (for example due to abrasion) down to the basal membrane. It heals without leaving a scar.

Excoriation: A change in the surface of the skin caused by scratching is called an excoriation. The tissue defect extends down to the stratum papillare.

Ulcer: An ulcer is a tissue defect that extends into the dermis or subcutis. It always heals with scarring.

5.3.3 Examination – manual assessment

Manual examination involves the targeted palpation and assessment both at rest and upon movement, e.g. while smiling, pouting, raising the brows, etc. Palpation of the skin comprises the assessment of:

- Elasticity/laxity (using the 'snap test', whereby a fold of skin is grasped between the thumb and index finger, held for a few seconds and then released. The speed at which the skin snaps back to its original state relates to the level of laxity and elasticity. Hence, a quick 'snap test' is associated with elastic and more youthful skin) (Fig. 5.2).
- Hydration (turgor provides an indication of the fluid-dependent tensile state of the tissue. To assess it, a 'snap test' is performed whereby a fold of skin is grasped between the thumb and index finger, held for a few seconds and then released. If the fluid content is reduced, the skin fold remains in place or disappears slowly).
- Surface texture and levels of oiliness and dryness.
- Surface relief (i.e. volume assessment and wrinkle depth).
- Wrinkle assessment (using the stretch test, where the wrinkle is stretched to assess its severity and presence of a residual crease. See section 5.3.4 for further details).
- Bony prominences (i.e. the upper and lateral orbital margin, the cheekbone, the lower jaw and the tip of the chin provide an anatomical guide for the planned injections) (Fig. 5.3).

Observation criteria for the frontal view

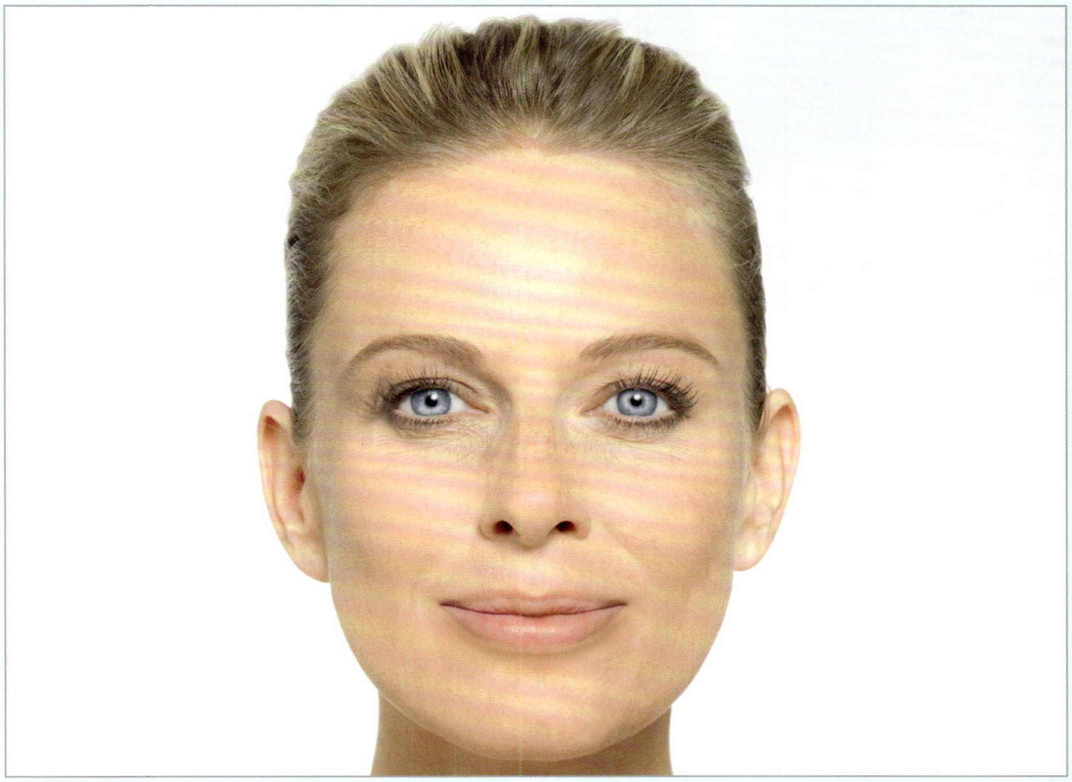

Fig. 5.7 Observation criteria for the frontal view

- Symmetry of the face
- Projection and facial harmony of the upper, mid and lower thirds of the face
- Skin pigmentation, texture, quality, laxity, presence of disease and injury
- Naevi, keratotic lesions and teleangiectasies
- Wrinkles and volume at rest
- Assessing the wrinkles and volume in dynamic activity, e.g. talking, laughing, frowning, etc
- Assessing individual key features and regions, e.g. temples, forehead, glabella, periocular region, cheeks, nasolabial folds, nose, lips, marionettes, chin and jawline, neck, décolleté, ears

Observation criteria for the lateral view

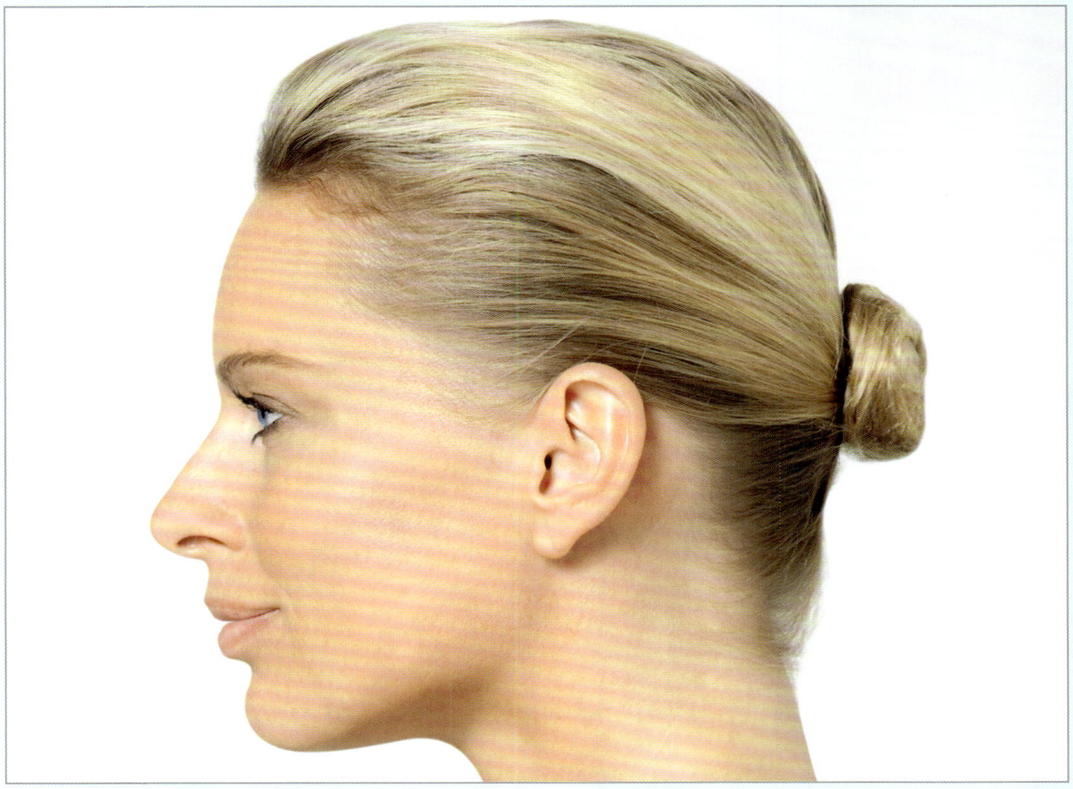

Fig. 5.8 Observation criteria for the lateral view

- Symmetry of the face
- Projection and facial harmony of the upper, mid and lower thirds of the face
- Skin pigmentation, texture, quality, laxity, presence of disease and injury
- Naevi, keratotic lesions and teleangiectasies
- Wrinkles and volume at rest
- Assessing the wrinkles and volume in dynamic activity, e.g. talking, laughing, frowning, etc
- Assessing individual key features and regions, e.g. temples, forehead, glabella, periocular region, cheeks, nasolabial folds, nose, lips, marionettes, chin and jawline, neck, décolleté, ears

Snap test

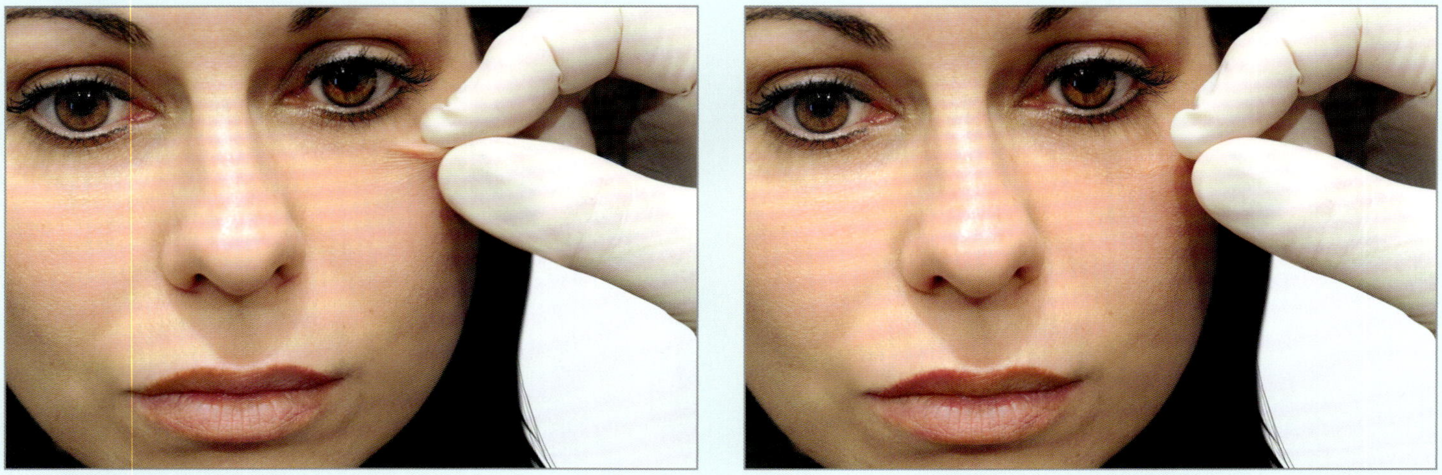

Fig. 5.9 Skin is grasped between the thumb and the index finger and tented upwards, held for a few seconds and then released. Youthful and well-hydrated skin should snap back right away into its normal position, indicating good levels of skin elasticity, hydration and turgor.

Bone prominences

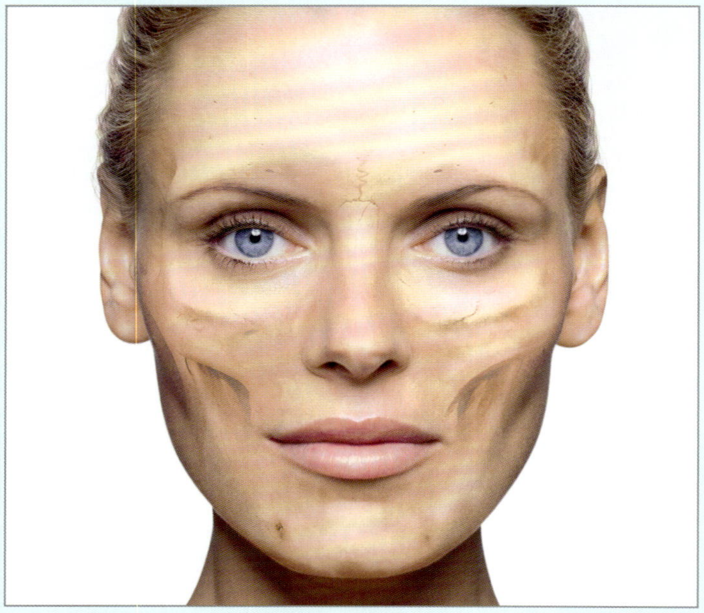

Fig. 5.10 Overview of the palpable bony prominences.

5.3.4 Evaluation of lines and wrinkles

When assessing lines and wrinkles, the first thing to observe is the surface relief. Palpation provides further clues on skin elasticity, thickness, texture and turgor. The evaluation of skin thickness is particularly important for augmentation procedures, as it determines factors such as the injection technique and depth required, alongside determining how to ensure the palpability and visibility of the injected substances in as natural a way as possible.

Fine wrinkles and puckering of the skin

Fine wrinkles and puckering of the skin due to its thinning need to be distinguished from the coarser lines left behind by subcutaneous tissue atrophy. The skin surface may also be altered by other disruption in its microrelief, such as scarring, nodules, milia, etc.

Lines and wrinkles due to sun damage

Sun damage causing the degeneration of the elastic fibres leads to slack lines and folds and, in extreme cases, to sagging of the superficial structures.

Facial expression lines

Lines caused predominantly by muscular activity are characterised by the fact that the skin still has few or no lines in zones where there is less expressive activity.

Lines caused by subcutaneous tissue atrophy

Shrinkage of the subcutaneous tissue, which acts as a foundation for the dermis, leads to stretching of the skin and resulting in the formation of lines and wrinkles.

Line caused by gravity

Lines and wrinkles caused by gravity markedly alter the macrorelief, i.e. the overall facial contours.

Sleep lines

Lines and wrinkles caused by sleeping habits are generally apparent on the face by virtue of their asymmetry, as almost every person has a preferred sleeping side. Retracting elements such as scars or ligaments, from which the sleep lines originate need to be identified by gently squeezing the areas of the skin where the sleep lines are located, in turn to target the injections directly to remedy the sleep lines. Palpation often provides further information about the skin's elasticity, thickness and turgor.

Table 5.3 summarises and highlights the available treatment options, based on the wrinkle type being corrected.

5.4 Objectification and Evaluation

Documenting the baseline findings is a crucial step during the consultation process. The notes in turn act as a reference for future consultations and treatments. Furthermore, documentation is an essential element for quality assurance and legal protection purposes.

Objective validated rating scales are a useful tool in the consultation process as well as in future assessment of treatment outcomes, as they allow assessment of the clinical picture alongside patient collaboration. A number of scales are available within the aesthetic arena, e.g. 'wrinkle severity rating scales' (WSRS), and the 'aesthetic scales' (see p. 259). These scales also allow both the baseline findings and the treatment outcome to be compared, evaluated and objectified.

Wrinkle type found	Augmentation with fillers	Alternative treatments
Fine lines, superficial wrinkles/ puckering and rough skin	Augmentation with non-cross-linked hyaluronic acid fillers	Superficial treatment with: • Topicals (e.g. retinoids, sunscreens) • Microdermabrasion • Chemical peeling • Laser resurfacing • Percutaneous collagen induction (dermal needling)
Facial expression lines caused by muscular activity	If deeply furrowed lines cannot be sufficiently smoothed with botulinum toxin type-A, the residual lines may be corrected with filler augmentation	Botulinum toxin type-A (first choice treatment)
Lines associated with solar elastosis are caused by degeneration of the elastic and collagenous fibres	• Biorevitalisation with non-cross-linked hyaluronic acid fillers • Augmentation with cross-linked hyaluronic acid fillers, initially as a combined treatment, to correct any residual lines left behind after other treatments	Procedures that stimulate collagen formation: • Non-ablative lasers • Flash lamp therapy • Radiofrequency • Percutaneous collagen induction (dermal needling) Depending on the quality of the uppermost skin layers: • Ablative laser treatments • Chemical peeling Other options: • Thread lifting procedures • Surgical lifting procedures
Sleep-induced lines and wrinkles, which are often fairly deep but localised	Suitable for augmentation with moderately and highly cross-linked hyaluronic acid fillers	If the lines are regional, extensive treatment with chemical peeling and mechanical dermabrasion are less suitable, unless the patient is happy to undergo a full-face treatment
Lines caused by subcutaneous tissue atrophy	Augmentation mainly in the subcutaneous tissues and in the submuscular region using cross-linked hyaluronic acid fillers	• Laser resurfacing or chemical peeling (gives greater smoothness to the more superficial skin layers) • Augmentation with autologous fat (also stimulates collagen formation) • Thread lifting • Surgical facelifting
Gravity-induced lines and wrinkles, caused by subcutaneous tissue atrophy and loss of SMAS* tone	Not a primary indication for augmentation with fillers	• Botulinum toxin type-A lifts heavy, sagging eyebrows (non-surgical brow lift) • Thread lifting • Surgical facelifting

Tab. 5.3 Type of wrinkling and the indicated treatment options. * SMAS (superficial musculo-aponeurotic system)

5

The former WSRS is used for wrinkle assessment, whereas the latter 'aesthetic scales' (see Tab. 5.4) have been introduced for volumetric assessment, and comprise validated ratings for the following areas:

- Forehead lines – at rest and dynamic
- Glabella lines – at rest and dynamic
- Brow positioning
- Lateral canthal lines – at rest and dynamic
- Infraorbital hollowness
- Upper cheek fullness
- Lower cheek fullness
- Marionette lines
- Nasolabial lines
- Lip fullness
- Lip wrinkles – at rest and dynamic
- Oral commissures
- Jawline
- Neck volume
- Ageing of the back of the hands

Aesthetic scale	
0	No wrinkles and volume changes
1	Mild wrinkles and volume changes
2	Moderate wrinkles and volume changes
3	Severe wrinkles and volume changes
4	Very severe wrinkles and volume changes

Tab. 5.3 Classification according to the 'aesthetic scales' (see pp. 259–267 also).

5.5 Treatment Planning

Once the patient's expectations have been evaluated, medical and aesthetic history taken, and the examination carried out, the next step is to create a treatment plan with the patient. The following points are worth considering:

- Does the patient wish for an immediate optimal result with one treatment, or one that involves a series of treatments to achieve a gradual improvement each time?
- Does the patient seek long-lasting or short-term results?
- How much downtime is the patient prepared to accept?
- How much potential risk is the patient able to accept?
- How does the patient feel about pre-treatment testing (if required)?
- What are the patient's financial considerations?

Importantly, if the above points are not thoroughly discussed at an early juncture, this may result in future misunderstandings and affect patient satisfaction with the treatment outcome.

Ultimately, the final choice of treatment depends on two parameters:

1. On the patient's wishes (provided there are no contraindications noted and the patient has understood the options available and the risk versus benefit of each possible treatment modality)
2. On the baseline findings and practitioner's proposed treatment choice.

Once an agreement has been reached between the practitioner and the patient, the patient can go ahead with written consent and be booked for a treatment.

5.6 Informed Consent

Informed consent (both verbal and written) is an essential component in every consultation and covers a variety of considerations, which should be addressed thoroughly with the patient, namely:

- Treatment options, including the pros and cons of each, whether they are off-label and the associated implications
- Why the selected treatment is the most appropriate option (the risks and benefits associated)
- Realistic expectations post-treatment
- Associated downtime and compliance
- Expected duration of the clinical outcome
- Long-term strategy
- Financial implications

The patient's psychological state alongside levels of compliancy should be carefully assessed during the consent process, as this can be detrimental to the treatment outcome and ultimate patient well-being and satisfaction. In particular, attention should be paid to:

1. Previous or existing history of psychiatric disorders, e.g. depression, body dysmorphic syndrome, psychosis, etc
2. Patients with unrealistic expectations
3. Patients requesting treatment for minimally visible and objectively quantifiable features
4. Patients who have seen many practitioners (known as 'clinic hoppers' or 'shoppers') and say they have not been fully satisfied by anyone previously
5. Patients who seek treatment to remedy a 'relationship' or 'solve all personal problems'
6. Patients seeking instant improvement and not apply to accept post-treatment associated downtime
7. Patients rushing with the treatment and not engaging with the full consultation, examination and informed consent process

Should the practitioner sense that the patient is not appropriate for a given treatment based on the initial consultation and consenting process, it is important to hold off any further treatment at this stage, while explaining and educating the patient as to why this is the case. This process can be unpleasant, particularly if the patient is adamant on having a treatment, but is necessary to avoid future problems.

5.7 Documentation

Written documentation is crucial and should detail the initial findings alongside any future consultations and interventions. Chapter 9, 'Aids for the Practitioner', contains a useful documentation form. It can be used to document the patient's details, baseline findings, treatment sites, filler products used (including batch number), the dosage per injection site/region, as well as other relevant information.

Photographic documentation is essential in all aesthetic procedures (see section 4.2 'Photographic Documentation').

6 Treatment

6 Treatment

The key aspects of a successful augmentation treatment are explored in this chapter. Importantly, key focus is placed on a detailed presentation of the variety of injection techniques used alongside their modifications by the authors. Furthermore, a thorough discussion will centre upon managing patients' comfort levels during the treatment itself, setting up the treatment area, and most importantly appreciating and respecting relevant anatomical considerations as factors constituting the basic platform for a successful augmentation treatment.

6.1 Pre-treatment Considerations

The following should precede the actual treatment:

- A detailed discussion including an evaluation of the patient's specific wishes and requests (see section 5.6)
- The signing of an informed consent form (see section 5.6)
- A thorough examination with photographic documentation of the baseline findings (see section 4.2)
- Drawing up a treatment plan as agreed with the patient (see section 5.5) alongside financial considerations

The treatment planning phase is guided by the wishes and needs of the patient. These are established jointly during the preliminary consultation (see section 5.2). In this context, the practitioner may need to explain sympathetically and put into perspective any unrealistic expectations or results that cannot be achieved fully. To avoid any misunderstandings, the practitioner should ask the patient to specifically point out with the help of a hand held mirror the areas that they would like to have treated and the issues associated with that perceived problem. The practitioner should also at this stage give their advice and suggestions, and then begin to explain the planned injection sites.

On the treatment day, the patient should be advised to either arrive without having applied any makeup, or remove it just before the treatment. An analgesic topical preparation is commonly applied before the augmentation treatment if the patient is particularly sensitive, especially if the planned injections are not invasive (see section 6.5). Otherwise, local blocks can be utilised with more invasive injections. The area to be treated is then thoroughly disinfected before any injections. Alcohol-free antiseptic solutions are preferred by this book's author G. Sattler, given there is less associated skin irritation, especially for sensitive skin types.

6.2 Treatment Setting

The treatment setting and the general atmosphere should be clinical, professional and comfortable. A bright, well-ventilated treatment room with a reclining treatment couch and appropriate space for moving around it is ideal.

The treatment itself should not be performed under any time pressure. Even with all the optimum preparatory consultations, the patient may still ask further questions, express concerns or put forward additional treatment requests immediately prior to the treatment. The practitioner should react to these enquiries openly, patiently and without haste. An optimum treatment result can only be expected with full patient compliance. In this respect, it is advisable to describe the planned treatment in detail one more time with the aid of the hand held mirror. The actual treatment follows only after all the outstanding questions have been answered and all uncertainties laid to rest.

Emotional and psychological care are also important factors to consider. Tactile stimuli (e.g. a stress ball), quiet background music and positive body language, alongside explaining the treatment process as it develops, can also prove helpful and reassuring to the patient.

6.3 Patient Positioning and Lighting

Correct patient positioning is essential not only for optimal treatment outcome but also for patient and practitioner comfort. A fully reclining and heigh-adjustable automated or manual treatment couch is ideal. During the treatment itself, the couch should be adjusted as per requirement. In some cases, it is ideal to have the patient fully reclined, whereas in others, an almost upright position is required to ensure the practitioner can visualise the true tissue positioning (Figs 6.1 and 6.2). This also enables the practitioner to assess the effects of the filler treatment, given that a supine position can displace the facial tissues and give a false impression of the treatment baseline and outcome. The height of the couch should be adjusted before the treatment to ensure the practitioner feels comfortable and to avoid straining the back.

A nearby good light source is also essential, alongside a well lit room. When considering which direction to place the light source from, it is generally accepted that the skin relief lines and wrinkles show up better if the face is lit more from above and the side.

6.4 Ergonomics

As discussed above, positioning the patient should also be in consideration to the ergonomics of the practitioner. An ergonomic posture, especially without back strain, allows the treatment to be conducted in a relaxed manner and ultimately allowing for optimal treatment outcomes (Fig. 6.3). Working with the upper body upright is one of the basic principles of an ergonomic posture; twisting movements between the pelvis and the pectoral (shoulder) girdle must also be avoided (Fig. 6.4). Any postural changes should involve the whole body.

The area to be treated should be at the appropriate height to ensure the practitioner does not need to bend over, hence automated couches prove very useful for the ease of adjustment.

6.5 Accessories

During the treatment, certain aids can be utilised to assist the patient and practitioner in the planning and conducting phase of the treatment.

6.5.1 Hand held mirror

During the treatment, the patient can find it reassuring to occasionally assess, with the guidance of the practitioner, the treatment results, to feel they are also in control of the process and when necessary to discuss and guide the practitioner during the process. Obvi-

Treatment positions

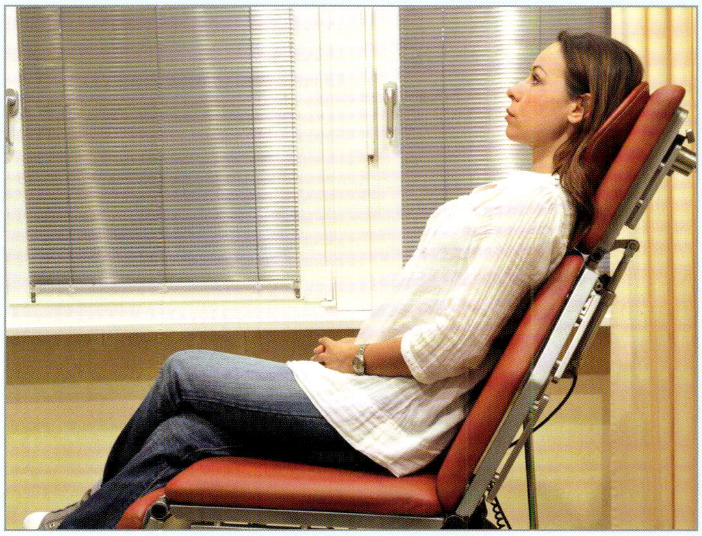

Fig. 6.1 Upright position Since the proportions of the face change with the patient's position, treatment planning takes place with the patient positioned upright.

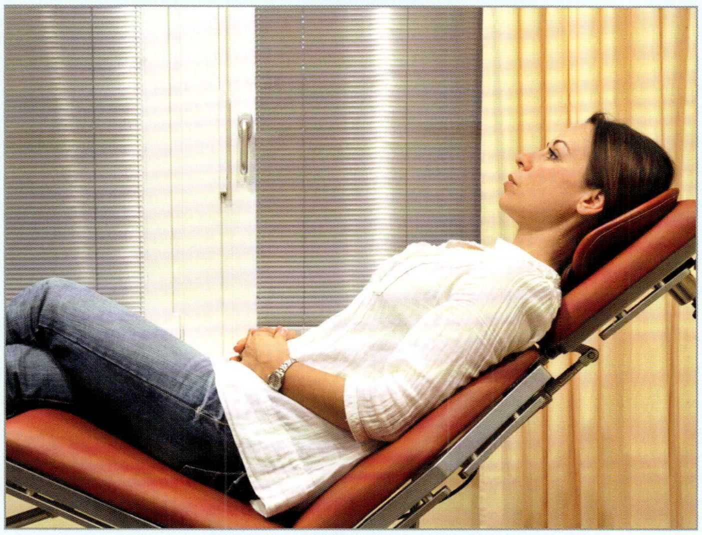

Fig. 6.2 Semi-supine position The semi-supine position makes it easier for the patient to relax and allows the practitioner to work more ergonomically, as all the areas of the face are easily accessible.

The practitioner's posture during the treatment

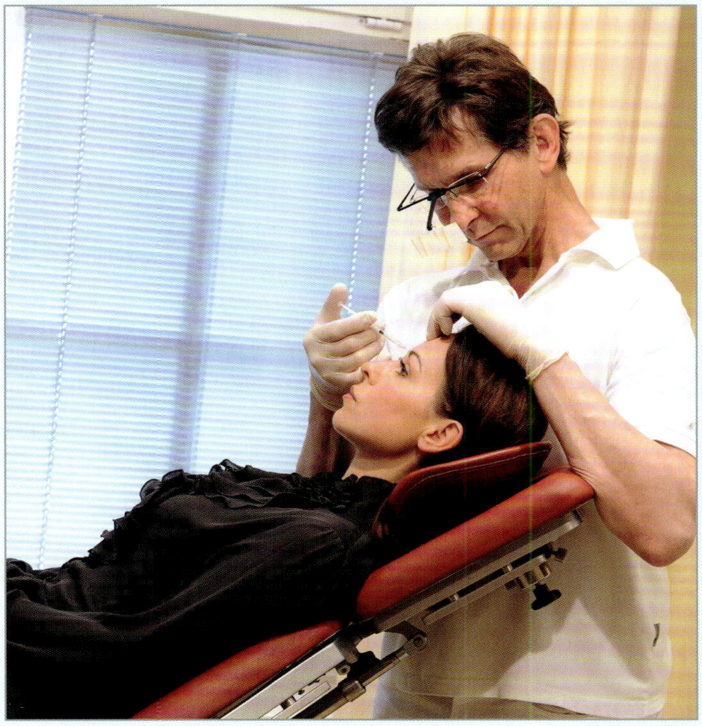

Fig. 6.3 Optimal posture In this posture, the practitioner's pelvis and shoulders are not twisted relative to each another, the back is straight and upright and the injection arm can be supported by the treatment couch if necessary.

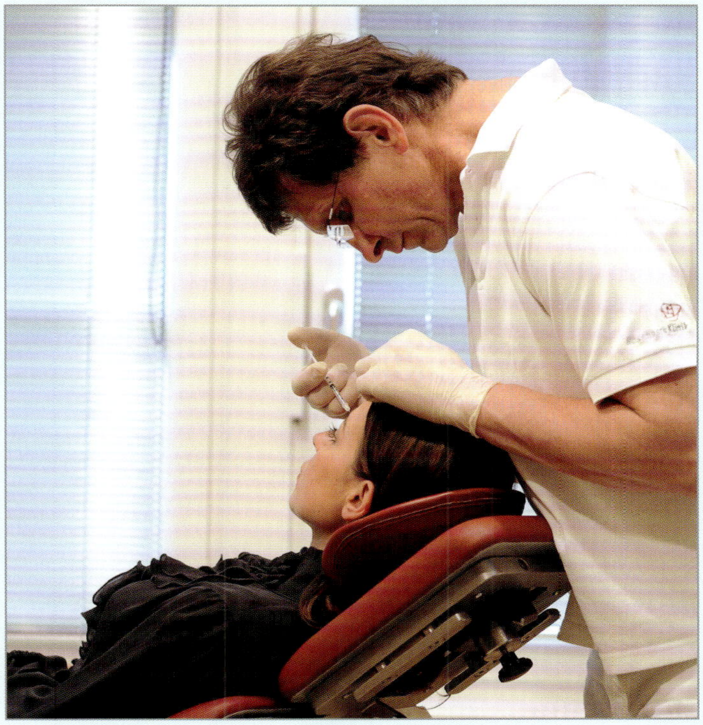

Fig. 6.4 Incorrect posture Here, the level at which the treatment is being performed is much too low: the practitioner needs to bend over, resulting in increased strain on the cervical spine. This position does not allow the treatment to be carried out in an effective, relaxed and safe manner.

ously, this needs to be managed well with the patient to ensure it does not become an interruption but rather an aid to the treatment outcome at several points during the treatment. In turn, this allows for an optimal treatment outcome alongside patient satisfaction.

6.5.2 Skin markers

Skin markers (similar to eyeliner pencils) are a useful but not obligatory pre-treatment tool to demonstrate and identify the key areas for injection. Patients often find this reassuring. However, given that infection control measures need to be upheld, it is recommended to remove the markings immediately pre-treatment.

6.5.3 Cold packs

Cold packs or ice packs can be utilised pre and post-treatment to manage some of the discomfort and pain associated with the treatment.

6.5.4 Topical anaesthetics

A number of anaesthetic options are available for aesthetic treatments (see section 6.8 for more details). Topical anaesthetic preparations are one of the most commonly used methods pre-treatment to allow for better pain management (Fig. 6.5), although many patients are satisfied with the anaesthetic containing fillers alone. Should a topical anaesthetic be offered, it is essential to screen the patient for any allergies or contraindications, and use the recommended volumes of the creams to avoid complications. These preparations should only be applied in the clinic and removed thoroughly prior to disinfecting the skin for treatment. It is important to note the speed of activation and the duration of effect of the chosen preparation.

6.5.5 Loupe glasses

Loupe glasses can be used by the practitioner, particularly when doing close-up injections (Fig. 6.6). The glasses have a wide visual field and give a sharp, undistorted image even at the margins. Furthermore, small blood vessels can be identified and avoided, particularly those around the eyes.

6.6 Needles and Cannulas

The chosen needle or cannula most suitable for augmentation with a given injectable filler product or injection technique may vary depending on the area being treated (see Tab. 6.1). To minimise the associated discomfort with injectable fillers, it is generally accepted that the smallest diameter (highest possible gauge) needles or cannula are used. However, lumen diameter is a variable that must be selected also according to the particle size and/or viscosity of the filler material. Very thin lumens can clog if used to inject a large-gel-particle hyaluronic acid (HA) product. In addition, higher injection pressure is needed to push 'stiff' fillers through a thin lumen. Furthermore, one should also use caution with regard to the risk of associated alteration of the filler material due to the mechanical stress associated with high pressure. For example, high-pressure injections can result in the liquefaction of autologous fat, and hence this needs to be taken into account. Most filler manufacturers advocate a particular gauge needle or cannula for a specific filler, which can be a good guide.

It is generally accepted that both needles and cannulas are essential tools in filler augmentation, and each have their advantages and disadvantages based on the specific area being treated, as well as for the specific injection depths and techniques used. Generally speaking, needles are commonly used for focal/point injections, whereas cannulas allow for a horizontal distribution of filler agents over larger surface areas.

Fine 30 to 32 gauge needles are ideal for conventional focal intradermal and subdermal augmentation. Thin needles can be used to inject low-viscosity HA products (see 1 Fillers for superficial injections, p. 62) under the skin surface with the accuracy needed to achieve

Treatment accessories

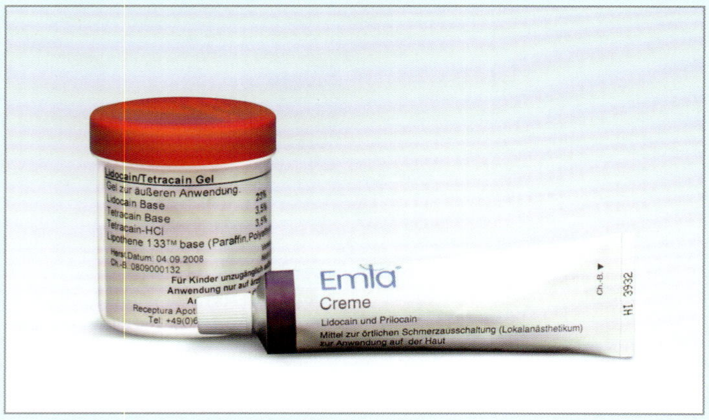

Fig. 6.5 Topical local anaesthetics Lidocaine or tetracaine-containing topical anaesthetics can be used for immediately pre-treatment in the clinic.

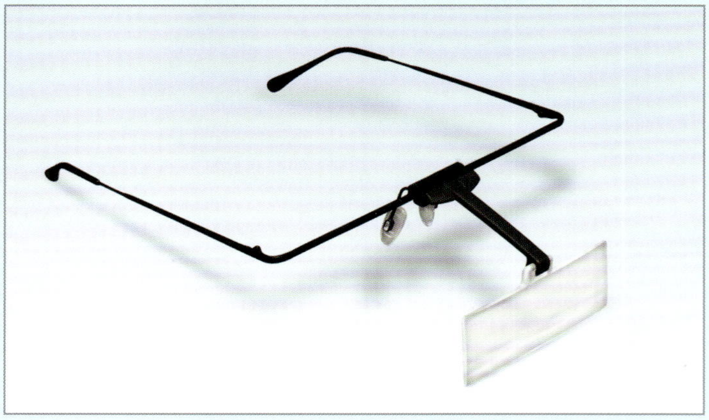

Fig. 6.6 Loupe glasses Loupe glasses like the ones shown here magnify the working area approximately four-fold and can be a useful aid to the practitioner when administering injections.

Needle specifications	Recommended uses			
Diameter (gauge)	**Depth of injection**	**Injection techniques**	**Filler products** (see section 3.2 for further descriptions)	**Clinical indications/ objectives**
30–32 G	Superficial to medium (intradermal and subdermal)	• Tunneling (linear) technique • Point technique • Vibrating technique • Sandwich technique • Fanning technique • Criss-cross technique • Deep mesotherapy	• 1, 2, A, B • Hyaluronic acid (HA) products with a small particle size, low degree of cross-linking and little tissue resistance (easily injectable)	• Superficial focal corrections • Surface irregularities • Correction of contours • Concealment of atrophy-related deficits
27 G	Medium to ultra-deep (subcutaneous, supraperiosteal, supramucosal)	• Vibrating technique • Sandwich technique • Fanning technique • Criss-cross technique • Vertical supraperiosteal depot technique (VSDT) • Tower technique (TT)	• 3, 4, B • HA products with a larger particle size, higher degree of cross-linking, greater tissue resistance (moderate ease of injection)	• Medium-depth augmentation, saturation, and concealment ('camouflage') of volume loss • Facial contouring
21–23 G	Ultra-deep (supraperiosteal)	Vertical supraperiosteal depot technique (VSDT)	• 4 • Very stiff HA products (difficult to inject) for longer-lasting volume augmentation	• Volume augmentation of deep structures • Facial contouring

Cannula specifications	Recommended uses			
Diameter (gauge)	**Depth of injection**	**Injection techniques**	**Filler products** (see section 3.2 for further descriptions)	**Clinical indications/ objectives**
27 G microcannula	Superficial to medium (intradermal, subdermal)	Superficial horizontal augmentation with cannula (SHAC)	• 1, 2, A, B • HA products with a small particle size and low degree of cross-linking (easily injectable)	• Skin surface regeneration • Mesotherapy
22–25 G	Deep (subcutaneous, supramucosal)	• Deep horizontal mobilising augmentation (DHMA) • Windmill technique	• 3, 4, B • HA products with a larger particle size and higher degree of cross-linking (moderate ease of injection)	• Widespread volume projection • Tissue mobilisation and homogenisation • Activation of fibrogenesis and tissue repair
18 G FAMI cannula	Deep (subcutaneous, supramucosal)	Autologous fat grafting	Autologous fat	• Volume augmentation via autologous fat grafting • Activation of fibrogenesis and tissue repair

Tab. 6.1 Overview of needles and cannulas recommended for vertical and horizontal injections.

6

Needles and cannulas

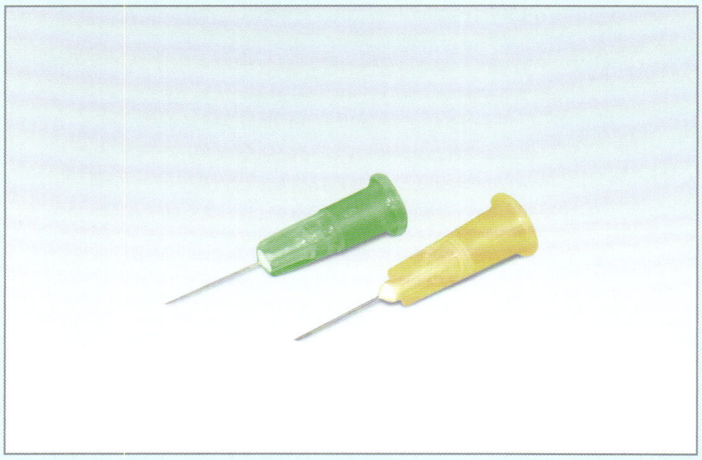

Fig. 6.7 Fine, sharp needles (30 and 32 gauge in this case) can be used for focal injections of filler into superficial tissue levels or for vertical injection onto bone or the mucosa. The lumen diameter is selected according to the viscosity of the filler material used (cf. Tab. 6.1).

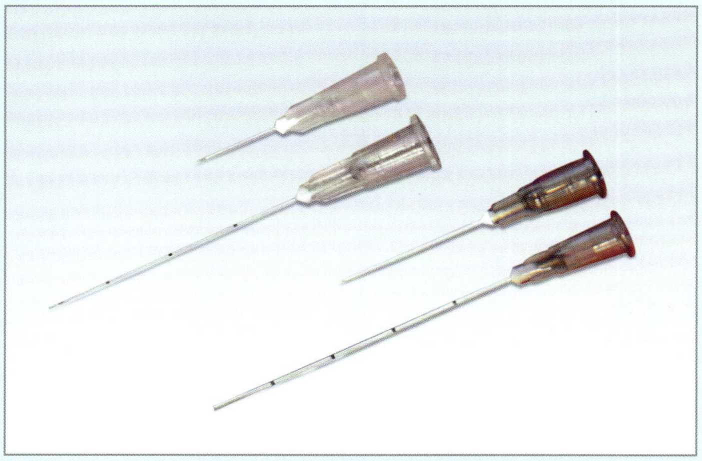

Fig. 6.8 Cannulas are used for horizontal injection with gentle tissue mobilisation. A 27 gauge microcannula (left) is recommended for superficial injections just below the skin. For deeper injections (e.g. for supramucosal treatment of nasolabial folds or marionette lines), it is best to use a 22 gauge needle (right) with a larger lumen diameter to reduce the risk of injury.

the fine focal corrections (Fig. 6.7). Vertical, volume-projecting augmentation with high-viscosity HA should be performed using needles with a larger lumen diameter (24 to 27 gauge) in order to prevent stress on the filler material and needle clogging.

If wide horizontal augmentation is to be performed, a cannula can be used to achieve tissue mobilisation with a reduced risk of injury (e.g. trauma to major blood vessels) and levels of discomfort (given the less injections required). The cannula is inserted into the respective tissue layer via an insertion point, which is made using a larger bore needle inserted into the desired depth to allow for easy penetration of the cannula. The selected lumen diameter of the cannula varies depending on the injectable filler product used and its specific properties. Thin 25 to 28 gauge microcannulas are used for injections just below the skin surface. Subcutaneous injections or supramucosal tissue mobilisation are also generally performed using 22 to 25 gauge cannulas (Fig. 6.8). Cannulas with larger lumen diameters have two main advantages in mid to deep injections: they facilitate the injection of medium-viscosity fillers (see 3 Fillers for deep injections, p. 66) and thus reduce risk of trauma to adjacent structures.

> **Vertical injections:** The smaller the lumen diameter of the needle, the less associated tissue trauma and discomfort.
> **Horizontal injections:** The greater the lumen diameter of the cannula (i.e smaller gauge size), the less tissue trauma and associated discomfort (smaller lumen diameter cannulas (larger gauge size) are sharper and thus carry a greater risk of trauma and injury).

Autologous fat grafting is routinely performed using a facial autograft muscle injection (FAMI) cannula.

6.7 Assisted Injection Systems

Although manual injections continue to be the most commonly performed, electronic injection systems are now being developed and marketed as an aid for administering hyaluronic acid-based fillers. These systems are favoured by some practitioners given they take care of most of the mechanical aspects of an injection, so that the practitioner no longer has to concentrate on the plunger pressure and the graduations on the syringe (Figs 6.9 to 6.11). The volume (ml/min) is controlled via the system's flow mode. In drop mode, defined amounts are administered per point. Flow mode is used for filling lines and drop mode for superficial revitalisation.

Assisted injection systems offer the following advantages (among others) to the practitioner:

- Reduced injector muscle fatigue during injections, as the operator's hand does not need to exert pressure on the plunger.
- Improved control of the injection speed and the injected volume allows the practitioner to concentrate fully on the injection depth and technique.
- Defined and continuous delivery of the filler material produces a homogeneous filling effect due to improved integration of the gel into the dermis.

Assisted injection systems also entail the following disadvantages, which should be considered:

- The practitioner cannot aspirate
- The practitioner cannot use cannulas effectively

Assisted injection systems

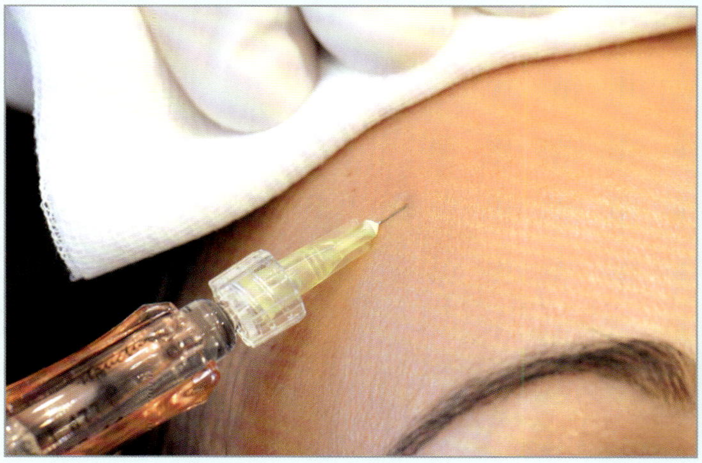

Fig. 6.9 An automated injection system used and recommended by some practitioners removes the need to maintain manual pressure on the plunger, as well as the need to continuously monitor the volumes injected. This enables the practitioner to concentrate fully on the injection depth and injection technique.

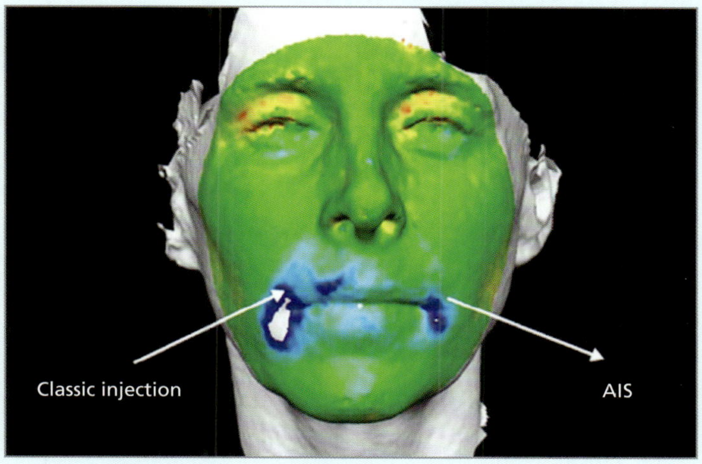

Fig. 6.10 This 3D photo analysis shows a more uniform injection result and less tissue irritation on the AIS-treated side.

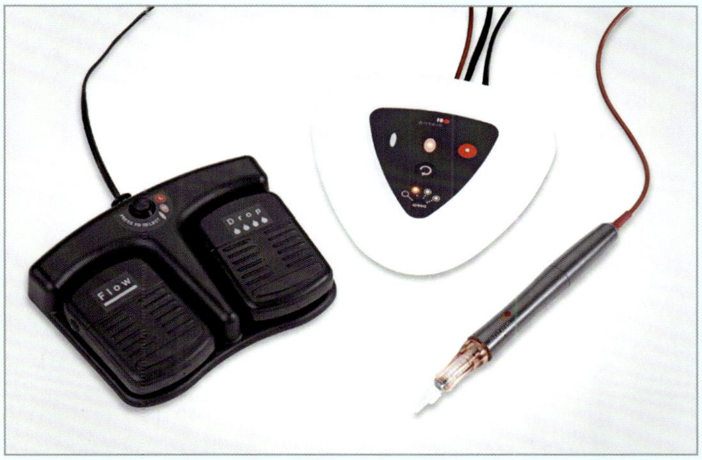

Fig. 6.11 The injection system consists of a foot pedal used to trigger the injection, a central unit and the hand piece.

6.8 Anaesthetic Methods

The onset of discomfort or pain during an augmentation treatment depends on a number of factors, namely:

- The patient's pain threshold, levels of stress, levels of tiredness, stage of a female hormonal cycle
- The practitioner's injection technique, steadiness and communication with the patient
- Region being treated (e.g. lips are highly sensitive)
- Level of invasiveness of the planned intervention

A number of anaesthetic methods exist, and the choice depends much on the practitioner's and patient's demands. They range from: doing nothing invasive but simply talking to the patient and reassuring them, i.e 'talkaesthesia'; application of focal cold stimuli; topical anaesthetic preparations; focal infiltration of local anaesthetics; regional nerve blocks; and finally more invasive oral central analgesics.

6.8.1 'Talkaesthesia'

Given that most injectable fillers contain in situ anaesthetic agents and some patients have a high pain threshold, in some cases it may be appropriate to negate topical or local anaesthetic methods. 'Talkaesthesia' is a term referring to the calming and reassuring effects achieved with simple education and communication to the patient in a clear and calm manner, before and during the treatment. Patients often find this works well, as they appreciate receiving instructions and explanations during the treatment, which allows them to manage their own levels of discomfort and anxiety.

6.8.2 Superficial anaesthesia with topical agents

Topical anaesthetic preparations may be applied before the treatment for particularly sensitive patients (Figs 6.12 and 6.13). A number of preparations are now available, mostly containing a combination of anaesthetic agents. One of the commonly used agents is a combination of lidocaine and prilocaine (EMLA®). For adequate analgesia, this anaesthetic should be applied at least 30 to 60 minutes before the procedure using the occlusion method. Another suitable and FDA-approved agent is Pliaglis®, a cream containing a mixture of lidocaine and tetracaine, which creates a self-adhesive layer that can be peeled away easily. Although these agents are considered generally safe and effective, care should be taken to ensure no contraindications for use are present, alongside maintaining dosage levels in the safe range with attention being paid to toxicity considerations.

6.8.3 Superficial anaesthesia with infiltration of local anaesthetics

Local infiltration of anaesthetics with small bore needles (30 to 32 gauge) can be used to either numb the needle insertion sites or to achieve a focal zone of anaesthesia where the filler will be placed. However, the superficial infiltration of the local anaesthetic may raise and smooth the tissue to be augmented, creating distortion and in turn lead to the effacement of lines. If this occurs, it may no longer be possible to locate and augment the lines or tissues accurately.

6.8.4 Nerve blocks

For particularly sensitive areas and for nervous patients, a nerve block may be offered (Figs 6.14 and 6.15). Local blockade of the mandibular and infraorbital nerves are the main options to be considered when treating the face. Almost complete anaesthesia can be achieved with minimal effort or time.

A special form of soft tissue anaesthesia can also be offered to the patient when treating lips, and is referred to as the annular 'mucosal' nerve block (Figs 6.16 and 6.17). It is performed at a distance of 2 cm around the mouth, and 1 cm from the inner lip margin in a line parallel to the lip line. The 'mucosal' block leads to abrupt anaesthesia of the lips (see Fig. 6.17). This technique does not distort the mouth. Its anaesthetic effect subsides after half an hour, when the patient is able to eat and speak naturally again.

6.8.5 Central analgesia

In some cases, especially where larger areas and larger volumes of fillers are to be injected, central analgesia can be employed using extremely short-acting agents such as remifentanil (Ultiva®); at a very low dose of between 25 and 50 µg, it may cause slight dizziness. Remifentanil is a selective µ-opioid agonist with a rapid onset of action and a very short duration of effect. The patient remains conscious in the presence of adequate analgesia. Furthermore, this can be combined with the administration of local anaesthetic depots at the access sites for the treatment. Subfascial autologous fat injec-

> **Caution**
>
> **Even short-acting opioids such as remifentanil, at the lowest doses, can lead to respiratory depression. Their use requires an emergency kit to be ready at all times, along with patient monitoring and an experienced administrator; these agents should only be administered by an anaesthetist.**

Occlusive methods

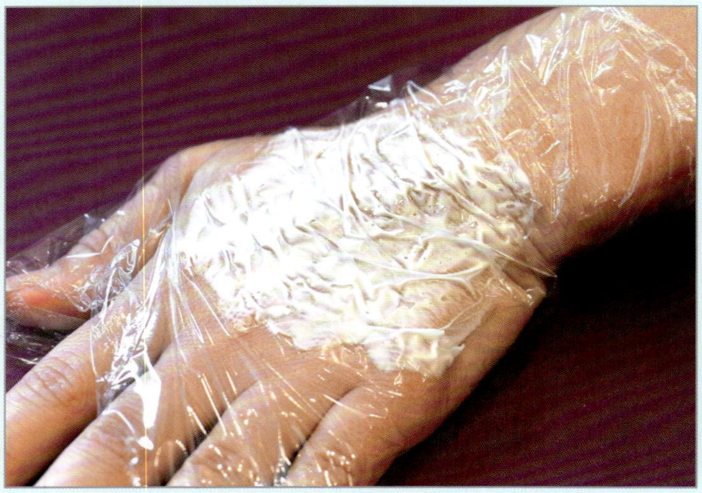

Fig. 6.12 The cream is spread out evenly across the treatment area and occluded with a film for the recommended time.

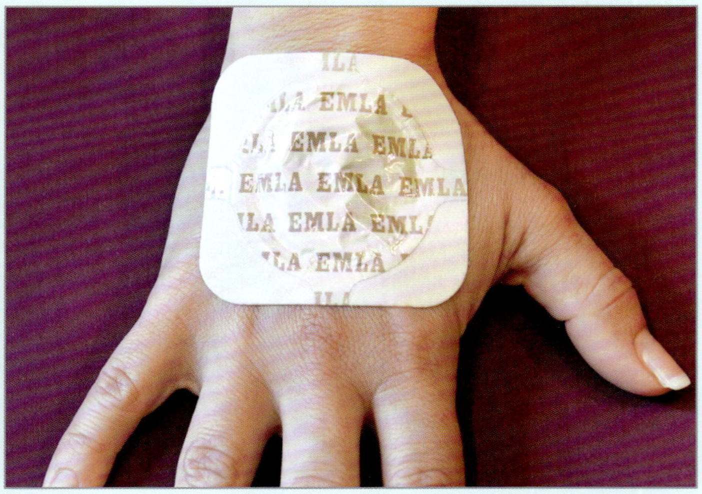

Fig. 6.13 Ready-to-use patches are also available, to be applied at least 30 minutes before the procedure.

tions can be administered in this manner, provided that the injection site is also anaesthetised. Following the administration of remifentanil, patients need to be observed for at least half an hour and driving restrictions apply as per recommendations.

6.8.6 Potential complications with anaesthesia

The administration of anaesthetic medicines should only be carried out by experienced practitioners who have the knowledge and experience in the aforementioned methods, particularly with regard to focal infiltration, local nerve blocks and central analgesia. Patients should be thoroughly consulted to ensure no contraindications are present and are furthermore advised of the associated risks.

Importantly, history of intolerance or allergy to the active substance or adjunctive preservatives should be discussed. For example, the preservative methyl 4-hydroxybenzoate is added to multiple-dose vials and sodium disulfite is found as a preservative in vials and am-

Infraorbital nerve block

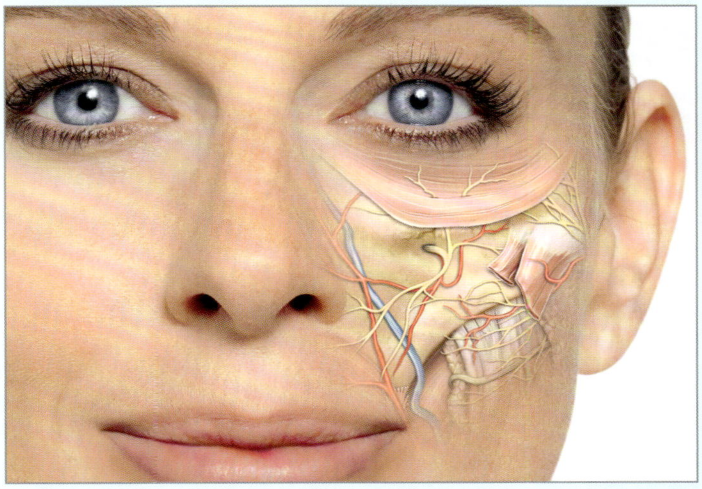

Fig. 6.14 The exit of the infraorbital nerve.

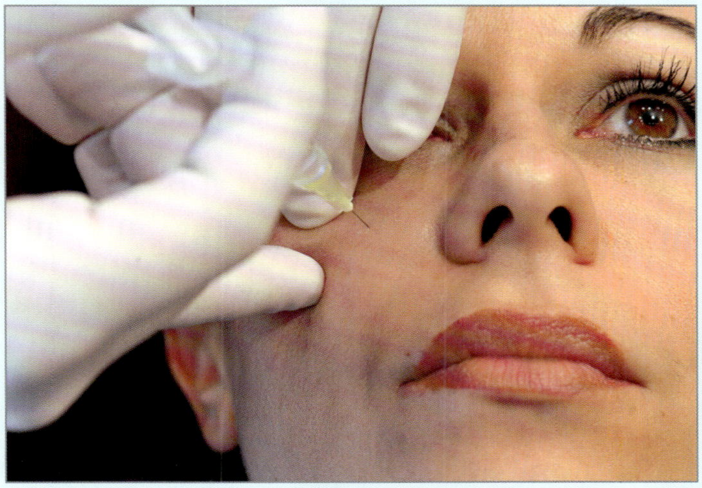

Fig. 6.15 Infraorbital nerve blocks can be achieved by infiltration of a local anaesthetic administered either intraorally or, as shown here, directly at the nerve exit.

'Mucosal' block

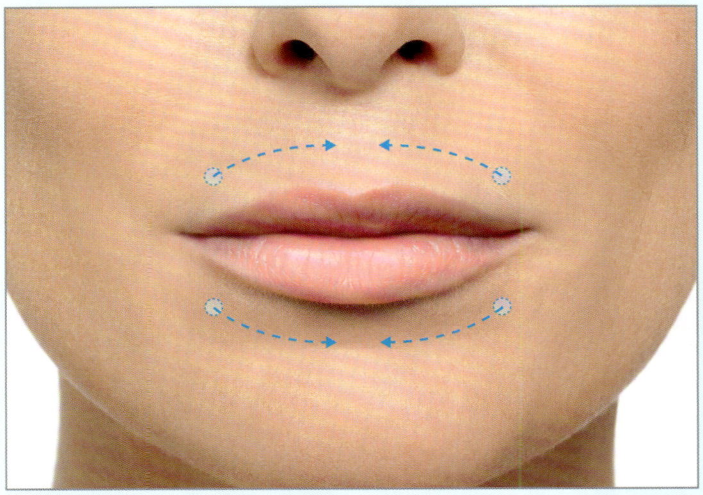

Fig. 6.16 Schematic representation of the injection points and direction of the injection for the 'mucosal' block.

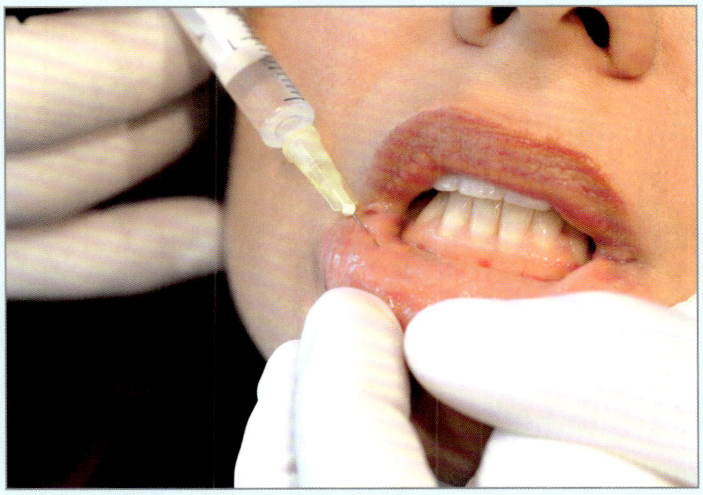

Fig. 6.17 The 'mucosal' block is performed intraorally. The practitioner grasps the lateral part of the lip with thumb and index finger, inserts the needle close to the angle of the mouth and advances the needle towards the middle of the lip. The anaesthetic is injected as the needle is being withdrawn.

poules containing added adrenaline. Acute warning signs of an allergic reaction include skin reddening, restlessness, anxiety and dyspnoea. The following may also occur: erythema; urticaria; fall in blood pressure; tachycardia; nausea; vomiting; abdominal pains; bronchospasm; respiratory arrest with hypoxia and circulatory arrest. The full clinical picture of this type of allergic reaction is known as anaphylactic shock.

Intoxication can occur if the local anaesthetic is accidentally administered into a blood vessel or at an excessive dose. Patients may report subjective signs of central intoxication, such as dizziness, a metallic taste in the mouth, tinnitus and sudden onset of anxiety. The objective warning signs of intoxication, including confusion, word repetition, restlessness and tremor can give the therapist an indication of the problem. Further administration of the anaesthetic must be stopped as soon as the first symptoms appear. Central nervous system excitation manifests as irregular breathing, muscle tics, nausea, vomiting, generalised seizures, as well as an increased pulse rate and blood pressure. Severe intoxication can lead to loss of consciousness, respiratory arrest, bradycardia, a fall in blood pressure and finally to cardiac arrest. The practitioner should have adequate knowledge and skills in managing such complications.

Furthermore, it is important to highlight to the patient that anaesthetic injections carry the risk of haematomas and focal oedema, which need to be expected and accepted by the patient in advance.

Nerve irritation caused by the needle itself is rapidly reversible, and is most common with conduction anaesthesia. If the desired numbing effect is insufficient or absent, this is usually due to a poor injection technique or perhaps due to anatomical variants in the course of a nerve.

6.9 Injection Techniques and Effects

A number of injecting techniques have been developed over the years, allowing a tailored approach to be used when delivering the filler to achieve a specific clinical outcome. This section explores the choice of injecting methods available for a practitioner.

6.9.1 Basic rules

When performing an injection, attention should be paid to the posture and positioning of the practitioner and the patient to ensure optimal safety and comfort. The basics of ergonomic working are explored in further detail in section 6.4. Furthermore, the syringe should be held in the dominant hand, and the non-dominant hand used for fixing and stretching the skin to aid the injection. A variety of holding positions are used and the authors particularly like the one whereby the filler syringe is held between the index and middle fingers, with the thumb resting on the plunger (Fig. 6.18). The anchor allowing stability of the injecting hand is achieved either by the little finger or the lateral side of the injecting hand firmly resting on the skin (Fig. 6.19).

6.9.2 Classic injection techniques

Tunneling Technique

Video: Tunneling Technique
http://www.kvm-tv.de/FIL/001.mp4

The tunneling technique is the currently practised technique derived from the basic techniques in augmentation therapy referred to as 'linear techniques' (Figs 6.20 to 6.23). This technique is suitable for the treatment of straight, narrow lines and wrinkles. The tunneling technique, in particular, aims at ensuring the filler does not spread

Hand position during injecting

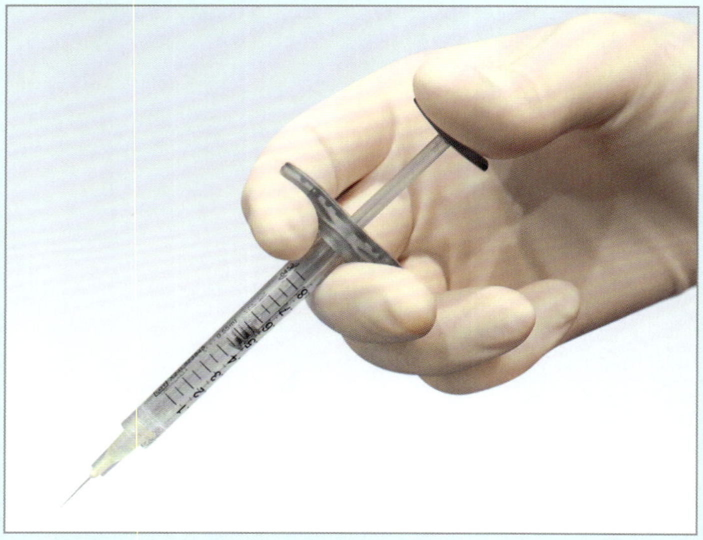

Fig. 6.18 Basic position The thumb rests loosely on the plunger. The injection hand is supported on its outer edge or by the little finger.

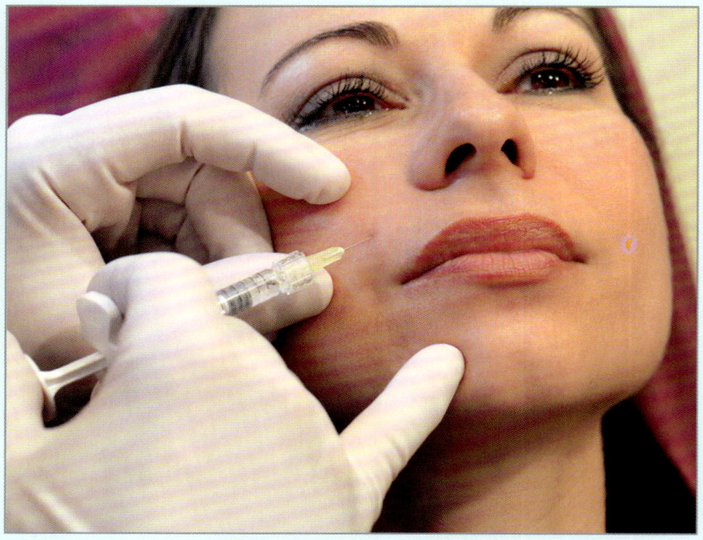

Fig. 6.19 When treating the face The injection hand is supported on its outer edge or with the little finger. This is the basic injecting position.

through the tissues, but rather remains exactly where it has been injected. This is particularly ideal when treating numerous small lines and wrinkles that lie close together. The tunneling technique is not restricted solely to injections into the middle dermis, but may be used for all skin layers.

Normally, the substance is injected as the needle or cannula is being withdrawn (also known as retrotracing or retrograde injections), but some also inject the filler when the needle or cannula is advanced forward (referred to as the 'push-forward' technique or anterograde injections). The retrograde technique is considered safer when using needles, as it alerts the injector should a vessel be transected upon

Caution

Too much pressure on the plunger can sometimes cause the needle or cannula to undo from the syringe itself. Overcorrection with more viscous, highly stabilised hyaluronic acid products should always be avoided in superficial line correction, as this can result in the unsightly Tyndall effect. This phenomenon results in bluish discolouration of the skin where the filler has been injected due to the light refraction.

Tunneling Technique

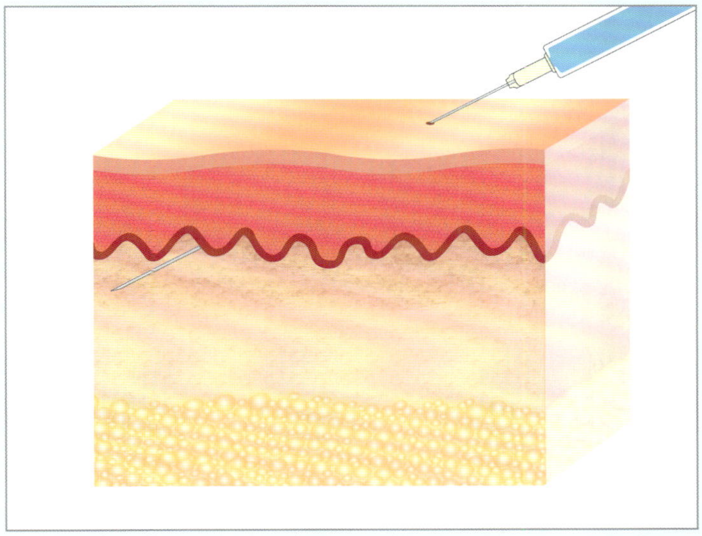

Fig. 6.20 Insert the needle at an acute angle or tangentially to the skin.

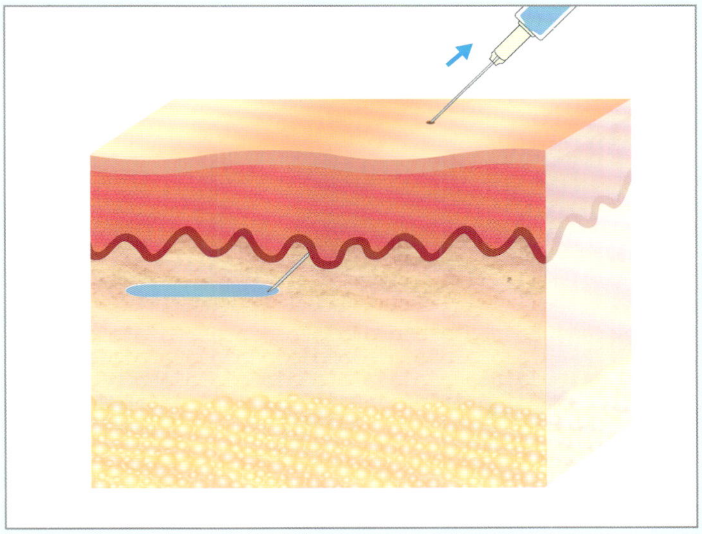

Fig. 6.21 Inject the substance while withdrawing the needle.

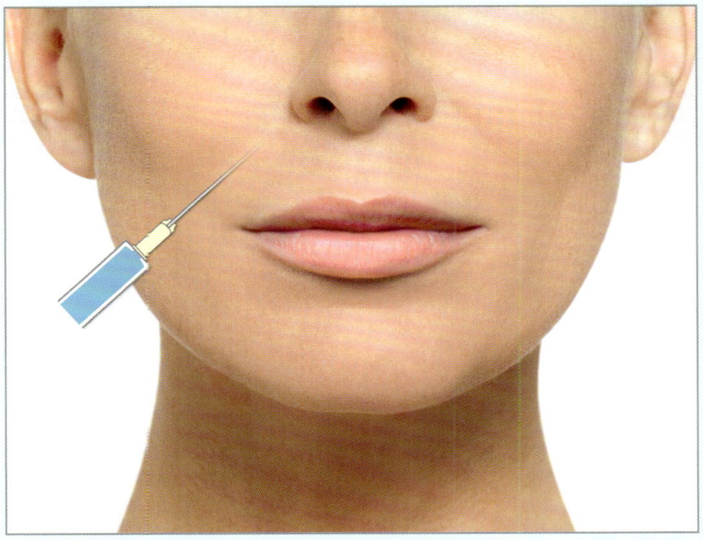

Fig. 6.22 The injection channel should follow the direction of the line or wrinkle.

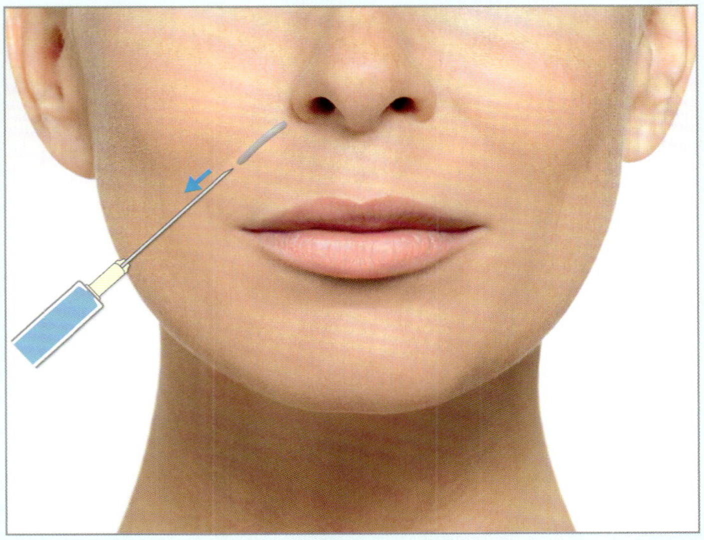

Fig. 6.23 The result should be full levelling or slight undercorrection of the defect.

positioning before the filler is delivered. Furthermore, retrograde injections allow a plane to be created in the desired level before the filler is delivered, which again ensures the correct plane of injection is achieved.

Tips and tricks: For deep lines caused by loss of subcutaneous tissue volume, further padding can be provided by injections into the deep dermis and more superficial subcutaneous planes (see p. 108, 'Sandwich Technique').

Point Technique

Synonyms: serial technique; droplet technique; micro-droplet technique; multi-puncture technique; multiple microinjections; microwheal injections; serial puncture technique. This technique involves deposition of small droplets of filler along a fine line or wrinkle in the upper dermis at a short distance from one another, e.g. 2 mm (Figs 6.24 to 6.27). Material wastage is minimal due to the short injection path.

This technique is also commonly used when performing mesotherapy to improve overall hydration and quality of the skin of a large surface area, as opposed to fine line and wrinkle correction.

Tips and tricks: A particularly good result can be achieved with small, superficial, fine lines if the needle is inserted with the bevel facing down. The point technique produces superficial augmentation, which is particularly suited for seborrhoeic skin.

Point Technique

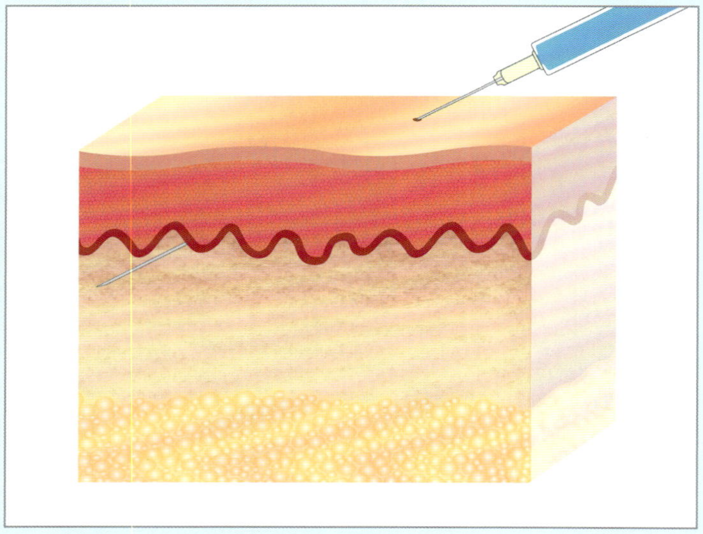

Fig. 6.24 Administer the filler into the upper dermis.

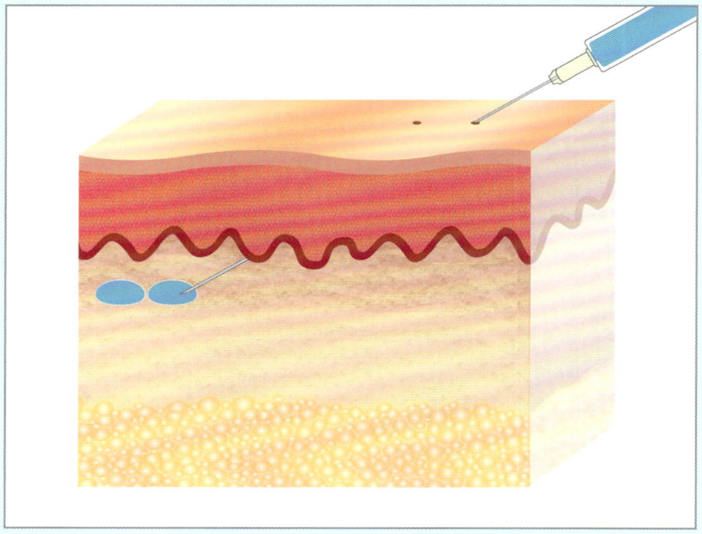

Fig. 6.25 Insert the needle at a 90-degree angle to the line or wrinkle being augmented.

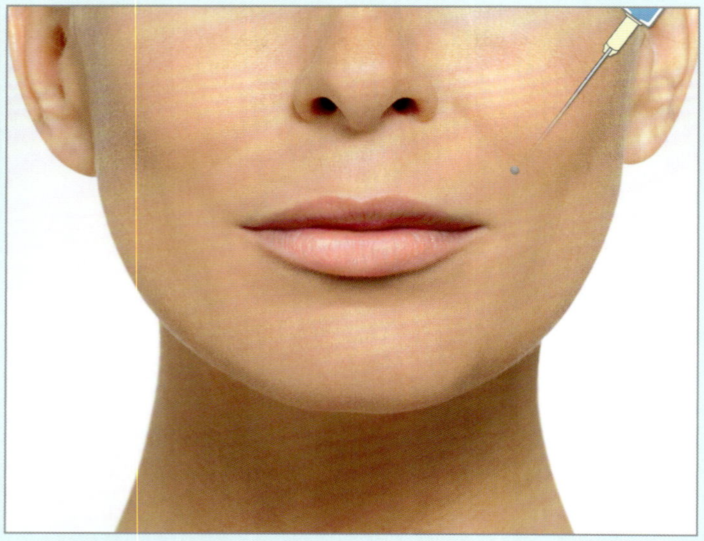

Fig. 6.26 The individual injection points should be close together, forming an almost continuous line.

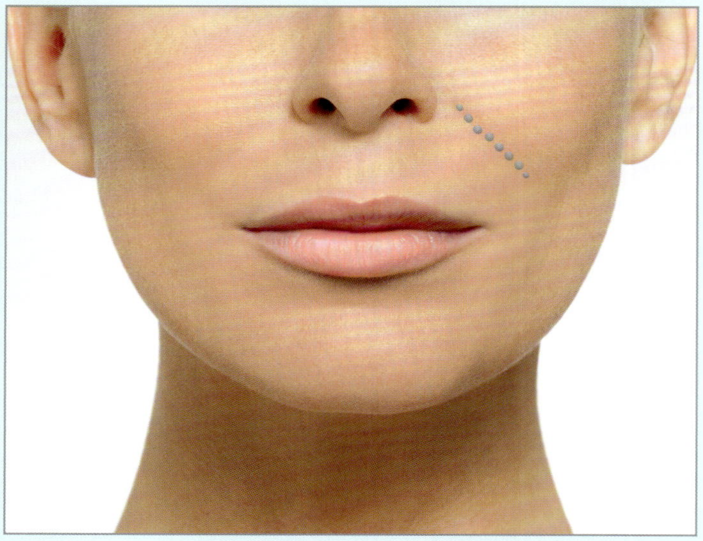

Fig. 6.27 The result allows for successful augmentation with reduced material consumption.

Caution

A bluish discolouration over the injected area known as Tyndall effect may be produced if excess material is injected or if the droplet is too close to the surface. This effect can occur with all superficial injections.

Stretching Technique

Video: Stretching Technique
http://www.kvm-tv.de/FIL/002.mp4

The stretching technique is a modified point technique, in which maximum stretching of the skin is used to alter the interstitial tissue pressure in preparation for the augmentation procedure (Figs 6.28 to 6.31). This influences substance distribution during the injection. The assisted stretching technique is suitable for fine lines on the upper lip or fine superficial lines on the forehead. It enables accurate augmentation to be achieved while reducing filler consumption.

Tips and tricks: The practitioner or their assistant stretches the patient's skin to a point where any excess filler is immediately visible below the skin. The interstitial tissue pressure determines the distribution of the filler in the tissues. This prevents bulges, particularly with horizontal lines on the forehead or radial lines around the

Stretching Technique

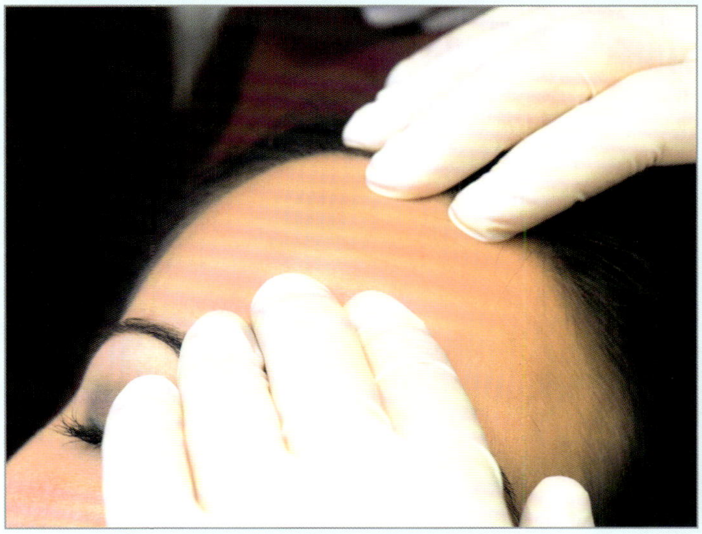

Fig. 6.28 An assistant stretches the skin transversely relative to the course of the line.

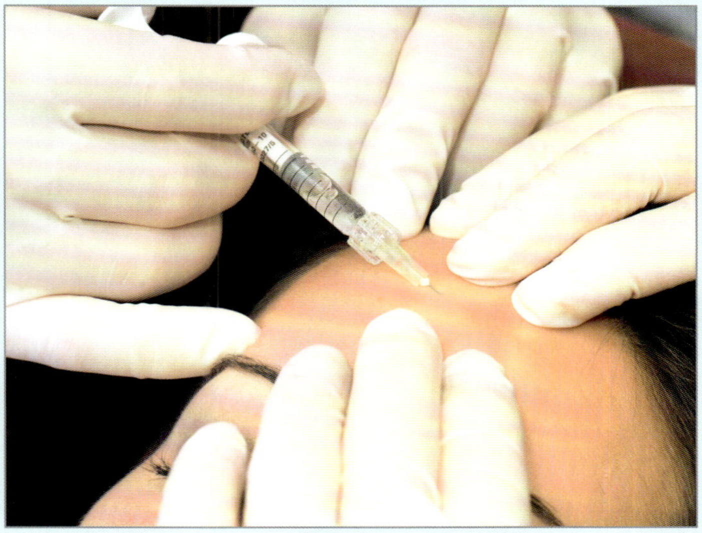

Fig. 6.29 With the skin stretched, advance the needle into the upper dermis in the augmentation area. The contours of the needle should be visible under the stretched skin.

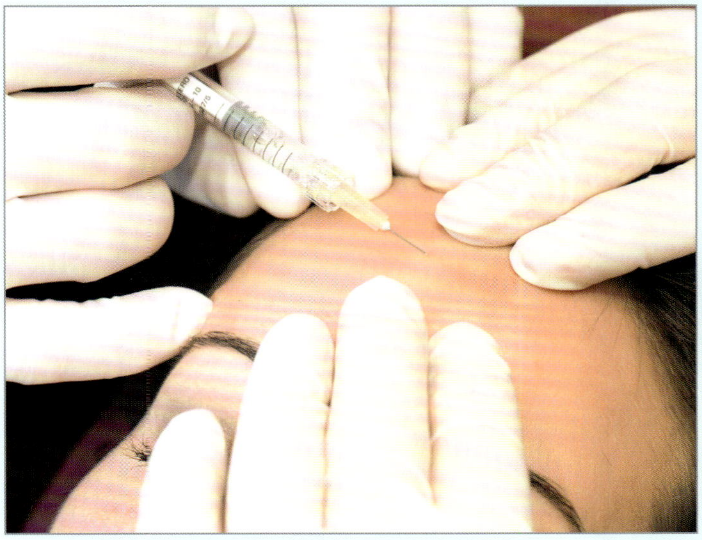

Fig. 6.30 Inject the substance into the upper dermis while withdrawing the needle.

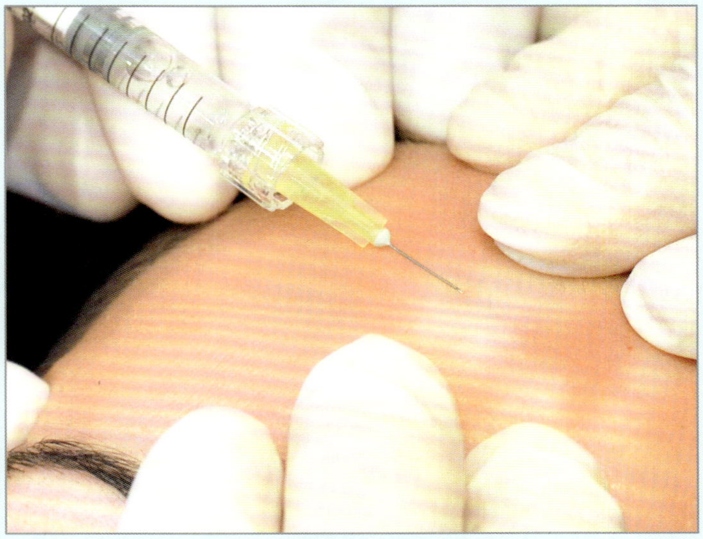

Fig. 6.31 The blanching effect produced by the stretching technique becomes clearly apparent.

mouth. Any reduction in the stretch becomes immediately apparent in the form of reduced resistance on the syringe plunger.

Compression Technique

Video: Compression Technique
http://www.kvm-tv.de/FIL/003.mp4

The compression technique is a modified point technique, in which maximum compression of the skin is used to alter the interstitial tissue pressure in preparation for the augmentation procedure (Figs 6.32 to 6.35).

This influences substance distribution during the injection.

> **Tips and tricks:** The non-injecting hand is used to grasp, lift and compress the skin around the target point as tightly as possible. The target point in the line is then injected with the needle. This enables targeted soft tissue augmentation, particularly at the mouth corners, the marionette and nasolabial lines, the glabellar region and the area around the eyes.

Compression Technique

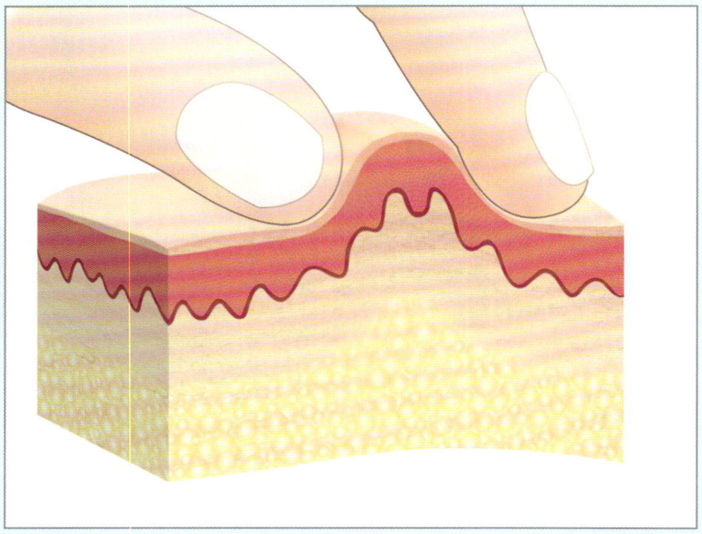

Fig. 6.32 Compress the skin around the target line between thumb and index finger.

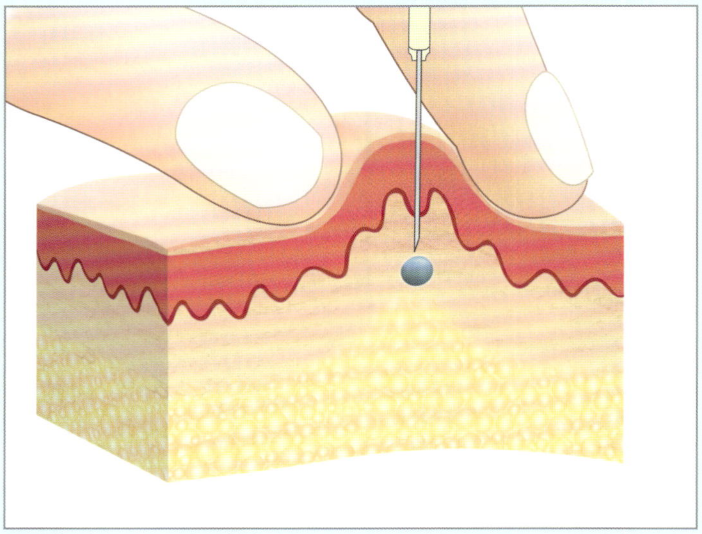

Fig. 6.33 Administer the injection with a point technique into the target area lifted by the non-injecting hand.

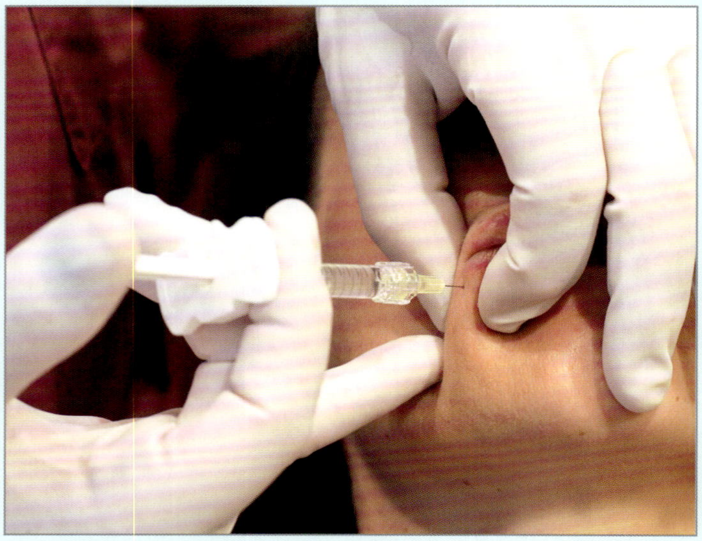

Fig. 6.34 Thumb and index finger compressing a marionette line.

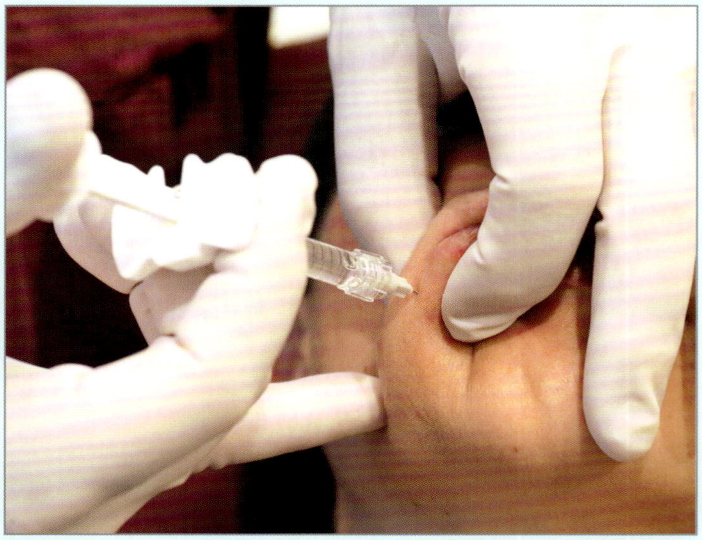

Fig. 6.35 The needle has been inserted into the target point along the line.

Vibrating Technique

The vibrating technique is a modification of the linear or the tunneling technique (Figs 6.36 to 6.39). Volume deficits, for example in the nasolabial area or in pitted acne scars, particularly benefit from the vibrating technique.

The desired modelling can be achieved with just a single treatment.

Tips and tricks: Targeted vibration leads to peripheral spreading of the augmentation material, and consequently to stabilisation of the dermis.
Use as little filler as possible, and repeat the treatment after 2 months if necessary.

Vibrating Technique

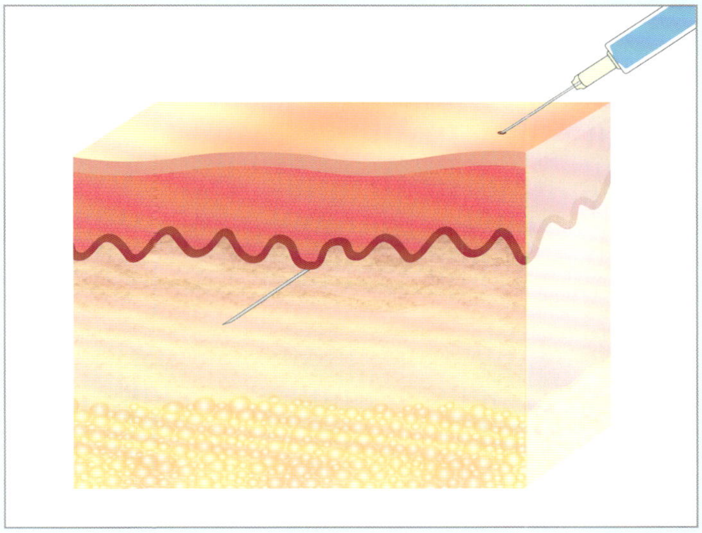

Fig. 6.36 Insert the needle into the course of the wrinkle at a shallow gradient.

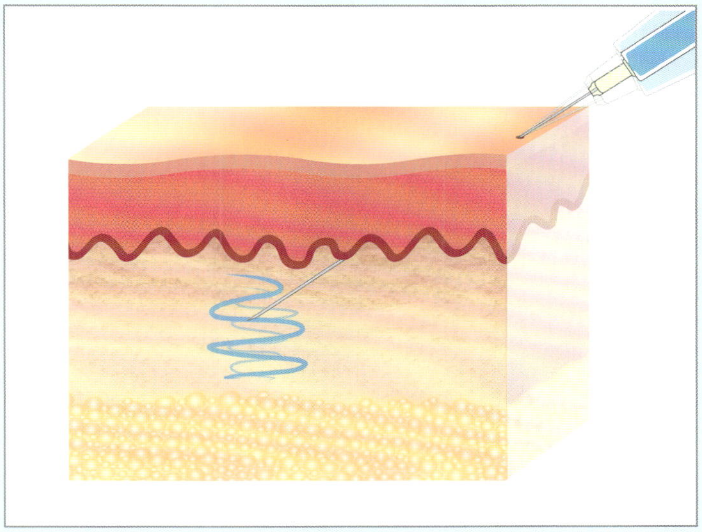

Fig. 6.37 Spread the substance diffusely through the upper, middle and deeper dermis.

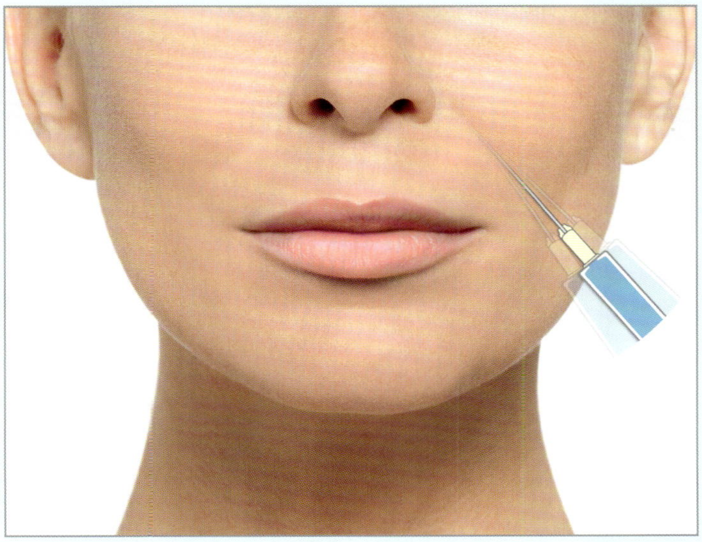

Fig. 6.38 Administer the injection with minimal pressure on the plunger, advancing and retracting the needle frequently and rapidly at various levels.

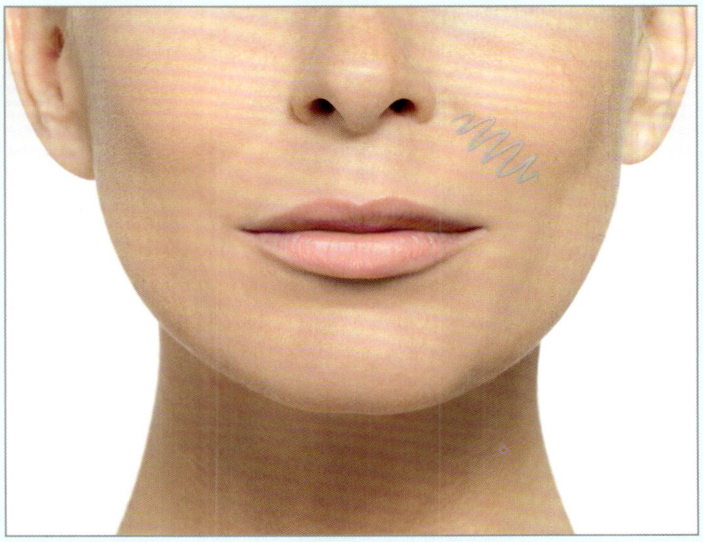

Fig. 6.39 This allows the tiniest amounts of the product to be placed diffusely below the line – thus avoiding visible, 'string of pearls' lines.

Sandwich Technique

Synonym: layering technique. The sandwich technique is used to fill pronounced skin defects and also for deeper, more rigid lines. It involves placing two or more layers of the augmentation material one on top of the other (Figs 6.40 to 6.43).

Hyaluronic acid products of differing viscosities can also be layered one above the other.

Tips and tricks: Various cross-linked hyaluronic acid products or autologous fat are suitable for the deep layers, while low cross-linked hyaluronic acid products are used more superficially.
The sandwich technique may be performed in several sessions, with intervals, or directly in a single session.

Sandwich Technique

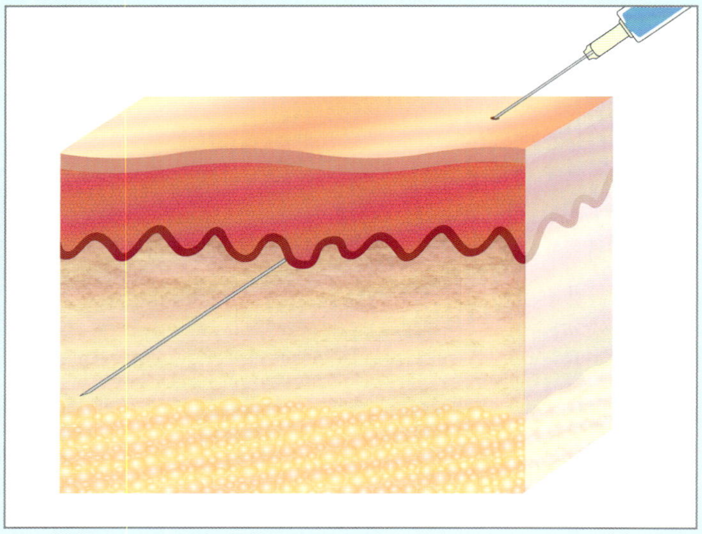

Fig. 6.40 Insert the needle at an angle of 30 to 40 degrees.

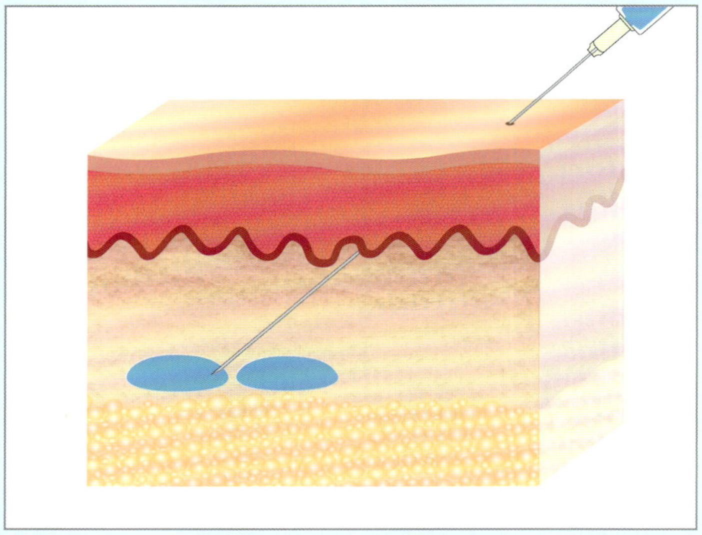

Fig. 6.41 The filler may be administered at all levels, starting with the injection into the deepest layer.

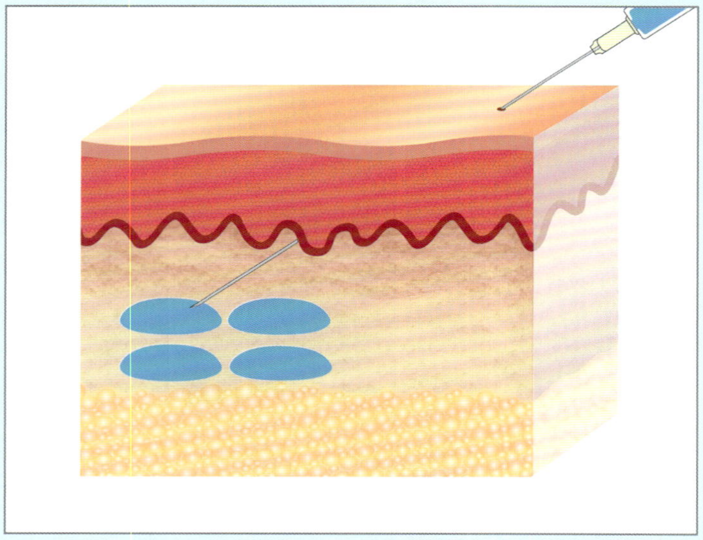

Fig. 6.42 This is followed by a second, shallower entry at an angle of 15 to 20 degrees.

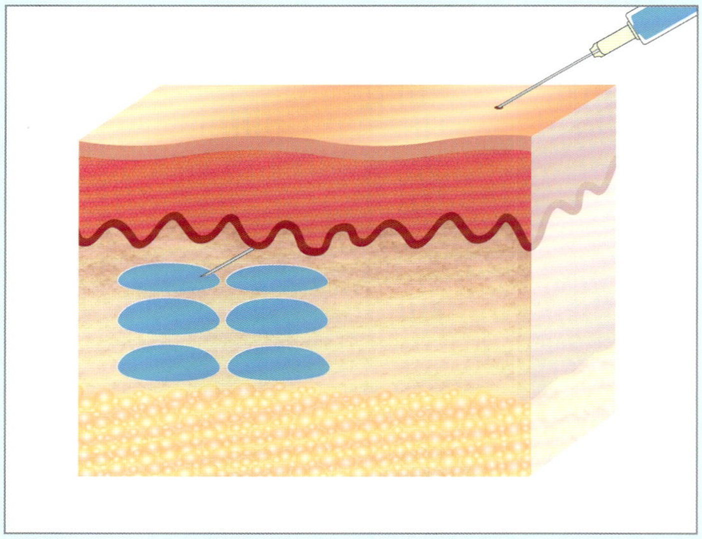

Fig. 6.43 If required, administer a third superficial injection into the dermo-epidermal junction zone.

Fanning Technique

The fanning technique involves sequential tunneling in a fanning fashion from a single puncture point (Figs 6.44 to 6.47).

The fanning technique is particularly suitable for the lateral regions of the face and cheeks, allowing large areas to be augmented efficiently.

Tips and tricks: When withdrawing the needle, ensure that the pressure on the plunger is reduced shortly before the needle returns to the puncture site, to avoid excess accumulation of material in this region, and also risking the Tyndall effect should the filler be deposited closer to the skin surface.

Fanning Technique

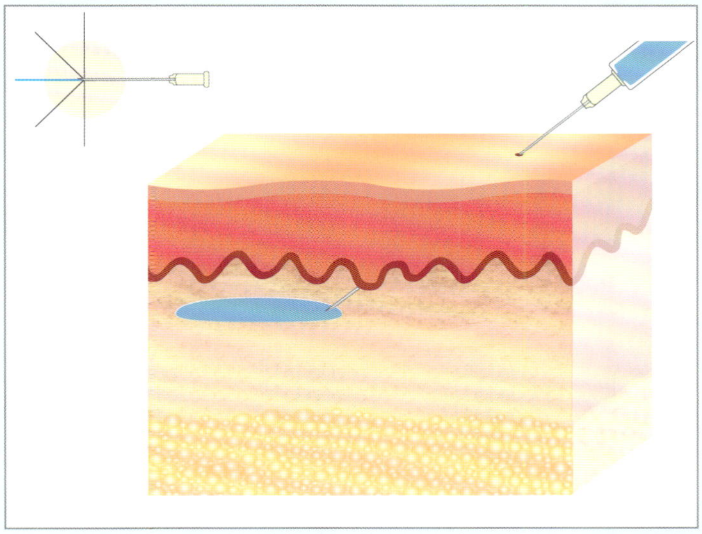

Fig. 6.44 Insert the needle at an angle of about 45 degrees.

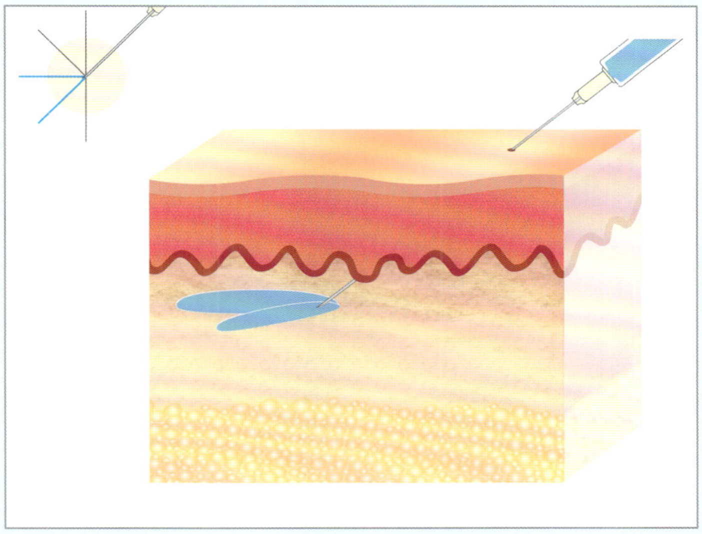

Fig. 6.45 Give the injection while withdrawing the needle.

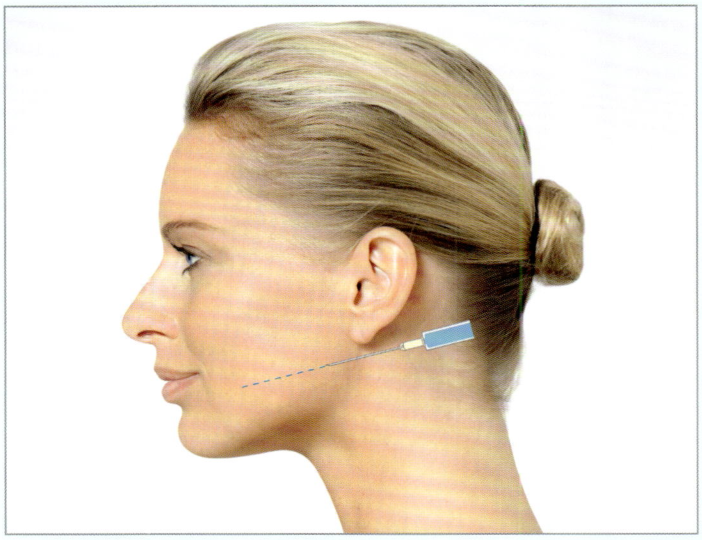

Fig. 6.46 Do not withdraw the needle fully from the skin …

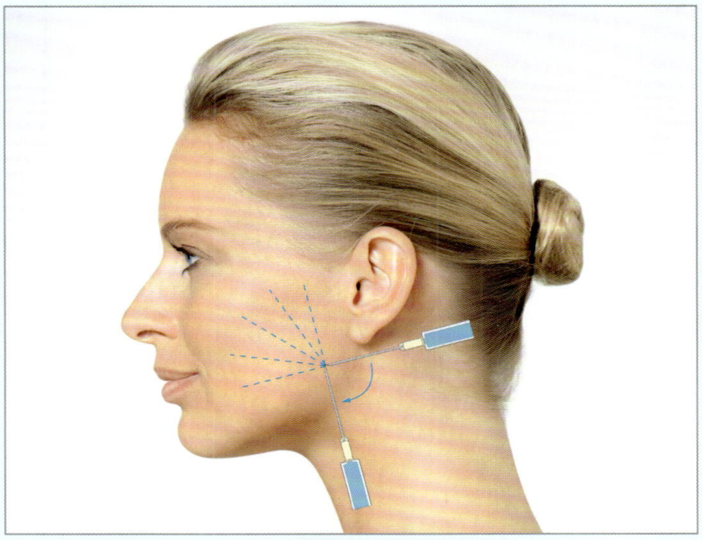

Fig. 6.47 … but advance it again at a different angle to the surface of the skin.

6

Criss-cross Technique

The criss-cross technique involves sequential adjacent tunneling in the same plane, in which the needle tracks form a grid (Figs 6.48 to 6.51). It can be used to treat superficial elastosis of ageing skin (biorevitalisation) and to remedy defects that cover a wide area, by laying down an extensive, supporting filler framework. This technique can be used not only for aesthetic treatments generally, but also specifically for the treatment of burns or weak connective tissue.

Tips and tricks: It is essential to ensure all injections are performed at the same level or plane to avoid any surface irregularities. All skin layers can be reached using the criss-cross technique:

- Biorevitalisation: superficial, using non-cross-linked hyaluronic acid fillers
- Fine wrinkles/puckered skin: mid-dermis with low cross-linked hyaluronic acid fillers
- Volume defects: deep dermis/subcutaneous tissue with higher cross-linked hyaluronic acid fillers or subcutaneously injected autologous fat

Criss-cross Technique

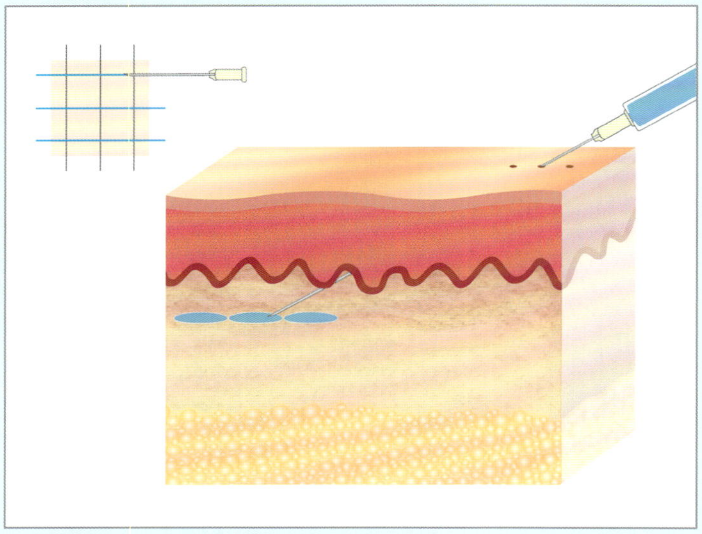

Fig. 6.48 First, administer linear injections at adjacent puncture points. Ensure light, even pressure on the plunger while withdrawing the needle and delivering the filler.

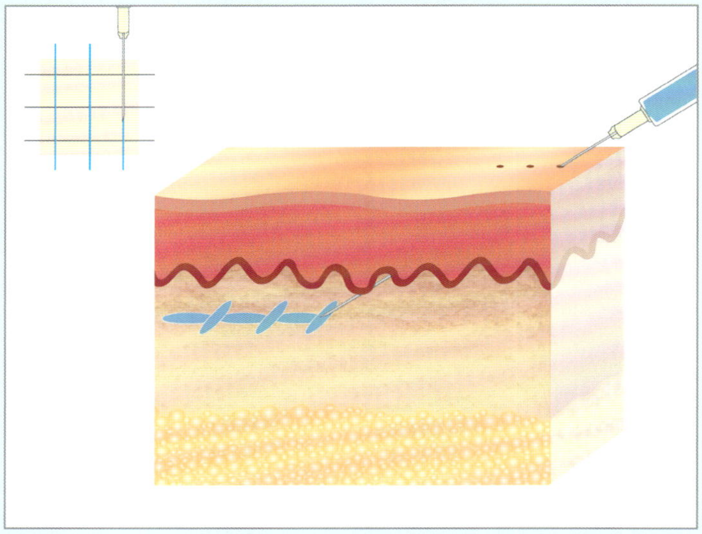

Fig. 6.49 Inject a second series of linear injections at 90 degrees to the first.

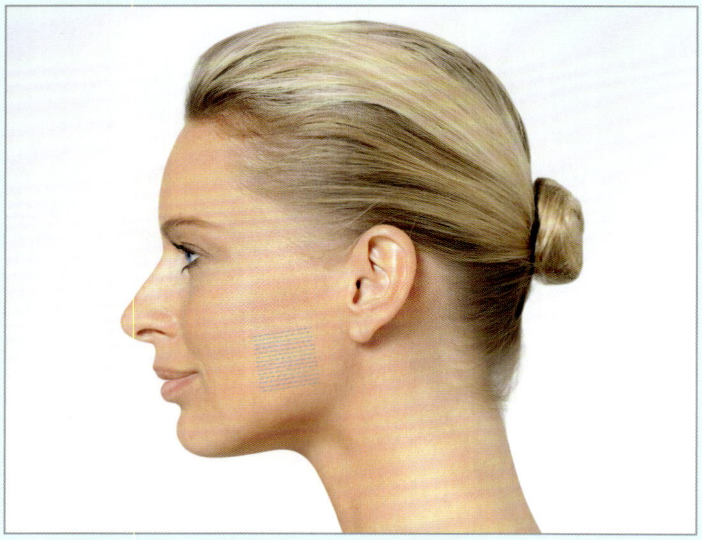

Fig. 6.50 Insert the needle into a new point for each line.

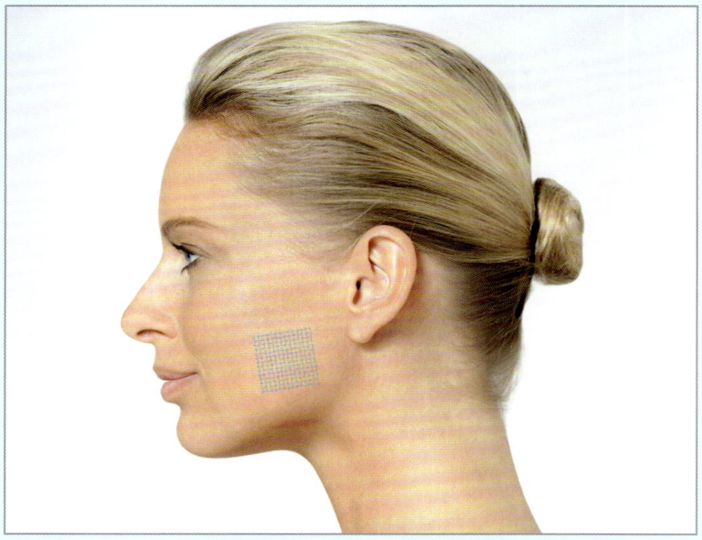

Fig. 6.51 The injections should cover a square grid of tissue at the same depth.

6.9.3 Vertical Injection Techniques

Vertical injection techniques can be regarded as a significant development in volumetric treatments with hyaluronic acid-based fillers. They involve focal treatment of the underlying defects in the deep subcutaneous adipose tissues. Vertical insertion of the needle on a mechanical base (periosteum or mucosa) ensures that the filler material is accurately deposited in the target area near the causal deep soft tissue deficit. The authors refer to this supraperiosteal injection point as the 'sweet spot'. A single supraperiosteal depot injection is sufficient to restore tension in the whole tissue complex from the base up. The projection effect achieved in this manner can induce a visible improvement of even severe soft tissue deficits without causing unnatural overprojection, and remove the need for further superficial correction with fillers (Fig. 6.52). At the same time, vertical needle insertion serves to prevent intravascular injections given that the vessels are more superficial.

Vertical injection techniques are performed using stabilised high-viscosity hyaluronic acid filler, which allow for minimal horizontal material distribution. Therefore, the most effective projection effect can be achieved at the base of the soft tissue deficit.

It is generally accepted that the vertical depot techniques have now replaced the HA column injection technique, which was originally taught and practised. This is primarily because unwanted static overprojection can now be negated. However, the column injection technique is still used for volume augmentation in other parts of the body.

Below we describe two vertical injection techniques: the vertical supraperiosteal depot technique (VSDT), and the tower technique (TT).

If the clinician hits the 'sweet spot' of volume loss, immediate elevation of the tissue structures will be seen due to the projection effect. If the filler is correctly injected in a true retaining ligament, an acoustic signal (grating sound) can be heard.

Practical tip: During vertical injection, the needle must always be completely inserted down to the periosteum or mucosa in order to prevent inadvertent intravascular injection.

6

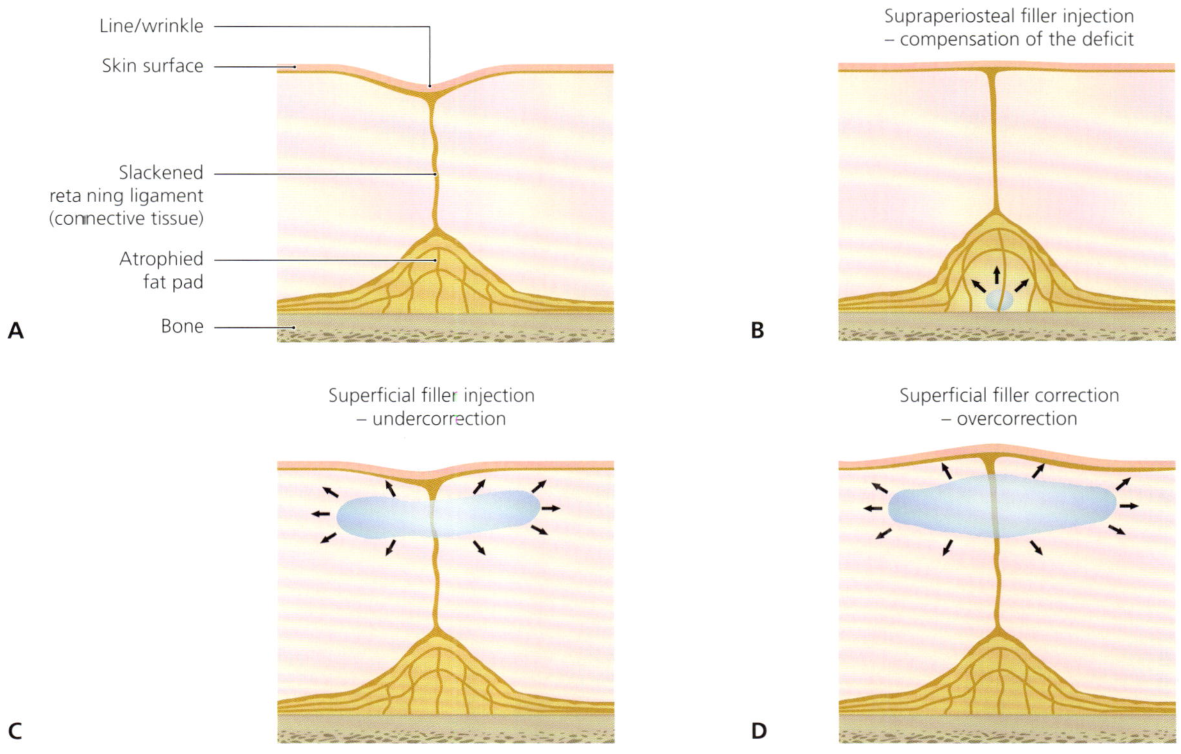

Fig. 6.52 (**A**) 'Sweet spot' of volume loss in the deep fat; comparison of projection effects of (**B**) vertical injection; and (**C/D**) superficial injection of the filler. Injection of a very small amount of a highly cross-linked hyaluronic acid gel at the supraperiosteal site, i.e. the origin of the volume loss ('sweet spot') increases tension in the retaining ligaments, resulting in natural elevation of the overall tissue complex. This technique allows for the treatment of deep wrinkles caused by severe fat tissue atrophy and produces an immediately visible effect. With superficial injections, on the other hand, masking of the intended projection effect occurs due to the strong horizontal spreading of the filler material. Therefore, superficial injection with a comparable amount of filler will result in undercorrection and unsatisfactory results. Attempts to resolve this apparent deficit by superficially injecting additional doses of filler often result in overcorrection with an unnatural, static and unsatisfactory appearance.

Vertical Supraperiosteal Depot Technique (VSDT)

Video: VSDT
http://www.kvm-tv.de/FIL/004.mp4

The vertical supraperiosteal depot technique (VSDT) allows the greatest projection effect to be achieved with the least amount of filler material (Figs 6.53 to 6.56). A similar technique over a supramucosal base can also be used.

A single supraperiosteal or supramucosal depot injection is placed in the 'sweet spot' of the volume deficit, preferably in the area of the involved retaining ligaments. This deep volume compensation depot is sufficient to restore tension in the retaining ligaments and to make the overall soft tissue complex 'rise up'. This results in a harmonious and smoothing effect, which is immediately visible. For treatment of extensive volume defects, such as deep nasolabial folds, a linear series of vertical depot injections can harmonise facial proportions.

> **Practical tip:** When treating nasolabial folds, the practitioner can insert the non-working thumb in the patient's mouth and place it beneath the injection site to create the support needed for the targeted administration of a supramucosal depot injection into the 'sweet spot' of the volume loss. Caution is advocated to avoid needlestick injuries.

Vertical Supraperiosteal Depot Technique

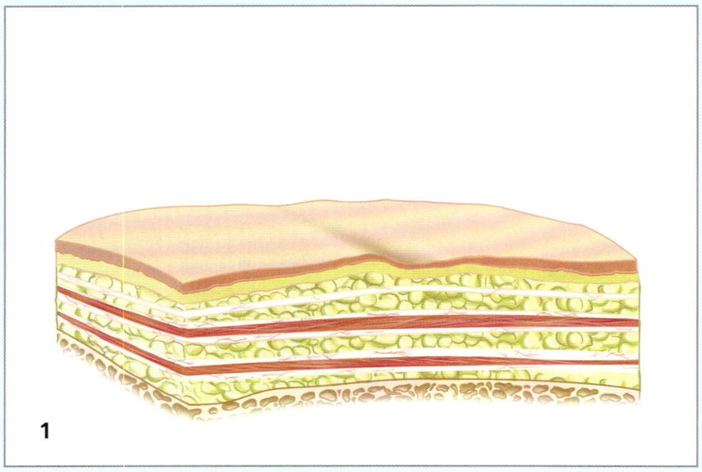

Fig. 6.53 The vertical supraperiosteal depot technique is performed using predefined anatomical landmarks, such as the bone in this case.

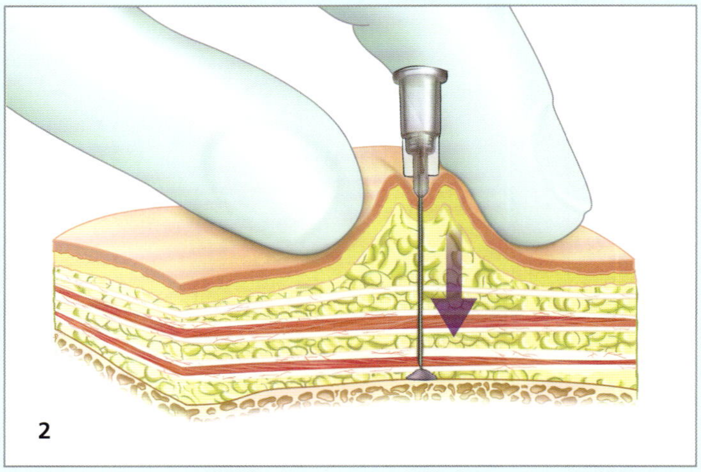

Fig. 6.54 When placing an ultra-deep injection, the target structure is compressed to ensure that the filler is injected directly above (i.e. supraperiosteum in this case). Proper technique can virtually exclude intravascular injection.

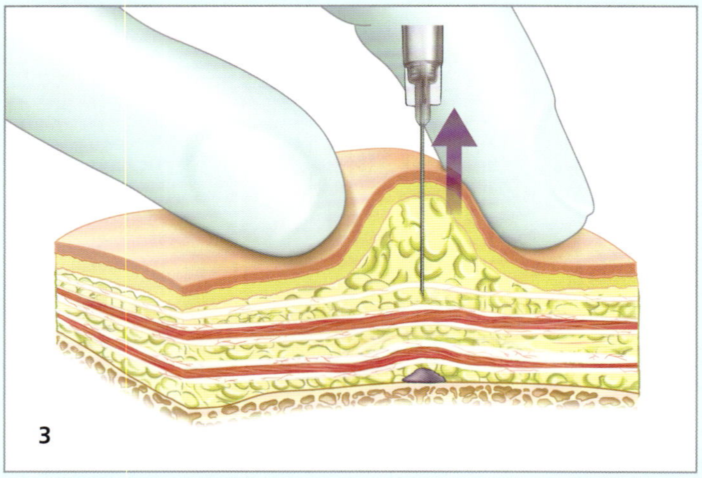

Fig. 6.56 Only a small amount of a suitable high-viscosity filler is administered before the needle is withdrawn.

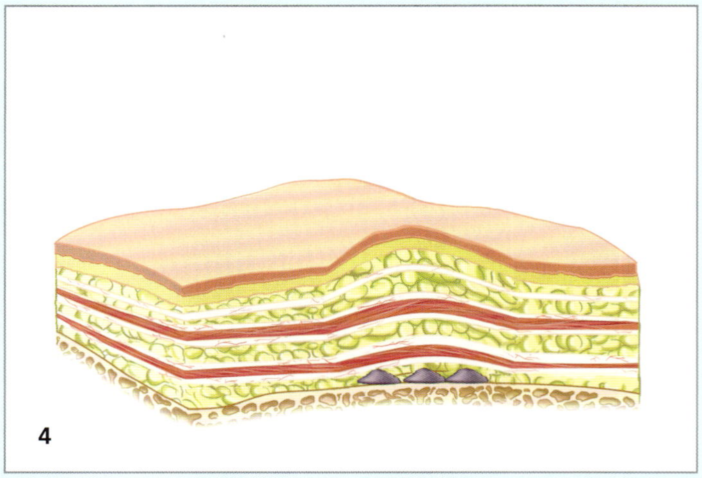

Fig. 6.55 The projection efficiency of a series of adjacent supraperiosteal depot injections is sufficient to eliminate severe soft tissue volume deficits.

Tower Technique (TT)

Video: Tower Technique
http://www.kvm-tv.de/FIL/005.mp4

The tower technique (TT) is a modification of the vertical depot technique. After placing an ultra-deep depot injection in the area of the 'sweet spot' of volume loss (Fig. 6.57), the needle is slowly retracted while placing additional depot injections at different tissue levels of decreasing depth, up to the subdermal plexus. This results in a series of depots, resembling a stack of coins (Figs 6.58 to 6.60). Additional static stabilisation and saturation of the tissue complex with fluids can be achieved in this manner. Because the overall projection effect induced at the deep tissue level is masked by the horizontal distribution of filler in the superficial tissue layers, the tower technique has lower projection efficiency than the vertical supraperiosteal depot technique (Figs 6.61 to 6.63).

> **Practical tip:** The tower technique is particularly effective in cases where mucosa, not bone, is the base structure below the target area. If located over a bony base, the effects of the tower technique may quickly lead to overprojection with static and unnatural results. It is recommended that one should first administer a single ultra-deep depot injection to assess the clinical effect and then decide if further injections are required. At times, a single ultra-deep injection can achieve the desired tissue projection in some cases without further injections.

Tower Technique

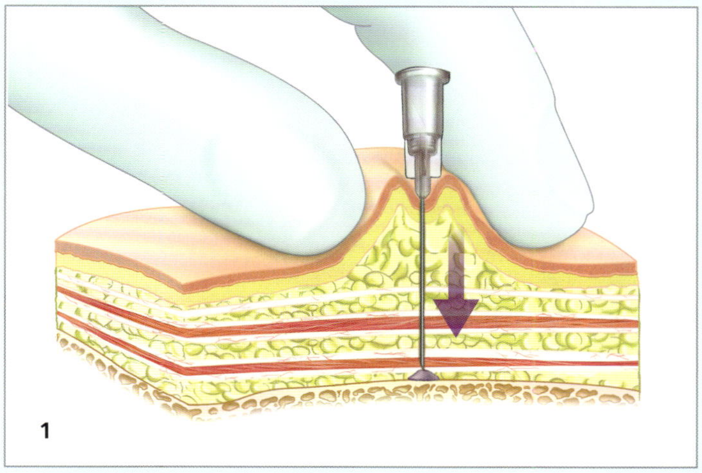

Fig. 6.57 The needle is inserted vertically through the skin to the underlying bone or mucosa. The first (ultra-deep) depot injection of filler material is administered there.

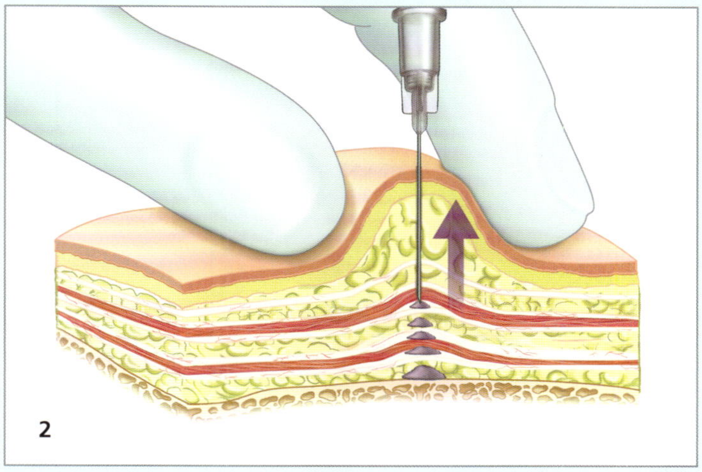

Fig. 6.58 Additional depots of filler are then injected at increasing tissue levels as the needle is being slowly retracted.

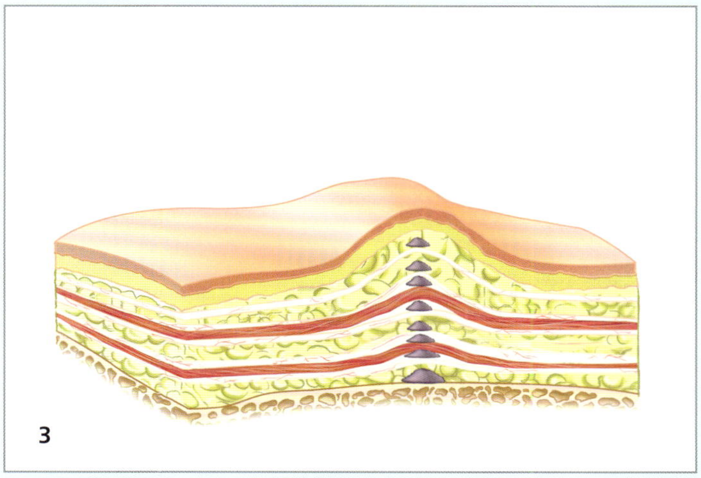

Fig. 6.59 This creates an accordion-like filler configuration that effectively augments and saturates the tissue complex with fluids.

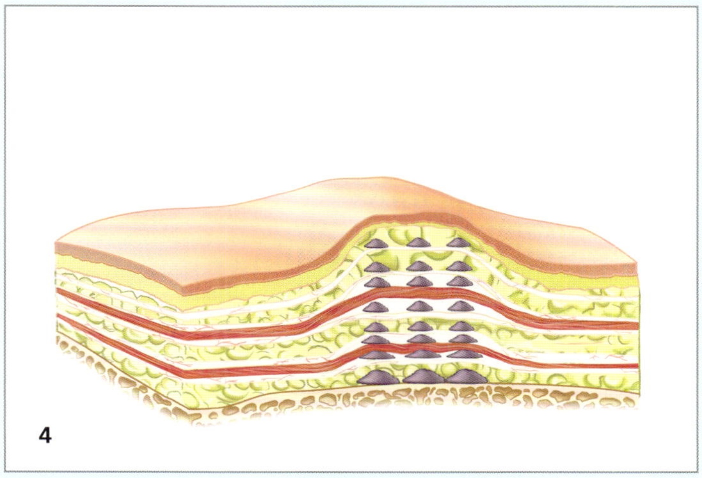

Fig. 6.60 When treating folds using the tower technique, it is recommended to leave between 3 to 7 mm between each depot, as this results in profound compensation of volume deficits and structural stabilisation of the atrophic tissue.

Volume augmentation by vertical injection techniques

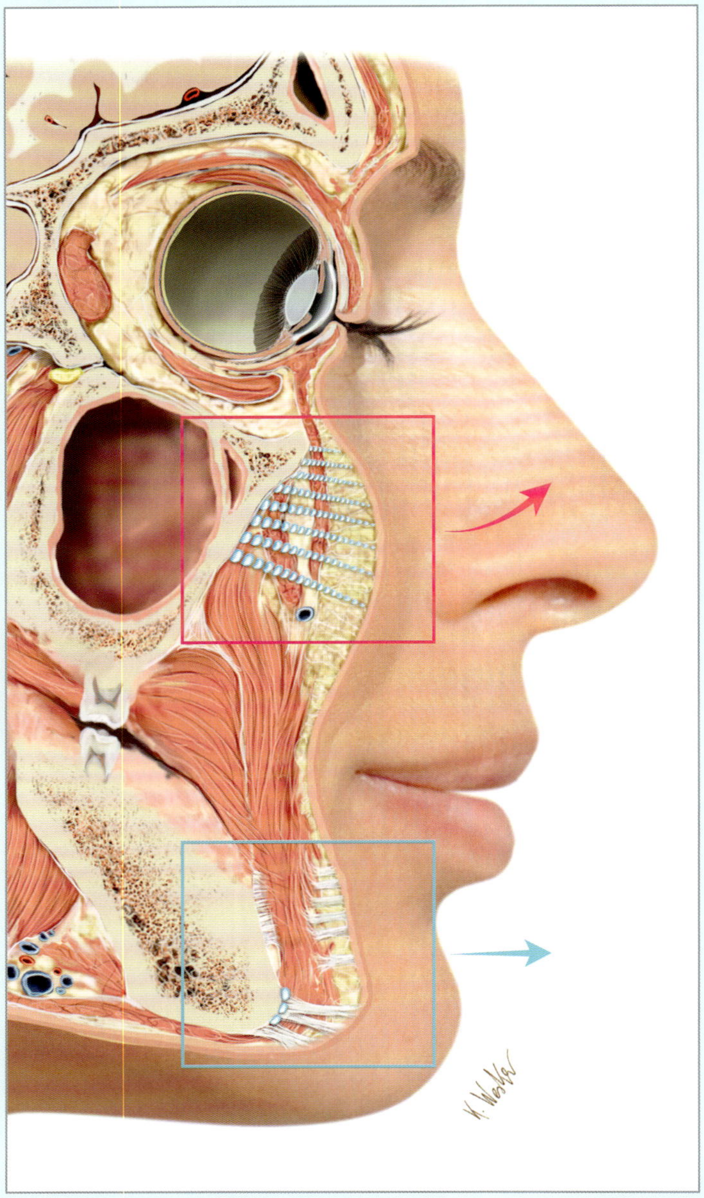

Fig. 6.61 Combined treatment using the vertical supraperiosteal depot technique (VSDT) for chin augmentation and the tower technique (TT) for the treatment of the midface and nasolabial folds.

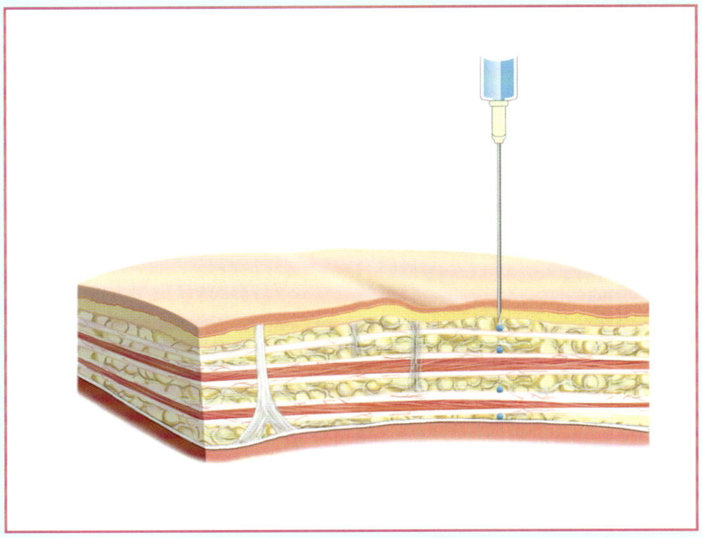

Fig. 6.62 The vertical **tower technique** is used for volume projection and static stabilisation, preferably above a non-bony base.

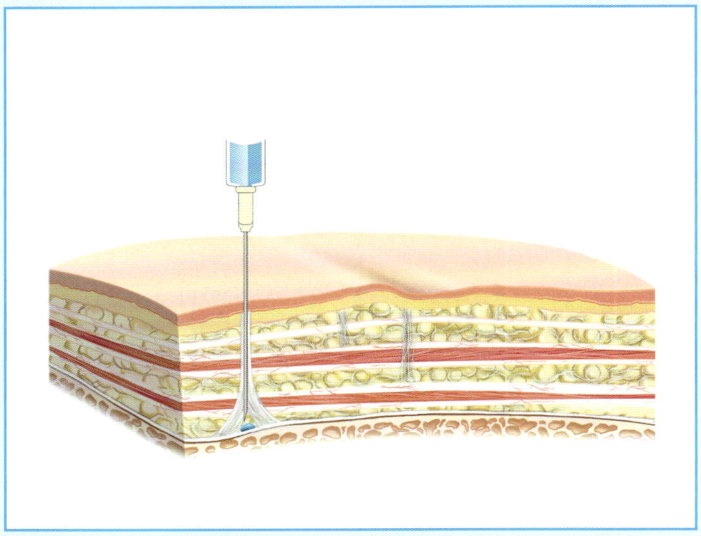

Fig. 6.63 The **vertical supraperiosteal depot technique** achieves the greatest projection effect with the least amount of filler material. It is useful for treating severe volume loss over a bony base, particularly in cases where true retaining ligaments are involved.

Deep Mesotherapy

The fluid supply and trophic state of the deep subfascial fat pads is crucial to the rate of tissue atrophy, which has implications for the elasticity and trophic state of the overall tissue complex. Therefore, mesotherapy in combination with augmentation therapy is indicated not only for superficial treatments just below the skin surface, but also and especially for treatments at deeper tissue levels, where the structural causes are located. In this treatment approach, serial vertical injections of an appropriate filler (see A Fillers for skin surface regeneration and mesotherapy, p. 69) are placed at the bone or the mucosa (Fig. 6.64). This results in rehydration and physiological support of atrophic subcutaneous tissue in combination with a small lifting effect, leading to proportional correction and overall harmonisation. Our clinical experience has shown that the improvements achieved by deep mesotherapy (e.g. homogenisation and revitalisation of the skin surface) are more significant than those achieved by standard (superficial) mesotherapy.

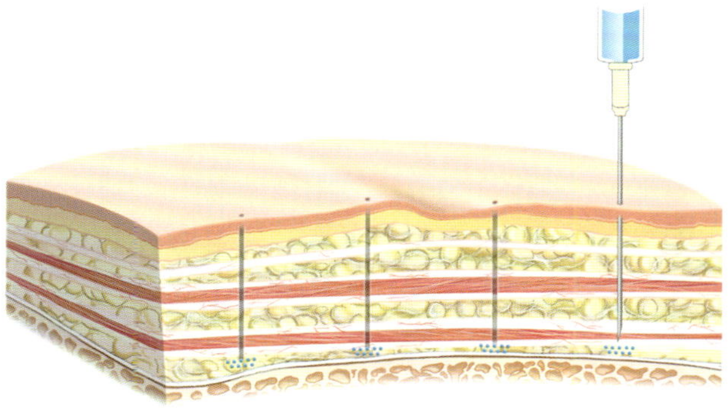

Fig. 6.64 Deep mesotherapy involves the supraperiosteal or supramucosal injection of a mesofiller. By improving the conditions resulting from fatty tissue atrophy, deep mesotherapy can harmonise the overall facial proportions at the physical, anatomical and clinical level more effectively than the superficial mesofiller injections recommended by the manufacturers.

Practical tip: Deep mesotherapy is useful, for example, for complete cheek treatment for general overall facial harmonisation in combination with a slight projection effect. To avoid inadvertent intravascular injection, the needle is inserted vertically and advanced down to the periosteum or mucosa. Typically for a full face, around 50 to 100 injections are made, spaced at a distance of a half a centimetre apart and depositing around 0.01 ml of the filler per injection.
Multi-injection systems developed by the manufacturers are useful for the uniform administration of serial injections.

6.9.4 Horizontal Augmentation Techniques

Video: HAC
http://www.kvm-tv.de/FIL/006.mp4

Extensive augmentation procedures are commonly performed using horizontal injection techniques with cannulas. As with vertical injection techniques, the range of applications has grown tremendously since the focus of attention has shifted from symptomatic therapy to causal treatment of individual target structures.

In atraumatic tissue mobilisation in the horizontal direction, the cannula homogenises the injection space and simultaneously activates fibrogenesis and tissue repair. Because this counteracts age-related deficiencies at the mechanical and material level (i.e. with HA filler injection), natural harmonisation of facial conditions can be achieved at different tissue layers. This technique is useful in cases where the objective of treatment is to achieve even augmentation of a large area, such as the cheek region. It is also indicated for the treatment of structures by which retaining ligaments or other possibly fibrotic tissues adhere to an atrophic base, resulting in the formation of wrinkles. A classic example of this is the marionette lines. An atraumatic technique can be used to release the anatomical anchors responsible for the tissue depressions from their base so that they can form better re-attachments. Relining the homogenised anchor surface with a mild to highly cross-linked HA filler creates a natural projection effect without the risk of nodule formation or static overprojection.

Depending on the indication, horizontal augmentation techniques may be performed at the superficial (intradermal or subdermal), medium (subcutaneous) or deep level (supramucosal or supraperiosteal). In any case, the target tissue area is evenly projected, saturated with new fluids and tightened via the induction of collagen and elastin synthesis in a single treatment session.

Horizontal injections of hyaluronic acid or autologous fat with atraumatic cannulas effectively create microlesions that activate fibrogenesis and tissue repair by stimulating neocollagenesis and new elastin synthesis. In the case of hyaluronic acid fillers, treatment results in tissue repair by two main mechanisms: the supply of fluids and by fibrogenesis.

Superficial Horizontal Augmentation with Cannula (SHAC)

Superficial horizontal augmentation with cannula (SHAC) is a horizontal mobilisation and augmentation technique employed for generalised improvement of facial skin texture via widespread rehydration and revitalisation of the cutis or just below in the immediate subdermal plane. A microcannula (27 G) is used to gently create a homogeneous horizontal injection plane in the intradermal or immediate subdermal plexus and reline it with a highly hydrophilic, low-viscosity injectable filler. This produces a uniform, water-binding support layer just below the skin surface. The resulting improvement of the subdermal skin condition improves the skin texture at the functional (elasticity, resilience, and strength) and aesthetic level (radiant complexion, suppleness, and homogeneity), as well as inhibits the progression of visible signs of skin ageing. The fibrogenesis and neocollagenesis induced by the fine microlesions also counteract UV-induced solar elastosis and can assist in tightening wrinkled skin.

Practical tip: Subdermal horizontal tissue augmentation and mobilisation is a useful method of skin surface regeneration, according to the authors. Alternatively, skin surface regeneration can be achieved by the serial puncture technique (with manual injection or with the assistance of an automated injection system), or using the criss-cross technique.

Horizontal Augmentation Techniques

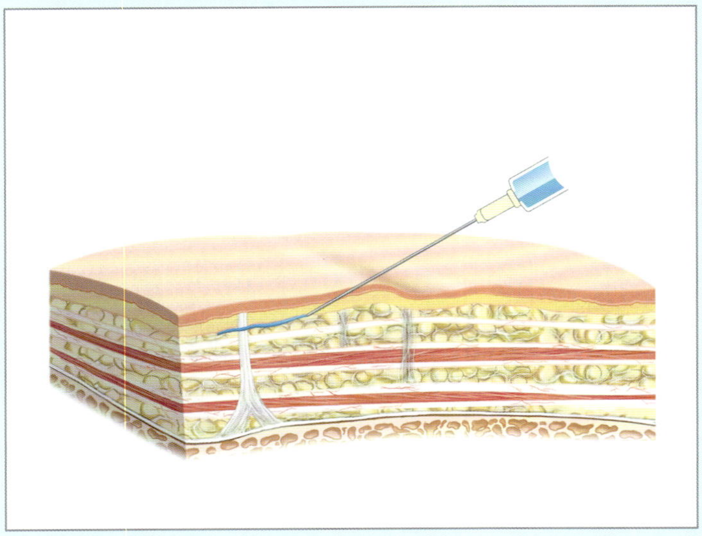

Fig. 6.65 A blunt-tip microcannula is used to create an intradermal or directly subdermal superficial water-binding layer. This results in large-scale rehydration and revitalisation of the skin surface.

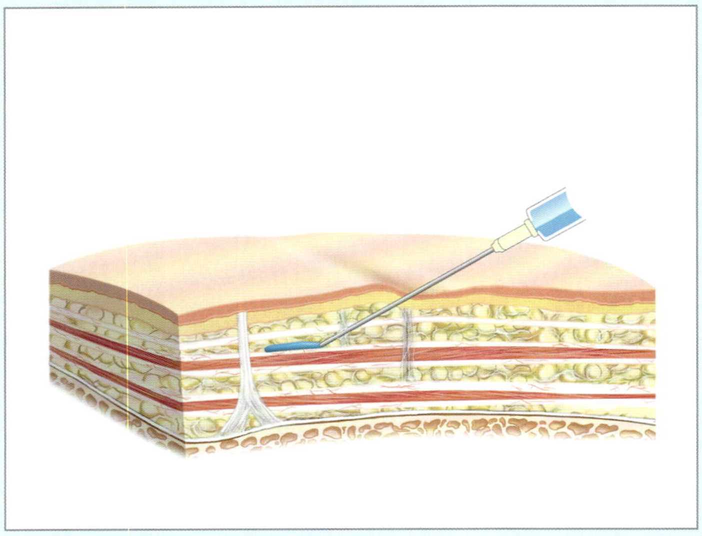

Fig. 6.66 Medium to deep horizontal augmentation with a cannula is useful for correcting large-scale volume defects in fatty tissues in order to restore a natural appearance and achieve overall improvement by addressing the root causes.

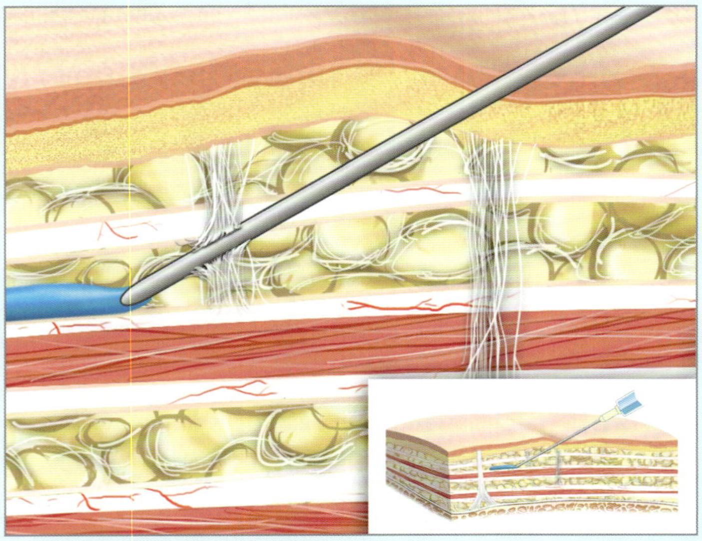

Fig. 6.67 When mobilising and homogenising the horizontal injection area, fine ligamentous anchors attached to the atrophic base are freed in a gentle and cautious manner. This, in turn, reduces the tensile forces on the skin that contribute to the severity of the wrinkles. At the same time, the atraumatically induced microlesions activate the clinically beneficial processes of fibrogenesis and tissue repair.

Deep Horizontal Augmentation with Cannula (DHAC)

Deep horizontal augmentation with cannula (DHAC), or subcutaneous horizontal mobilisation and augmentation, is used to harmonise facial proportions and to achieve overall improvement of atrophic volume defects over large areas (Figs 6.65 to 6.67). In DHAC, the injection depth is dependent on which target structure is to be treated. This technique is used, for example, for supraperiosteal injections in the forehead and the temple region, or for supramucosal injections for the treatment of nasolabial folds and marionette lines. The tissues are gently mobilised in the horizontal direction in order to release fibrotic structures that might be adhering to the base, as well as to reduce tensile forces on the skin. This induces the reduction of wrinkles caused or aggravated by induration of skin over an atrophic area. At the same time, the base is slightly relined with a medium-viscosity HA filler, which produces an additional, harmonious projection effect and saturates the tissues with additional fluids. The atraumatic microlesions created in the tissues not only activate fibrogenesis and tissue renewal but also lead to physiological improvement of the treated structures.

Practical tip: By inserting the non-injecting forefinger or thumb in the patient's mouth and positioning it below the region of the marionette lines or nasolabial folds, the practitioner can stabilise the mucosal base, which facilitates the horizontal augmentation procedure.

Windmill Technique

The windmill technique is a special variant of the deep horizontal augmentation with cannula (DHAC) technique. It is used for harmonising volume augmentation throughout the entire cheek area. The practitioner uses one singular insertion point from which radiating injections are made in all suitable directions for a harmonising mobilisation and augmentation of the entire cheek region, e.g. infraorbital, nasolabial, periorbital and posterior (temporal) areas. Importantly, overall improvement of facial proportions can be achieved in a single treatment session. (For a detailed description of the method, see Ch. 7, p. 171.)

6.9.5 Injection-dependent effects

Blanching effect

The blanching effect describes the whitening seen on the skin surface caused by the pressure exerted by a superficially injected filler, with appropriate visco-elastic properties. The spread and displacement of the filler leads to compression of the superficial vessels, with resultant whitening of the skin.

The appearance of blanching is an indication that an injection has been placed into the upper layer of the dermis.

Caution

The desired blanching effect should not be confused with the Tyndall effect, where a highly cross-linked hyaluronic acid filler is injected too superficially by mistake, which results in persistent bluish discolouration alongside surface irregularities.

Correction level

The desired correction level depends on the filler being used. However, overall we advocate undercorrection for most fillers, as top-ups are a much easier and safer option than having to remedy an overcorrection.

Overcorrection

Overcorrection is to be strictly avoided with fillers that are not broken down in the tissues (Fig. 6.68). Care should also be taken with hyal-

Correction level

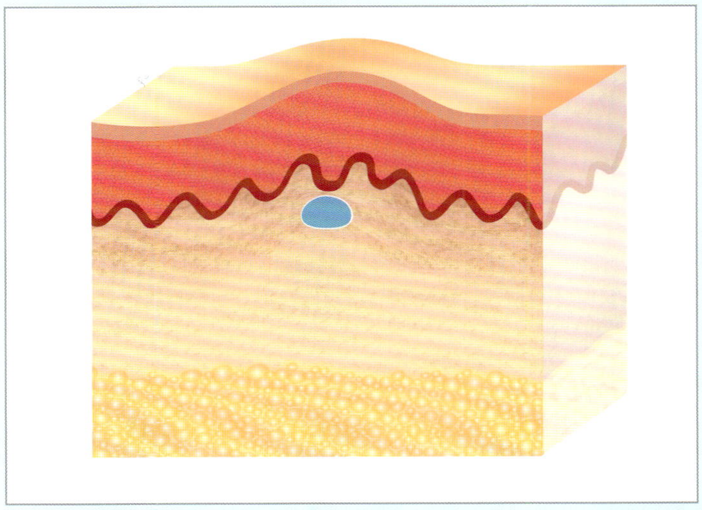

Fig. 6.68 Overcorrection. Overcorrection can be necessary with filler agents that quickly degrade within the tissues.

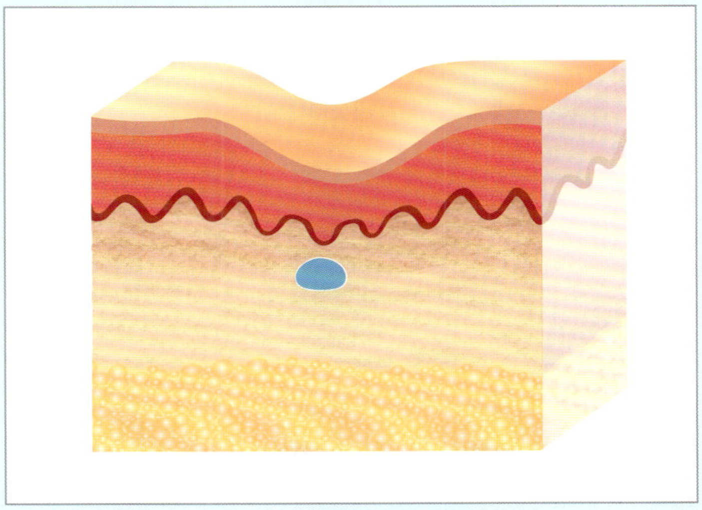

Fig. 6.69 Undercorrection. Undercorrection is necessary when using non-degradable filler agents.

uronic acid fillers, as they tend to hydrate post-treatment and therefore slight undercorrection is also advocated (Fig. 6.69). Furthermore, semi-permanent fillers should also be injected with care, as it is far easier to top-up at a later stage rather than have to try to resolve overcorrection. In summary, undercorrection is the preferred choice with most fillers, followed by further augmentation after a treatment break of at least 6 weeks if required.

In some cases, particularly with the use of autologous fat or collagen, overcorrection may be a good idea or at times even necessary. Failure to overcorrect in such cases can result in the patient being disappointed with the clinical outcome and notably its duration of effect, given the volume will decrease to the desired level within a relatively short period of time.

Marked resorption takes place particularly after the first injection. Resorption is not only influenced by the filler properties themselves, but is also affected by several factors relating to the patient, including the blood supply within the injected area, alongside level of mechanical stress within the tissues, etc. It is frequently much less pronounced following subsequent injections. Regular treatments to upkeep the effects allow less filler to be used and achieve natural progressive improvements.

Long-term treatment and the 'pillow face'

Long-term treatment with hyaluronic acid fillers should never result in disproportionate overvolumisation of the face. This phenomenon, known as the 'pillow face', most commonly occurs in very slim people as an unfortunate consequence of poor overall planning with volumisation therapy. Instead of addressing the actual structural causes, some practitioners attempt to correct focal deficits by injecting excessive amounts of filler into the superficial tissue plane, resulting in subsequent accumulation of the filler. After three to five filler treatments, the face starts to look unnaturally inflated. Ultimately, the face is blown out of proportion to the rest of the body, in turn resulting in disharmony. To prevent this, the general rule is to use the smallest amounts of filler required to specifically treat only those structures in need of treatment (i.e. the structures responsible for the patient's key complaints) in order to restore natural facial harmony. The right augmentation technique can even create the visual impression of tissue deflation, as evidenced by the ovalisation of the overall face after chin volumisation.

> **Caution**
>
> **If not placed within the correct anatomical plane, filler material settles in the subcutaneous tissues in a disproportionate manner a few months after the hyaluronic acid filler treatment. This distorts the treatment outcome, and further injection is needed for correction.**

> **Practical tip:** To achieve successful long-term augmentation with hyaluronic acid fillers, not only should the individual proportions of the face, but also the volume ratio between the face and rest of the body be considered at all times. Generally, the practitioner should only treat the specific causes of age-related loss of attractiveness in the patient and restore the affected structures to a form specific to the individual patient. Causal treatment of the underlying subcutaneous tissue loss is the most filler-sparing way to avoid disproportionate overvolumisation of the face over the long term.

6.10 Complications and Their Management

6.10.1 Expected injection-related effects and complications

During and post-treatment a number of side effects can occur, which are not considered complications as they are a common aspect seen with injections. As such, patients should be advised of these and accept the risks involved. They include:

- Pain can occur during the injection; its intensity depends on the area being treated and the practitioner's injection technique. The perioral region, including the lips, and the periorbital region are regarded as highly sensitive areas. Patients should be advised in advance of the possibility of some discomfort, and offered anaesthesia to improve comfort levels.
- Erythema and swelling are commonly noted and fully reversible within a few hours to a few days post-treatment. Again, patients should be pre-warned and be willing to accept these effects.
- Itching and mild irritation in the treated areas may also be noted and can typically persist for a few days after the treatment, but is a rare feature overall.
- Small haemorrhages in the skin or larger haematomas can occur and typically subside within a few days to a couple of weeks. As such, sun exposure and visits to the solarium are not recommended during this time to avoid further hyperpigmentation.
- Acneiform papules, cysts and milia can develop as a result of superficial injections of the products into the dermis; some of these eruptions may need to be removed mechanically.

Bacterial infections and abscesses are very serious complications but are not common. If the infection control guidelines are adhered to, the risks are greatly reduced. With regard to viral herpes simplex, patients with a previous history should be managed with prophylactic oral antivirals should they have a positive past history of cold sores. A variety of protocols exist, some advocating initiation on the day of the treatment, whith others advising 2 days prior to treatment, for a duration of 5 days. Importantly, treatment should be withheld should a cold sore be present in or near the treatment site.

> **Injecting slowly, gently, with minimal filler volumes, good infection control measures and aspiration pre-injection are some of the key measures to reduce the risk of complications.**

6.10.2 Specific complications related to deep injection

The growing use of subcutaneous augmentation techniques to correct the causative deficiencies in the deep fat compartments makes it necessary to discuss the additional complications associated with these procedures. Inserting a needle into deeper tissue layers where larger blood vessels are located poses the risk of intravascular injury, which is associated with the risk of serious complications such as tissue necrosis and blindness (cf. p. 57). This can and should be avoided with the use of lower risk related injection techniques, described below.

When administering a deep vertical injection, it is imperative to advance the sharp-tip needle down to the bone slowly and in a controlled manner, accompanied by aspiration pre-injection. Furthermore, when planning horizontal injections, a cannula is an ideal injection tool as it reduces the risk of intravascular puncture compared to a needle. Importantly, the gauge of the cannula should be considered, as the thinner the cannula, the sharper the tip, and therefore can also act like a sharp needle. Cases of 27 gauge cannulas have been reported in medical literature to result in intravascular injection and for this reason we recommend larger bore cannulas (22 to 25 gauge) to be used in the vicinity of major blood vessels, when placing injections in deeper tissue planes, as well as when providing horizontal augmentation techniques.

However, in the unlikely event of accidental intravascular injection when using hyaluronic acid fillers in spite of proper technique, the following emergency treatment measures should be followed:

- Immediately infiltrate hyaluronidase (maximum dose, and depending on the injected volume of the filler) at the site of the suspected occlusion. Due to the increased vascular permeability, the hyaluronidase will reach the intravascular filler without having to be injected into the vessel.
- Keep the skin area warm (with warm compresses) coupled with the application of nitropaste to stimulate circulation and promote vasodilatation. NEVER apply ice or cold packs!
- Gently massage the area without applying too much pressure.
- If available, perform a radiological vascular investigation to try to locate the site of the occlusion.
- Send the patient to a medical facility where the blocked vessel can be re-opened (surgically, if necessary) as quickly as possible. Furthermore, consider the use of a hyperbaric oxygen chamber.

Caution should be taken to avoid intravascular injections of the filler by careful planning with regard to the safe injection plan, slow injection technique coupled with aspiration when using a needle, slow and gentle injection techniques, alongside the deposition of small volumes. Furthermore, cannulas are particularly useful in high risk zones and when performing deep injections.

6.10.3 Filler-specific complications

Resorbable fillers

Below we shall discuss some of the key complications with regard to the commonly used resorbable fillers in today's medical aesthetic market (see section 3.2, 'Filler Types', p. 57 onwards).

Hyaluronic acid is regarded as the most commonly used filler in the international arena today, due to its safety and efficacy profile. Because of the biological degradability of hyaluronic acid, many potential complications associated with it are also, on the whole, fully reversible. Below, we briefly consider some key complications worth noting, namely: intolerance and allergy, infection, lumps and irregularities, as well as filler migration.

With regard to intolerance or allergy, it is essential to screen all patients for any history of hyaluronic acid and lidocaine allergy or sensitivity. Intolerance or allergic reactions, including foreign body granulomas, rarely occur following the use of hyaluronic acid fillers, namely in about 0.42 % of cases. According to the manufacturers' information, prior skin testing of hyaluronic acid fillers for all patients is not necessary, but is still being discussion within the industry. However, if a patient is known to have an allergy to chicken egg albumin, only hyaluronic acid products obtained by fermentation in Streptococcal cultures should be used.

The issue of bovine spongiform encephalopathy (BSE) and prion infection needs to be kept in mind with all filler agents derived from animal origin. However, manufacturers guarantee strict controls have been applied to sourcing animals and assure that the fillers have been manufactured in ways that minimise the infection risk.

Sterile hyaluronic acid abscesses have rarely been observed; they heal without complication following a point incision to relieve the pressure and express the filler. These skin reactions can develop regardless of the origin of the filler (i.e. Streptococcal fermentation). In fact, these sorts of tissue reactions depend on several aspects, i.e. the cross-linking degree and technology, the cross-linker used as well as the concentration of the hyaluronic acid being incorporated.

Visible and palpable nodules and linear ridges can develop with hyaluronic acid fillers following superficial injections into the dermis, even when overcorrection is avoided. Depending on the viscosity and chemical modification (cross-linking) of the filler used, these irregularities can resolve on their own within a few hours to days without any further intervention. However, the patient should be advised to thoroughly massage the area should they notice these surface irregularities, and thereafter visit the practitioner should they not resolve soon after.

In volume augmentation with highly viscous cross-linked hyaluronic fillers, some migration of the filler can present a few days to weeks after the treatment. Even if this material is injected correctly into the desired subcutaneous or supraperiosteal planes, the substance still exhibits some movement in response to external manual pressure. As discussed previously, patients should be advised to avoid extremes of temperature and persistent pressure at the site of the injection for the 1 to 2 days and ideally 2 weeks post-treatment. Furthermore, particular care is needed to ensure that the filler is not injected in the undesired plane when the needle or cannula is being withdrawn, so as not to deposit filler in a superficial plane with the resultant visible nodule or Tyndall effect. Should this happen immediately after the injection, it is advisable to either squeeze or express the filler through a small hole created with a 21 G needle.

With regard to collagen fillers, although generally they are not used much these days, for those that still use them a number of considerations should be noted, namely: intolerance and allergy; discolouration; nodules and irregularities; and infection.

Given that lidocaine is added to bovine collagen fillers, all patients should be screened for lidocaine intolerance and allergy pre-treatment. Furthermore, all patients undergoing collagen treatments should receive a skin test. Around 3 to 4% of patients who are tested react positively to bovine collagen and therefore should not be treated with this filler. However, even if the test is negative, there is still the potential for sensitisation to the animal derived filler during the course of the treatment, which should always be considered. The probability of this is estimated to be around 1.5%. Furthermore, severe granulomas at the injection site can occur because of an antigen–antibody reaction, but are fully reversible after several months due to the biological degradability of the filler. Autologous human collagen and pooled human cadaveric collagen can be used even if the patient reacts positively to animal collagen products when tested.

The skin may take on a whitish discolouration due to the opalescent, whitish colour of the collagen fillers, particularly if the filler is injected too close to the skin surface. This impairs the aesthetic result for a prolonged period and reduces patient satisfaction.

Nodules, ridges or cord-like protuberances may be visible and palpable for a few hours to a few days post-treatment, particularly in the event of overcorrection, which in itself should be avoided. Thorough moulding massage immediately after the injection reduces these complications significantly.

Despite strict controls, the risk of viral or prior infection needs to be kept in mind when using collagen products of animal origin or pooled cadaveric collagen fillers.

Regarding poly-L-lactic acid (PLLA), given pre-mixing with lidocaine occurs, patients should be screened for intolerance or allergy to lidocaine and the filler itself pre-treatment. Key factors for a complication-free treatment include the proper reconstitution of the lyophilisate in the vials, ensuring that the suspension is homogenised as thoroughly as possible with a shaker immediately before the injection, and a correct injection technique coupled with thorough massage is performed. Although practitioners may have their own variants with regard to the dilution protocols used, this book's author Gerhard Sattler commonly uses: 10 ml of water for injections when injecting the face, and 20 ml of water for injections when injecting the body. Furthermore, the author also highlights that an optional 2 ml of a local anaesthetic can be added immediately before the injection.

This protocol ensures greater dilution of the filler substance. Maximum homogenisation of the suspension is achieved by leaving the suspension to rest for up to 48 hours following the addition of 5 or 20 ml of water for injections, and by shaking it repeatedly in each phase of the reconstitution. An incorrect injection technique, particularly a far too superficial injection into the dermis, as well as administering too much filler in one site can produce visible nodes and ridges, which are also palpable deep inside the skin. In a small percentage of cases, foreign body granulomas may develop in the treated areas even many months after the filler augmentation. These foreign body granulomas generally subside very slowly over several months, and tend to disappear completely with time. This process can be accelerated considerably with repeated intralesional administration of small amounts of a crystalline suspension of steroids, or a mixture of 5-fluorouracil and triamcinolone 10 mg/ml (9:1) every 2 to 6 weeks. Abscess-forming inflammations, perforation or migration of the substance into other tissues, and allergic reactions have not been observed to date.

Non-resorbable, permanent fillers

The use of non-resorbable, permanent fillers is not a subject of discussion in this book. The continuing development of appropriate resorbable alternatives with associated fewer side effects has rendered the use of permanent materials highly questionable from both the medical and aesthetic points of view.

The wish for a permanent soft tissue augmentation effect, as expressed by many patients, originally led to the emergence of non-resorbable, permanent fillers, such as polymethyl methacrylate (PMMA), hydroxy-ethyl methacrylate (HEMA), ethyl methacrylate (EMA), and polyacrylamide gel or liquid silicon (PMS 350).

Aside from their associated complications, permanent fillers also fail to adjust to the natural, individual ageing processes. A very prominent shape that becomes unnatural in later years, for example following lip volume augmentation, cannot be changed and ultimately will not fit harmoniously with the rest of the face. Hence, permanent augmentation in a youthful face may represent a complication in its own right many years later.

Today we are aware that the risk of serious complications with permanent fillers is higher than with the use of degradable substances, including the development of granulomatous foreign body reactions, abscess-forming inflammations, perforations, and the migration or dislocation of the filler implant in the tissues months or even years after they are injected.

With regard to foreign body granulomas a variety of treatment options are possible, and include some of the following:

- Surgical resection (achieves complete resolution but unfortunately is related to unsightly scars)
- Crystalline steroid suspension injections
- Oral allopurinal, with or without steroid cream application, fluorouracil and triaminolone 10 mg/ml (9:1) injections

With regard to liquid silicone, chronic inflammatory reactions and granulomatous foreign bodies are well known, presenting with erythema, swelling, induration, scarring and the formation of hard nodes in the treated tissue. These reactions can still occur years after the administration of silicone, and even with the correct injection techniques being used. Long-term complications and aesthetically unsatisfactory permanent effects typically result from an incorrect injection technique, e.g. the injection of excessive amounts, injecting the substance too superficially into the dermis, overcorrection of a line or a defect, vascular injury and embolisation. Lymph node enlargement in the relevant drainage zone can also occur, alongside life-threatening systemic reactions (acute pneumonia, granulomatous hepatitis), which have also been reported following the administration of large amounts of this filler. Many of the complications and side effects associated with the use of liquid silicon, PMS 350 (polydimethylsiloxane; viscosity 350 centistoke) are attributable primarily to its improper use.

Furthermore, a resorbable filler is often added to permanent injectable fillers as a lubricant to improve their injection properties. Collagen and hyaluronic acid are typical additives used with acrylic compounds, for example PMMA (e.g. Artecoll®). Of course, complications can also be triggered by these resorbable substances or by the addition of lidocaine to the collagen vehicle.

6.11 Post-treatment Advice

6.11.1 Dos and don'ts for the patient following augmentation treatment with hyaluronic acid fillers

The treatment area should be gently but thoroughly massaged immediately after completion of the treatment, to mould the filler to achieve a smooth plane. Some practitioners, including G. Sattler, also use antibiotic cream or ointment during the massage. Patients should be taught how to perform gentle focal moulding massage for the next couple of weeks post-treatment, should they encounter an irregularity. However, should irregularities persist for longer or be challenging to manage, patients are advised in advance to contact the practitioner immediately for further advice.

Immediately post-treatment, patients should be advised to avoid touching, exerting focal pressure and applying any topical preparations at the injection sites for a further 8 hours to avoid infection, and prevent migration of the filler from its placement site. Excessive exercise is also to be avoided for 8 hours to reduce the risk of bruising. If necessary, herpetic prophylaxis is to be initiated immediately after treatment. Otherwise, patients should be advised that they can resume their everyday and occupational activities. Cooling of the treated area can be performed in the case of swelling or a haematoma; however, as previously mentioned, extremes of temperature are to be avoided for the following 2 weeks post-treatment to ensure appropriate filler integration.

Furthermore, during the initial post-treatment period, the patient should be advised:

- Not to apply excessive pressure to the treatment area for 1 to 2 weeks post-treatment.
- To avoid excessive exercise giving rise to increased heat and sweating for 1 to 2 days post-treatment.
- To avoid exposure to excessive strong sunlight, heat (e.g. saunas, steam baths) and cold temperatures for 1 to 2 days post-treatment.
- To cautiously massage the injected area should an irregularity be noted within 1 to 2 weeks post-treatment, while making sure the risk of infection is minimised by ensuring clean conditions when massaging the skin. Otherwise, massage is not indicated when no irregularity is noted, and patients should be advised to avoid this so as not to inadvertently redistribute the filler.

7 Regional Applications

7 Regional Applications

7.1 Global Approach

For many years, aesthetic medicine has mainly focused on treating the obvious visual manifestations of ageing rather than the root causes themselves, primarily due to the lack of detailed anatomical knowledge. In recent years, advances in the understanding of atrophy-related tissue volume loss and the beneficial volume compensating effects achieved with hyaluronic acid filler injections has allowed for a more complete rejuvenation and augmentation approach.

> **Evidence from clinical studies showing that hyaluronic acid fillers achieve predictable and reproducible results has confirmed the new hypothesis that the initial signs of facial ageing respond well to reversible and thus minimally invasive treatments.**

According to current knowledge, the following factors are responsible for the appearance of the visible signs of ageing in the face:
- Degenerative changes in the skin and connective tissues (i.e. elastosis, fibrosis)
- Loss of skin tone and elasticity in the overall tissue complex due to the effects of ligament laxity
- Decreased supply of fluids and nutrients to the skin and the subcutaneous tissues
- Atrophic volume loss in the deep fat pads (which act as biomechanical support structures to the overlying skin envelope)
- Descent of the destabilised soft tissues and the skin due to the effects of gravity
- Hypertonia and volume loss of the muscles of facial expression
- Shift in the balance of power between the depressor and elevator muscles, in favour of the depressor muscles

Volume augmentation with hyaluronic acid fillers plays a key role in counteracting the age-related atrophic changes in the face with a holistic and global approach.

> **Treatments designed to restore aesthetic harmony, especially in the facial region, should consider the following four key considerations of aesthetic harmony:**
> - **Assessment of the age-related changes**
> - **Three-dimensional assessment of the anatomical structures**
> - **Assessment of the dynamics of the tissues (driven by muscular activity)**
> - **Assessment of the patient's psychological levels relating to motivation and compliance with the proposed treatment**

A variety of injection techniques are discussed in this chapter to manage specific indications with the aim of achieving safe and effective treatment outcomes, while addressing the four key considerations of aesthetic harmony (see box above). In the following section, we present a strategic approach to filler injections, which allows for satisfactory and reproducible results. However, we appreciate that there are alternative methods with equally satisfactory clinical outcomes.

Filler injections not only allow for an immediate visible lifting and volumising effect due to the gel's viscoelastic properties, but we should also bear in mind the fibrogenetic (related to the mechanical mobilisation effects, especially when using cannulas) and fluid-related effects of hyaluronic acid fillers. Therefore, in this book we shall refer to such treatments as 'Minimally Invasive Augmentation Surgery' (MIAS).

The next section outlines the key strategies of the MIAS approach. Detailed descriptions of the treatment techniques (both conventional and innovative) and filler options suited for a variety of facial indications are discussed below.

> **The key principle to adhere to when attempting to restore facial harmony and enhance attractiveness with filler augmentation is to minimise the damage to the natural tissue structures. As previously mentioned, the aim of such treatments is to treat the root cause of the age-related defects while respecting the anatomy. Furthermore, the aim of the treatment should also be to use the least volume of filler possible to achieve the desired outcomes, and in a manner that optimises biological tissue regeneration. Hence, choosing the correct filler is also a vital element to ensuring successful clinical outcomes.**

7.1.1 Treatment goals and procedures of MIAS

Minimally Invasive Augmentation Surgery (MIAS) is a holistic approach to restoring facial harmony at the physiological, anatomical and clinical level. It encompasses five practical techniques, which can be used together where appropriate and applied at different planes of the tissue complex, depending on the objectives of the treatment (see Tab. 7.1, p. 126). They include:

I **Superficial Augmentation Techniques (SAT):** These entail the older or 'classic' methods of concealment or camouflage of volume deficits of various degrees of severity.

II **Vertical Augmentation Techniques (VAT):** Methods used for focal compensation of defects in the deep fat compartments.

III **Deep Horizontal Augmentation with a Cannula (DHAC):** Methods used for overall improvement of larger surface areas and in regions with high dynamic muscular activity associated with soft tissue atrophy.

IV **Skin Surface Regenerating Augmentation (SSRA):** Methods used for rehydration and revitalisation of the skin surface.

V **Deep Mesotherapy:** Methods used to increase the supply of fluids and nutrients to the atrophic subcutaneous tissues.

Treatment entailing the use of the five therapeutic techniques allows for optimal rejuvenation of all of the tissue planes, and represents maximum utilisation of the different hyaluronic acid fillers. The following sections in this chapter discuss a variety of indications and suitable techniques, as well as suitable filler agents. However, it is ultimately up to the practitioner to select the optimal technique in accordance with the clinical findings, the patient's wishes, and one's practical experience.

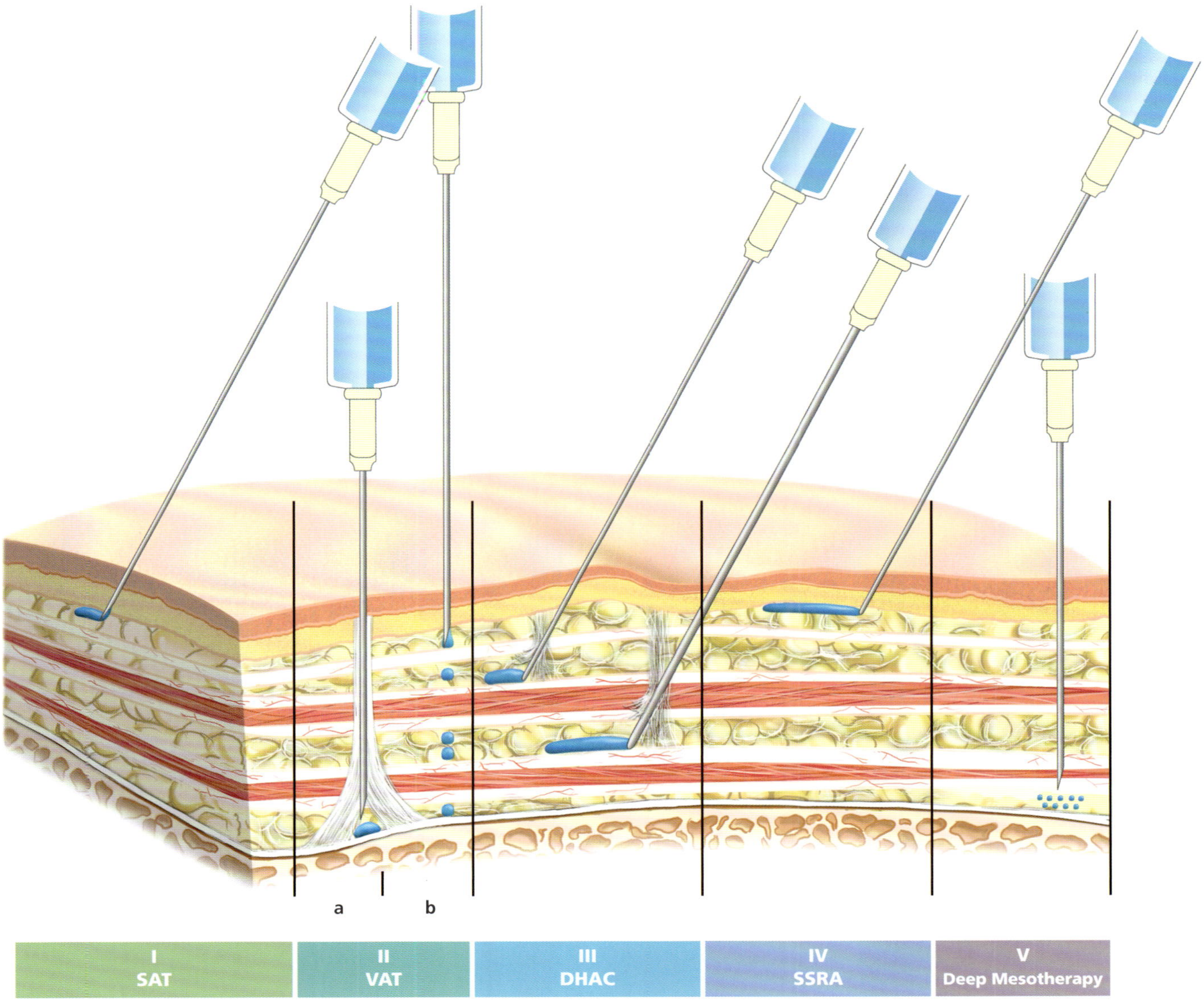

Fig. 7.1 Five techniques of MIAS according to Sattler: I Superficial Augmentation Techniques (SAT) for decorative concealment or camouflage; II Vertical Augmentation Techniques (VAT) for targeted focal compensation of volume defects; III Deep Horizontal Augmentation with a Cannula (DHAC) for large-scale volume augmentation; IV Skin Surface Regenerating Augmentation (SSRA) techniques; V Deep Mesotherapy.

Treatment goals and procedures of Minimally Invasive Augmentation Surgery (MIAS)				
Procedure	**Depth of injection**	**Injection techniques**	**Suitable filler products** (see section 3.3, 'Filler Navigator', p. 60 ff.)	**Clinical indications and objectives**
I **Superficial Augmentation Techniques (SAT)** 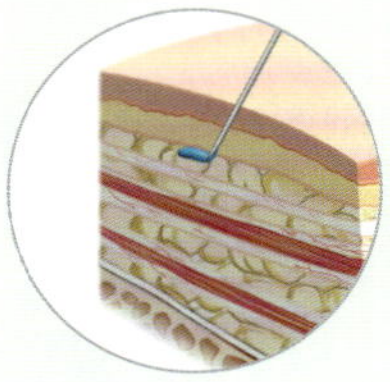	• Dermal • Subdermal • Subcutaneous	• Tunneling technique • Spot technique • Fanning technique • Criss-cross technique • Vibrating technique • Sandwich technique	1, 2	• Correction of fine wrinkles • Decorative concealment of the various signs of ageing due to soft tissue atrophy (particularly due to elastosis) • Precise and detailed contouring
II **Vertical Augmentation Techniques (VAT)** 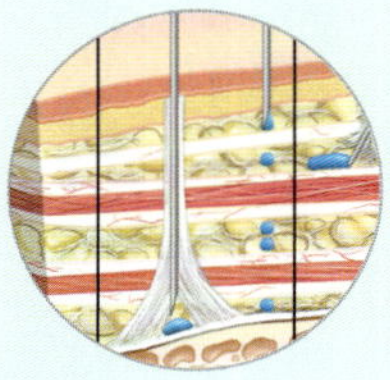	• Supraperiosteal • Supramucosal • Through all the planes of the tissue complex (with filler depots stacked one on top of each other)	• IIa Vertical Supraperiosteal Depot Technique (VSDT) • IIb Tower technique	3, 4	• Correction of deep wrinkles • Tissue projection • Contouring • Severe volume loss correction • Volume augmentation of the deeper structures
III **Deep Horizontal Augmentation with a Cannula (DHAC)** 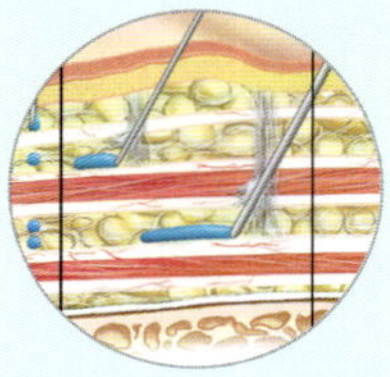	• Subcutaneous • Supraperiosteal • Supramucosal	• Deep Horizontal Augmentation with a Cannula (DHAC) • Windmill technique	2, 3, 4	• Large-scale volume projection • Medium and deep wrinkle correction • Anatomic release of adherent structures • Activation of fibrogenesis • Correction of the muscle-related signs of ageing
IV **Skin Surface Regenerating Augmentation (SSRA)** 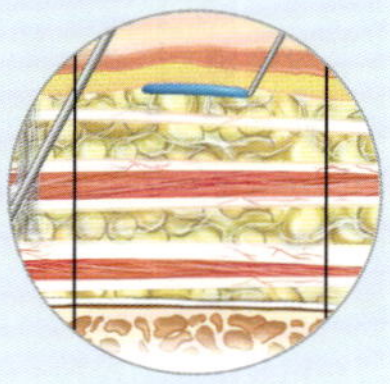	• Intradermal • Subdermal	• Superficial Horizontal Augmentation with a Cannula (SHAC) • Serial puncture technique • Criss-cross technique	1, A, B	• Improvement of skin texture • Skin surface rehydration and homogenisation • Correction of skin surface defects • Improvement of advanced skin ageing
V **Deep Mesotherapy** 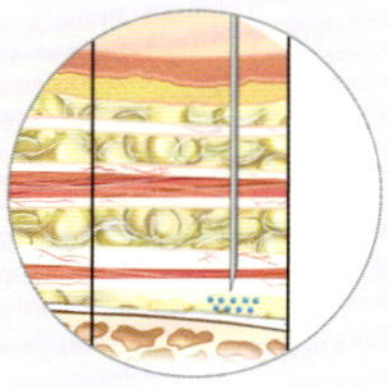	• Supraperiosteal • Supramucosal	Serial VSDT	A	Improving the supply of fluids and nutrients to the deep tissues (to achieve global improvement in tissue quality)

Tab. 7.1 Overview of Minimally Invasive Augmentation Surgery (MIAS) as proposed by Sattler et al, enabling the achievement of a holistic and causal augmentation treatment approach.

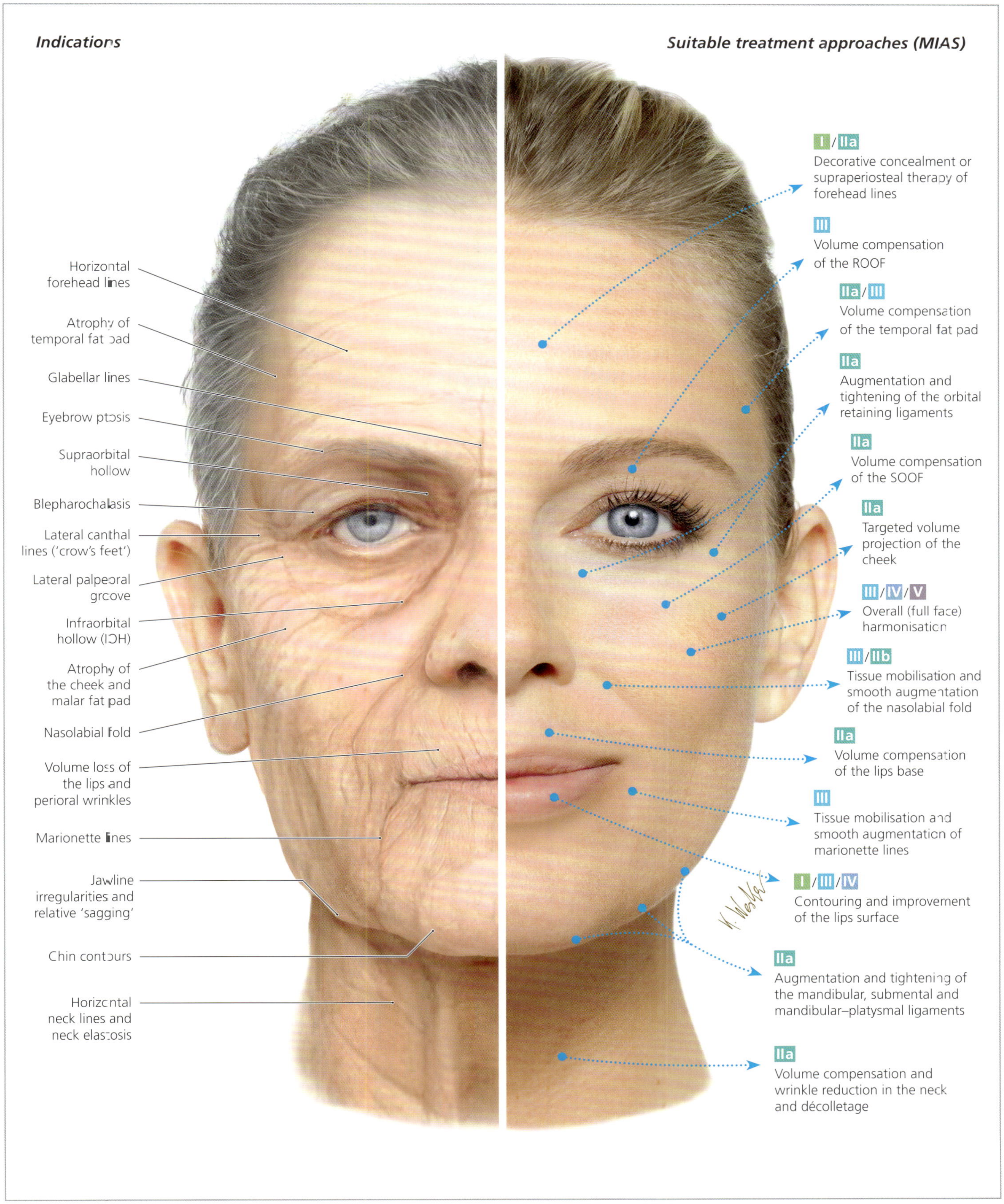

Fig. 7.2 Overview of the clinical indications and practical approaches of MIAS.

I Superficial Augmentation Techniques (SAT)

Indications

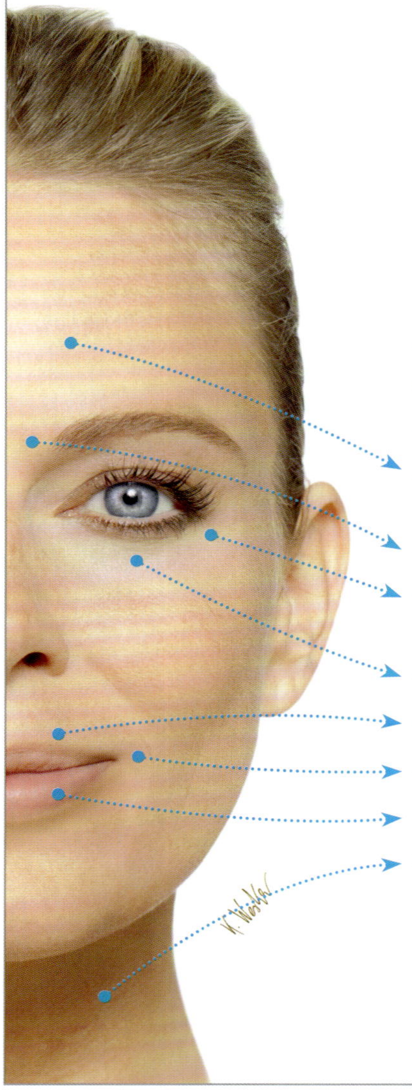

Treatment indications/ areas:

- Skin surface defects
- Fine lines on the forehead
- Mild glabellar lines
- Fine periorbital and lateral canthal wrinkles
- Lower eyelid wrinkles
- Fine perioral wrinkles
- Corners of the mouth
- Lips
- Neck lines

Treatment

Depth of injection: intradermal; subdermal; superficial subcutis

Injection techniques: Linear tunneling technique; Spot technique; Fanning technique; Criss-cross technique; Vibrating technique; Sandwich technique

Filler choice: 1 (p. 62), 2 (p. 63)

Tool: 30 gauge needle

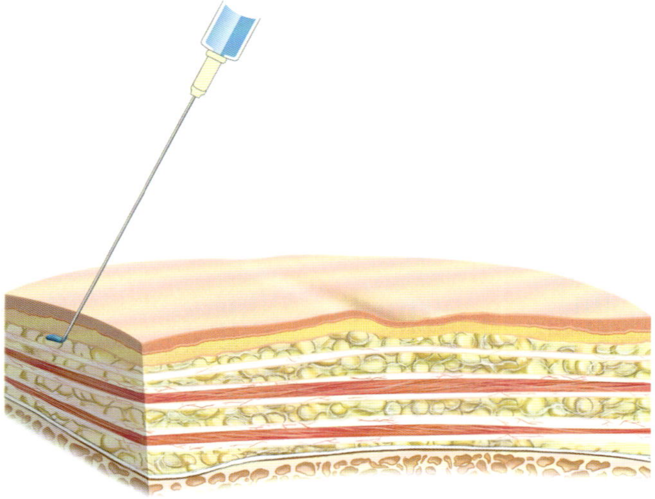

I
OAT

Treatment objectives

- Improvement of the skin texture
- Correction of fine lines and wrinkles caused by elastosis
- Decorative concealment or camouflage of the surface deficits of variable severity without treatment of the deeper structures (considered as the causal or trigger factors)
- Smoothing and detailed contouring of the skin surface relief
- Saturation of the subcutaneous supporting layer
- Enhancement after deeper treatment of the causal ageing factors (e.g. post deep volume compensation due to fat pad atrophy or post botulinum toxin type-A injections in dynamic wrinkles)

Post-treatment outcomes

Primary clinical improvement: Initial improvement occurs immediately post-injection due to the 'plumping' effect within the superficial tissues. The maximum effect is observed between 2 and 3 weeks post-treatment.

Secondary effects of the treatment: Secondary biological regeneration of the skin surface can be expected as a result of the improvement of the dermal and subdermal fluid conditions. Within 2 to 5 months of treatment, the integration of the filler material can be considered virtually complete.

Transient side effects: Puncture-related swelling, inflammation and bruising (ecchymosis) at the injection site may last up to 5 days post-treatment.

II Vertical Augmentation Techniques (VAT)

Indications

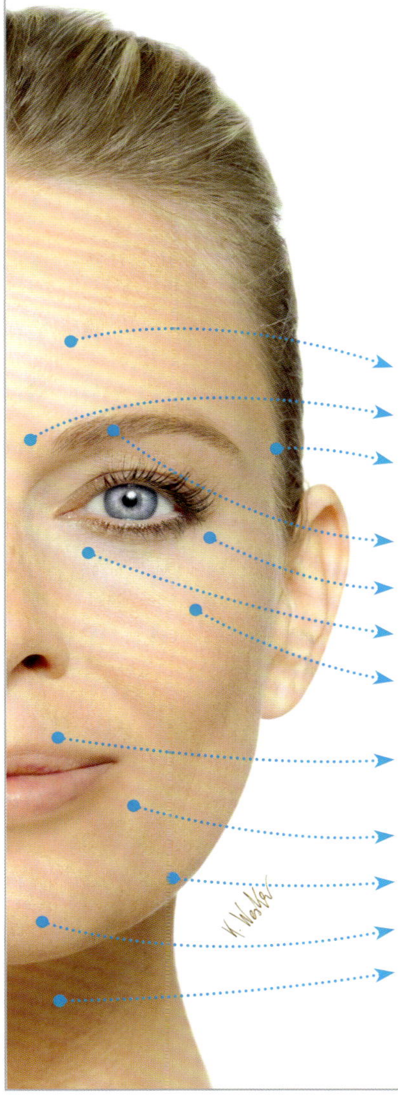

Treatment indications/ areas::

- Deep forehead wrinkles
- Deep glabellar lines
- Atrophy of the temporal fat pad
- Eyebrow ptosis
- Lateral canthal wrinkles
- Infraorbital hollow
- Malar fat pad and bucco-maxillary ligament
- Lip atrophy and perioral wrinkles
- Marionette lines
- Jawline contour
- Chin atrophy and contour
- Neck/décolletage

Treatment

Depth of injection: supraperiosteal or supramucosal injection into the 'hot spots' of the target atrophic structure, either as a single depot injection (VSDT) or as multiple 'stacked' depot injection extending from the underlying supraperiosteal or supramucosal base up to the dermal plexus (tower technique [TT])

Injection techniques: Vertical depot or tower technique

Filler choice: 3 (p. 66), 4 (p. 67)

Tool: 21–27 gauge needle

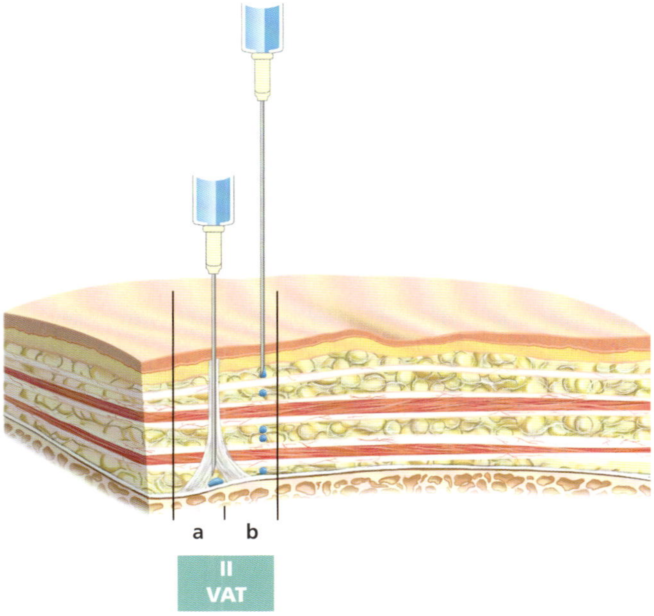

Treatment objectives

- Compensation for the underlying deep fat loss (trigger factor)
- Targeted focal tissue projection with the least amount of filler required
- Restoration of the ligament's tensile strength in order to stabilise and augment the soft tissues

Post-treatment outcomes

Primary clinical improvement: When the filler is correctly placed in the 'hot spots', the projection and 'plumping' effect can be observed immediately within the target tissues. The optimal clinical harmonising outcome is observed between 2 and 3 weeks post-treatment.

Secondary effects of the treatment: Particularly with the tower technique (TT), augmentation treatments improve the water-binding capacity of the underlying soft tissues. This results in the secondary biological regeneration of the fluid-dependent conditions in the global tissue complex. Within 2 to 5 months post-treatment, the integration of the filler can be considered virtually complete.

Transient side effects: The most common are transient injection-related sequelae (see p. 57), such as swelling and ecchymosis at the injection site and generally subside within 5 days post-treatment. Vertical insertion of the needle down to the bone or mucosa, in a slow and gentle manner with the patient's cooperation, alongside aspiration, reduced the risks of vascular trauma and intravascular injection.

III Deep Horizontal Augmentation with a Cannula (DHAC)

Indications

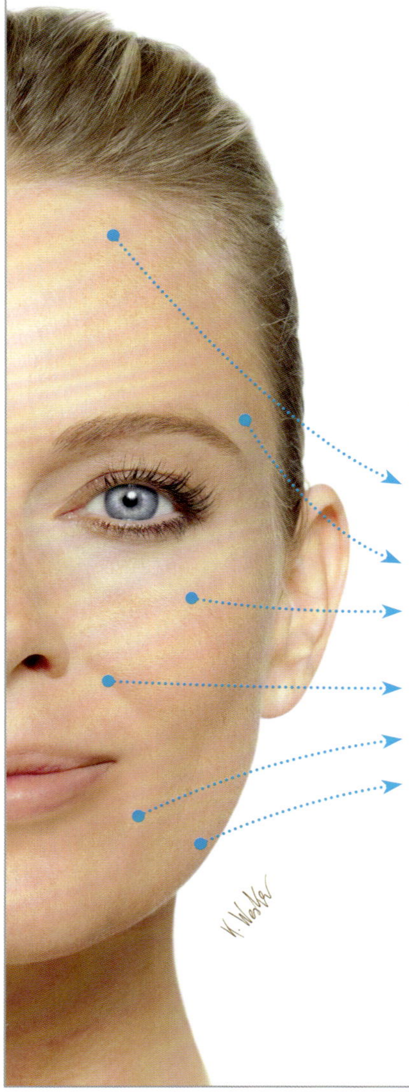

Treatment indications/ areas:

- Atrophy of the forehead and forehead lines
- Temporal atrophy
- Overall volume loss and elastosis
- Nasolabial fold
- Marionette lines
- Jawline contour

Treatment

Depth of injection: subcutaneous; submuscular; supramucosal; supraperiosteal

Injection techniques: DHAC; windmill technique

Filler choice: 3 (p. 66), 4 (p. 67), B (p. 70)

Tool: 22–25 gauge cannula

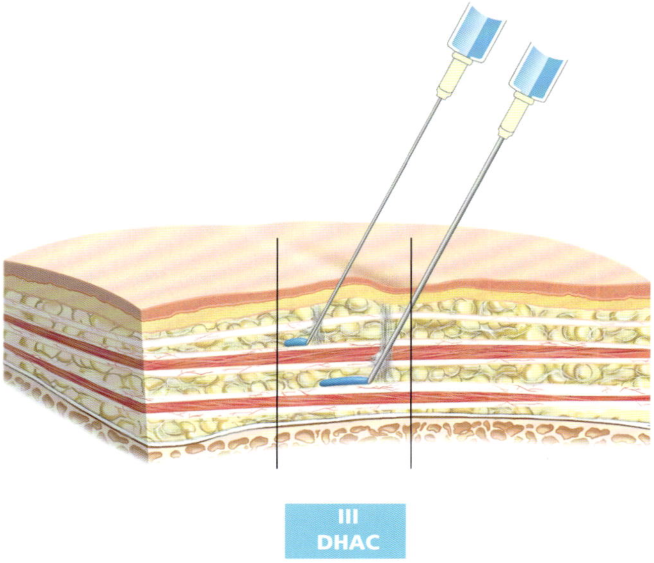

Treatment objectives

- To improve the skin surface quality and treat superficial skin defects
- To saturate the subdermal tissues supporting the skin
- To increase the supply of nutrients to the skin and to improve the epidermal barrier function
- To enhance the physiological and clinical features of the skin (degree of hydration, suppleness and complexion)

Post-treatment outcomes

Primary clinical improvement: Depending on the target structure and the depth of injection, clinical improvement can be observed on the whole immediately after tissue mobilisation. Thereafter, the practitioner can decide whether further filler injections will be necessary, e.g. to allow for a vertical projection effect. The maximum degree of harmonisation is generally observed between 2 and 3 weeks post-treatment.

Secondary effects of the treatment: Augmentation using cannulas allows for improvement in skin hydration, regeneration and activation of fibrogenesis. Within 2 to 5 months post-treatment, the integration of the filler can be considered virtually complete.

Transient side effects: The most common transient sequelae post-injection (see p. 57), such as swelling and ecchymosis at the injection site generally subside within 5 days post-treatment. The use of a large bore cannula (22 gauge) alongside gentle and slow manipulation of the tissues enables reduction in the risk of vascular trauma.

IV Skin Surface Regenerating Augmentation (SSRA)

Indications

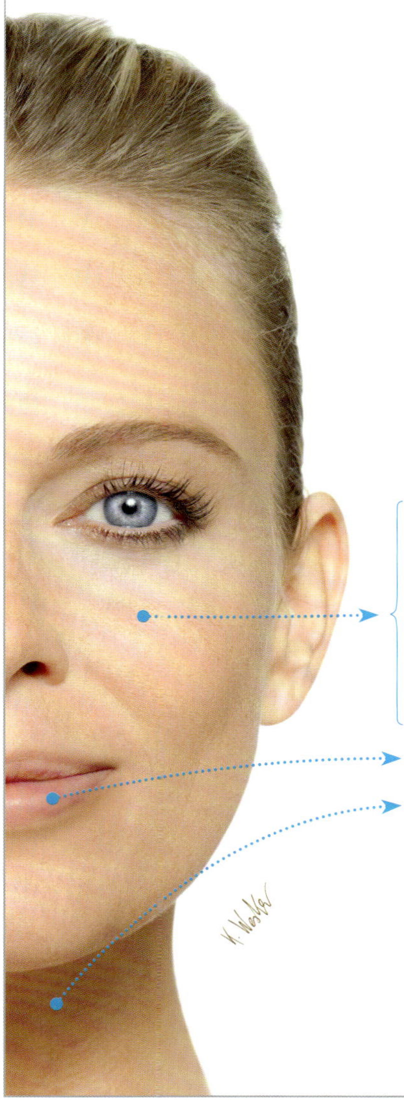

Treatment indications/ areas:

- Overall improvement of skin texture and glow
- Diverse skin defects due to photodamage, stress and ageing e.g.: skin dryness, poor blood supply, elastosis
- Lip surface
- Neck and décolletage
- Hands

Treatment

Depth of injection: intradermal; subdermal

Injection techniques: SHAC; Serial puncture; Criss-cross technique

Filler choice: 1 (p. 62), A (p. 69), B (p. 70)

Tool: 30–32 gauge needle; 27 gauge cannula (SHAC)

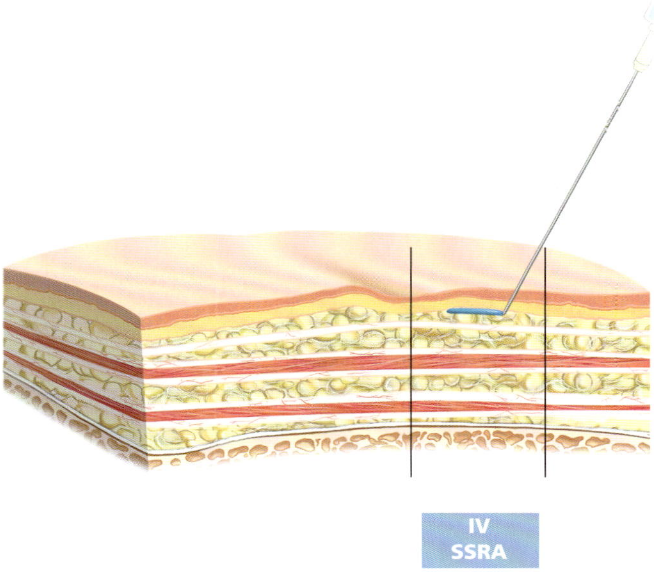

Treatment objectives

- To improve the skin surface quality and treat superficial skin defects
- To saturate the subdermal tissues supporting the skin
- To increase the supply of nutrients to the skin and to improve the epidermal barrier function
- To enhance the physiological and clinical features of the skin (degree of hydration, suppleness and complexion)

Post-treatment outcomes

Primary clinical improvement: Mild superficial enhancement may be observed immediately post-injection. The skin regenerating effects generally become apparent between 2 and 3 weeks post-treatment.

Secondary effects of the treatment: Secondary effects include tissue regeneration, hydration and activation of fibrogenesis, neocollagenesis and neoelastogenesis (depending on the technique used). In turn the skin quality and texture appears improved, and prevention of further skin ageing can be expected subsequent to the primary effects described above.

Transient side effects: The most common transient sequelae post-injection (see p. 57), such as swelling and ecchymosis at the injection site generally subside within 5 days post-treatment. In the context of fibroblast activation, the formation of small haematomas at the puncture sites is even considered by some to be desirable.

V Deep Mesotherapy

Indications

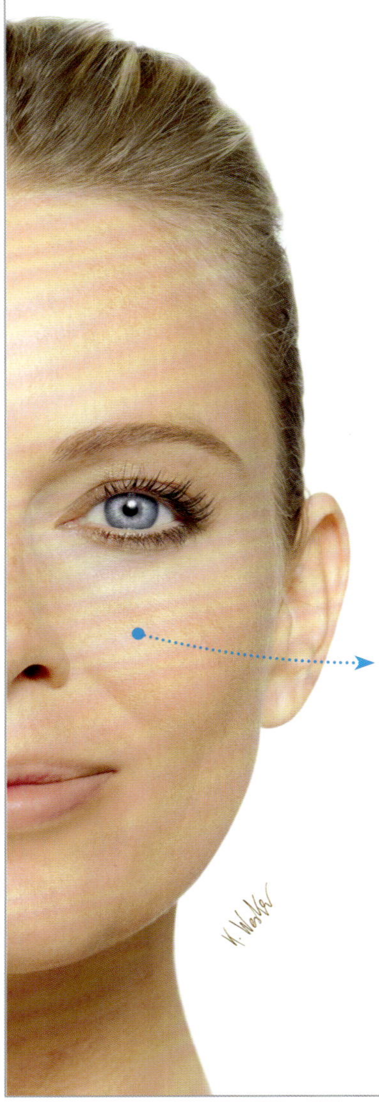

Treatment indications/ areas:

- Overall improvement of volume proportions, skin texture and glow
- Diverse skin defects due to photodamage, stress and ageing, e.g. skin dryness, poor blood supply, elastosis
- Proportional harmonisation of the full face

Treatment

Depth of injection: supraperiosteal; supramucosal

Injection techniques: serial VSDT

Filler choice: 1 (p. 62), A (p. 69)

Tool: 27 gauge needle

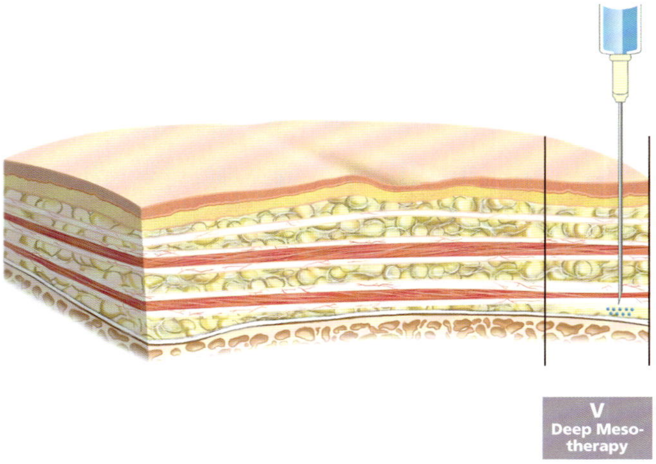

Treatment objectives
- Fluid and physiological support to the atrophic underlying soft tissues
- Natural tissue regeneration
- Slight lifting effect

Post-treatment outcomes
Primary clinical improvement: A slight lifting effect can generally be observed immediately post-treatment. The effects of the skin regeneration mechanisms usually become apparent a few weeks post-treatment.

Secondary effects of the treatment: Skin hydration and fibroblast-dependent tissue regeneration can be viewed as the primary intention of deep mesotherapy. These processes require several months to set in.

Transient side effects: The most common transient sequelae post-injection (see p. 57), such as swelling and ecchymosis at the injection site, generally subside within 5 days post-treatment. Gentle, slow, vertical injections onto the bone are recommended to reduce the risks of vascular trauma and intravascular injection.

7.2 Forehead Region

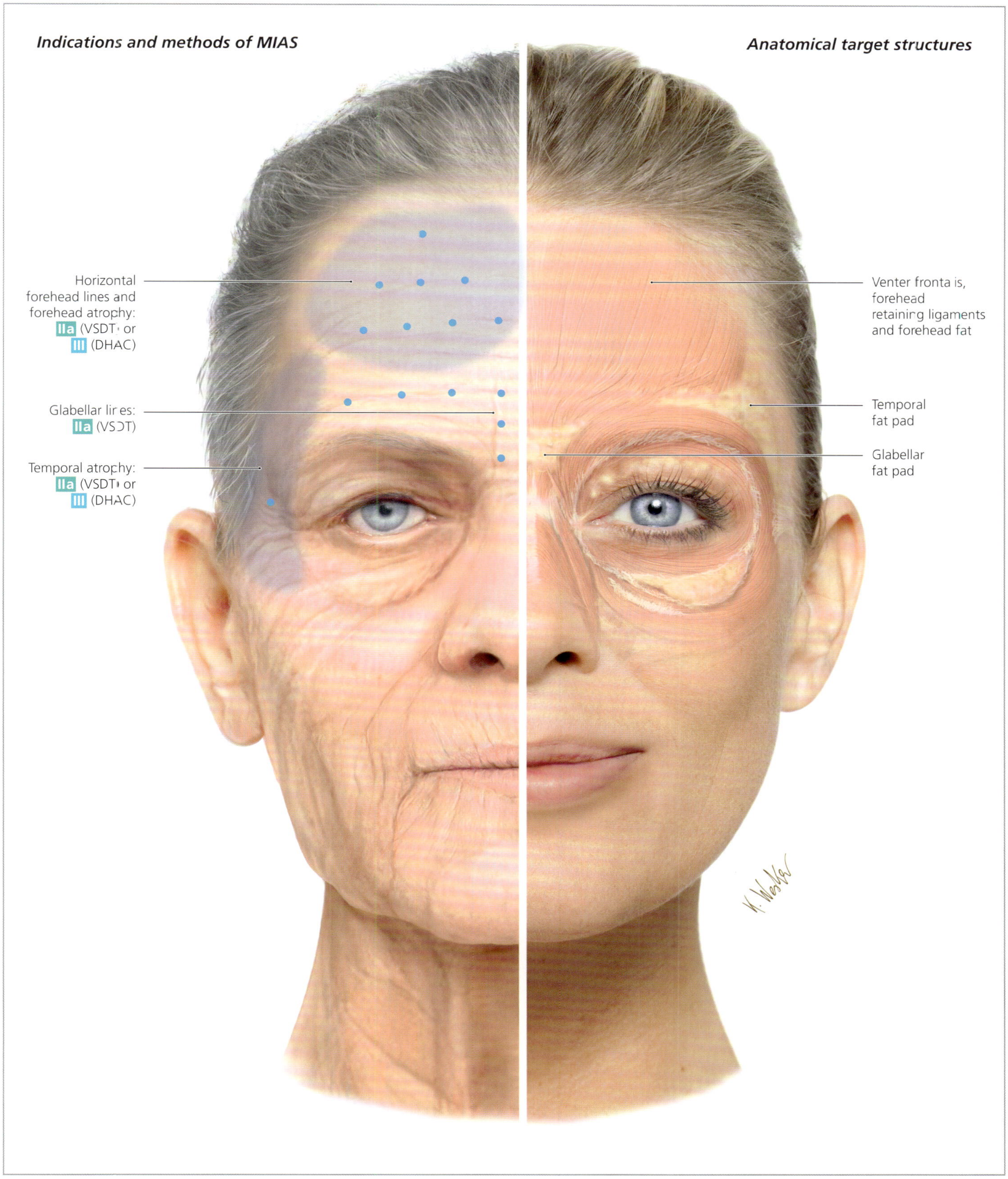

Fig. 7.3 Overview of the target treatment areas and recommended treatment techniques.
• VSDT (or, alternatively, SAT for camouflage purposes); DHAC.

7.2.1 Horizontal lines and volume loss of the forehead

The horizontal forehead lines are a common aesthetic concern particularly for female patients, predominantly when they are visible at rest and when they run deep. These lines arise due to the contraction of the frontal belly of the epicranius muscle, and are typically associated with emotions associated with being surprised. Furthermore, natural ageing processes alongside photodamage lead to elastotic changes in the skin, and manifest as a reduction in the skin's resilience and elasticity, which in turn results in static forehead wrinkles.

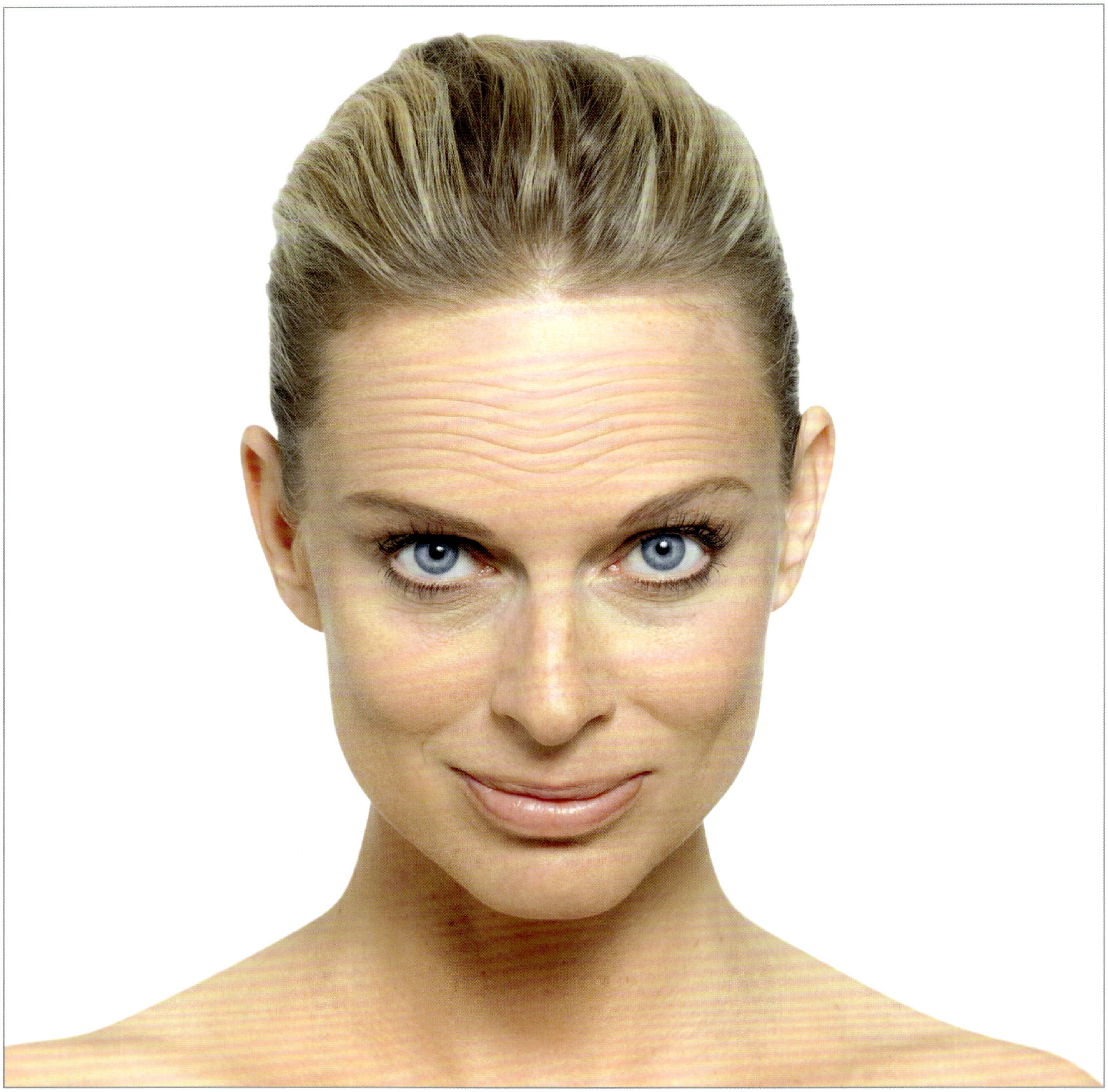

Patient selection/assessing the indication

Horizontal lines which are elicited upon muscle contraction (i.e. dynamically), and which the patient perceives as unsightly, can best be treated with chemical denervation using botulinum toxin type-A. Fine horizontal lines that persist at rest (i.e. are static) are best managed with filler augmentation. Vertical injections into the forehead ligaments also allow for a more general volumising effect in this region, and as a result achieve compensation for the age-related volumes loss.

Combined botulinum toxin treatment and filler augmentation is often jointly recommended.

Anatomy

The occipitofrontalis muscle and the temporoparietal muscle are referred to jointly as the epicranius muscle. The epicranius upon contraction raises the eyebrows, producing horizontal lines across the forehead.

There are no deep fat pads located below the epicranius muscle. The superficial fat layer is minimal, particularly on the lateral aspect of the forehead.

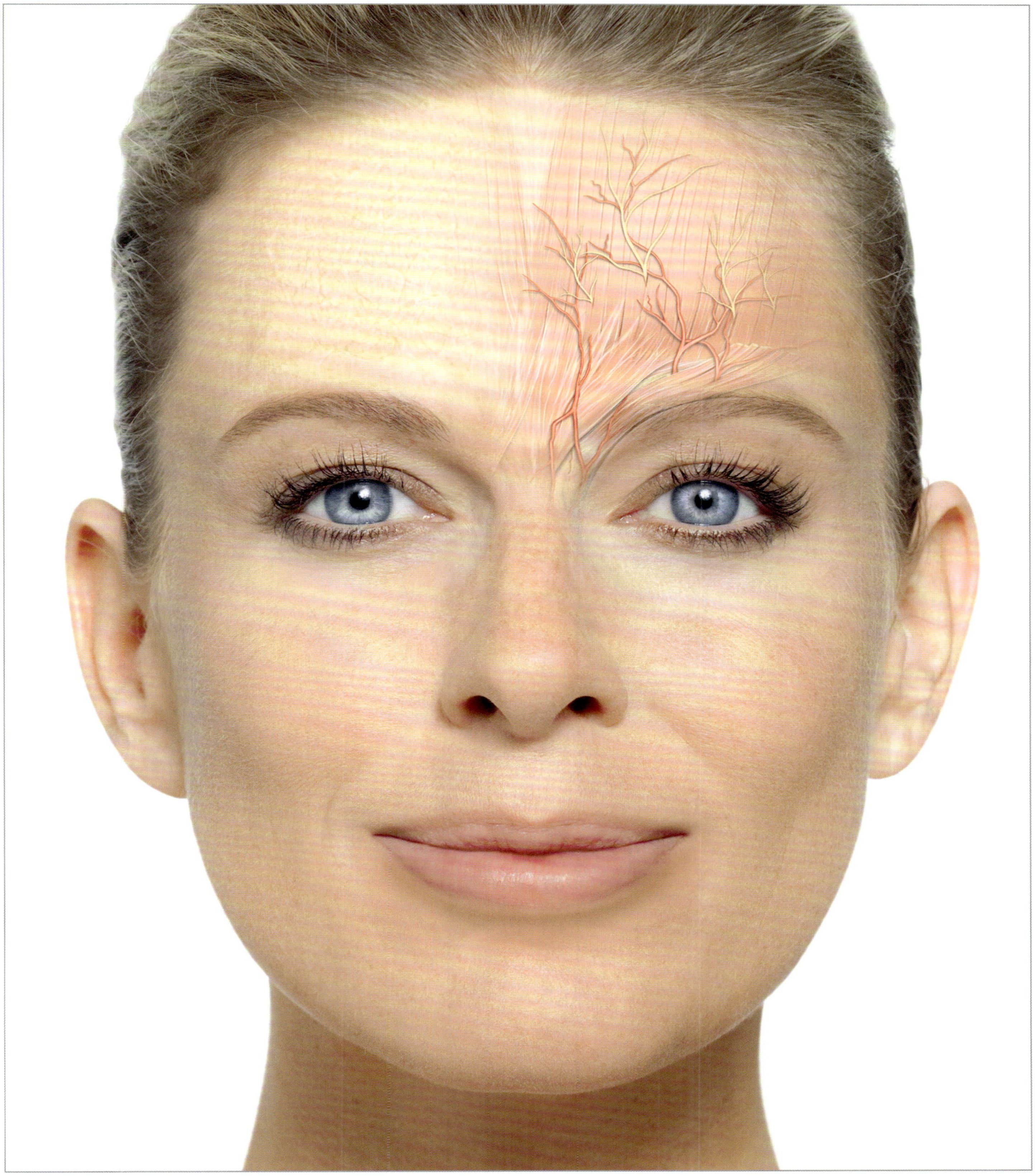

Treatment planning – Superficial wrinkle correction
Superficial filler augmentation techniques on the forehead allow the smoothing out of the fine horizontal lines on the forehead that persist when the face is at rest. Optimal treatment outcomes are achieved when a combination approach is used with botulinum toxin type-A in the forehead and the glabella.

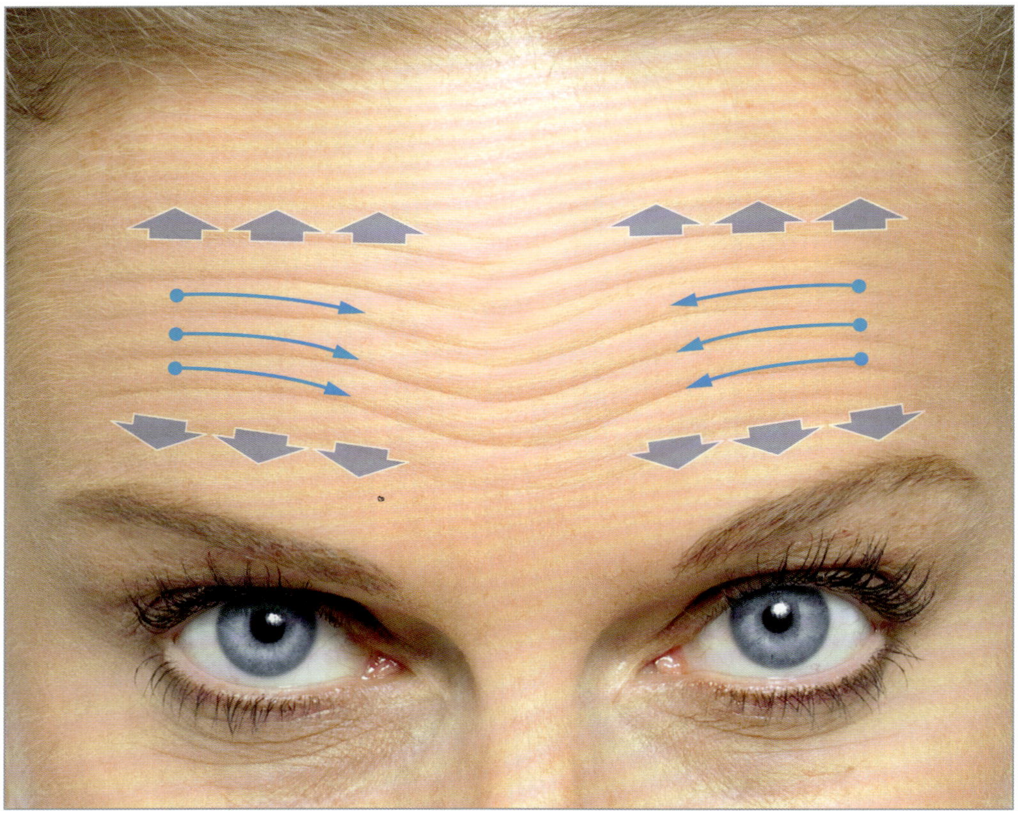

Technique: linear technique; stretching technique
Injection sites: one to two points per line
Depth: intradermal

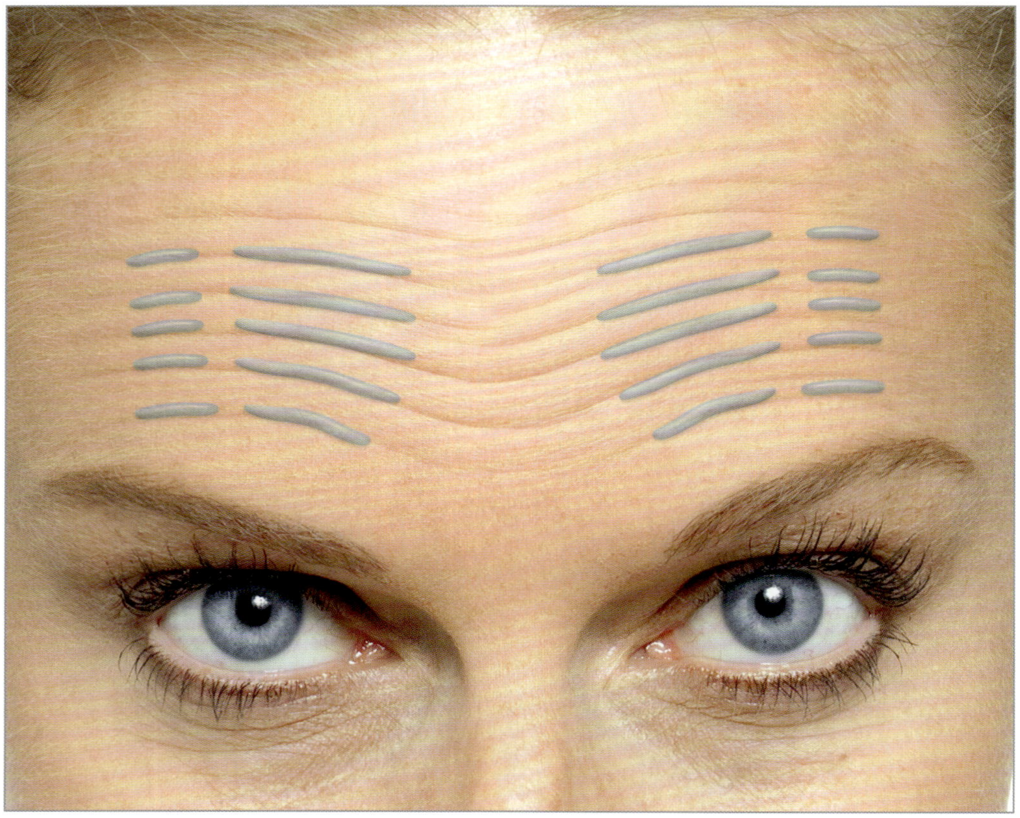

Volume: 0.01–0.02 ml/injection
Tool: 30 gauge needle

Treatment – Superficial wrinkle correction

Linear technique/stretching technique

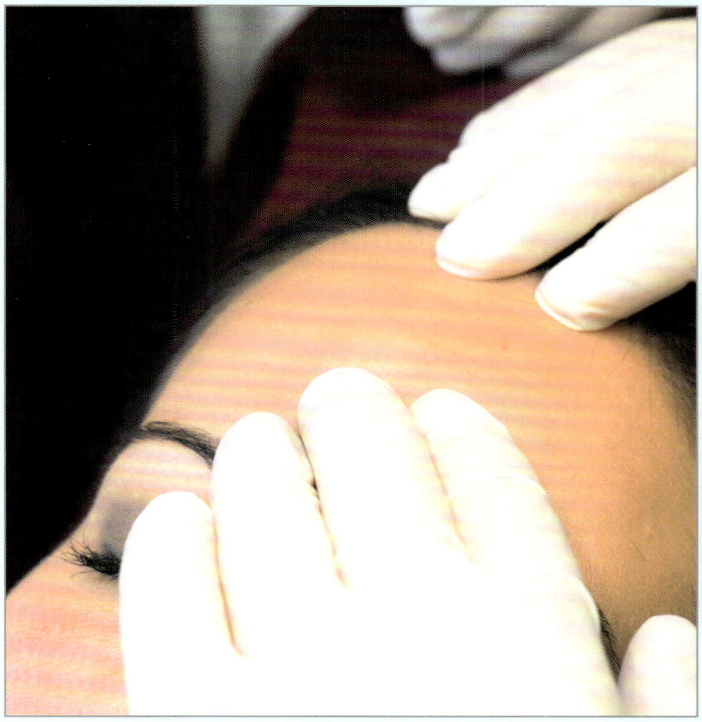

Fig. 7.4 The assistant stretches the skin optimally at right angles to the lines and holds it steady during the injections.

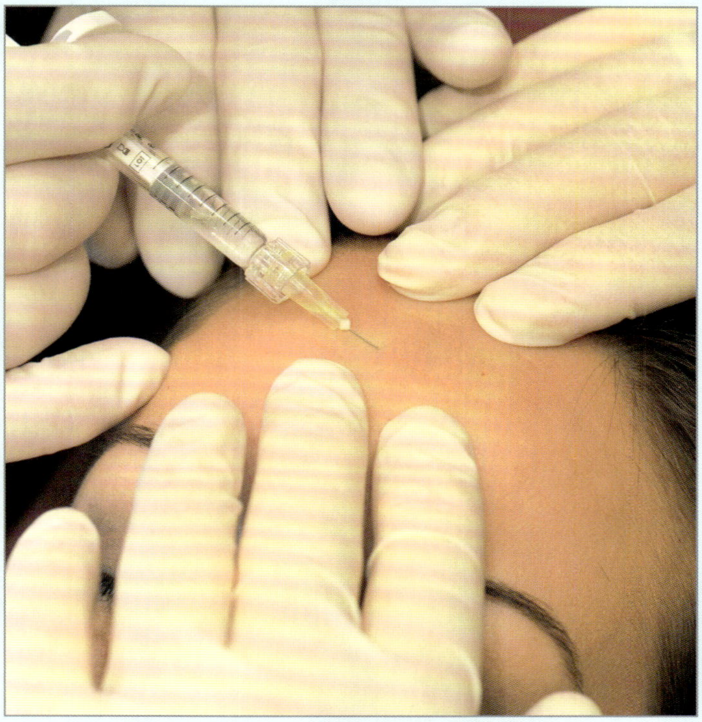

Fig. 7.5 Using the linear technique, the needle is inserted superficially and advanced along the course of the line. The filler is injected as the needle is being withdrawn. Administration of the filler leads to clearly visible skin blanching at the injection sites. This blanching effect should be distinguished from the whitening effect produced when the skin is held at maximum stretch.

Treatment steps

- Remove makeup
- Disinfection
- Anaesthesia (optional)
- Injection: linear technique/stretching technique
- Massage and mould (ensure appropriate distribution of the filler)
- Inform patient about post-treatment dos and don'ts
- Arrange a follow-up appointment

Practical tip

Dynamically produced forehead and frown lines should be treated before filler augmentation with chemical denervation using botulinum toxin type-A in the relevant muscles.

Filler selection

1 Superficial injection (p. 62)

2 Medium injection (p. 63)

Combined treatment options

In cases of dynamic forehead wrinkles, chemical denervation of the forehead and the glabella is recommended 1 to 2 weeks before filler augmentation.

Complications/Managing complications

- Overcorrection in the thicker forehead skin should be avoided at all times, and the stretching technique is useful in that respect.
- Palpable nodules may form due to the aggregation of the filler used. Thorough massage and moulding of the injected filler directly after the treatment ensures uniform distribution.

Treatment planning – Volume correction of the forehead
Volumising filler treatments in the forehead allow to compensate for the profound volume loss, and simultaneously smooth out the static forehead wrinkles. This treatment involves either focal vertical depots into the ligaments, along the skin folds, with a needle or horizontal cannula augmentation techniques.

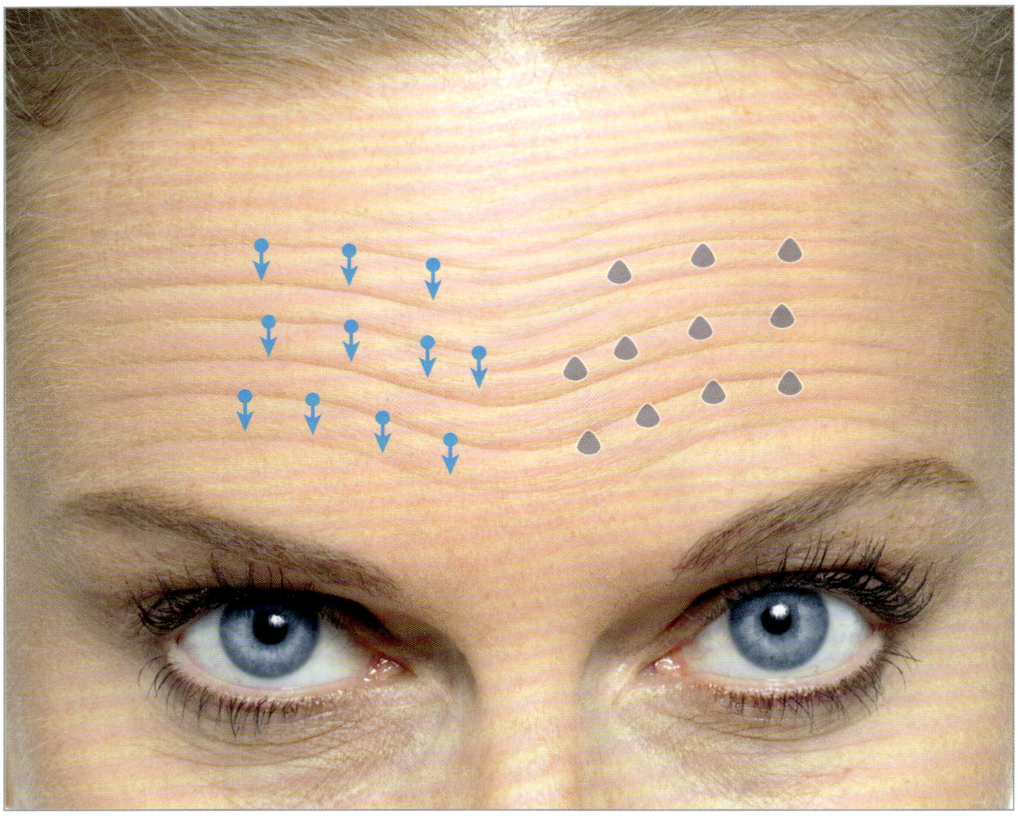

Technique: VSDT
Injection sites: three to four injection sites or 'hot spots' per line; approximately 30 injection sites in total in the forehead
Depth: supraperiosteal
Volume: 0.02–0.05 ml/point; approximately 1 ml in total for the forehead
Tool: 27 gauge needle

Caution: Injections should be done carefully and under close continuous monitoring of the augmentation effect to avoid overcorrection. The injected filler needs to be thoroughly massaged in and distributed immediately post-treatment.

Video: Forehead VSDT
http://www.kvm-tv.de/FIL/007.mp4

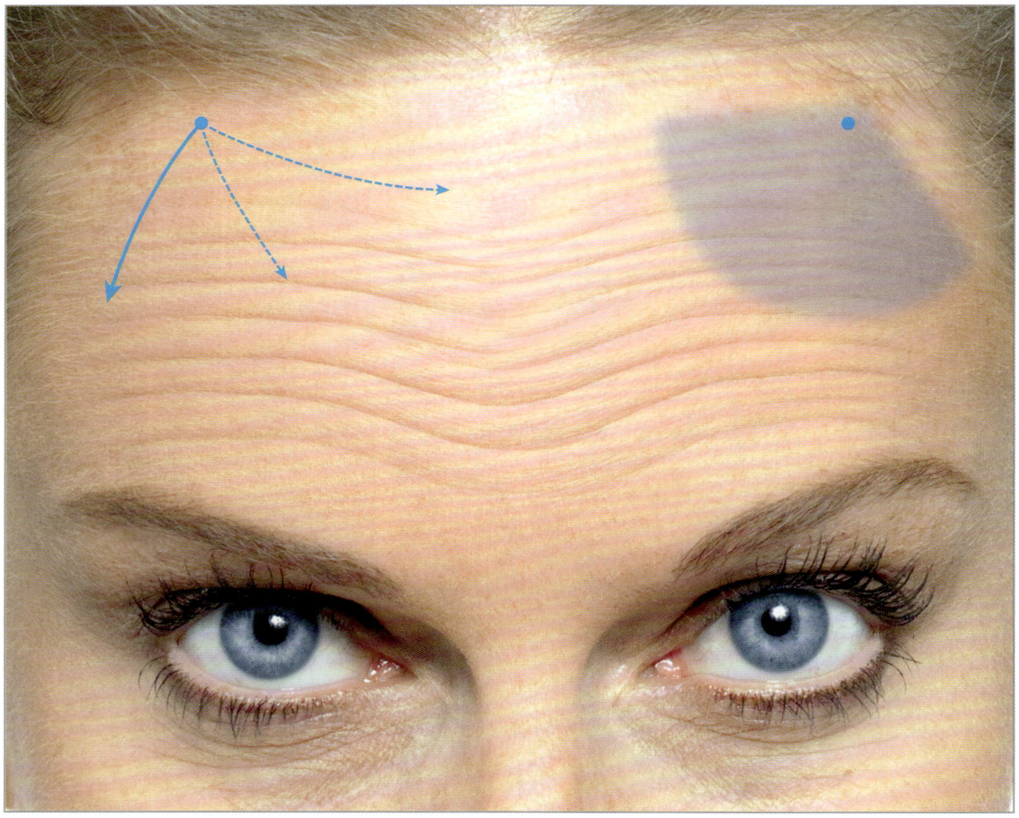

Technique: DHAC
Insertion site: close to the hairline in the lateral third of the forehead
Volume: 0.2–0.5 ml/side
Depth and direction: subcutaneous, in a fan-like fashion from the hairline radiating inferiorly
Tool: 22 gauge cannula

Caution: Horizontal wrinkles running parallel to each other are defined by ligaments, which in turn result in the formation of compartments created in a horizontal fashion, making it challenging to distribute the filler in a horizontal plane with horizontal augmentation techniques.

Treatment – Volume correction of the forehead

VSDT

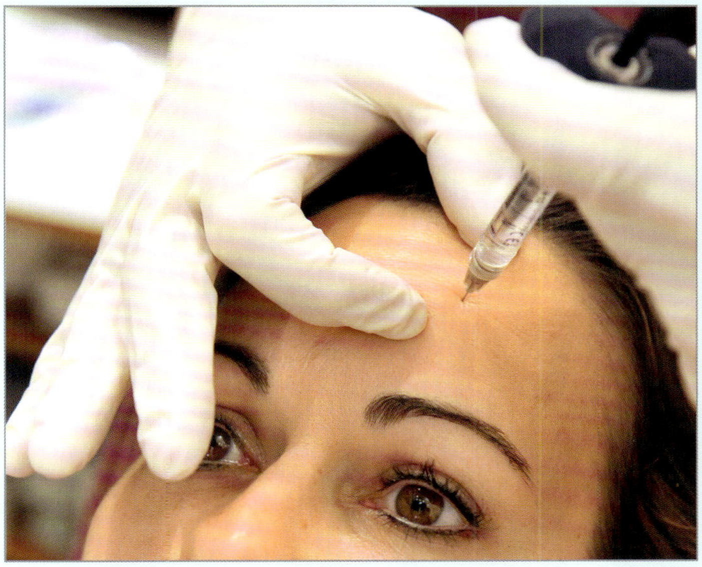

Fig. 7.6 Upon forehead contraction, the injections are made along the horizontal lines into the forehead ligaments with vertical injections aiming to raise the ligaments. Take care to insert the needle slowly and gently into the 'hot spots' of the line and down to the bony base to deliver 0.02–0.05 ml/depot. When injecting the filler, monitor the volumising effect closely to determine the correct volume and to avoid overcorrection. To achieve greater precision, slight stretching can be provided with the non-injecting hand during the injection.

DHAC

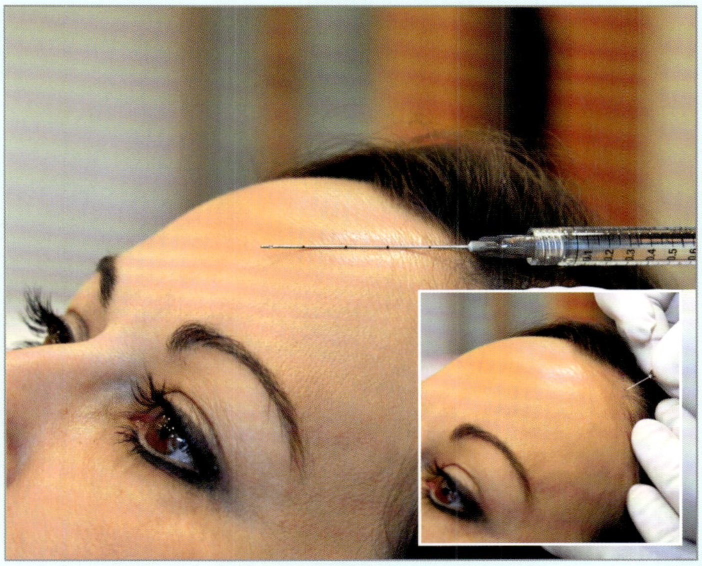

Fig. 7.7 Alternatively, the cannula can be used to inject the filler in a horizontal direction. A point insertion with a needle is made at the hairline (small picture). The cannula then inserted and moved in a fanning fashion and 0.2–0.5 ml is injected.

Treatment steps

- Remove makeup
- Disinfection
- Anaesthesia (optional)
- Injection: VSDT or DHAC
- Massage and mould (ensure appropriate distribution of the filler)
- Inform patient about post-treatment dos and don'ts
- Arrange a follow-up appointment

Filler selection

3 Deep injection (p. 66)
4 Ultra-deep injection (p. 67)

Practical tip

Because of the vertical ligamentous septation of the forehead, it is challenging to uniformly distribute the filler with horizontal augmentation techniques. Therefore, serial vertical depot injections (VSDT) followed by thorough massage and moulding may prove a more effective approach to restoring forehead volume. The results can be further optimised with botulinum toxin type-A injections a couple of weeks before filler treatment.

Select a filler with adequate viscoelastic properties, allowing it to be moulded after injection.

Combined treatment options

Dynamic wrinkles are best treated with botulinum toxin type-A 1 to 2 weeks before filler augmentation. Typically, the glabella is treated simultaneously with the forehead wrinkles.

Complications/Managing complications

- Overcorrection in the thicker forehead skin should be avoided at all times, and the stretching technique is useful in that respect.
- Palpable nodules may form due to the aggregation of the filler used. Thorough massage and moulding of the injected filler directly after the treatment ensures uniform distribution.

Caution

The regions around the temples and the glabella have a highly dense network of vessels, and hence care should be taken to avoid traumatising these structures when performing deeper injections. Therefore, it is recommended to perform vertical injections with a needle onto the supraperiosteal plane. When using a cannula, it is recommended to utilise a large bore 22 gauge cannula to gently mobilise the tissues.

7.2.2 Glabellar lines

Both the forehead and the glabella are extremely expressive regions of the face, and reflect an individual's mood to a great extent. The glabella in particular often expresses negative emotions of disagreement or unhappiness. As such, it is an area often sought for rejuvenation treatments.

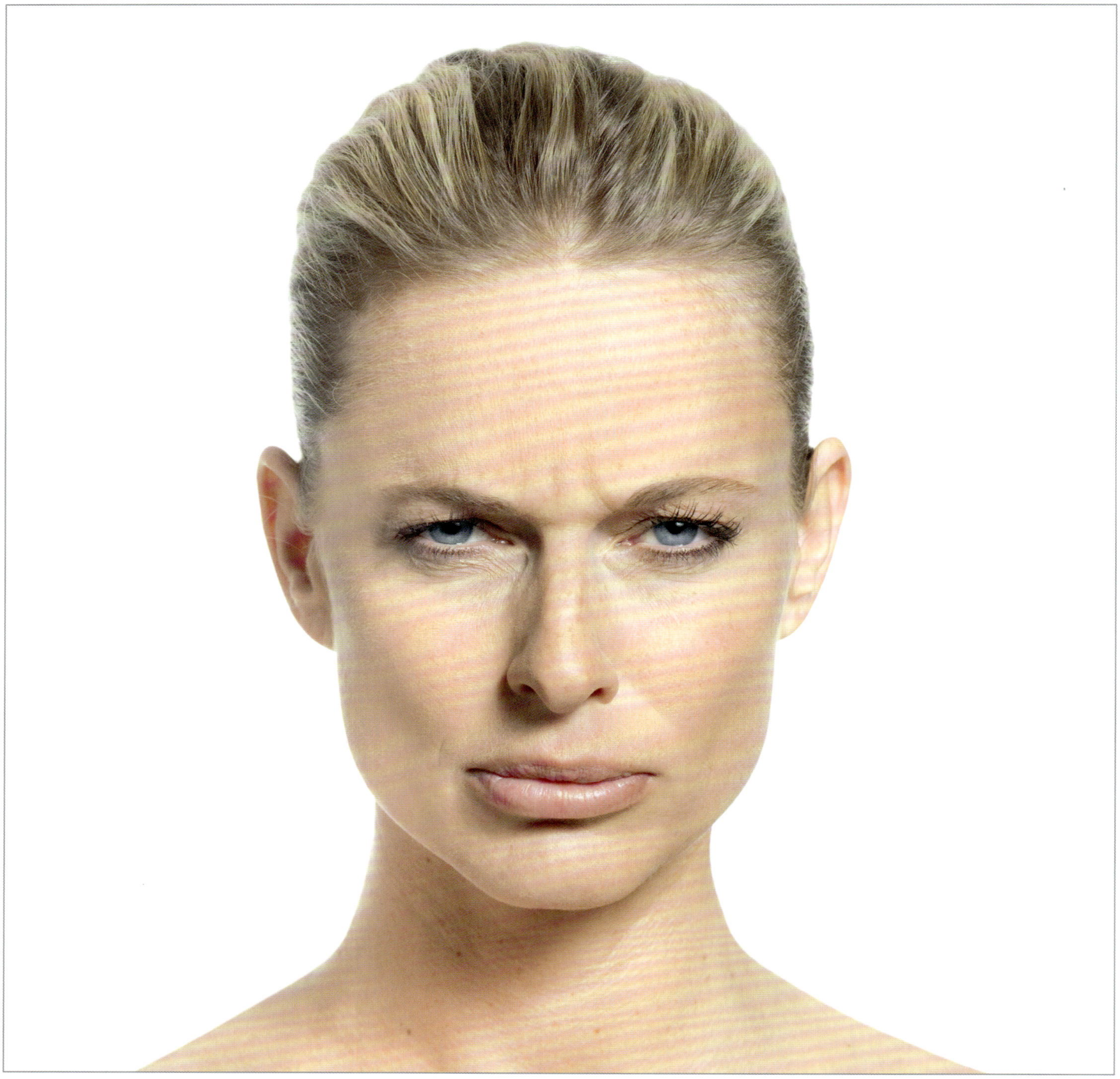

Patient selection
Patients who present with dynamic frown lines in the glabellar region should ideally be treated with botulinum toxin type-A prior to undergoing filler augmentation. Filler augmentation should be reserved for residual static lines that are not resolved with chemical denervation.

Assessing the indication
Frown lines can be smoothed out satisfactorily with a combination treatment approach using botulinum toxin type-A followed by filler augmentation (at 2 weeks after chemical denervation). Repeat maintenance treatments should be recommended to achieve an optimal and lasting result.

Anatomy

Frown lines are produced largely by the contraction of three muscles, namely:

- Procerus (1)
- Corrugator supercilii (2) and
- Depressor supercilii (3).

The procerus muscle, together with the corrugator supercilii muscle, draw the medial aspect of the eyebrow down towards the root of the nose, thus producing the transverse lines in the glabella.

The corrugator supercilii muscle, together with the depressor supercilii muscle, draw the medial aspect of the eyebrows medially and downwards, producing vertical lines in this region, which can be also seen over the root of the nose.

The glabella fat pad, situated below the muscles, atrophies with age and this in turn leads to more pronounced glabellar lines due to a decrease in the underlying support structure and the associated lifting forces.

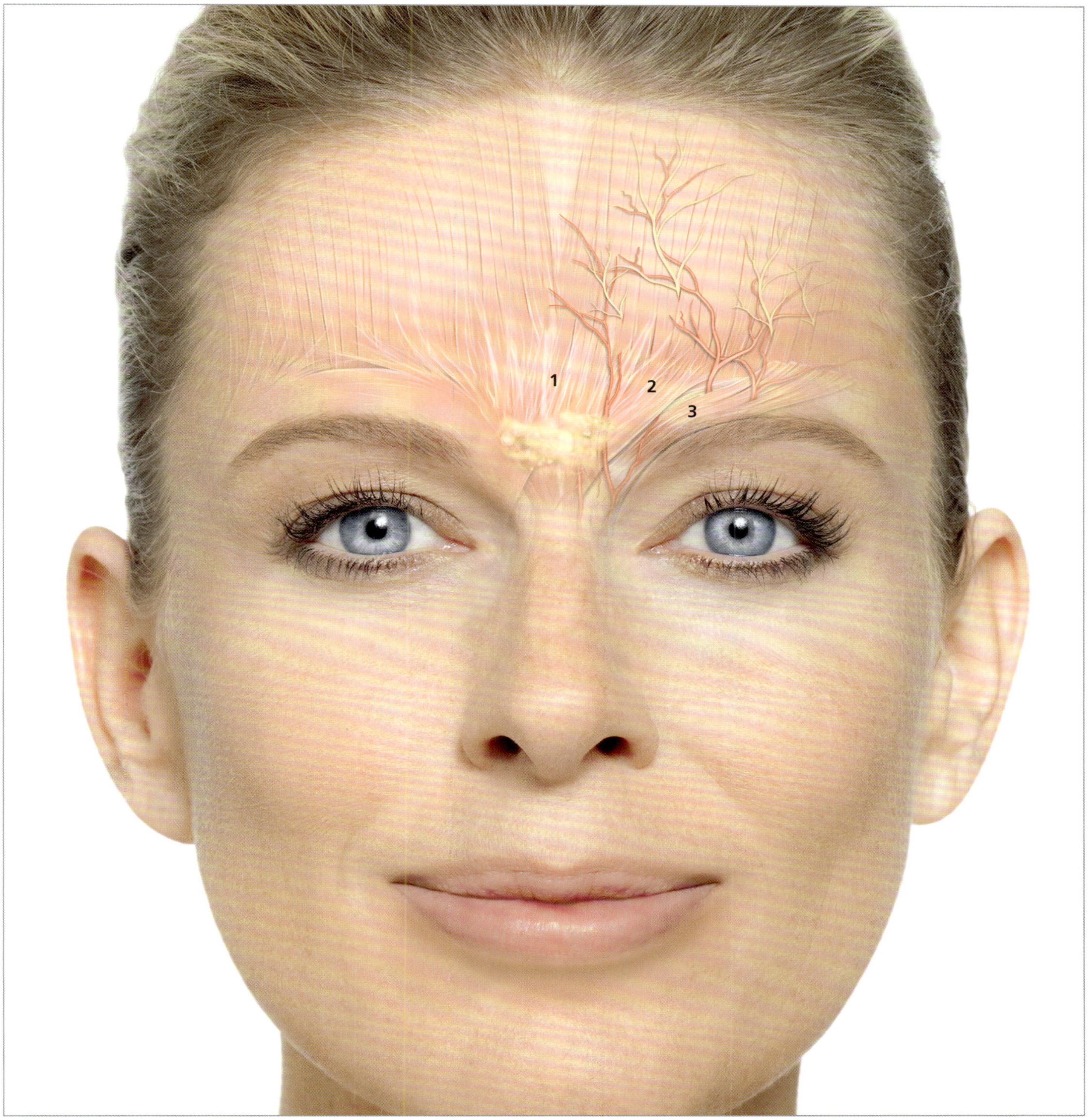

Treatment planning – Superficial augmentation

The aim of superficial augmentation is to achieve a gentle masking effect of the static glabellar lines following chemical denervation with botulinum toxin type-A.

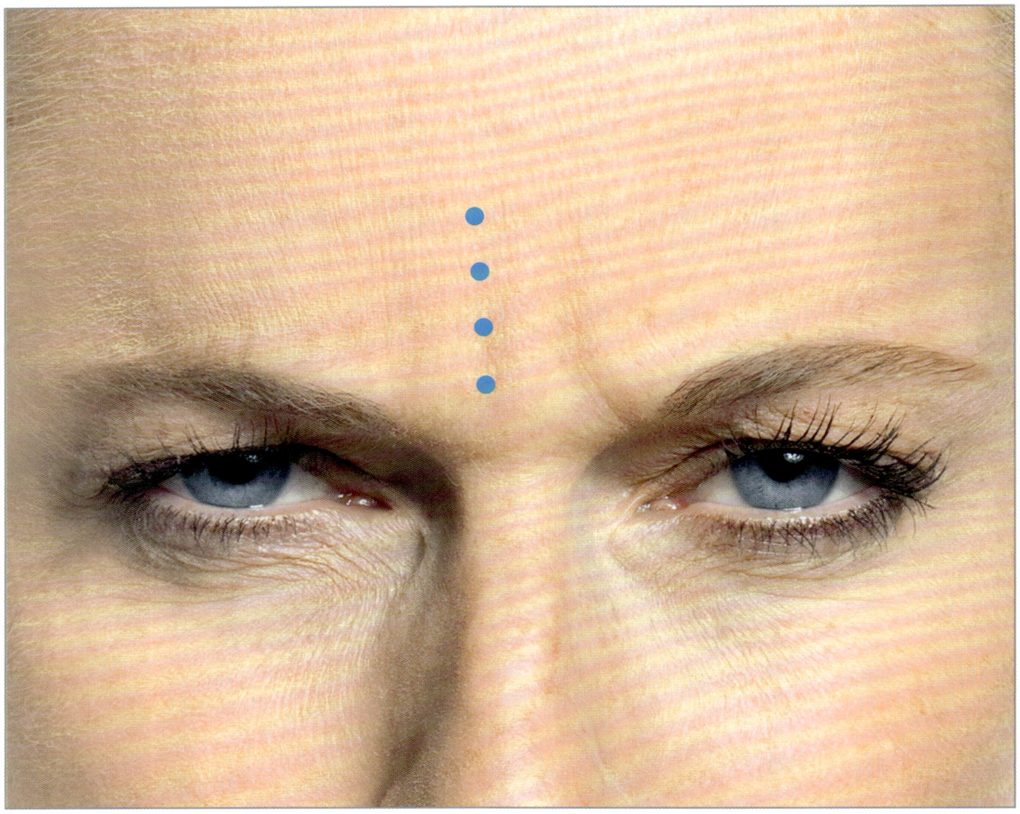

Technique: ● ● ● point technique, especially in cases with seborrheic skin
Injection sites: ● several injection sites per line, depending on individual findings
Volume: 0.05 ml/point
Tool: 30 gauge needle

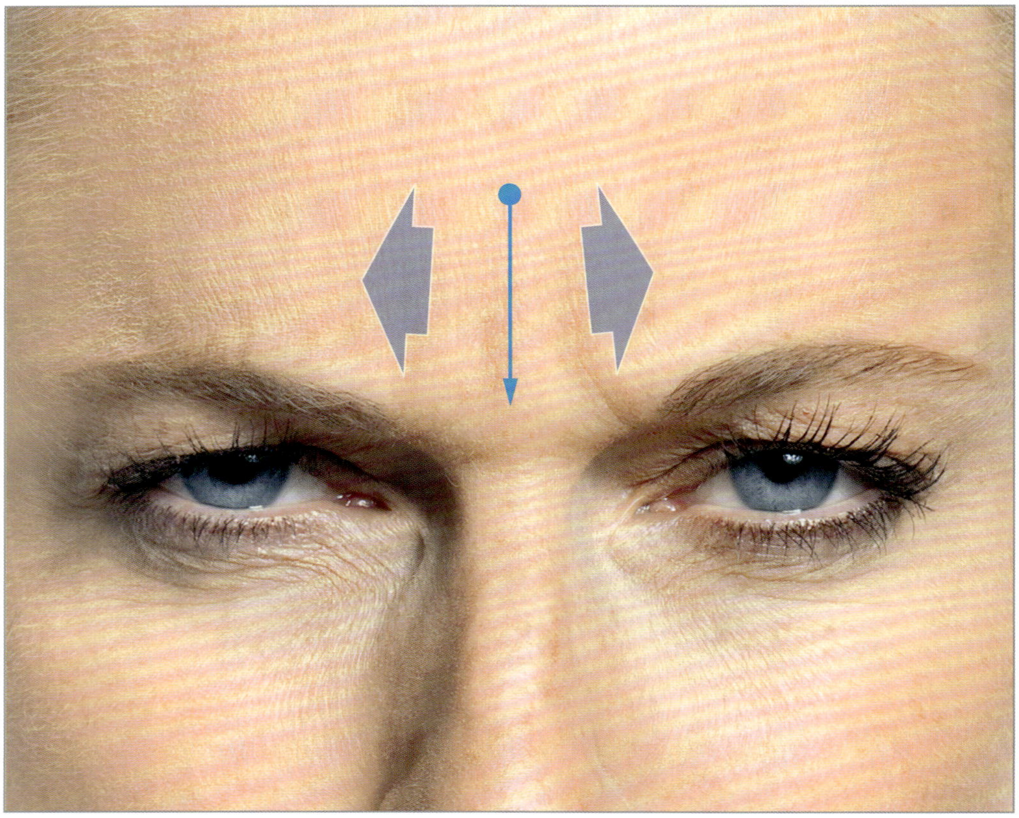

Technique: linear technique with stretching
Injection site: ● one injection point at the proximal end of the line
Volume: 0.05–0.1 ml/line
Tool: 30 gauge needle

Treatment – Superficial augmentation

Linear technique with stretching

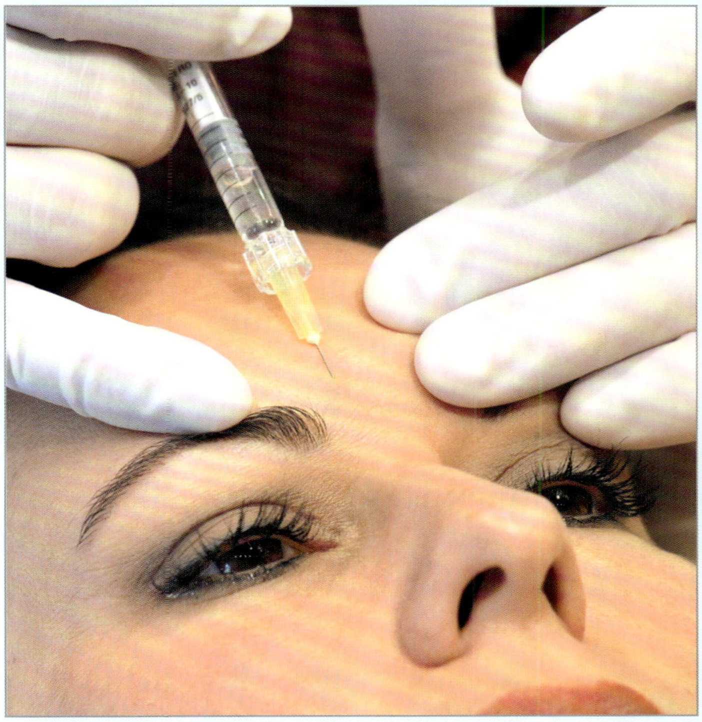

Fig. 7.8 The injection is done while the skin is stretched. The needle is inserted from the cranial direction. It is gently advanced in the cranial direction following the direction of the wrinkle. The filler is injected while the needle is withdrawn.

Point technique

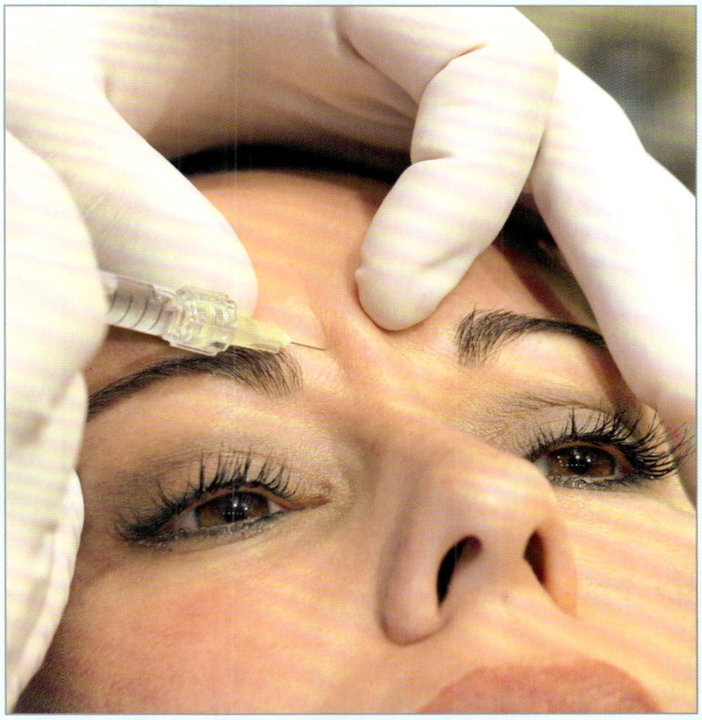

Fig. 7.9 The injection is made with the point technique, following the direction of the line. A blanching effect should be observed upon injection.

Treatment steps

- Remove makeup
- Disinfection
- Anaesthesia (optional)
- Injection: linear technique/point technique
- Massage and mould (ensure appropriate distribution of the filler)
- Inform patient about post-treatment dos and don'ts
- Arrange a follow-up appointment

Filler selection

1 Superficial injection (p. 62)
2 Medium injection (p. 63)

Combined treatment options

Chemical denervation of the glabellar muscles 1 to 2 weeks before filler augmentation.

Complications/Managing complications

Palpable nodules may form due to the aggregation of the filler used. Thorough massage and moulding of the injected filler directly after the treatment ensures uniform distribution.

Practical tip

Glabellar lines should ideally be first treated with botulinum toxin type-A. Lines that persist even after chemical denervation are suited to filler augmentation. Successful outcome, however, is usually achieved with several repeat augmentation treatments.

Caution

The glabella region has a rich vascular network and hence care should be taken to avoid intravascular injections when injecting at a deeper plane. Reports, although rare, exist of filler related necrosis and blindness after filler injections into the glabella. For that reason, vertical injections need to be done carefully on a supraperiosteal plane.

Treatment planning – Deeper augmentation
The goal of the treatment is to compensate for the atrophy-related volume deficit in the glabellar fat pad, manifesting as static glabellar lines, which remain pronounced even after botulinum toxin type-A treatment.

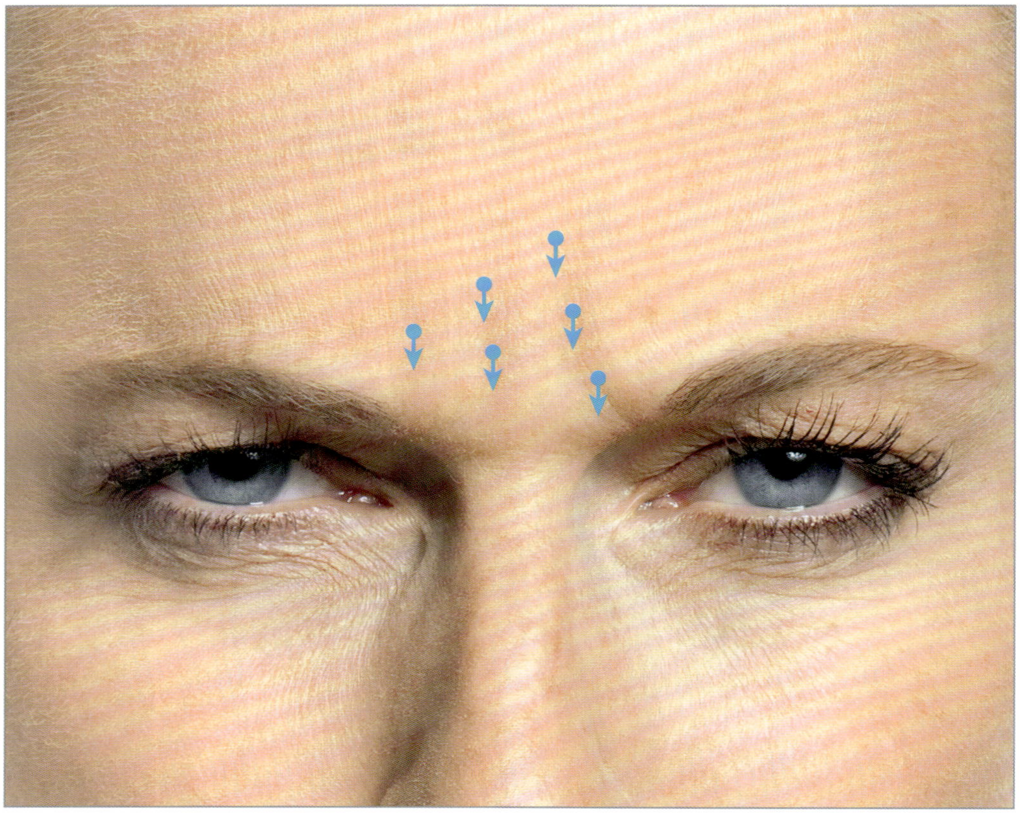

Technique: VSDT
Injection sites: several 'hot spots' per line

Caution: reduce the risk of intravascular injection by carefully and slowly injecting down to the bone before delivering the injection. It is also useful to ask if the patient feels any unusual onset of discomfort or sensations at any point during the injection, which will warn the practitioner to stop, observe, and in turn reduce the risk of vascular trauma.

Video: Glabella VSDT http://www.kvm-tv.de/FIL/008.mp4

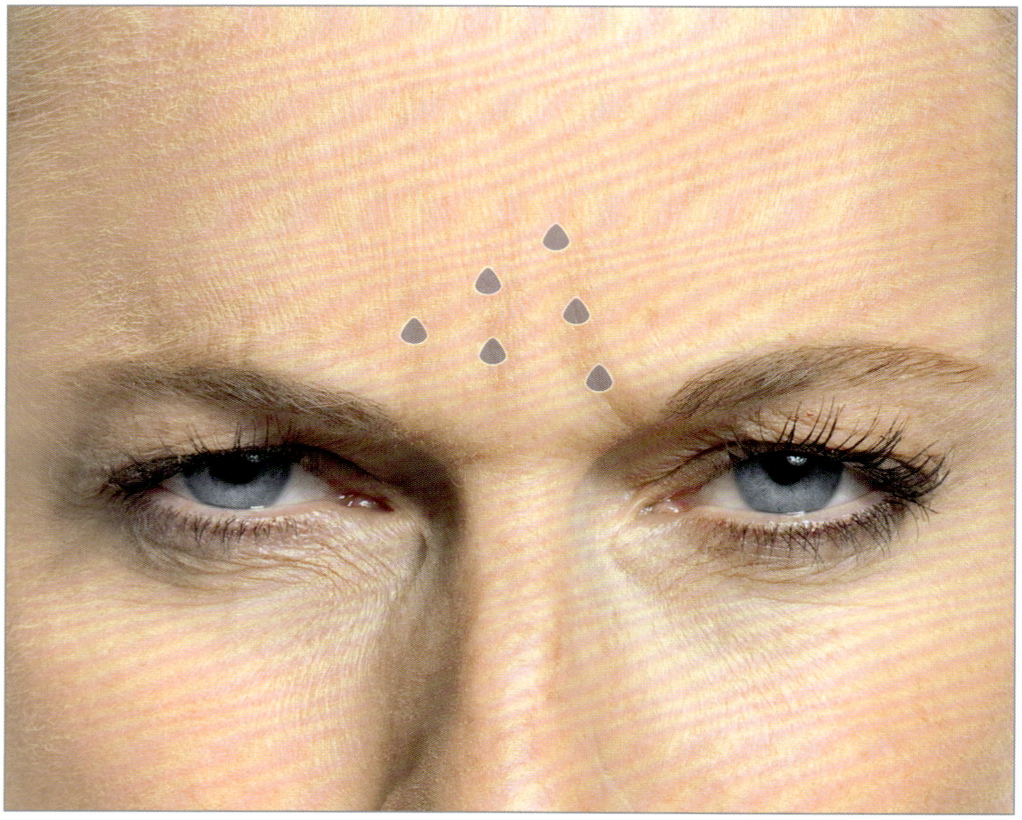

Volume: 0.05 ml/point
Tool: 27 gauge needle

7

Treatment – Deeper augmentation

VSDT

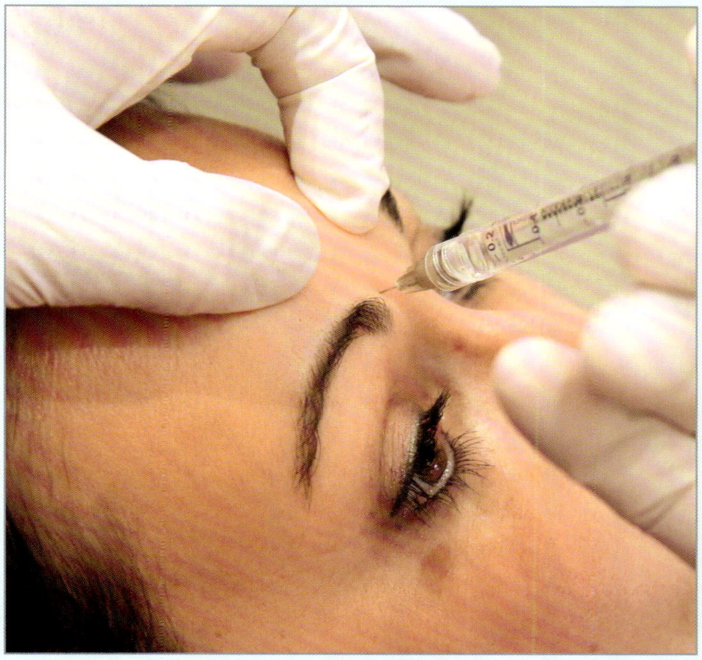

Fig. 7.10 During the treatment, the non-injecting hand palpates and gently compresses the treatment site.

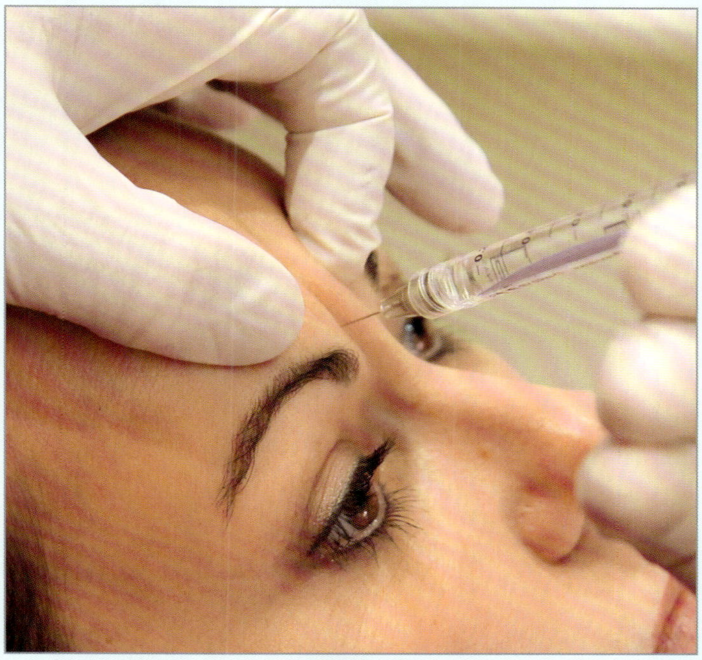

Fig. 7.11 The needle is carefully and slowly inserted vertically down to the supraperiosteal plane. It can also be useful to ask the patient if they experience any unusual levels of discomfort or odd sensations during the injection, which can be an indicator of an intravascular trauma and would alert the practitioner to stop immediately and assess the situation. Ultimately, the needle should be sited at the supraperiosteal plane prior to injection for maximum safety.

Treatment steps

- Remove makeup
- Disinfection
- Anaesthesia (optional)
- Injection: VSDT or DHAC
- Massage and mould (ensure appropriate distribution of the filler)
- Inform patient about post-treatment dos and don'ts
- Arrange a follow-up appointment

Practical tips

- Filler augmentation should be performed as an adjunctive treatment after chemical denervation using botulinum toxin type-A (at 2 weeks post-treatment). Furthermore, it should be noted that in most cases, several repeat treatments are required for optimal clinical outcome.
- Slow penetration speed and patient cooperation while inserting the needle down to the supraperiosteal plane decreases the risk of vascular trauma and intravascular injection.

Filler selection

3 Deep injection (p. 66)

4 Ultra-deep injection (p. 67)

Combined treatment options

Chemical denervation using botulinum toxin type-A in the glabellar muscles 2 weeks before filler augmentation.

Complications/Managing complications

Palpable nodules may form due to the aggregation of the filler used. Thorough massage and moulding of the injected filler directly after the treatment ensures uniform distribution.

Caution

The glabella region has a rich vascular network and hence care should be taken to avoid intravascular injections. Reports, although rare, exist of filler related necrosis and blindness after filler injections into the glabella. For that reason, vertical injections need to be done carefully on a supraperiosteal plane.

7.2.3 Temples/Temporal region

Atrophy of the temporal fat pad is considered the key reason for the early onset loss of volume and manifestation of visible blood vessels in the temple region. Although temples do not feature as a primary area of concern for the majority of patients seeking rejuvenation, it is important to treat this area as it contributes to an overall harmonisation of the upper third of the face.

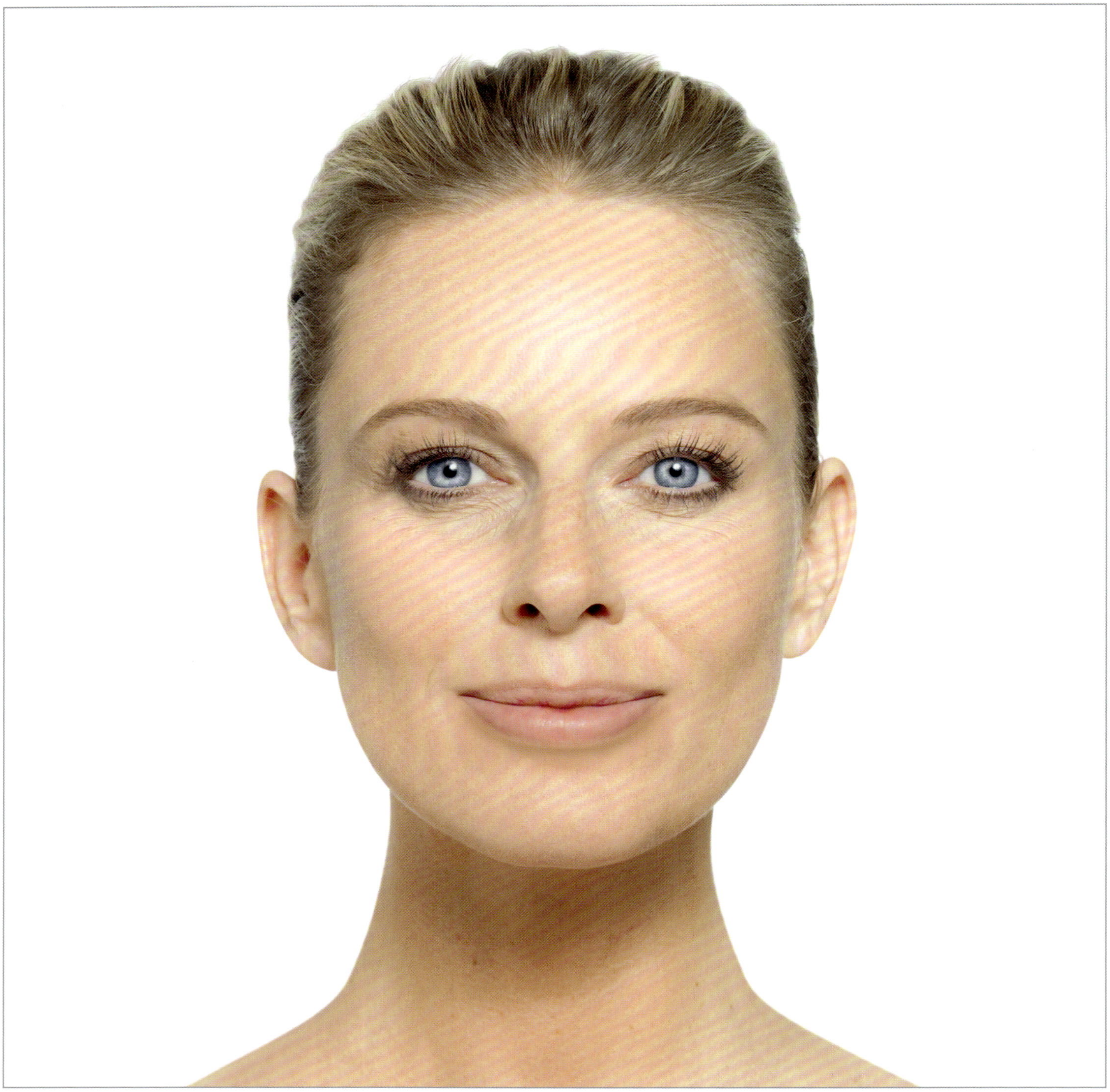

Patient selection
Patients presenting with visible blood vessels and hollowness in the temple and forehead region can benefit from filler augmentation in the temples. This treatment simultaneously treats the lateral periorbital canthal lines.

Assessing the indication
Filler augmentation of the temples can be performed with deep filler placement using either vertical or horizontal augmentation techniques. Repeat maintenance augmentation enables optimal and long-lasting treatment results.

Anatomy

The temporal region has minimal superficial fat. Atrophy-related loss of the deep temporal fat pad results in volume loss of the temples. As a result, blood vessels, which are numerous in this region, become more visible. Importantly, during filler injection, care should be taken to avoid intravascular injection of the deep *A temporalis,* particularly when using a needle, and hence gentle, slow, supraperiosteal injections are advocated.

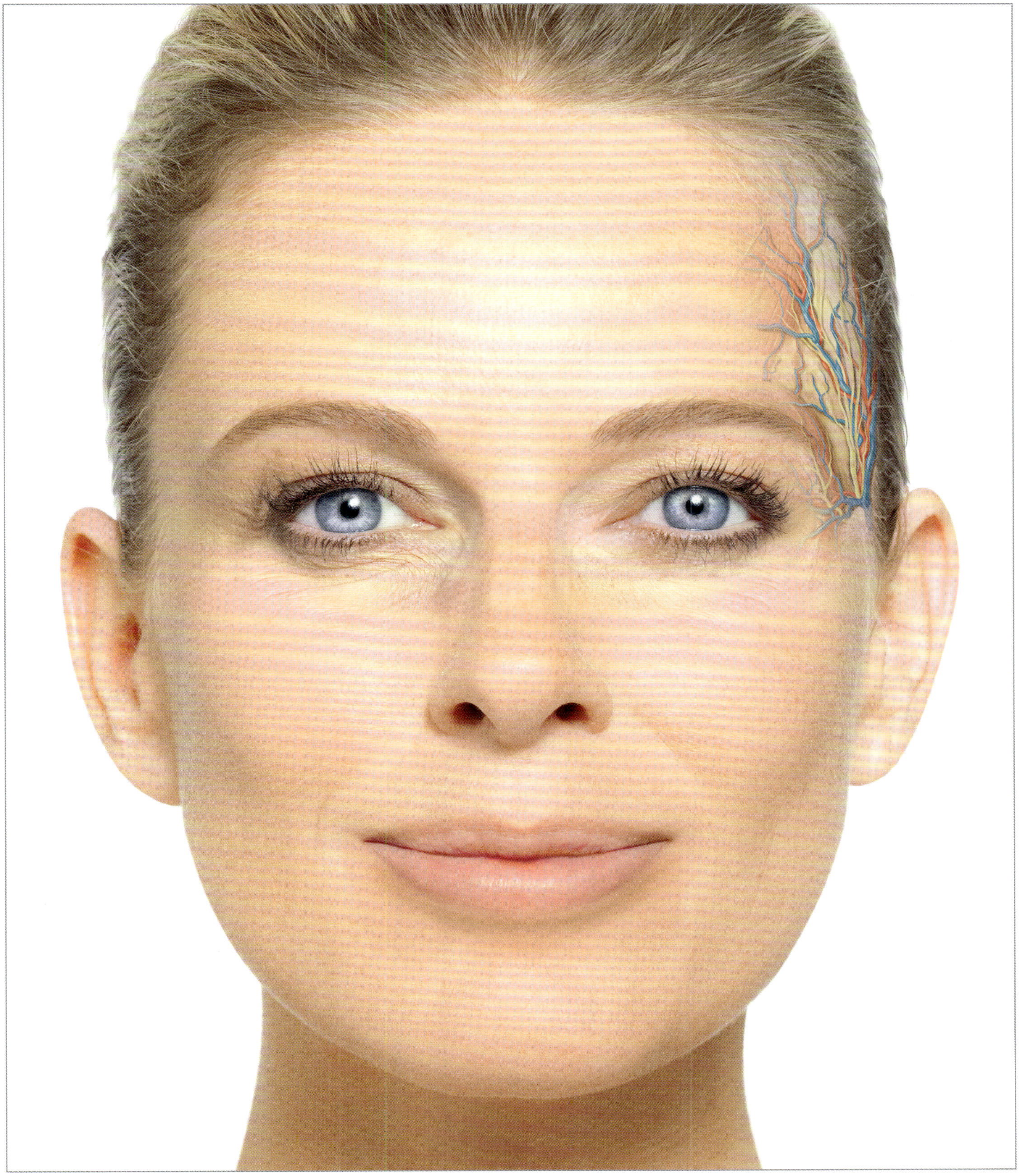

Treatment planning – Volume therapy of the temples
The aim of this treatment is to re-volumise the atrophy-related volume deficits in the temporal fat pad. Either a vertical supraperiosteal focal depot technique with a needle, or a deep horizontal mobilisation technique with a cannula can be used.

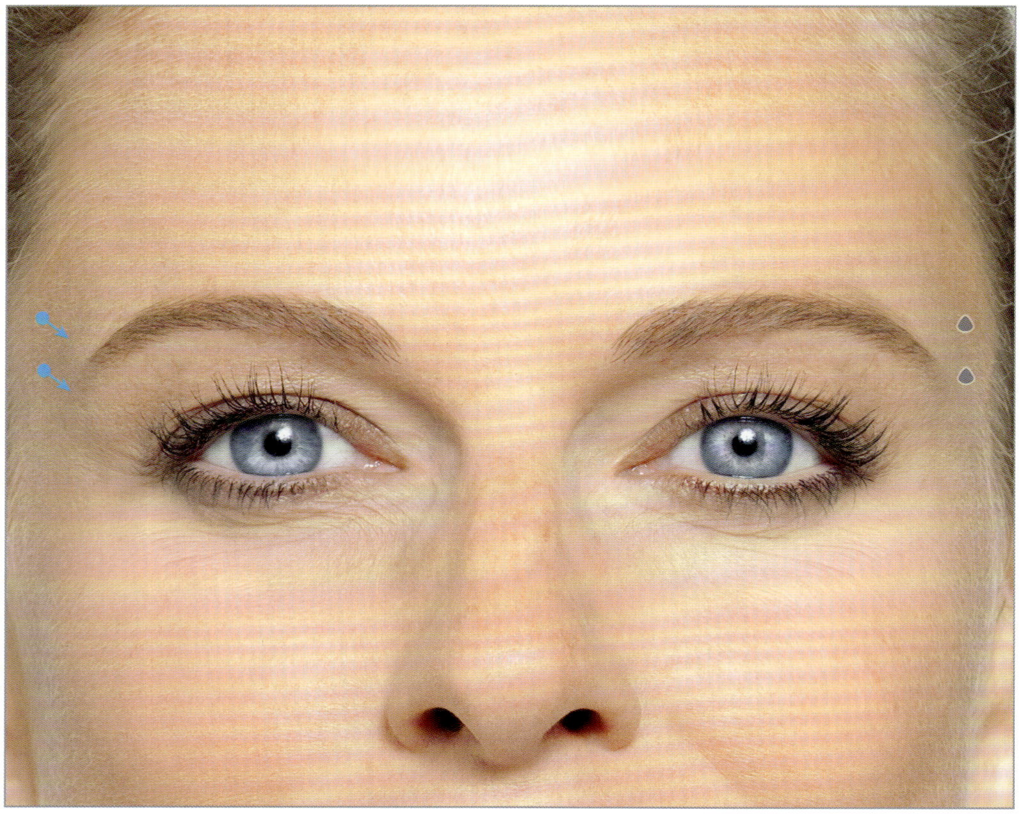

Technique: VSDT
Injection sites: one to two 'hot spots' close to the lateral hairline, slightly above the lateral border of the eyebrow

Caution: Avoid injury to the *A temporalis* by careful penetration to the supraperiosteal plane

Volume: 0.1–0.3 ml/point
Tool: 27 gauge needle

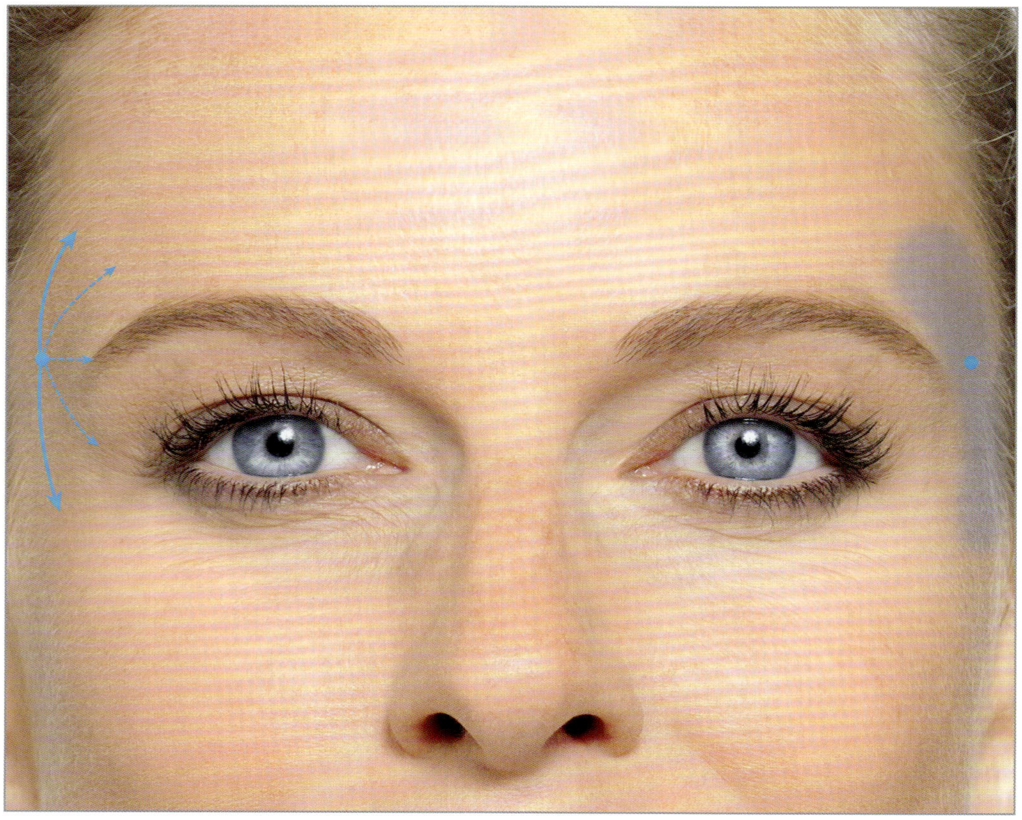

Technique: DHAC
Insertion site: at the temporal hairline, approximately at the level of the lateral border of the eyebrow
Volume: 0.2–0.5 ml per side
Depth and direction: Subcutaneous injection, distributing the filler in a caudal, medial and cranial direction
Tool: 22 gauge cannula

Video: Temples DHAC
http://www.kvm-tv.de/FIL/009.mp4

Treatment – Volume augmentation of the temples

VSDT

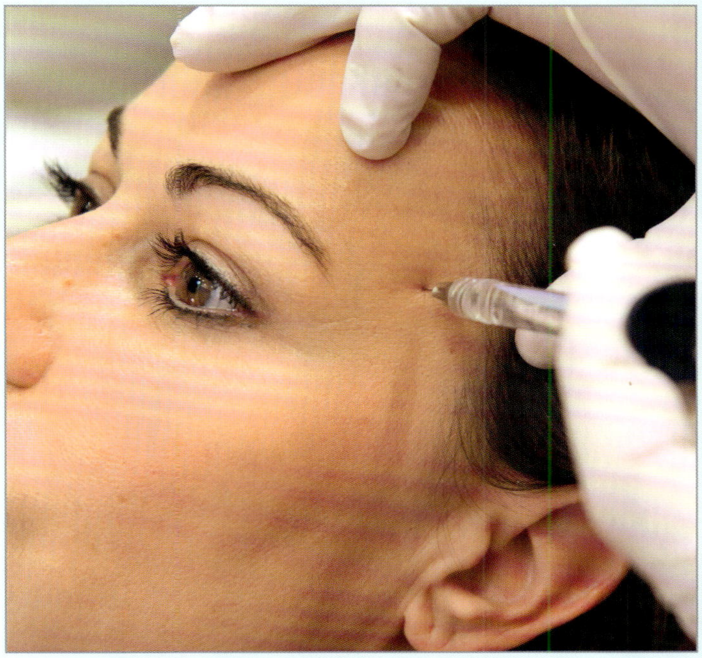

Fig. 7.12 The needle is vertically inserted with slow penetration speed down to the bone. If the patient does not feel any pain, a supraperiosteal depot is then injected slowly.

DHAC

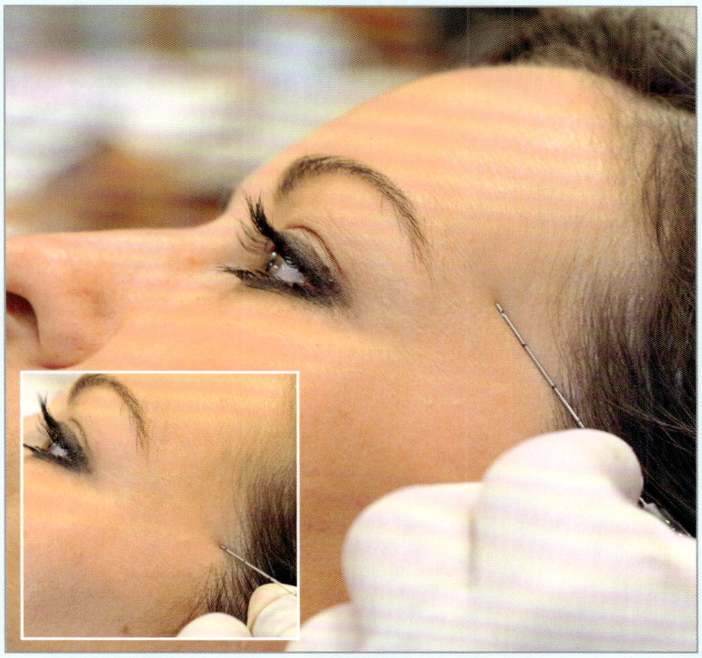

Fig. 7.13 A 22 gauge cannula is advanced through an insertion point at the lateral hairline. When in the subcutaneous plane, the cannula is gently advanced and retracted to mobilise the tissues in a superior, medial and inferior direction while the filler is injected (0.2–0.5 ml per side), followed by thorough massage and moulding to achieve an even distribution.

Treatment steps
- Remove makeup
- Disinfection
- Anaesthesia (optional)
- Injection: VSDT or DHAC
- Massage and mould (ensure appropriate distribution of the filler)
- Inform patient about post-treatment dos and don'ts
- Arrange a follow-up appointment

Filler selection

3 Deep injection (p. 66)

4 Ultra-deep injection (p. 67)

Combined treatment options
- Chemical peeling
- Laser resurfacing
- Medical needling

Complications/Managing complications

Palpable nodules may form due to the aggregation of the filler used. Thorough massage and moulding of the injected filler directly after the treatment ensures uniform distribution.

Practical tips

- The most homogenous distribution of the filler can be achieved with a vertical injection technique.
- Careful penetration of the needle down to the bone in cooperation with the patient reduces the risk of intravascular injection of the temporal vessels.
- For less experienced practitioners it may be safer to use a large bore cannula, e.g. 22 gauge, to deliver horizontal augmentation.

Caution

The temple region has a rich blood supply, and hence care should be taken to avoid vessel injury when performing deep injections. Therefore, vertical injections with needles should be done carefully while placing the filler on the supraperiosteal plane.

7.3 Periorbital Region

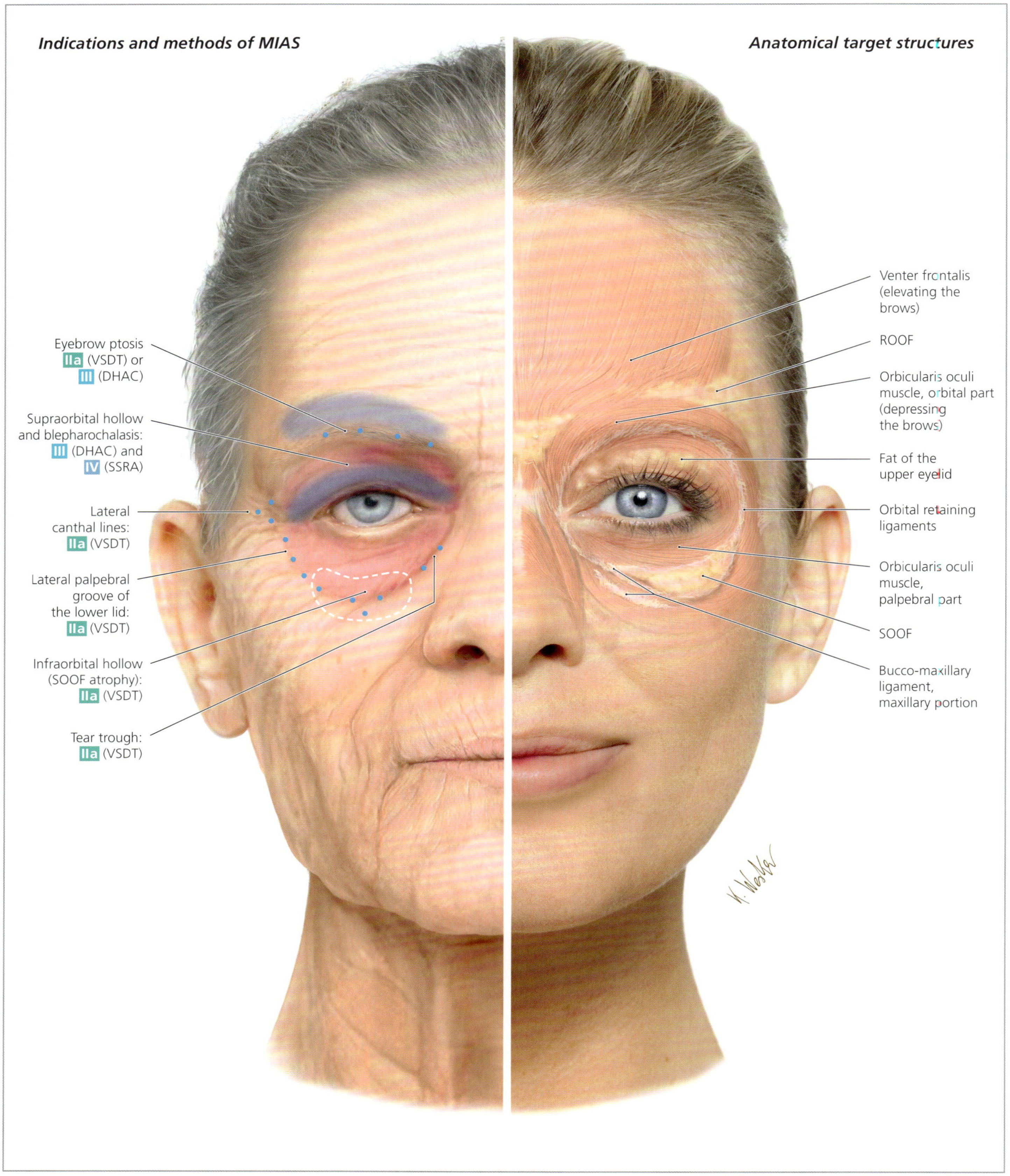

Fig. 7.14 Overview of the anatomy, target structures and cause-related augmentation techniques in the periorbital region.
• VSDT (or, alternatively, SAT as a camouflage technique); DHAC; SSRA

7.3.1 Supraorbital region (eyebrows and the upper eyelid)

Eyebrows are key facial landmarks, and their colour, position, curvature and thickness dictate the aesthetics of the upper face to a great extent. Low set brows communicate a tired and weary expression. High set, shapely brows make the face appear fresher, younger and more alert.

Eyebrows together with the upper eyelid are often considered as a single unit. With ageing, the underlying fat pads in this region atrophy and give rise to brow ptosis. The declining structural support beneath the thin skin envelope of the brow region also results in the formation of wrinkles and at times blepharochalasis. Upper eyelid hollowness can also present with advanced ageing, a feature that is commonly sought for within the non-surgical aesthetic arena.

Eyebrows are often divided into three thirds, for the purposes of having reference points when describing the ideal eyebrow shape. In a female face, the first two thirds of the eyebrow should rise gently from the medial aspect to the uppermost peak, after which they should slope downwards gently in the final third. The reference points can be illustrated using three imaginary lines.

Furthermore, when assessing this part of the face, the ideal eye position should also be noted, whereby the distance between the eyes should ideally equate to that of the length of the eye itself.

- **Eyebrow origin:** Originating at the site marked by a vertical axis drawn from the outermost point of the wing of the nose.
- **Eyebrow peak:** Situated at the point whereby the line connecting the wing of the nose and the pupil intersects the brow.
- **Eyebrow end point:** Situated at the point where the line connecting the wing of the nose and the lateral corner of the eye intersects with the end of the brow (particularly in females it is considered that any brow hairs growing past this point may disrupt the overall harmony of the face).

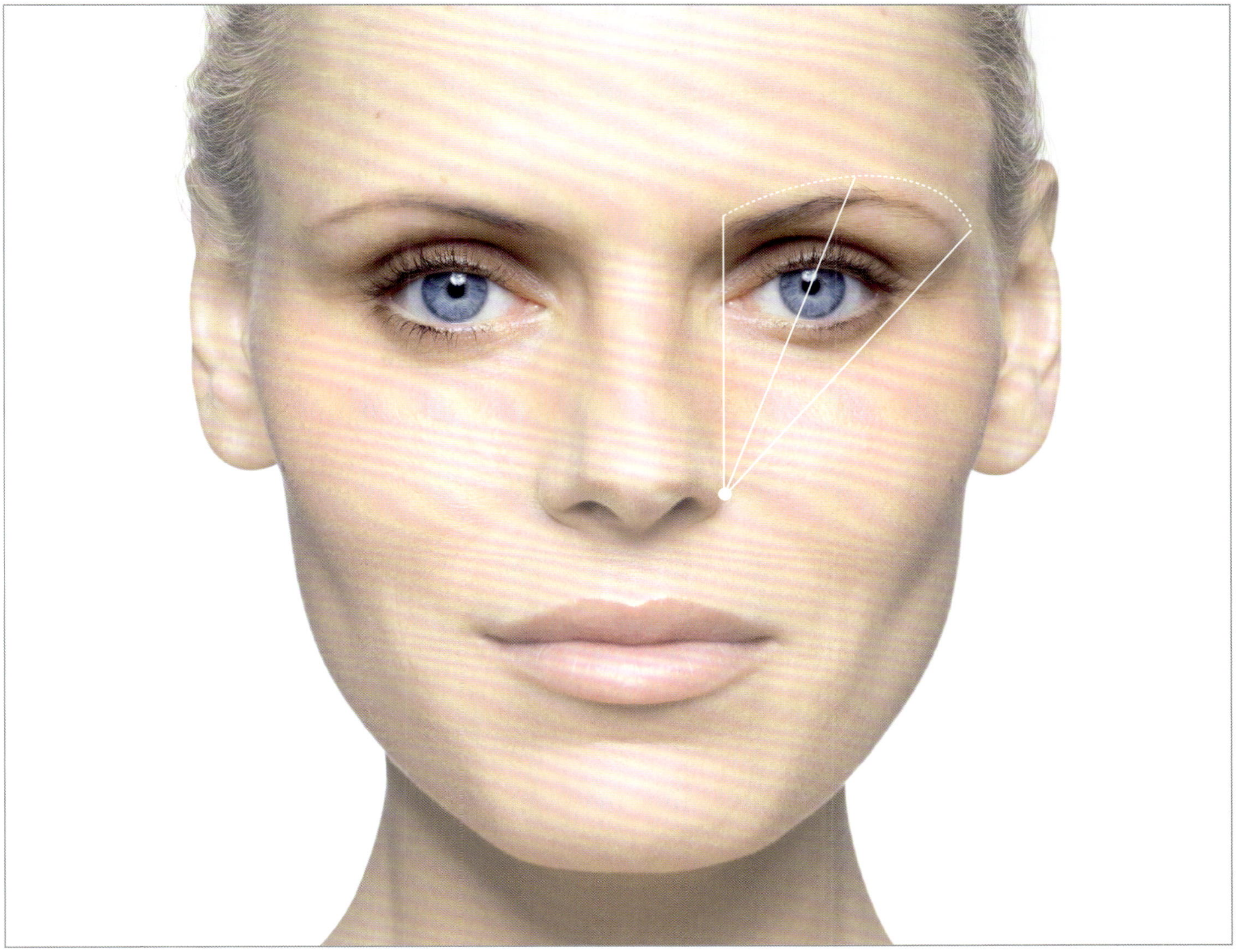

Anatomy

The supraorbital region does not contain significant quantities of superficial fat. Hence, the orbicularis oculi muscle lies directly under the skin. Its pars orbitalis functions together with the corrugator supercilii and the procerus as an eyebrow depressor, contributing to skin wrinkling and progressive ageing of the upper eyelid.

Below the musculature, a deep fat pad is found – the retro-orbicularis oculi fat pad (ROOF, 1). In youth, it forms the volumising and supporting soft tissue base of the supraorbital region. With age, it slowly diminishes due to a combination of decreased perfusion alongside tissue atrophy. This results in reduced tension forces in the entire tissue complex and leads to visible laxity and sagging in this region. Below the supraorbital foramen, advancing fat atrophy provokes the manifestation of the supraorbital hollowness.

The ageing processes of the supraorbital region are reinforced by skin changes and a slowly progressing imbalance of the forces between the hypertonic depressor muscles and the only levator muscle of the eyebrow region, namely the venter frontalis muscle, which also progressively gets weaker with age.

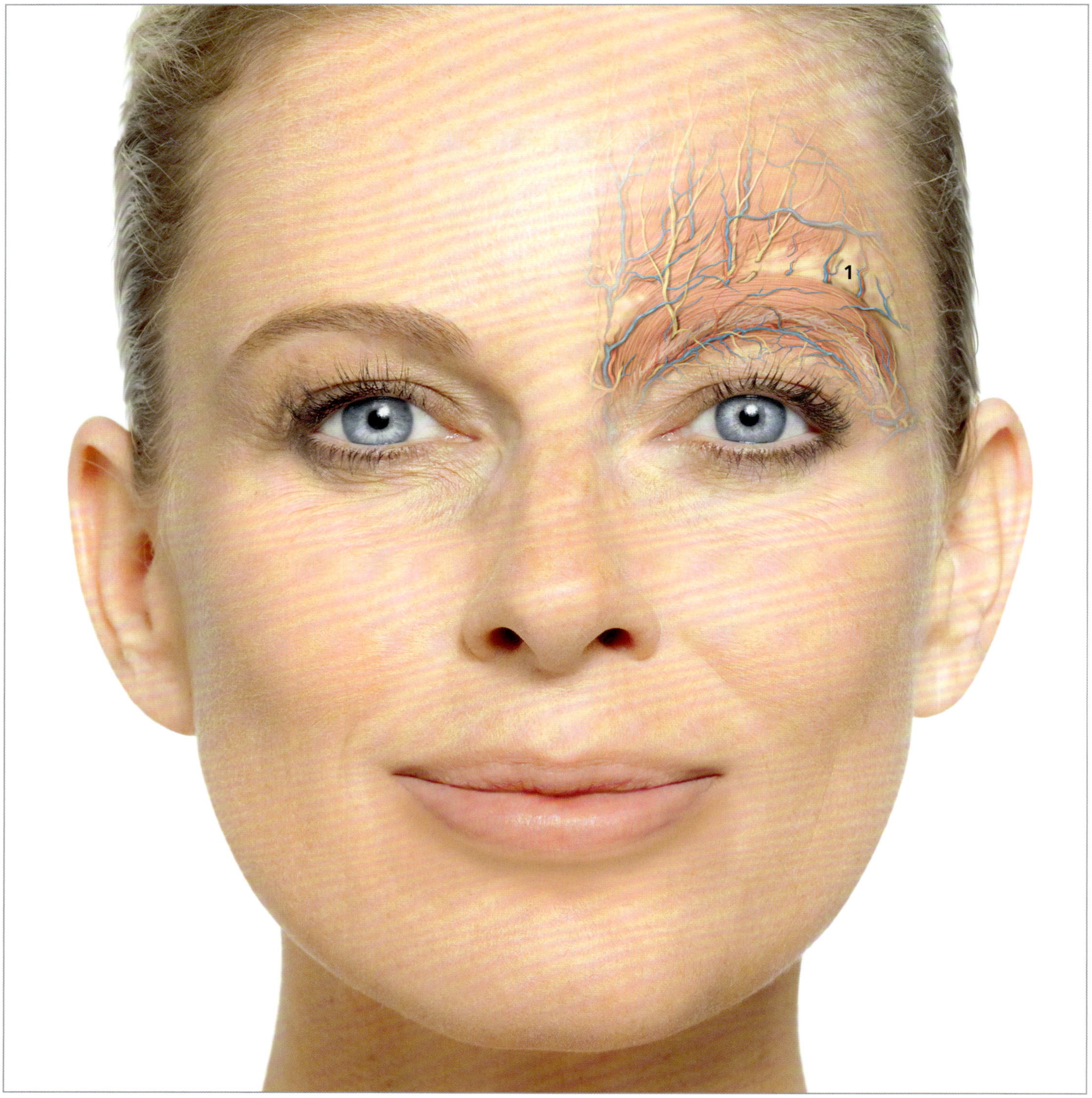

Progressive age-related changes in the eyebrows and the upper eyelids

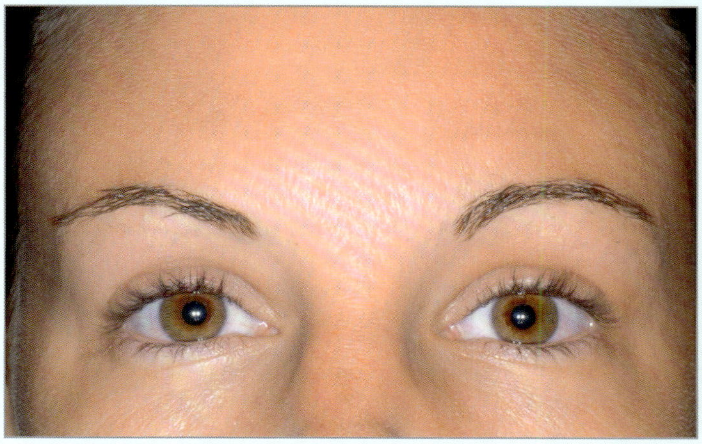

Fig. 7.15 High arch of the brow.

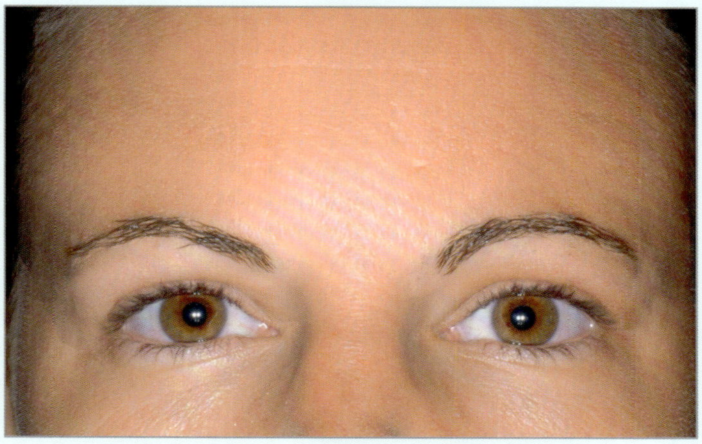

Fig. 7.16 Medium arch of the eyebrow.

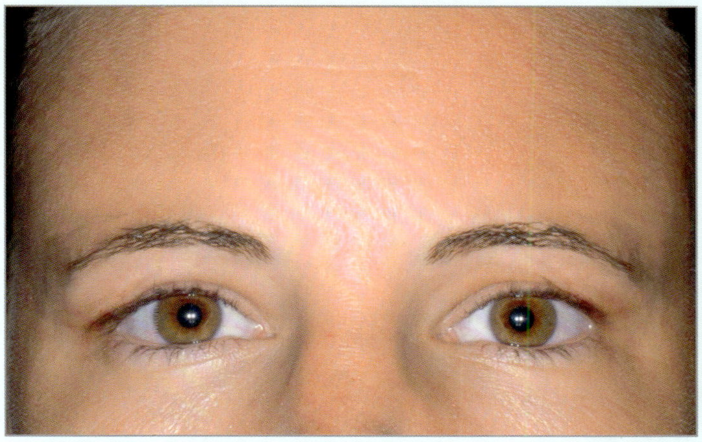

Fig. 7.17 Flat arch of the eyebrow.

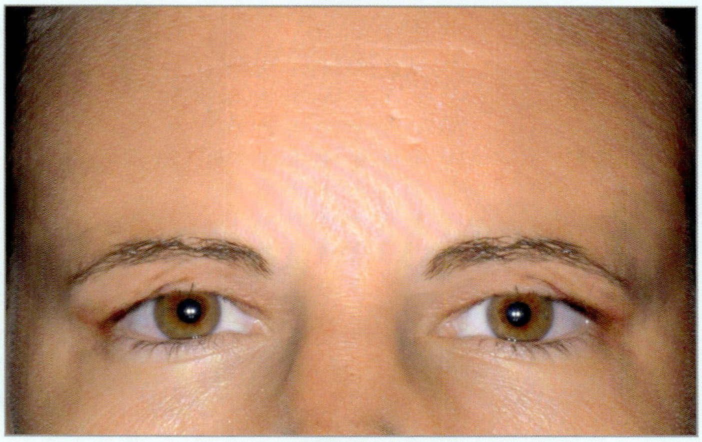

Fig. 7.18 Sunken arch of the eyebrow.

Findings and patient selection

When assessing and planning a treatment in this region, eyebrow shape and position should be discussed with the patient with regard to the fashion doctrine at the time, i.e. the desired thin eyebrows of the 1920s differ greatly to the arched and thicker brows preferred today. Furthermore, gender-specific differences and preferences also need to be taken into account. Females generally prefer arched brows with a higher peak, whereas men prefer straighter eyebrows. A thorough discussion with the patient will elucidate the desired aesthetic outcome being sought.

It is important to note that with progressive ageing, the eyebrows descend, particularly in the lateral segment. In addition, there is progressive loss of the eyebrow arch. With regard to the upper eyelids, progressive ageing manifests in the formation of skin wrinkling, blepharochalasis and/or hollowness.

Injectable fillers can be used to manage these age-related changes given they can replace the soft tissue that has shrunk with time. Particularly if the clinical findings elucidate atrophy-related changes, filler augmentation can be sufficient to achieve satisfying clinical results. In some cases, filler augmentation can even eliminate the need for a chemical or surgical brow lift. However, in severe cases of eyebrow ptosis or blepharochalasis, surgery remains the only optimal intervention and this should be discussed with the patient in advance.

Assessing the indication

Age-related volume deficits of the retro-orbicularis oculi fat pad can be compensated with deep injections using hyaluronic acid fillers. In doing so, augmentation therapy can achieve a natural improvement in brow ptosis and/or hollowness of the upper eyelid. It is however advisable to combine augmentation therapy with botulinum toxin type-A treatment of the depressor muscles in order to achieve optimal results, which should ideally be done prior to filler augmentation. Furthermore, superficial augmentation techniques with hyaluronic acid fillers can be used for fine-correction of the eyebrow shape, as well as for a general improvement in skin quality.

Treatment planning – Eyebrow augmentation

The primary goal of eyebrow augmentation is to compensate for the volume loss of the atrophied ROOF. The deep depot injections into the upper orbital ligaments fill the fat pad, which in turn increases the stabilising forces arising from the ligaments. This promotes the stabilising forces of the eyebrows and the upper eyelid, while harmonising the entire supraorbital complex. Filling techniques can either involve vertical supraperiosteal depots using a needle or horizontal tissue mobilisation using a cannula. Superficial injections can further assist in elevating the lateral part of the brow arch.

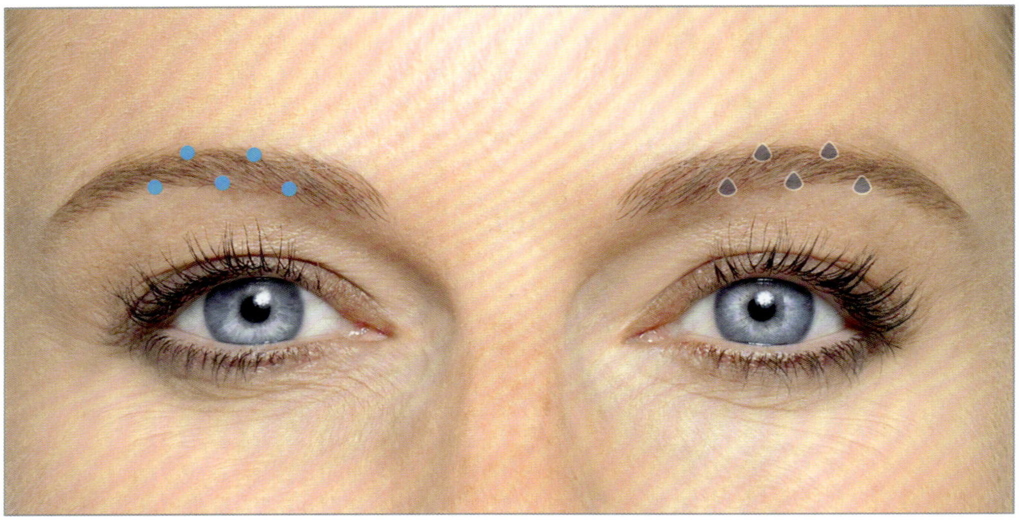

Technique: VSDT
Injection sites: five to six 'hot spots' along the brow at the site of the upper orbital ligaments (when injecting a 'hot spot' a crunching sound should be heard)
Volume: 0.02 ml/injection
Tool: 27 gauge needle

Caution: Insert the needle slowly down to the bone and inject as much filler as is required to achieve the desired visual lifting effect.

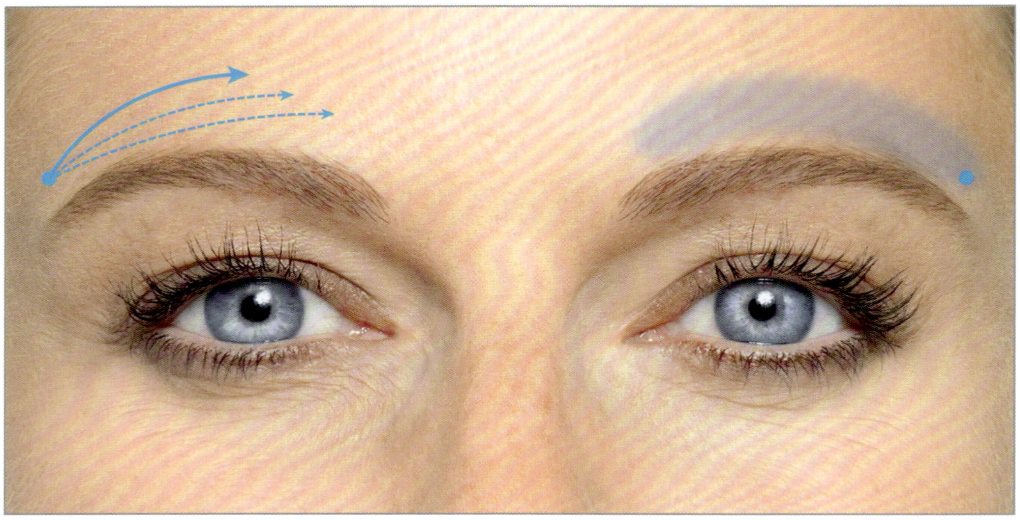

Technique: (DHAC)
Insertion point: superior to the lateral end of the eyebrow
Injection depth and direction: subcutaneous into the ROOF above the ligaments, from lateral to medial
Volume: 0.2–0.3 ml/side
Tool: 22–25 gauge cannula

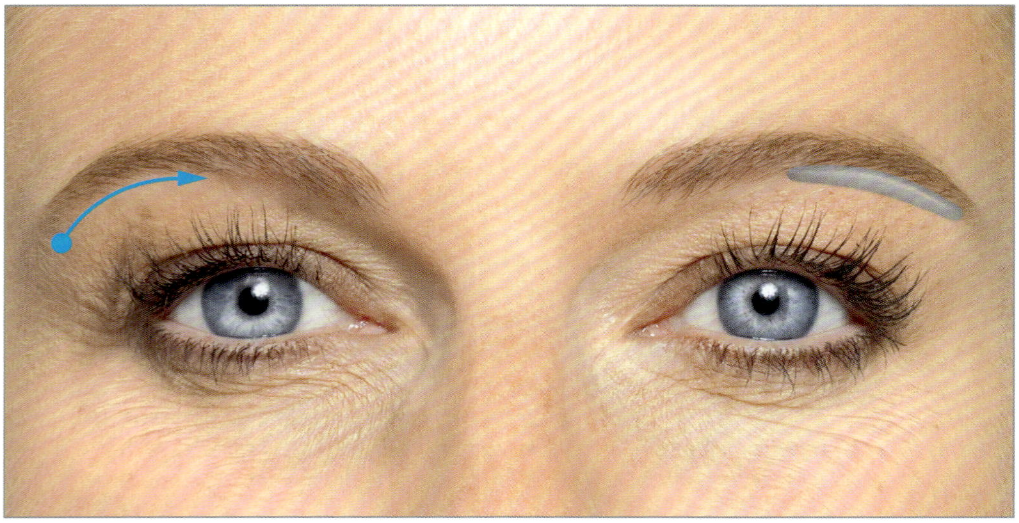

Technique: tunneling technique
Injection site: lateral aspect of the eyebrow
Volume: 0.2–0.5 ml/side (depending on findings)
Tool: 30 gauge needle

Treatment – Eyebrow augmentation

VSDT

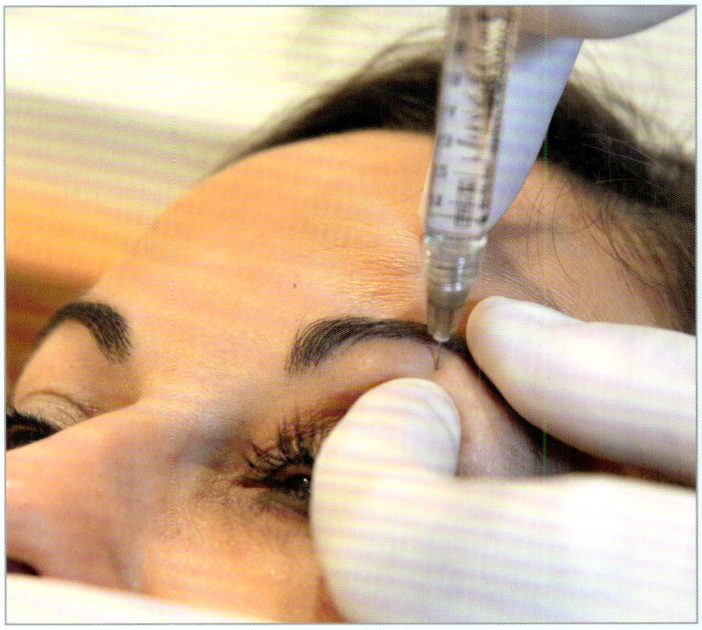

Fig. 7.19 The needle is inserted vertically into the retro-orbicularis oculi fat pad. A lifting effect is achieved by injecting several vertical depots of approximately 0.02 ml next to each other along the eyebrow length. Thereafter, a cannula is inserted into the fat pad and approximately 0.2–0.3 ml is injected per eyebrow in a horizontal direction while mobilising the soft tissues gently.

DHAC

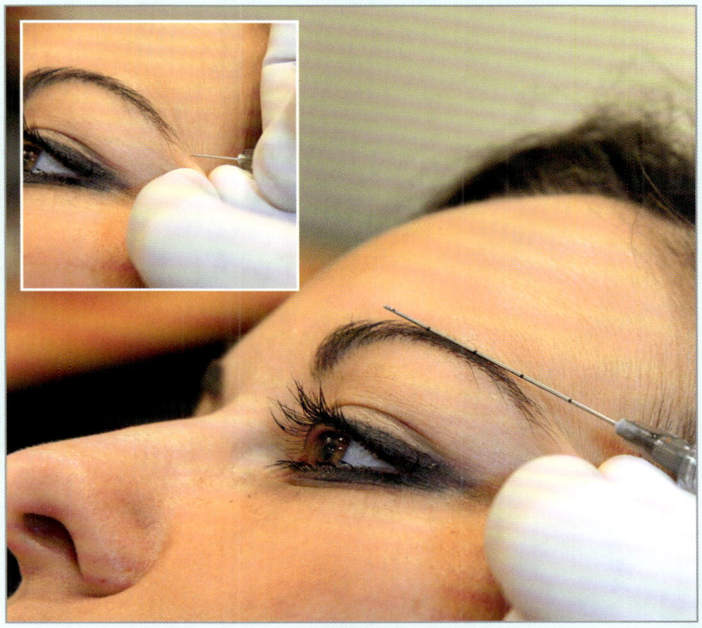

Fig. 7.20 The practitioner grasps the skin at the lateral end of the eyebrow and creates an insertion hole with an introducer needle.

Treatment steps

- Remove makeup
- Disinfection
- Anaesthesia (optional)
- Injection: VSDT or DHAC, eventually with superficial correction
- Massage and mould (ensure appropriate distribution of the filler)
- Inform patient about post-treatment dos and don'ts
- Arrange a follow-up appointment

Filler selection

1 Superficial injection (p. 62)
2 Medium injection (p. 63)

Fillers with lower water-binding capacity are ideal in this region, given this area is prone to oedema.

Combined treatment options

Chemical denervation (using botulinum toxin type-A) of the orbicularis oculi muscle 1 to 2 weeks before filler augmentation.

Complications/Managing complications

Palpable nodules may form due to the aggregation of the filler used. Thorough massage and moulding of the injected filler directly after the treatment ensures uniform distribution.

Practical tips

- When treating the upper eyelid region, it is advisable to use a filler with a limited water-binding capability to avoid swelling and an undesired distribution of the filler.
- If the eyebrows are asymmetric from the outset, take care and highlight this to the patient before treatment. It may be appropriate to only treat the one eyebrow that is lower to achieve bilateral alignment.
- The outcome of the augmentation treatment can be optimised with adjuvant botulinum toxin type-A treatment ('chemical brow lift'), which should ideally be conducted before filler augmentation.
- Should accidental eyebrow ptosis develop as a result of botulinum toxin type-A treatment in the orbital region, the ptosis can be improved with filler augmentation to achieve a lifting effect.

Treatment planning – Upper eyelid

The aim of the treatment is to volumise the upper eyelid to improve the manifestation of a supraorbital hollow and/or skin wrinkling. A two-level cannula technique can be used to minimise the risk of bleeding. At first, an injection of a small volume of filler is made into the deep subcutaneous supraperiosteal plane directed to the medial crease of the upper eyelid, to improve the hollowness. Subsequently, a superficial subdermal injection is delivered over the entire upper eyelid in order to support, regenerate and tighten the skin surface.

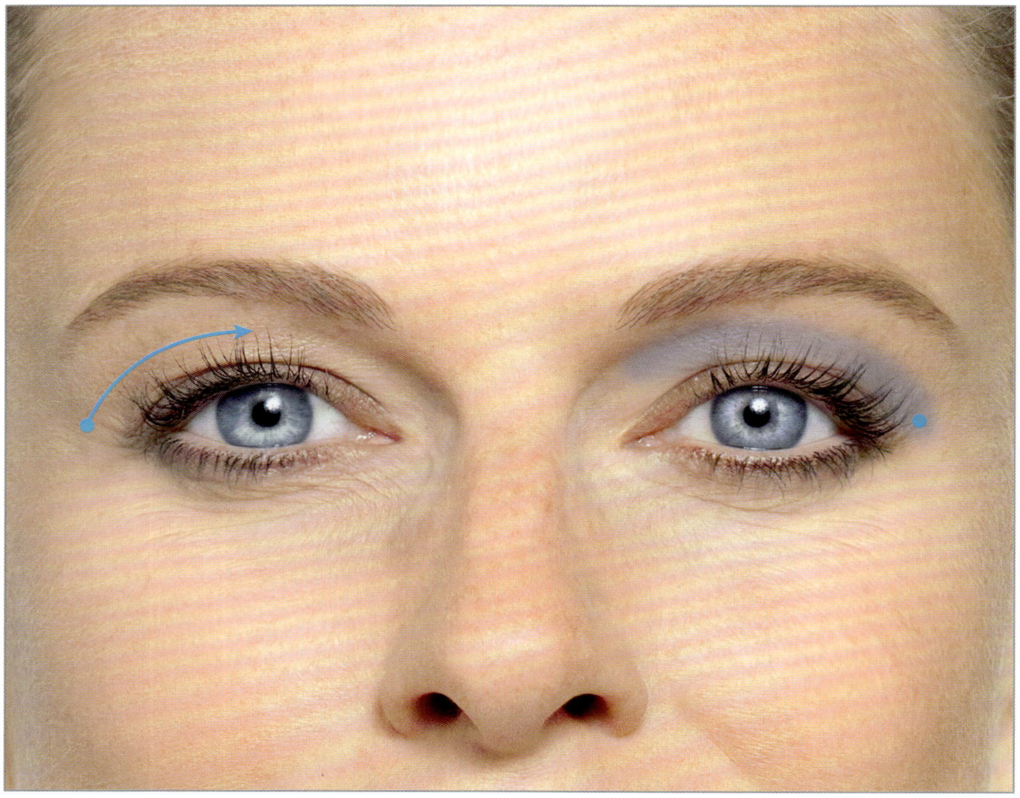

Technique: DHAC
Insertion site: lateral rim of the orbit close to the lateral canthus
Injection depth and direction: subcutaneous, following the course of the upper eyelid fold, from lateral to medial into the supramuscular fat plane
Volume: 0.05–0.1 ml/side
Tool: 22–25 gauge cannula

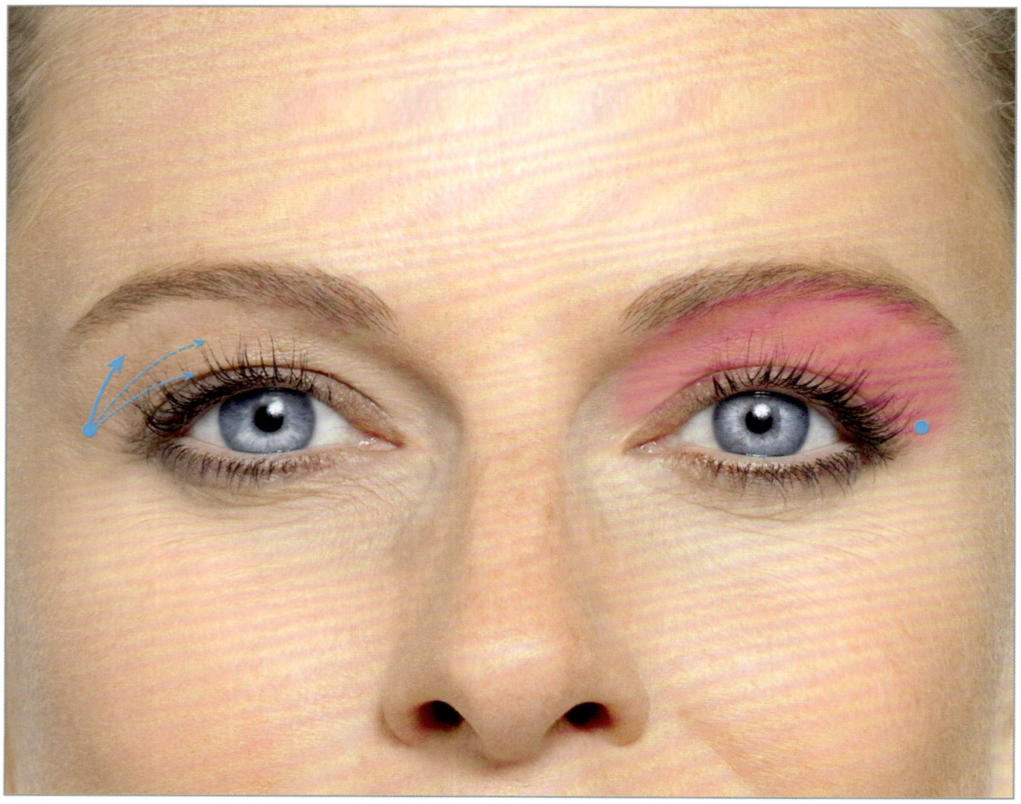

Technique: SHAC
Insertion site: lateral rim of the orbit close to the lateral canthus
Injection depth and direction: subdermally from lateral to medial, covering the entire upper eyelid
Volume: 0.1–0.2 ml/side
Tool: 22–25 gauge cannula

Treatment – Upper eyelid

DHAC

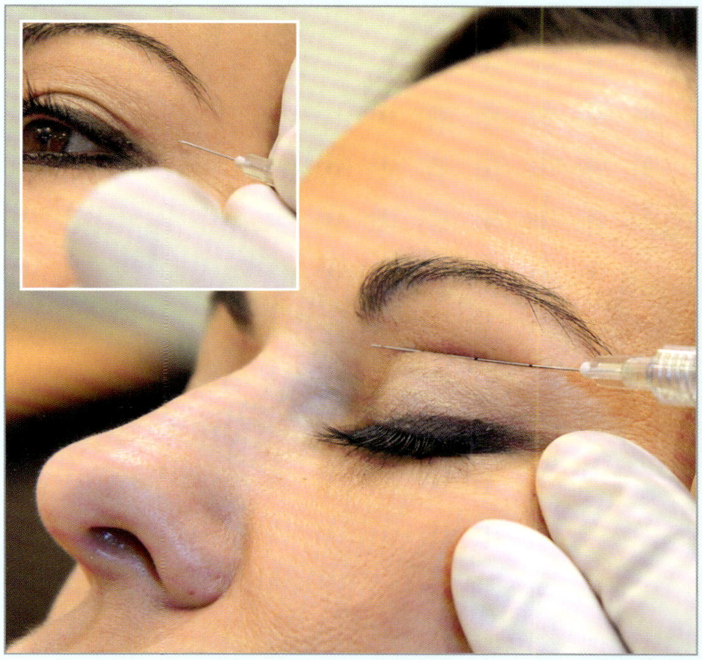

Fig. 7.21 An insertion point is made at the lateral end of the upper eyelid fold using an insertion needle. The cannula is then inserted into the entry hole and directed towards the medial aspect of the upper eyelid in the deep (subcutaneous) plane, by gently advancing it forwards and then retracting back in order to mobilise the soft tissues, while delivering 0.05–1 ml per eyelid.

SHAC

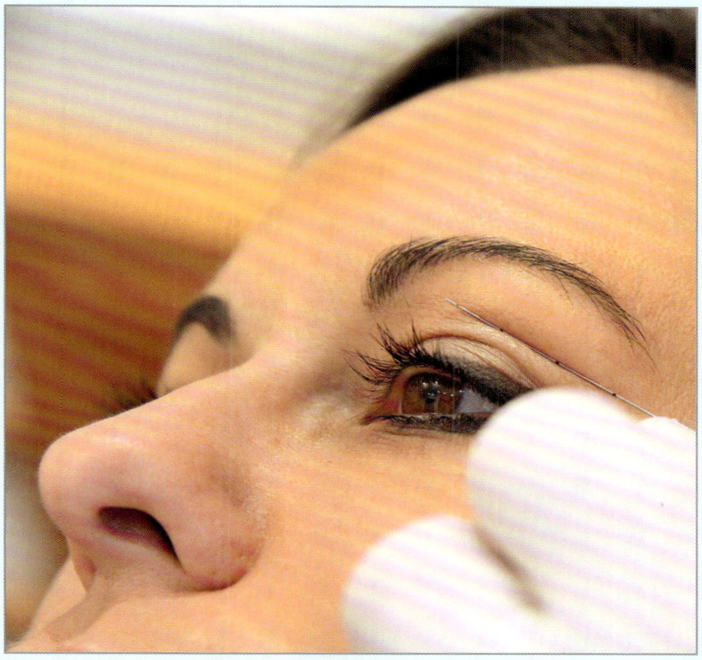

Fig. 7.22 In the next step, the cannula is brought into the superficial (subdermal) plane, and the skin surface is supported with 0.1–0.2 ml of the chosen filler, which is then injected and distributed over the entire eyelid region.

Treatment steps

- Remove makeup
- Disinfection
- Anaesthesia (optional)
- Injection: DHAC and SHAC
- Massage and mould (ensure appropriate distribution of the filler)
- Inform patient about post-treatment dos and don'ts
- Arrange a follow-up appointment

Filler selection

1 Superficial injection (p. 62)
2 Medium injection (p. 63)

Fillers with lower water-binding capacity are suitable in this region, as it is prone to oedema.

Combined treatment options

Chemical denervation using botulinum toxin type-A in the orbicularis oculi muscle 1 to 2 weeks before filler augmentation.

Complications/Managing complications

- When injecting subdermally, a 22–25 gauge cannula is optimal, as the large bore size allows navigation around the vessels and reduces the risk of bleeding.
- Palpable nodules may form due to the aggregation of the filler used. Thorough massage and moulding of the injected filler directly after the treatment ensures uniform distribution.

Practical tips

- It is advisable to use fillers with limited water-binding capacity in the upper eyelid region in order to avoid swelling.
- The dual technique utilises two planes of injection, and hence this allows for a more natural clinical outcome, while also promoting fibrogenetic regeneration of the treated area. In turn, this enables management of the age-related tissue atrophy, as well as achieving improvement in skin quality.

7.3.2 Lateral canthal lines (crow's feet)

The region around the lateral aspect of the eyes plays a significant role in the face, as dynamic contraction of the orbicularis oculi muscle here communicates positive emotions, with the resultant formation of dynamic fine lines, e.g. when smiling. However, with progressive ageing this region also begins to display static wrinkles, which can be a significant aesthetic concern for many patients.

Furthermore, skin thickness also plays a key role in the formation of the lateral canthal wrinkles, whereby thicker skin is commonly associated with deeper wrinkling, whereas thin skin exhibits finer and more superficial wrinkling.

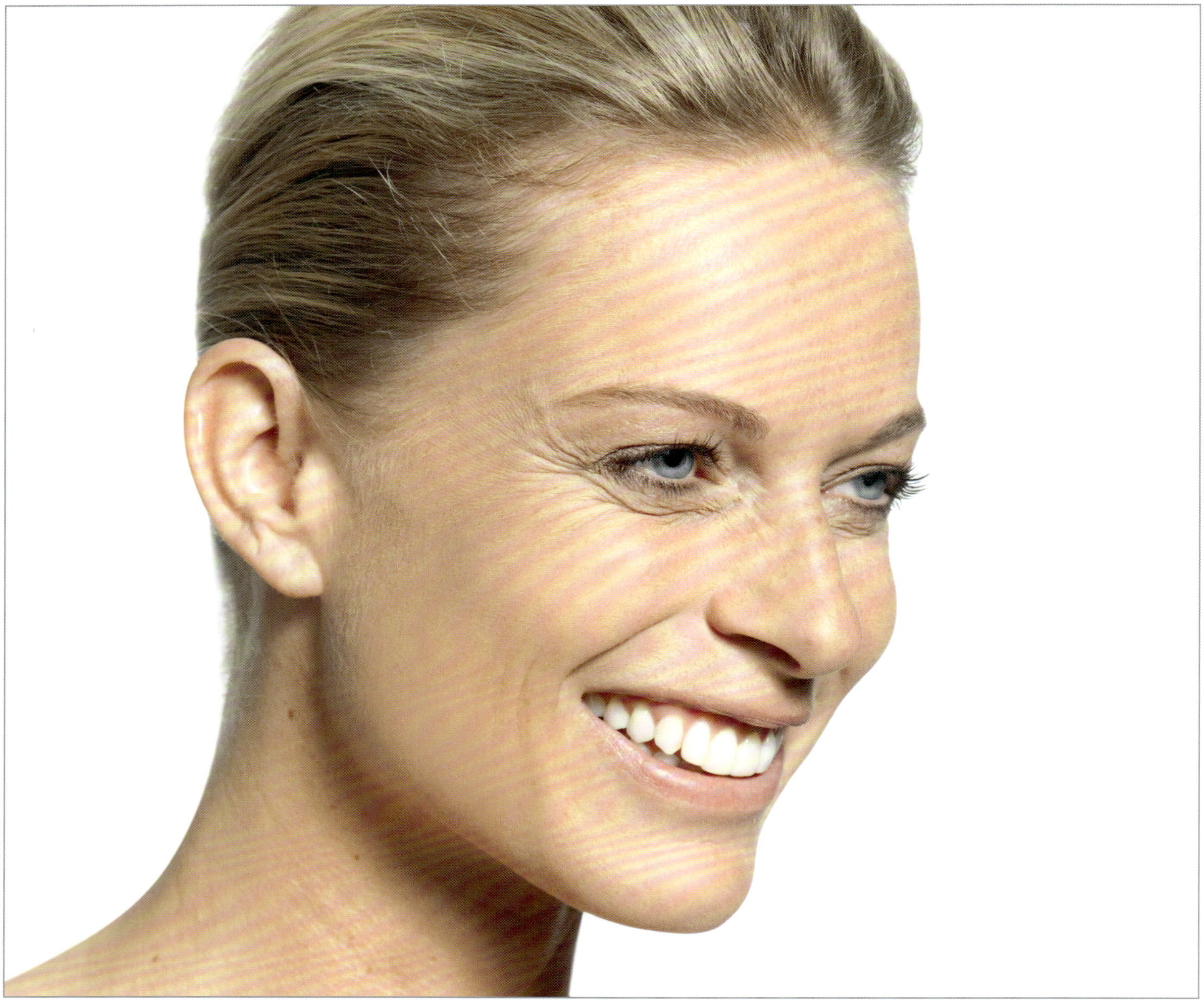

Patient selection
First and foremost it is essential to ascertain the extent of the dynamic and static lines present. Dynamic lines, activated by muscular contraction (e.g. smiling) are an indication for botulinum toxin type-A treatment. However, static lines are best treated with filler augmentation, and furthermore, ideally pre-treated with chemical peeling, laser resurfacing or dermal needling to improve the quality of the skin. Combining botulinum toxin type-A and fillers is also appropriate in many cases; with the muscle relaxation treatment ideally performed 2 weeks before augmentation with hyaluronic acid fillers.

Interestingly, the extent of the desired wrinkle correction in this region depends greatly on the gender of the patient. Typically, male patients request a partial reduction of the lateral canthal lines, whereas women often seek complete eradication.

Assessing the indication
Static lines respond well to treatment with filler augmentation, as discussed above. Deeper lines can be treated with vertical injections to restore the lost volume below the orbital ligaments. Very superficial wrinkles can be corrected with injections into or directly below the dermal plexus.

Anatomy

Upon contraction of the orbicularis oculi muscle (1), e.g. when smiling, radial lines form from the lateral canthus and radiate as far as into the cheek itself.

The space between the bone and the orbicularis oculi muscle is padded with volumising subcutaneous fat tissue. The orbital retaining ligaments (2), which connect the orbital rim with the skin, lose their tension forces when this fat tissue begins to shrink as a consequence of age-related tissue atrophy. The declining traction forces on the skin further provoke periorbital wrinkling, which as discussed previously primarily results from muscular activity and later on in life from actinic elastosis of the skin.

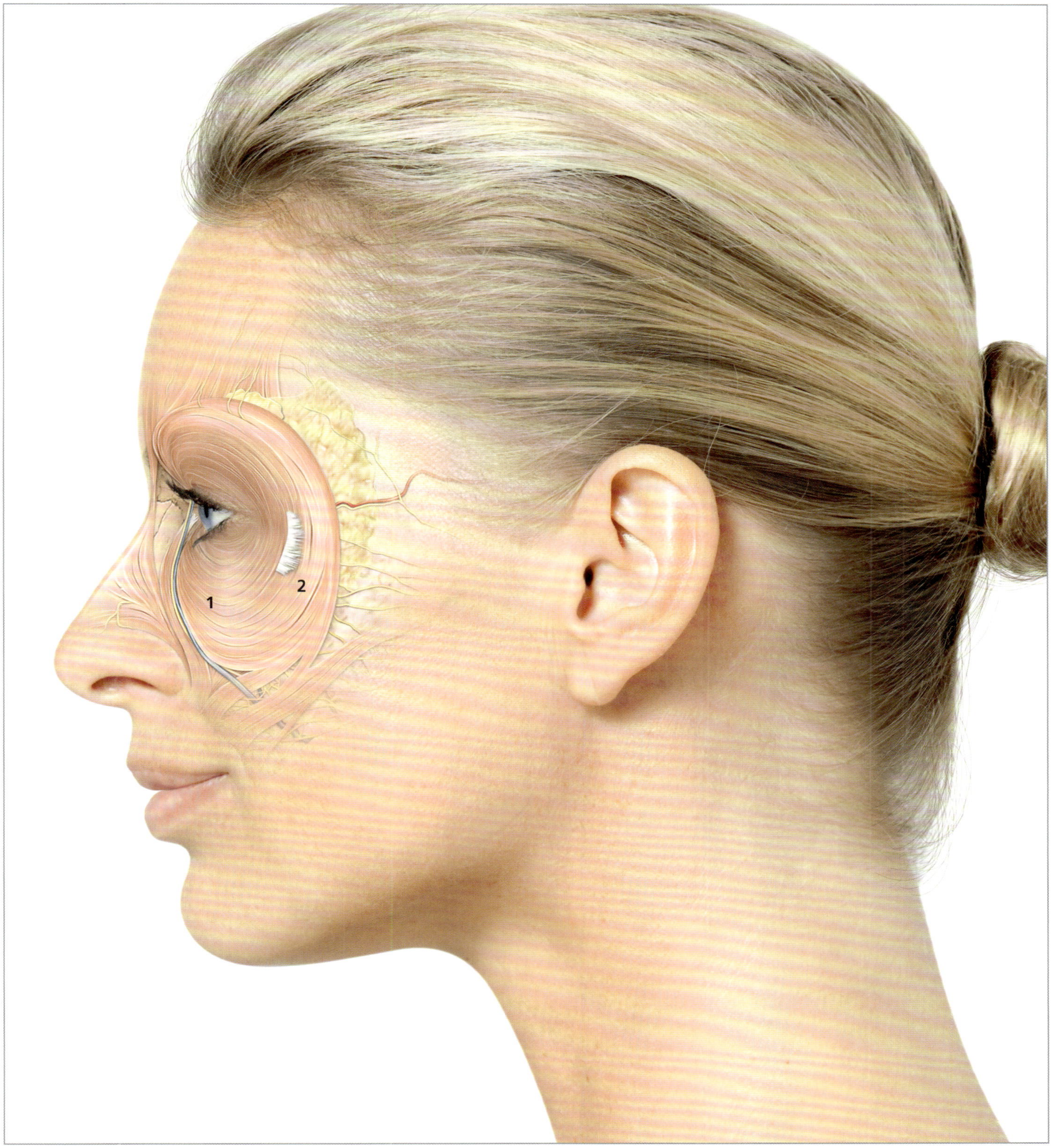

Treatment planning – Superficial wrinkle correction
The aim of the treatment is to target the superficial dermal or immediately subdermal plane to achieve correction of the static lateral canthal lines. The treatment is indicated in patients presenting with static lines, and when seeking to optimise the results after botulinum toxin type-A treatment.

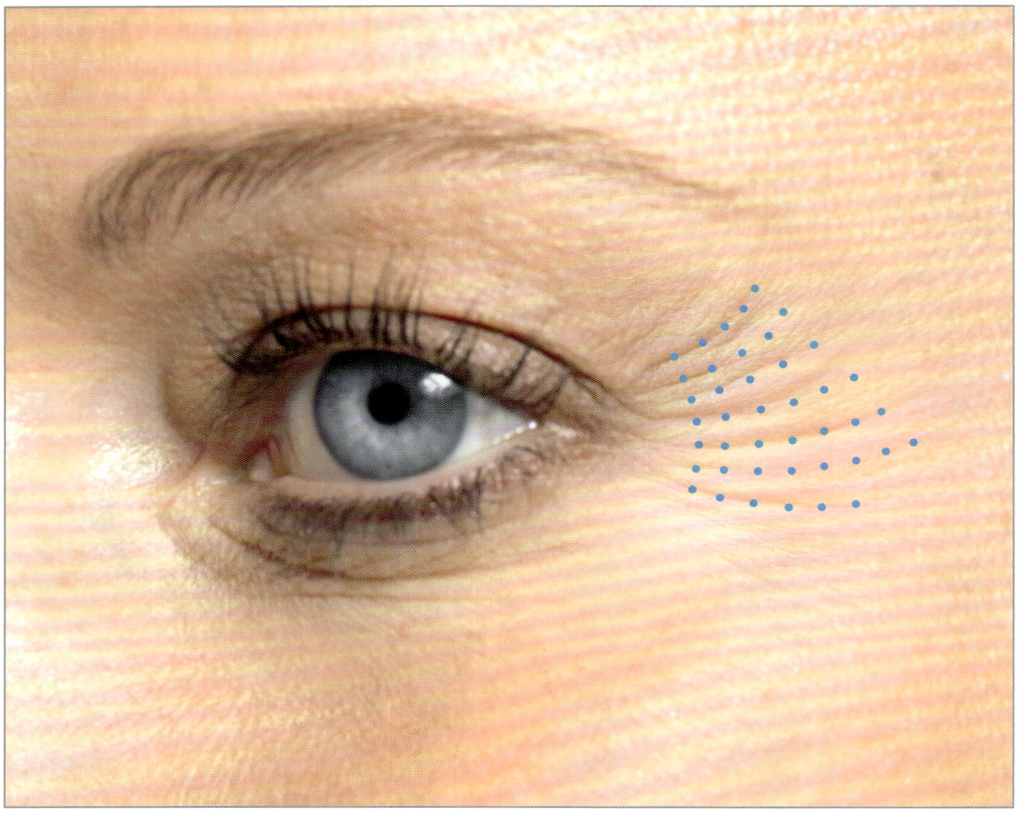

Technique: point technique with gentle stretching
Injection sites: three to five injection points per wrinkle (lateral to the orbital rim)
Injection depth: intradermal or immediately subdermal
Volume: minimum dose possible
Tool: 30–32 gauge needle

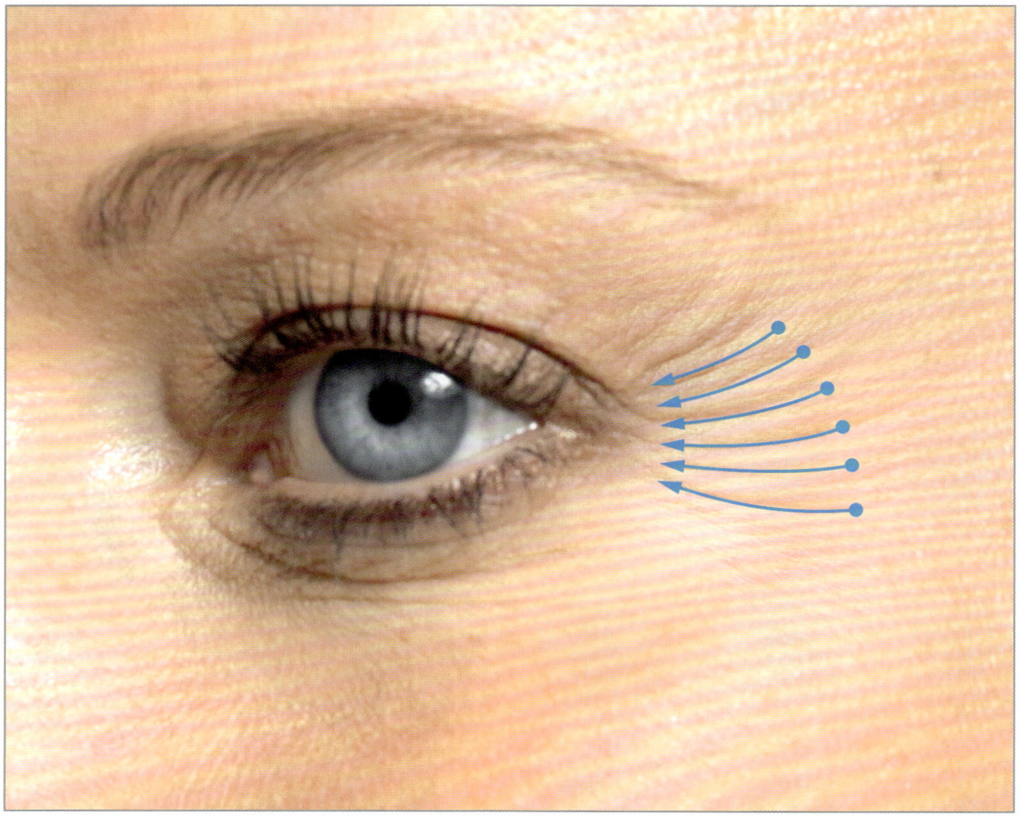

Technique: tunneling technique with gentle stretching
Injection site: from the lateral end of the wrinkle (not injecting past the lateral orbital rim)
Injection depth: intradermal or immediately subdermal
Volume: < 0.05 ml/thread
Tool: 30–32 gauge needle

Video: Lat-can tunneling http://www.kvm-tv.de/FIL/010mp4

7

Treatment – Superficial wrinkle correction

Point technique

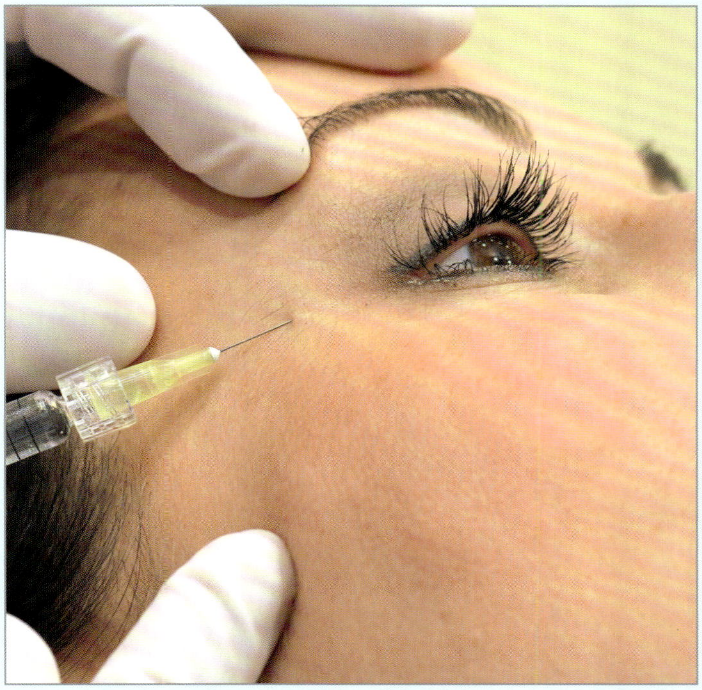

Fig. 7.23 The skin is gently stretched until the selected wrinkle remains just visible and the minimum possible depot volume is injected intradermally or immediately subdermally along the length of the wrinkle.

Tunneling technique

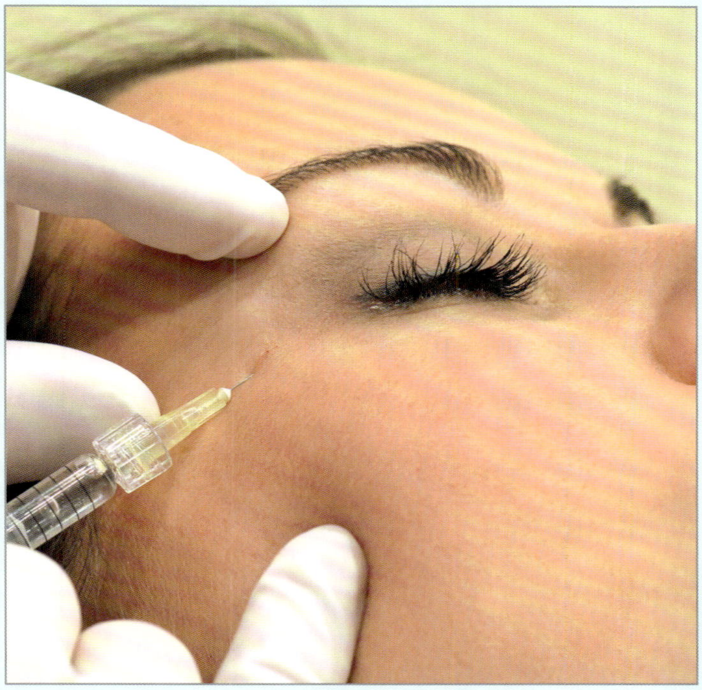

Fig. 7.24 While stretching the skin gently, the needle is inserted at the lateral end of each wrinkle and tunnelled under the skin using the linear technique. Small amounts of filler, approximately 0.05 ml, are administered as the needle is being withdrawn in the intradermal or immediate subdermal plane to deliver a thread.

Treatment steps
- Remove makeup
- Disinfection
- Anaesthesia (optional)
- Injection: point technique/tunneling technique
- Massage and mould (ensure appropriate distribution of the filler)
- Inform patient about post-treatment dos and don'ts
- Arrange a follow-up appointment

Filler selection

1 Superficial injection (p. 62)

2 Medium injection (p. 63)

Combined treatment options
- In cases of elastosis/sun damage: chemical peeling; laser resurfacing; medical needling
- In cases of orbicularis oculi muscle overactivity: botulinum toxin type-A
- In case of fat atrophy: filler augmentation of the temples and lateral cheeks

Complications/Managing complications
- Injections should be delivered no closer than the lateral aspect of the orbital rim.
- The lateral canthal and temple regions are highly perfused: take care to assess and avoid traumatising (i.e. by aspirating, injecting gently and slowly) any blood vessels.
- Palpable nodules may form due to the aggregation of the filler used. Thorough massage and moulding of the injected filler directly after the treatment ensures uniform distribution.

Practical tips
- Overcorrection is to be avoided at all times. Importantly, patients should be advised that the initial treatment may not be able to achieve optimal correction, so undercorrection is to be expected. Patients should therefore be advised in advance that several treatments may be required to achieve natural and satisfying clinical results.
- In case of dynamic lines, a muscular denervation therapy with botulinum toxin type-A should ideally be conducted prior to (ideally 2 weeks before) filler augmentation for optimal results.
- The manifestation of lateral canthal lines can further be reduced with adjacent volume restoration of the temples and the lateral cheeks.

⚠ Prior to injecting any filler, please refer to the latest manufacturer guidelines for specific instructions for use.

Treatment planning – Volume compensation
The aim of the treatment is to restore the volume lost at the lateral canthal region due to the soft tissue atrophy in the submuscular plane. The treatment entails vertical depot injections into the lateral orbital ligaments in the 'sweet spots' of the lateral canthal lines. In doing so, the deeper crow's feet can be improved with minimal filler volumes.

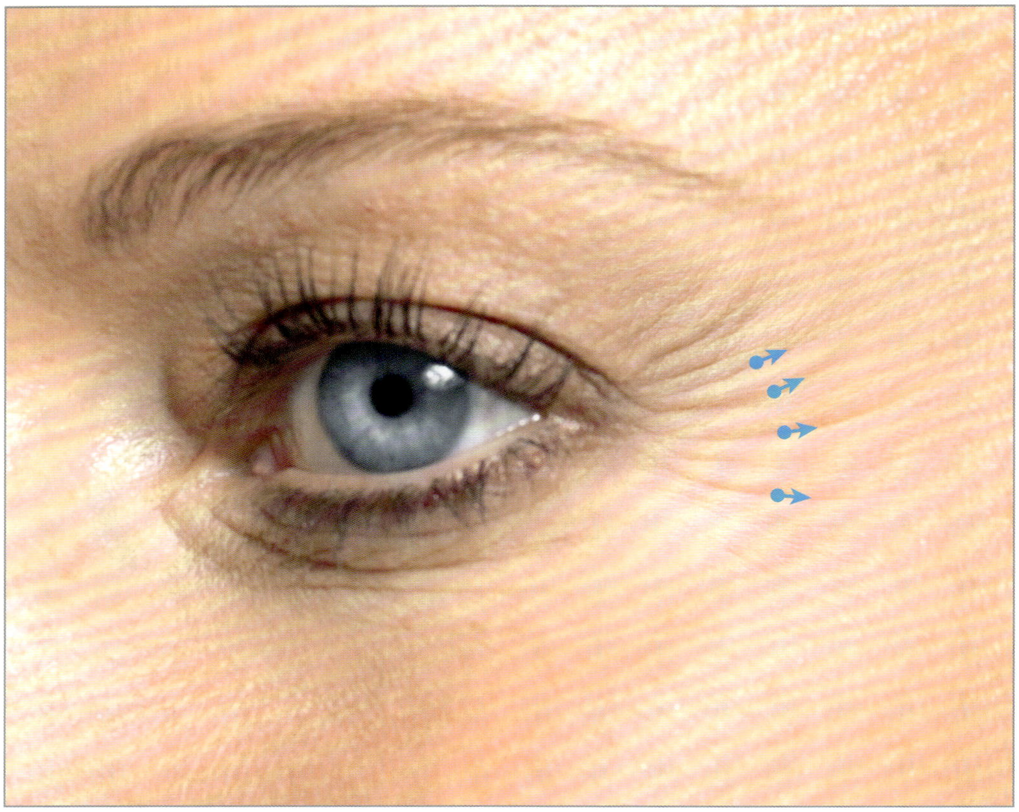

Technique: VSDT
Injection site: one 'sweet spot' per wrinkle into the orbital ligaments at the lateral rim of the orbit

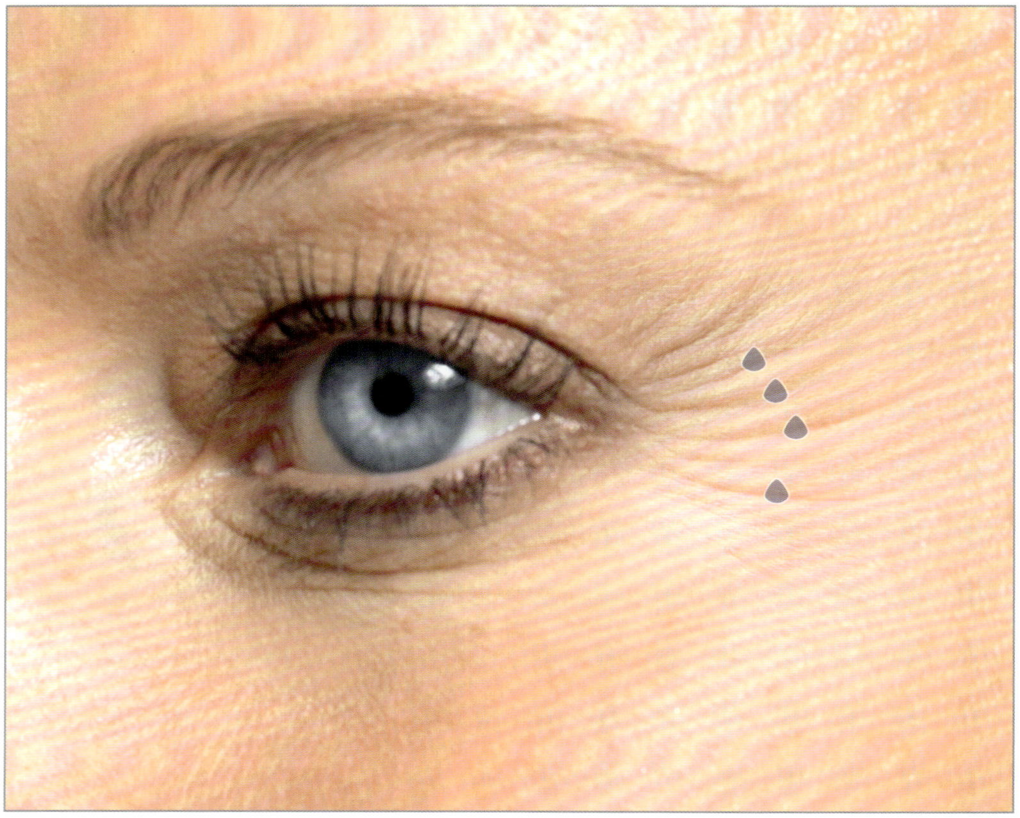

Volume: 0.01–0.02 ml/injection point
Tool: 27–30 gauge needle

Treatment – Volume compensation

VSDT

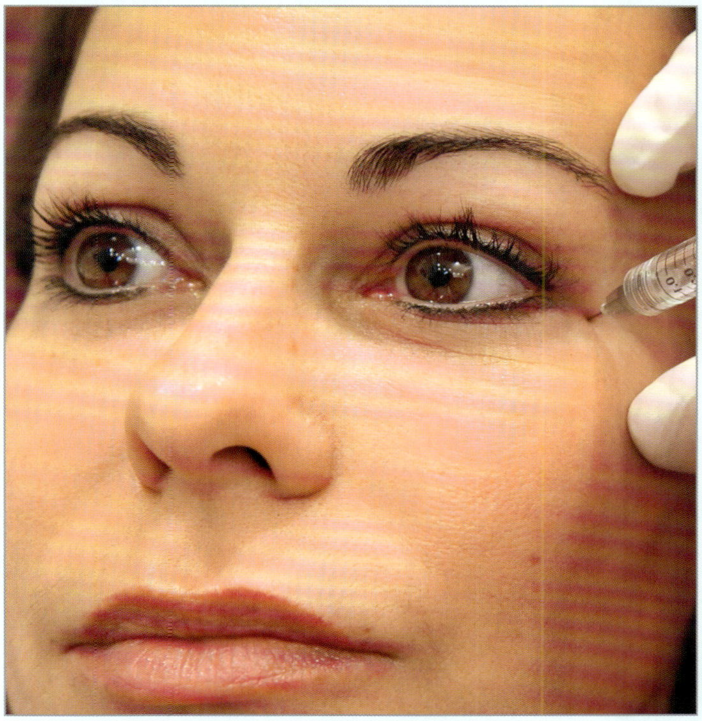

Fig. 7.25 The deep injection is performed while gently stretching the skin. The needle is inserted vertically into one of the 'hot spots' in the wrinkle at the lateral orbital rim where the orbital ligaments are located.

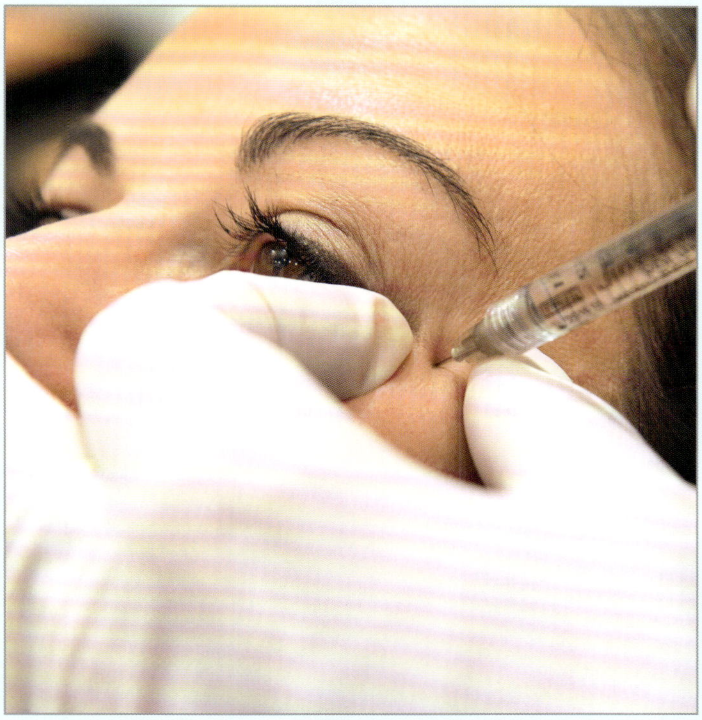

Fig. 7.26 If the injections reach the 'hot spots', where the ligaments are located, a crunching sound should be heard. Minimal amounts of filler volume per depot are adequate to achieve the desired clinical outcome.

Treatment steps
- Remove makeup
- Disinfection
- Anaesthesia (optional)
- Injection: VSDT
- Massage and mould (to ensure appropriate distribution of the filler)
- Inform patient about post-treatment dos and don'ts
- Arrange a follow-up appointment

Filler selection

2 Medium injection (p. 63)
3 Deep injection (p. 66)
4 Ultra-deep injection (p. 67)

Due to the thin skin around this region and the delicate structures below, it is advisable to use a soft filler for optimal results.

Combined treatment options
- In cases of elastosis/sun damage: chemical peeling; laser resurfacing; medical needling
- In cases of orbicularis oculi muscle overactivity: botulinum toxin type-A treatment
- In cases of fat atrophy: volume augmentation of the temples and lateral cheeks

Complications/Managing complications
- Injections should be delivered no closer that the lateral aspect of the orbital rim.
- The lateral canthal and temple regions are highly perfused: take care to assess and avoid traumatising (i.e. by aspirating, injecting gently and slowly) any blood vessels.
- Palpable nodules may form due to the aggregation of the filler used. Thorough massage and moulding of the injected filler directly after the treatment ensures uniform distribution.

Practical tips
- If the 'hot spot' is injected correctly, a crunching sound can be heard when the injection is made into the ligaments.
- Overcorrection is to be avoided at all times, even if the result of the first treatment is not optimal. Patients should be advised in advance that several treatments might be required to achieve best results.
- In cases of dynamic wrinkles, botulinum toxin type-A injections should ideally be carried out 2 weeks before filler augmentation.
- Lateral canthal lines can also be improved with filler augmentation of the temples and the lateral cheeks.

7.3.3 Infraorbital region (infraorbital hollowness)

The infraorbital region is affected quite early on in the ageing process and is a significant concern for many patients. As such, patients commonly seek improvement within the non-surgical arena. Dark shadows at the lower eyelid, accentuation of the tear trough, fine wrinkling and enlarged lower eye bags are a major concern as they are often associated with a tired, haggard and burned-out appearance.

A perfusion-dependent atrophy of the sub-orbicularis oculi fat pad (SOOF) alongside the infraorbital hollowness (IOH) are considered the key factors to the aforementioned features. (In this book we shall refer to the infraorbital hollow [IOH] as the U-shaped depression under the eyes comprising of the tear trough, nasojugal fold, and the palpebromalar groove.) More superficial dermal ageing particularly associated with photodamage, as well as the deeper skeletal changes also affect the aforementioned features. Both intrinsic factors such as genetics and general health, as well as extrinsic factors such as smoking, stress, diet, cold temperatures and wind (to name a few) play a key role in these processes.

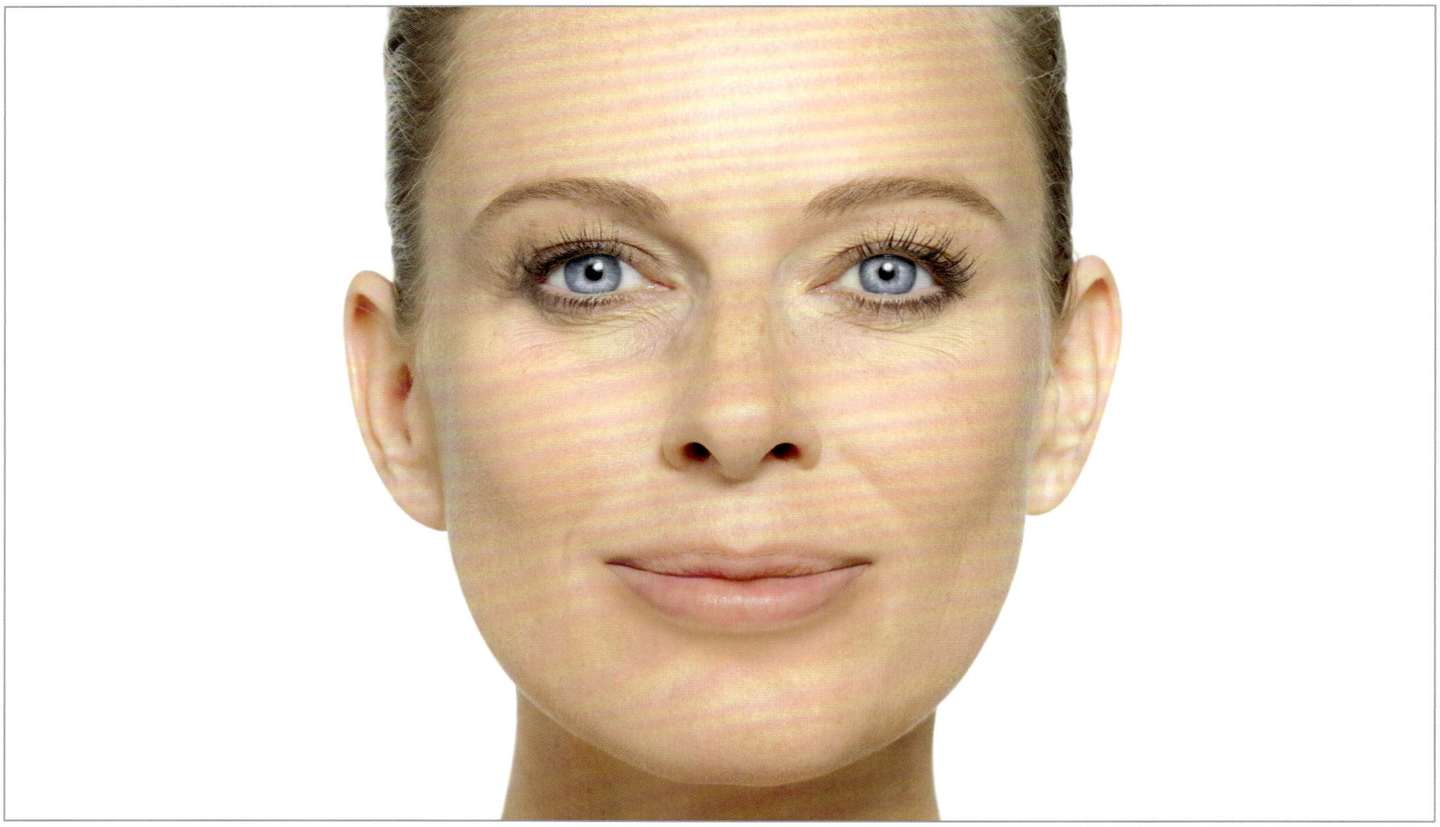

7

Patient selection

It is important to distinguish between patients who present with age-related fat pad atrophy resulting in infraorbital hollowness, versus those with a natural predisposition to infraorbital hollows. In the former case of age-related fat loss, deep vertical filler injections are indicated. However, in patients presenting with buccal fat situated more inferiorly, and independent of the age-related fat atrophy, the orbital rim may appear prominent, and hence volume compensation of the SOOF is not indicated. Instead, the transitional zone between the cheek and lower eyelid should be harmonised with low volume, medium-depth filler augmentation.

Given that the IOH emerges from volume loss in the midface, it can be treated with vertical filler injections into the SOOF. Further injections into the medial and lateral orbital ligaments can help to harmonise the appearance of the tear trough and the lower eyelid shadows. Furthermore, fine wrinkling and other defects of the lower eyelid, relating to skin ageing, can be improved with superficial filling techniques.

Assessing the indication

Augmentation with hyaluronic acid fillers offers an effective non-surgical solution for rejuvenation of the infraorbital region. Many consider that results with hyaluronic acid treatment compared to those with autologous fat transplantation are comparable with regard to the reproducibility of the treatment outcomes.

Rejuvenation of the infraorbital region with hyaluronic acid fillers encompasses four aspects to the treatment:

- Volume compensation in the SOOF
- Tightening of the adherent orbital retaining ligaments via restoration of their soft tissue base
- Enhancement of the superficial fat layer and blending in the buccal-infraorbital junctional zone
- Improvement of the skin quality

The infraorbital region is prone to swelling following filler augmentation treatments with water-binding hyaluronic acid fillers, and hence: patients should be made aware of this prior to the treatment; the correct filler chosen; alongside great care taken during the injections to avoid overcorrection.

Anatomy

This region represents a junctional zone between the infraorbital superficial fat-deficient zone and the fat-rich cheek region. Below the orbital fat-deplete zone lays the orbicularis oculi muscle (1). Its pars orbicularis is directly connected to the skin. The infraorbital skin is particularly thin and hence minimal muscular activity elicits fine wrinkles, which ultimately persist at rest with advancing age. This is further enhanced by skin elastosis and skin dryness, both associated with advanced ageing.

Below the orbicularis oculi muscle, the sub-orbicularis oculi fat pad (SOOF, 2) is positioned. In youth, the SOOF is a major volumising element, which fills and elevates the infraorbital and the midface region. Its atrophy-related reduction leads to an infraorbital hollow and accentuation of the orbital rim. This provokes the prominence of the 'tear trough' at the medial aspect and the lateral palpebral groove at the lateral aspect of the eye circle. The orbital retaining ligaments (3), which are anchored along the orbital rim and retract the skin towards the atrophied base, contribute to the manifestation of the atrophy-related IOH.

In the infraorbital region, the minimal infraorbital superficial fat transitions into the fat-rich cheek region, which is dynamically elevated by the zygomaticus muscle during laughing and smiling. Depending on individual disposition, the junctional zone can be more or less pronounced leading to a non-atrophy-related predisposition to IOHs. In cases of atrophy-related IOH the recommended injection technique is VSDT, whereas in cases of non-atrophy related IOH the recommended treatment approach involves intra- or subdermal injections.

The infraorbital foramen is situated medially and below the orbital rim, through which a rich neurovascular bundle emerges. Care should be taken to avoid traumatising these structures when injecting.

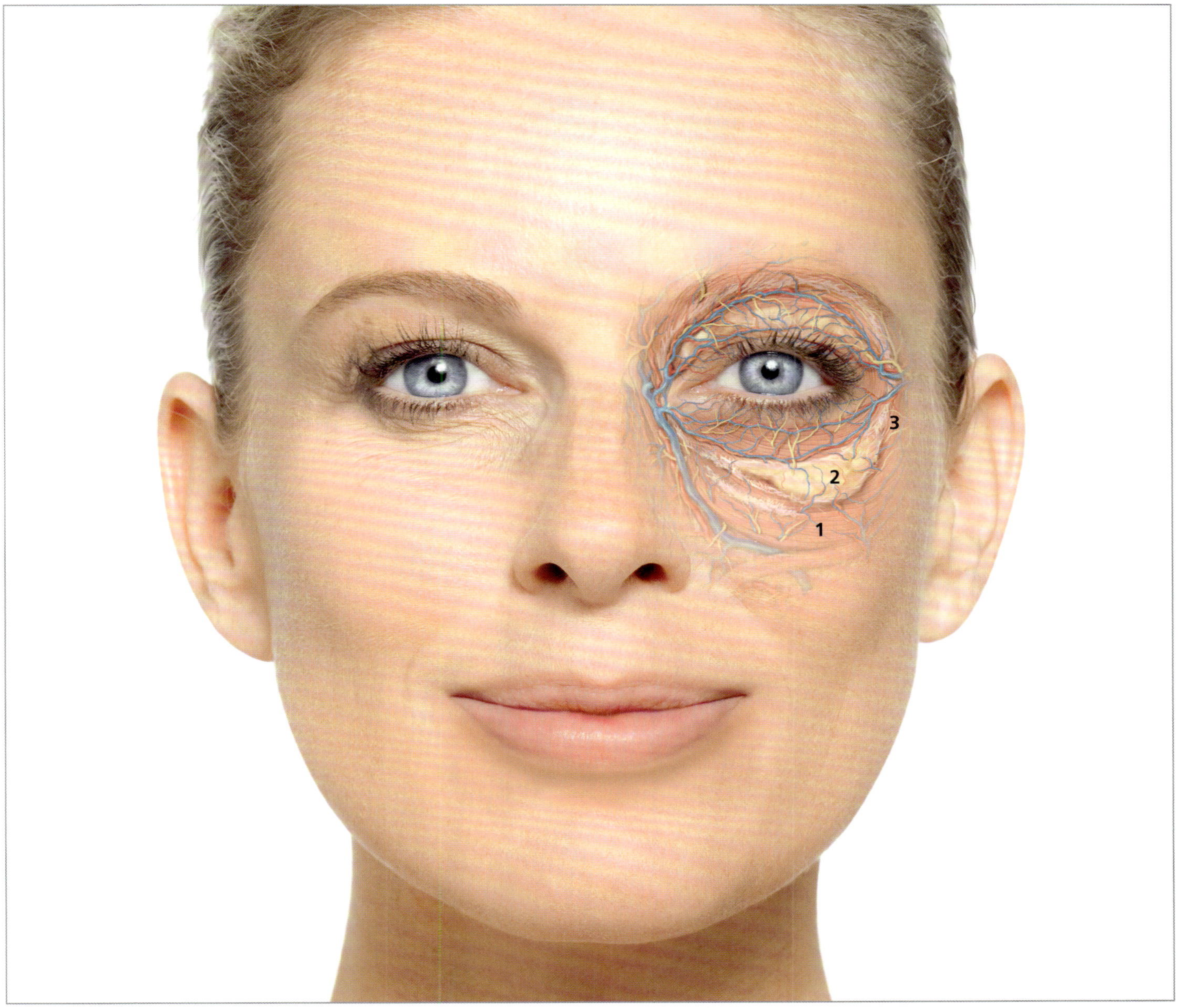

Treatment planning – Superficial correction
The aim of filler treatment is to augment and harmonise the non-atrophy-related changes in the infraorbital region. Superficial filler augmentation using a cannula enables reduction of the fine static wrinkles, as well as enhancement of the general skin quality. Furthermore, the non-atrophy-related visibility of the IOH could be improved with medium-depth filler augmentation in the infraorbital junction zone between the lower eyelid and the cheek.

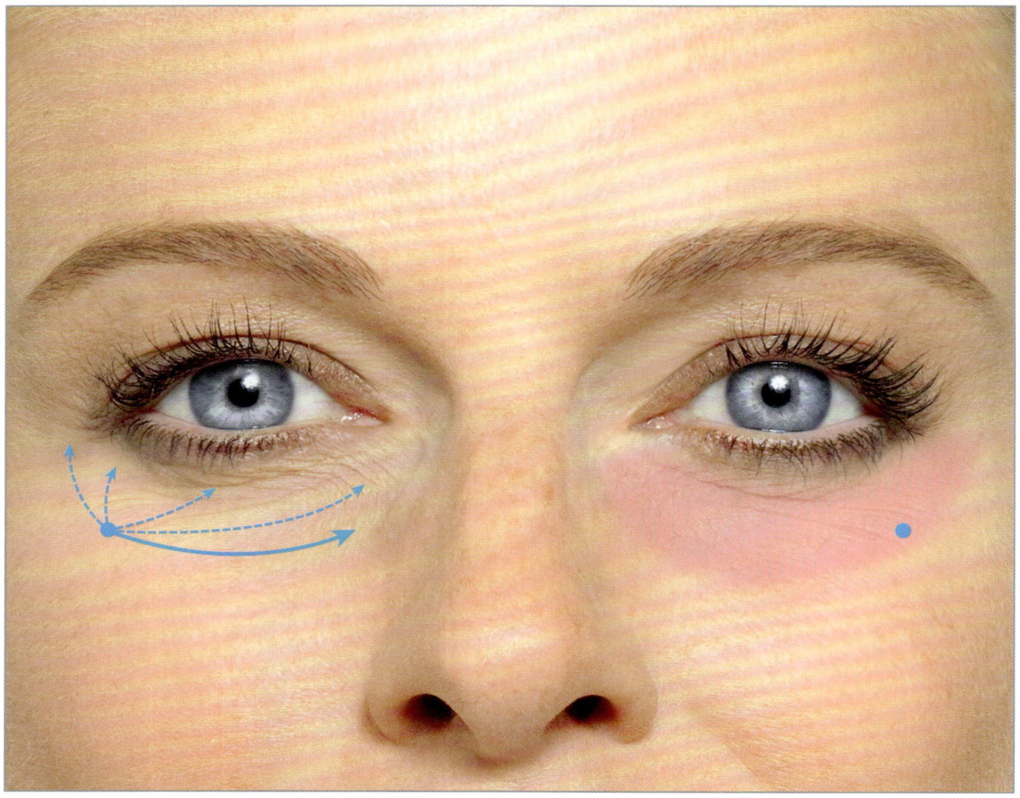

Technique: SHAC or serial point technique
Insertion site: at the lateral border of the lower orbital rim
Injection depth and direction: into the dermal or subdermal plane, working from the lateral to the medial aspect as well as superiorly, to cover the entire lower eyelid
Volume: 0.05–0.1 ml total per side
Tool: 25–27 gauge cannula (SHAC), or 30–32 gauge needle (serial point technique)

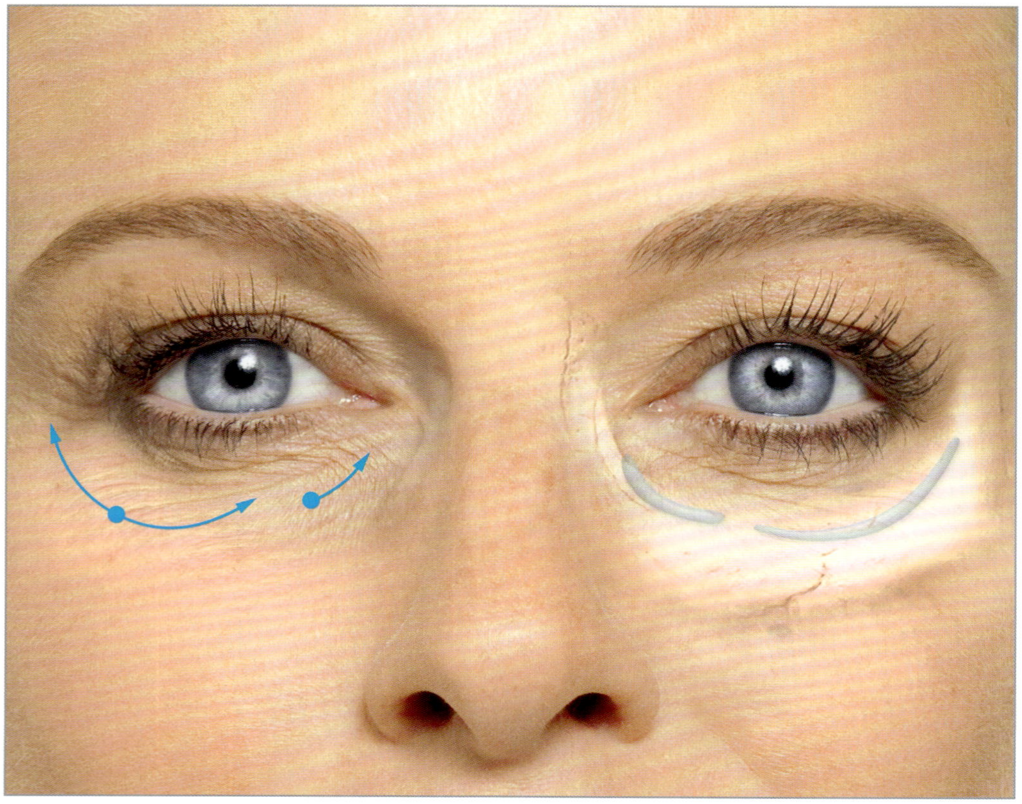

Technique: tunneling technique
Injection site: above the orbital rim
Injection depth: medium-depth into the subdermal plane
Volume: depending on the findings, 0.1–0.2 ml total per side
Tool: 30 gauge needle

Treatment – Superficial correction

SHAC

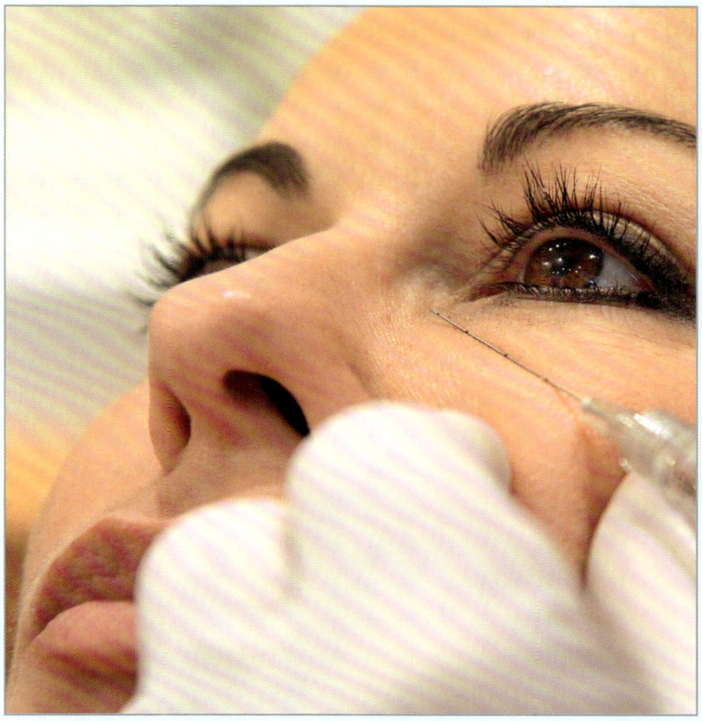

Fig. 7.27 The cannula is brought into the infraorbital dermal plexus via an insertion point at the lateral border of the lower orbital rim. The subdermal tissue is then gently mobilised and filled with 0.1–0.2 ml of the hyaluronic acid filler, depending on the patient's individual needs.

Tunneling technique

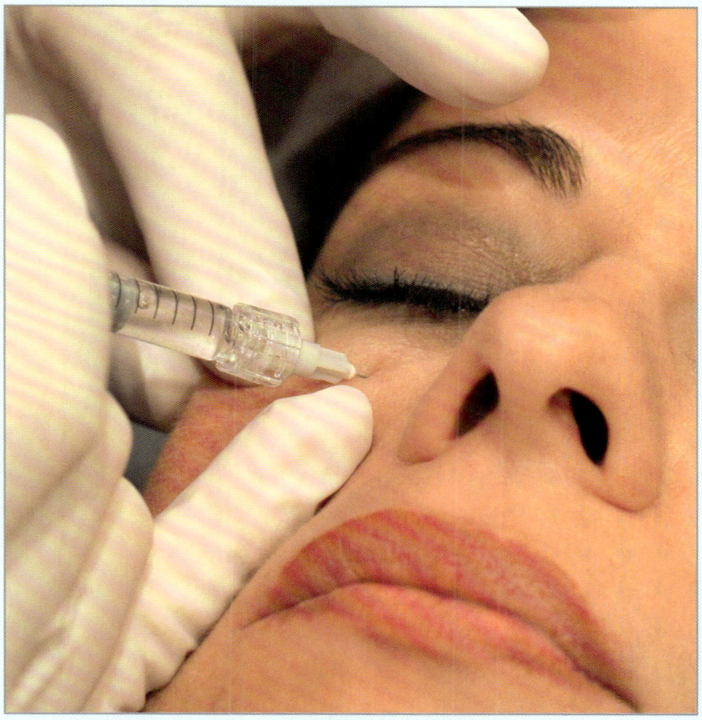

Fig. 7.28 The needle is inserted at an angle of 45 degrees to the skin surface. The filler is placed into the superficial subcutaneous tissue covering the appearance of the IOH.

Treatment steps
- Remove makeup
- Disinfection
- Anaesthesia (optional)
- Injection: SHAC/tunneling technique
- Massage and mould (ensure appropriate distribution of the filler)
- Inform patient about post-treatment dos and don'ts
- Arrange a follow-up appointment

Filler selection

1 Superficial injection (p. 62)

2 Medium injection (p. 63)

Since this region is prone to swelling after filler augmentation, it is advisable to use hyaluronic acid fillers with lower water-binding capacity.

Combined treatment options
- In cases of elastosis/sun damage: chemical peeling; laser resurfacing; medical needling
- In cases of orbicularis oculi muscle over activity: botulinum toxin type-A

Complications/Managing complications
- Palpable nodules may form due to aggregation of the hyaluronic acid filler used. Thorough massage and moulding of the injected filler directly after the treatment ensures uniform distribution.
- The infraorbital region is highly perfused: avoid traumatising blood vessels (e.g. by either using a cannula or by injecting ultra-deep with a needle).

Practical tips
- For the infraorbital region, the authors recommend using a hyaluronic acid filler with limited water-binding capacity to avoid severe swelling.
- If the IOH does not result from the atrophy of the SOOF but rather from an inherent inferior location of the cheek fat, the SOOF should not be treated with fillers, as this can lead to swelling of the fat pad.

Treatment planning – Volume compensation

The aim of the treatment is to reduce the prominence of the infraorbital hollow (IOH). A deep volumising injection into the atrophied medial part of the SOOF is made. After visible projection of the fat pad, the medial aspect of the IOH (i.e. the tear trough) can be treated with further vertical depots into the adherent orbital ligaments if necessary. The same technique can be applied to the lateral aspect of the IOH at the lateral orbital rim. In doing so, the stabilising ligaments arising from the deep fat pads to the skin are provided with new tension forces, making the infraorbital fat elevate in a natural fashion. However, the result is highly dependent on the ultra-deep supraperiosteal positioning of the filler.

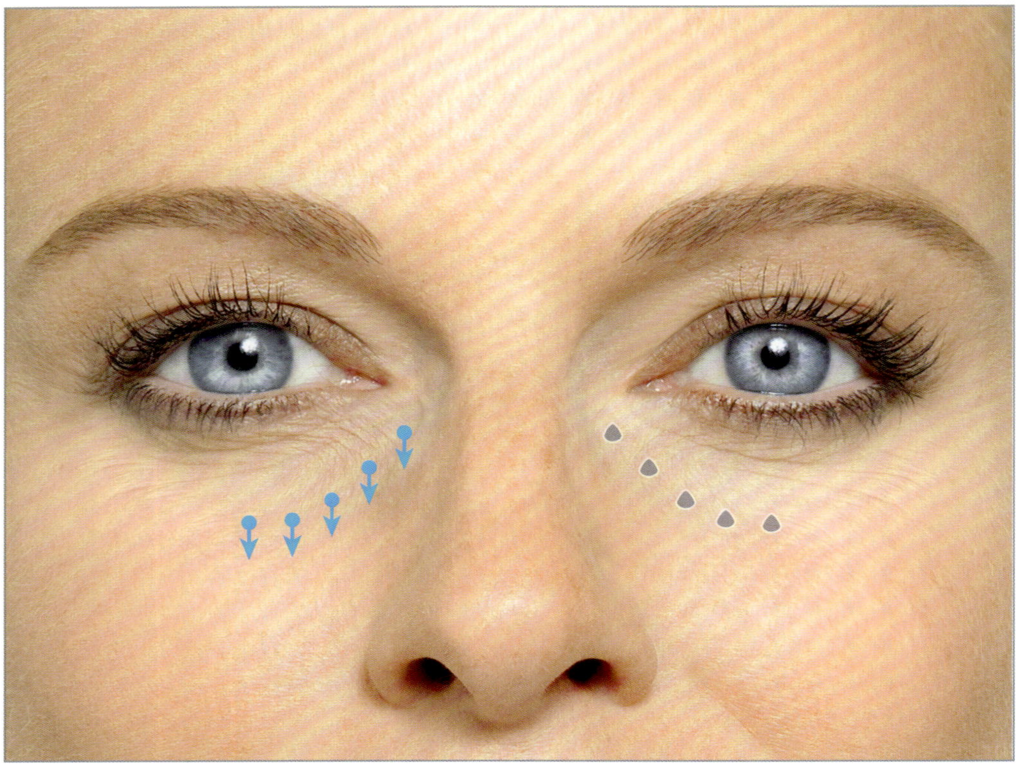

Technique: VSDT
Injection points: • SOOF volumisation: one to two injections at the medial aspect of the SOOF into the point of the deepest depression (i.e. 'hot spot')
Tear trough: an additional three or so injections at the medial orbital rim into the orbital retaining ligaments (a crunching sound should be heard when the injection makes contact with the 'hot spot')
Volume: 0.2–0.3 ml/depot into the SOOF; 0.05–0.1 ml/depot into the orbital retaining ligaments
Tool: 27 gauge needle

Caution: When treating the SOOF, avoid the infraorbital neurovascular bundle and take care when inserting the needle carefully and slowly in the vertical direction down to the bone.

Video: IOH medially
http://www.kvm-tv.de/FIL/011.mp4

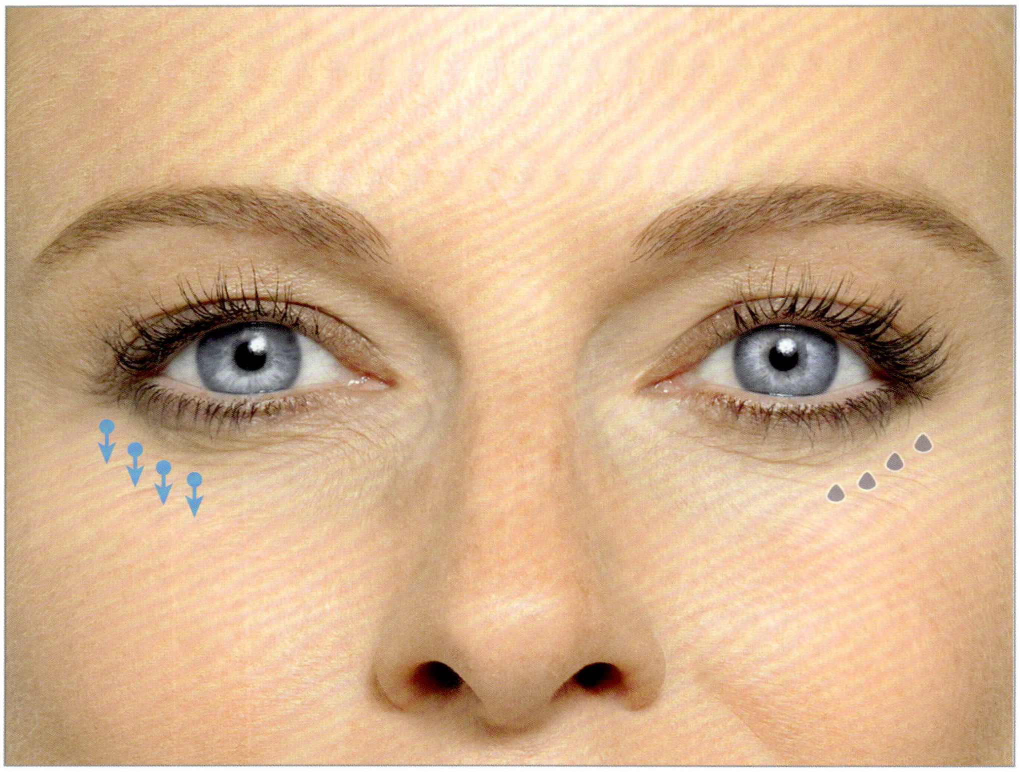

Technique: VSDT
Injection points: • three to four 'hot spots' into the orbital ligaments along the lateral lower orbital rim to harmonise the lateral palpebral groove (a crunching sound is heard when the injection makes contact with the 'hot spot')
Volume: 0.05–0.1 ml/injection point
Tool: 27 gauge needle

Video: IOH laterally
http://www.kvm-tv.de/FIL/012.mp4

7

Treatment – Volume compensation

VSDT medial

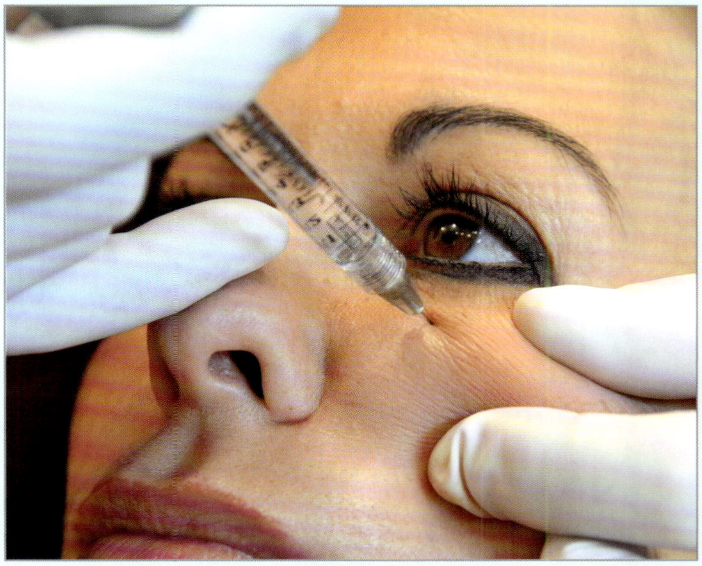

Fig. 7.29 The first injection is made by gently elevate the tissues with the non-injecting hand and injecting vertically into the medial part of the atrophied sub-orbicularis ocular fat pad. The injection should be done slowly and gently, away from the infraorbital neurovascular bundle. If the injection makes contact with the 'hot spot', the fat compartment is visibly lifted. Further vertical injections of smaller depots along the medial lower orbital rim will tighten the ligaments leading to an improvement in the medial IOH.

VSDT lateral

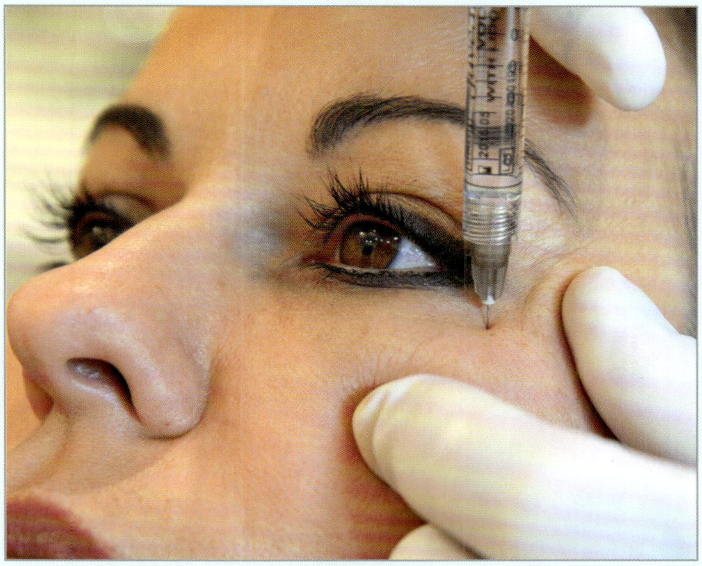

Fig. 7.30 The lateral part of the IOH is treated with vertical injections of small depots (0.05–0.1 ml) into the orbital ligaments at the lateral lower orbital rim.

Treatment steps
- Remove makeup
- Disinfection
- Anaesthesia (optional)
- Injection: VSDT
- Massage and mould (ensure appropriate distribution of the filler)
- Inform patient about post-treatment dos and don'ts
- Arrange a follow-up appointment

Practical tips

- Additional superficial filler augmentation, using a blunt cannula technique (SHAC), improves the static fine wrinkling, which in turn ensures a more global and optimal outcome.
- Fillers with limited water-binding capacity should be used in the infraorbital region to avoid severe swelling.
- If the IOH does not result from atrophy of the SOOF but rather from an inherent inferior location of the cheek fat, the SOOF should not be treated with fillers, as this can result in swelling of the fat pad and an unattractive clinical outcome.

Filler selection

2 Medium injection (p. 63)
3 Deep injection (p. 66)
4 Ultra-deep injection (p. 67)

Since this region is prone to swelling after filler augmentation, it is advisable to use fillers with lower water-binding capacity.

Combined treatment options
- In cases of elastosis/sun damage: chemical peeling; laser resurfacing; medical needling
- In cases of orbicularis oculi muscle overactivity: botulinum toxin type-A

Complications/Managing complications
- The infraorbital region is highly perfused, and hence care should be taken to avoid traumatising any blood vessels when vertically inserting a needle to an ultra-deep supraperiosteal level.
- Avoid the infraorbital foramen and its neurovascular bundle, and when treating around the area take great care, aspirate and inject slowly.
- Palpable nodules may form due to the aggregation of the filler used. Thorough massage and moulding of the injected filler directly after the treatment ensures uniform distribution.

7.4 Midface

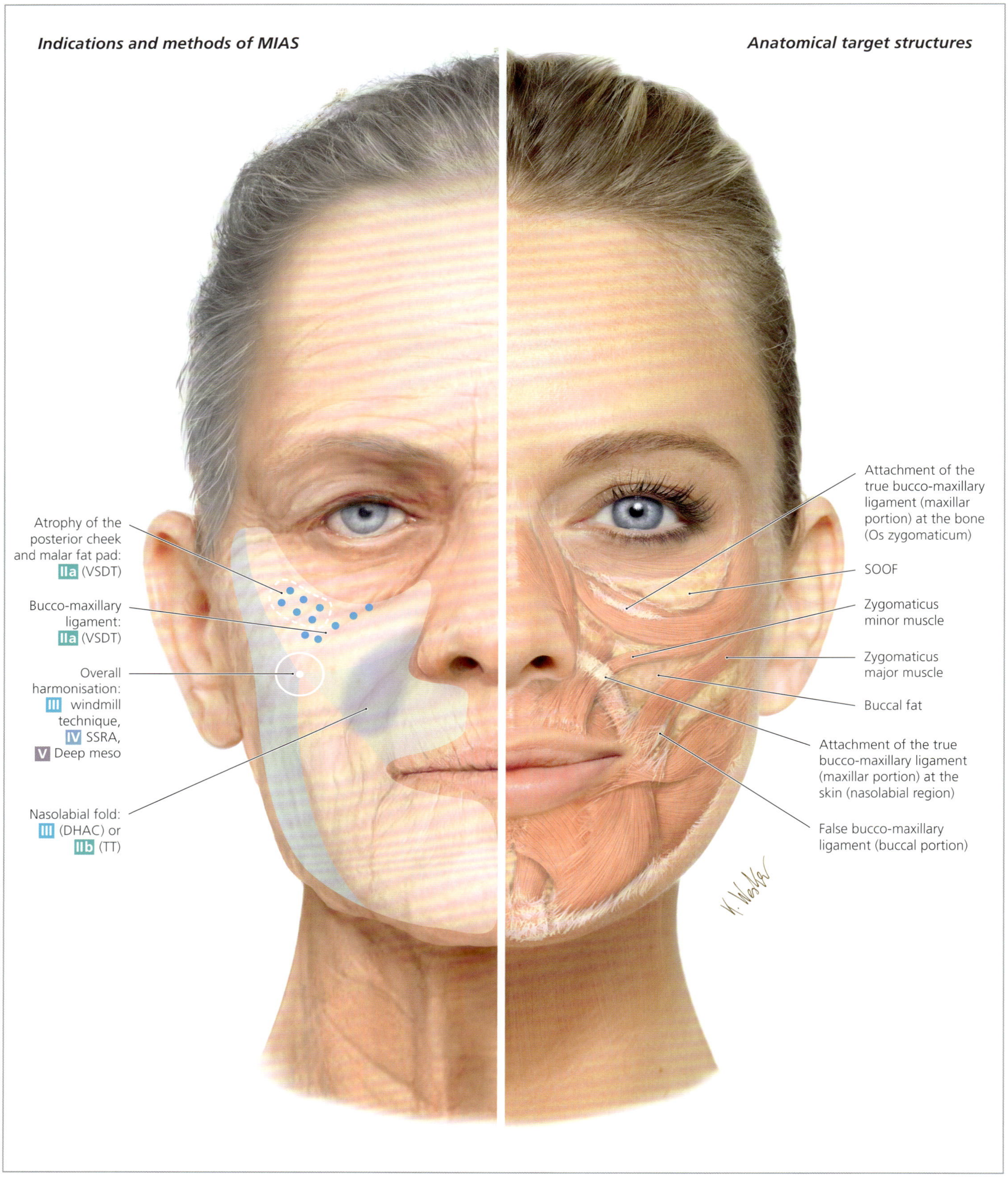

Fig. 7.31 Overview of the anatomy, target structures and cause-related augmentation techniques in the midface.
• VSDT (or, alternatively, SAT for camouflage purposes); DHAC; ⊙ windmill technique, SSRA or deep mesotherapy for an overall harmonisation.

7.4.1 Overall harmonisation of the midface (Windmill technique)

One of the key characteristics of a youthful, attractive face is the mid-face region. Adequate fat pad support is essential for a pronounced and well contoured mid and lateral cheek region. Furthermore, a homogenous and smooth skin surface is also important to optimise the aesthetics of this region.

During the natural course of ageing, these features diminish as a result of limited perfusion, advancing atrophy of the soft tissues, alongside bony resorption and skin ageing. With the declining tensile forces combined with the effects of gravity, the upper fat compartments of this region together with their overlying skin slowly slip off their bony support and migrate downwards towards the lower half of the face. This gradually leads to an inversion of the facial shape from an 'upright triangle' to the 'inverted triangle' associated with ageing. Furthermore, intrinsic and extrinsic skin defects accumulate leading to an increasing inhomogeneity of the skin surface with dryness, pigmentary changes and wrinkles.

Filler treatment in this region allows us to restore the harmony of the midface region. The windmill technique (a variant of the deep horizontal augmentation with a cannula technique [DHAC]) can be a useful strategy to achieve this. Importantly, it allows the practitioner to use just one insertion point to achieve multi-directional augmentation of the midface region, including the entire infraorbital, periorbital and posterior (temporal) cheek regions. Furthermore, should there be a need to treat the more superficial wrinkling and uneven skin surface relief, the superficial horizontal augmentation with a cannula (SHAC) or the deep mesotherapy techniques can also be used to achieve optimal clinical results.

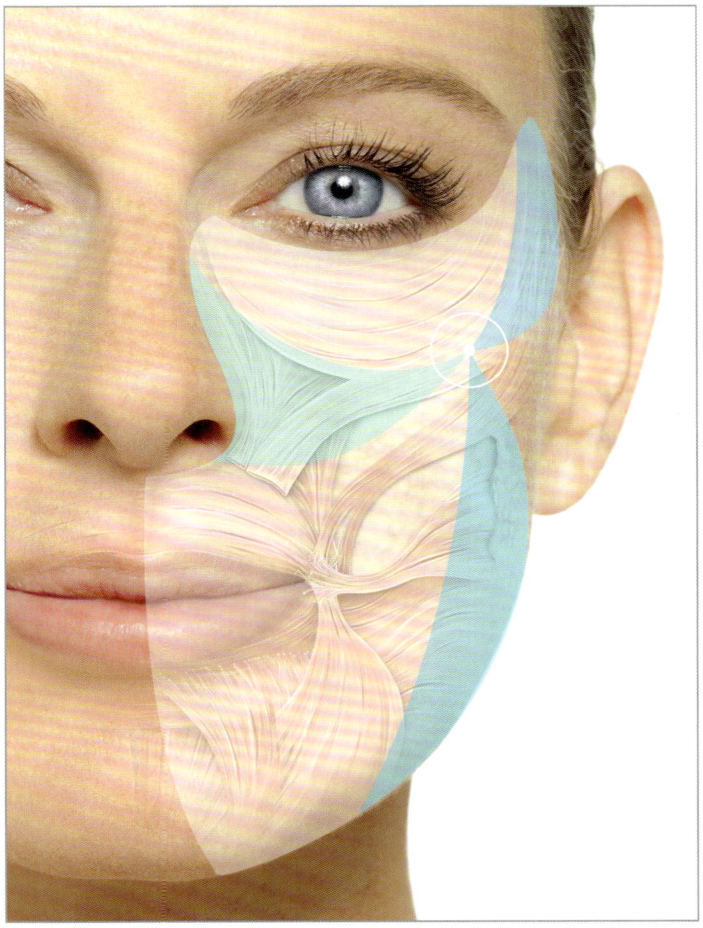

Treatment steps
- Remove makeup
- Disinfection
- Anaesthesia: local anaesthesia around the insertion point is mostly offered, but more invasive anaesthetic methods can also be used if required
- Injection: a combination of horizontal augmentation techniques (DHAC, Windmill, SHAC) or deep mesotherapy
- Massage and mould (ensure appropriate distribution of the filler)
- Inform patient about post-treatment dos and don'ts
- Arrange a follow-up appointment

Filler selection
Windmill technique:
2 Medium injection (p. 63)
3 Deep injection (p. 66)

SHAC or deep mesotherapy:
A Special indications: skin surface regeneration augmentation (SSRA) and deep mesotherapy (p. 69)

7

Practical tips
- With the aid of the windmill technique, the practitioner is able to achieve an overall harmonisation of the midface with a single insertion point. This makes it very attractive for the patient, given the limited injections required. The method can also be performed with autologous fat transplantation.
- Additional harmonising augmentation options can be achieved by combining the above with the full-face application of SSRA or deep mesotherapy.

Combined treatment options
Chemical peeling, medical needling, laser resurfacing.

Complications/Managing complications
- Palpable nodules may form due to the aggregation of the filler substance used. Thorough massage and moulding of the injected filler immediately after the injection ensures uniform distribution.
- The blunt 22 gauge cannula needs to be inserted gently and carefully, using minimum force. Care is required when encountering any resistance, to avoid unnecessary tissue trauma and vascular injury. Haematomas can occur and as a result impair the patient's appearance for up to a couple of weeks. It is therefore essential to ensure that the procedure is performed in as atraumatic manner as possible. To date, there have been no reports of trauma affecting the nerves; in theory however, it is possible if excess force is used to advance the cannula.
- Overcorrection should be avoided. If the filler is administered too superficially, this may cause unexpected and undesirable skin irregularities, which should be avoided.

Treatment planning (1)

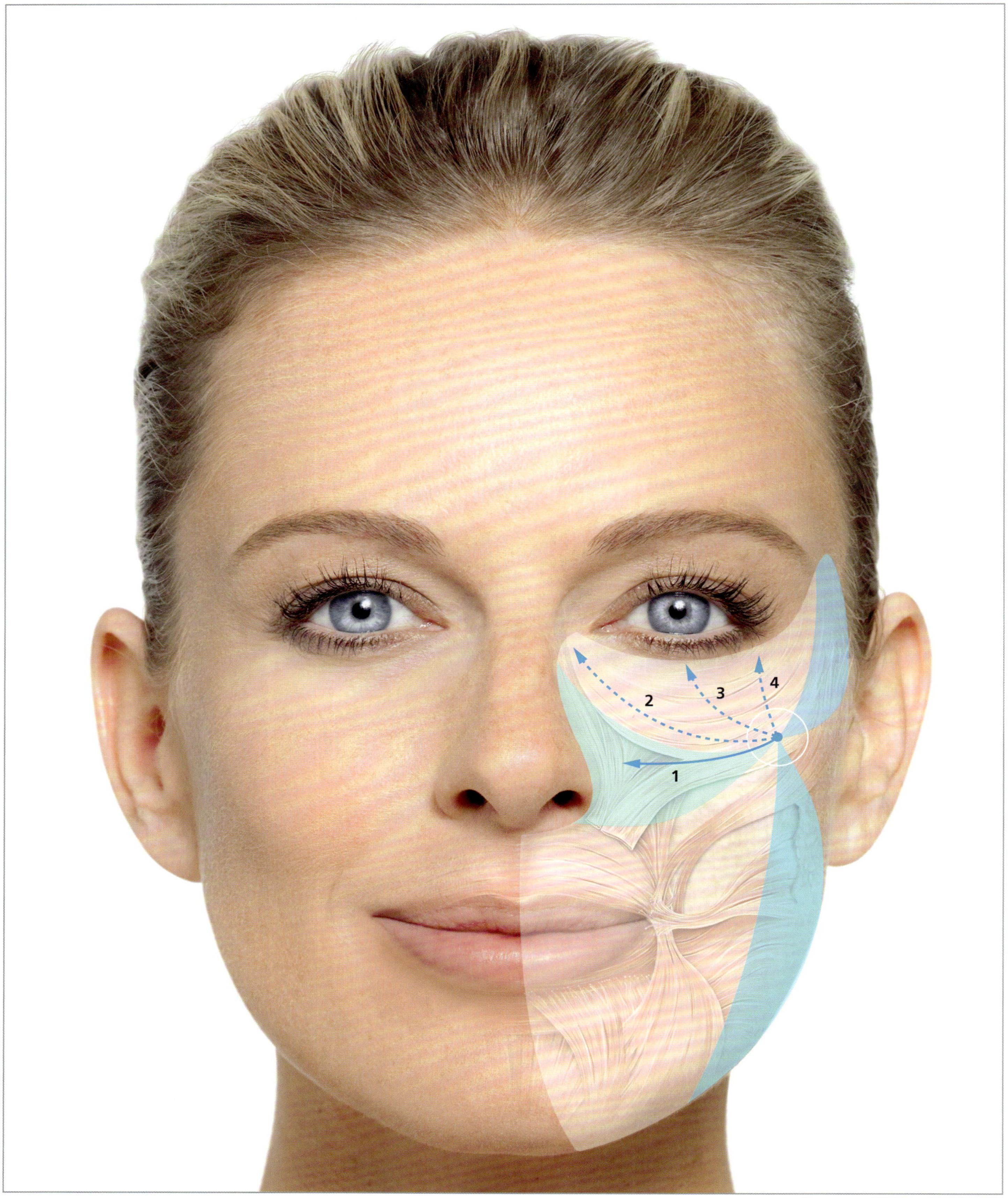

Fig. 7.32 The filler should be injected below the orbicularis oculi muscle.

Treatment (1)

Injections below the M. orbicularis oculi

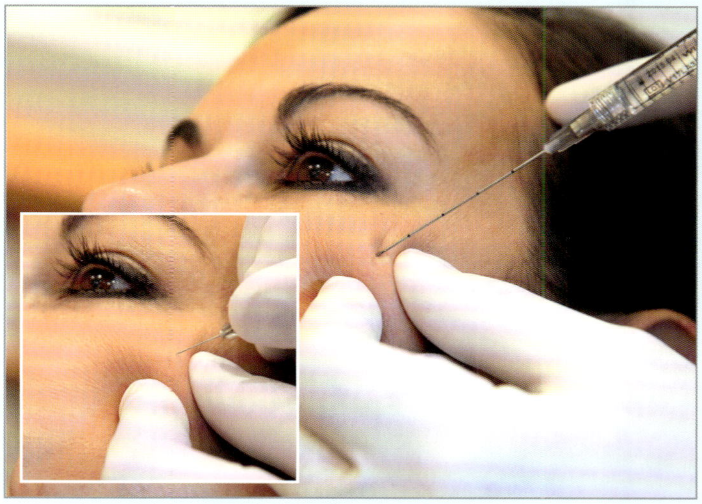

Fig. 7.33 An insertion point is made with a larger bore needle on the Os zygomaticum (zygomatic bone), to allow for the insertion of the cannula. A blunt 22 gauge cannula is then gently inserted into the subcutaneous plane below the orbicularis oculi muscle and advanced towards the centre of the face.

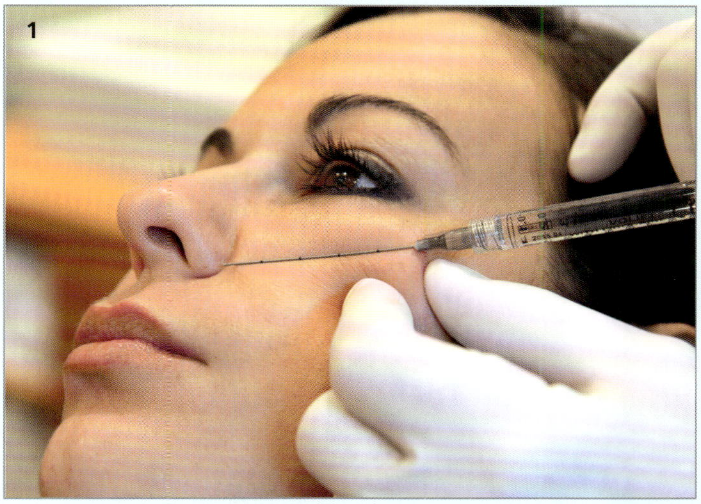

Fig. 7.34 By carefully mobilising the tissue in a horizontal direction, the practitioner can then inject around 0.5 ml into the SOOF in a retrograde linear thread.

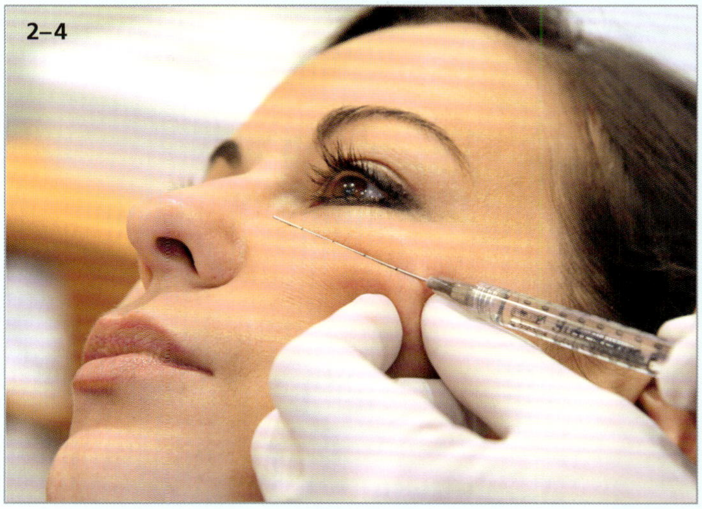

Fig. 7.35 The cannula is then retracted to half its length or so and rotated around towards the forehead. It is brought below the orbicularis oculi muscle in the medial aspect of the infraorbital hollow (tear trough). The filler is then slowly injected (between 0.1 and 0.2 ml) in another retrograde thread. Thereafter, the cannula is again retracted, rotated and brought into another soft tissue space more laterally. Around 0.1–0.2 ml of the filler is injected below the orbicularis oculi muscle in yet another retrograde thread. The procedure is repeated at the most lateral aspect of the orbicularis oculi muscle.

⚠ Prior to injecting any filler, please refer to the latest manufacturer guidelines for specific instructions for use.

Treatment planning (2)

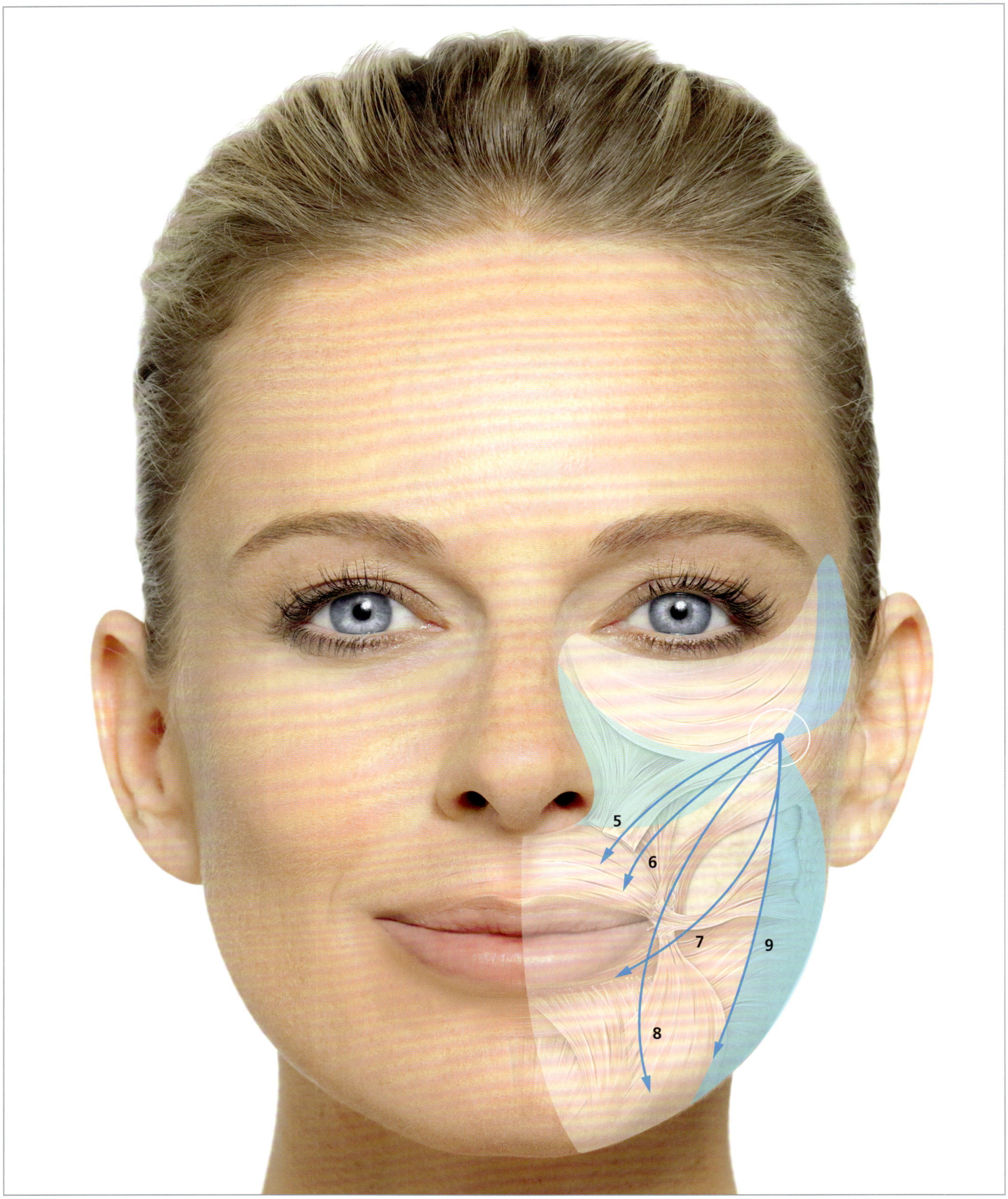

Fig. 7.36 Injection into the medial-inferior cheek (nasolabial fold, mental fold and mandibular region).

Treatment (2)

Injections in the medial and inferior cheek

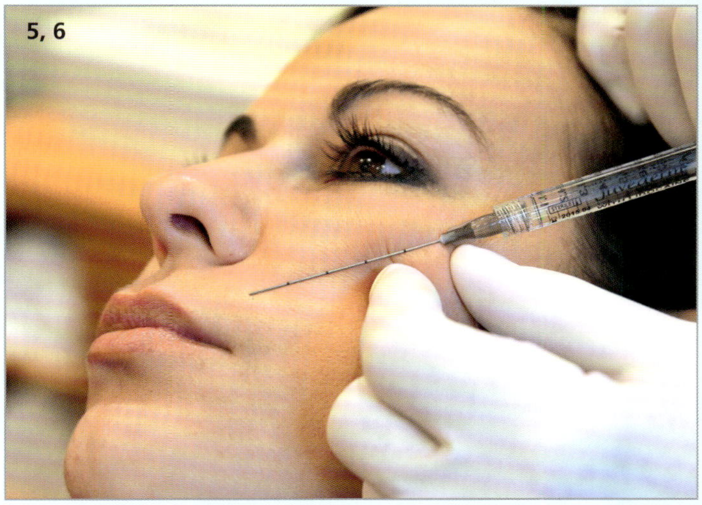

Fig. 7.37 The cannula is redirected towards the inferior aspect of the face and towards the nasolabial fold. The cannula is carefully moved backward and forward to mobilise the adherent tissue below the nasolabial fold. Subsequently, 0.2–0.3 ml of the filler is injected in a retrograde linear thread. The same mobilising technique can also be applied to the inferior part of the nasolabial fold. Here, the anchoring layer is filled with 0.1–0.2 ml of the filler in a retrograde thread.

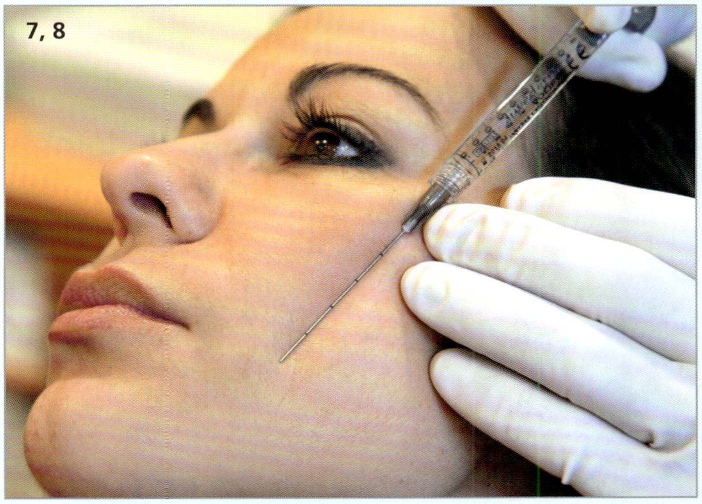

Fig. 7.38 In the next step, the cannula is again withdrawn but not fully removed from the insertion point. It is then advanced forward, but this time in the direction of the lower lip and the marionette line. The filler needs to be injected below the depressor anguli oris muscle, allowing for the mobilisation of the supramucosal space with an injection of 0.2–0.4 ml of the filler. Thereafter, the cannula is withdrawn again and brought into the subcutaneous layer as close as possible to the lateral chin border. A further 0.3–0.5 ml of the filler is injected here.

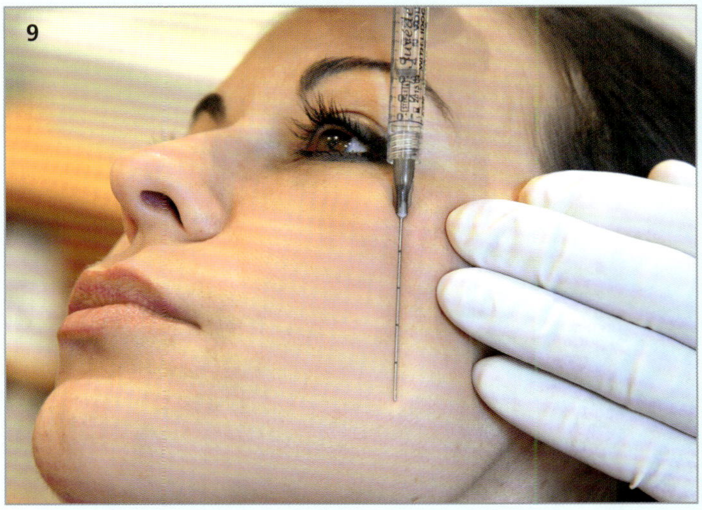

Fig. 7.39 After once more withdrawing the cannula, it is inserted from medial to lateral following the jawline contour. Depending on individual findings of the soft tissue deficit in the caudal region (the amount to inject can vary greatly from 0.4 to 2 ml).

Treatment planning (3)

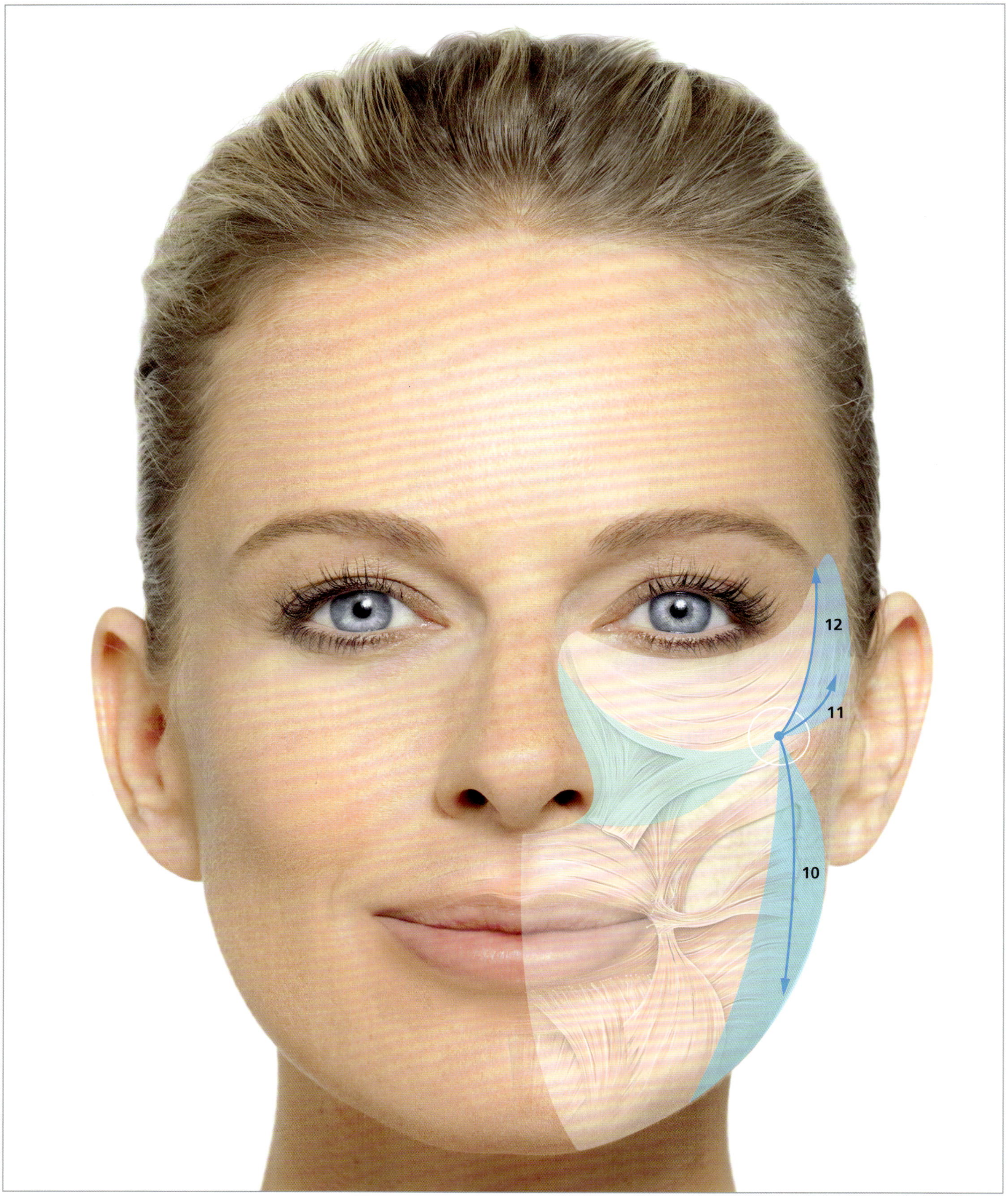

Fig. 7.40 Injections into lateral region (lateral cheek, lateral mandible and temples).

Treatment (3)

Injections into the lateral cheek, lateral mandible and towards the temples

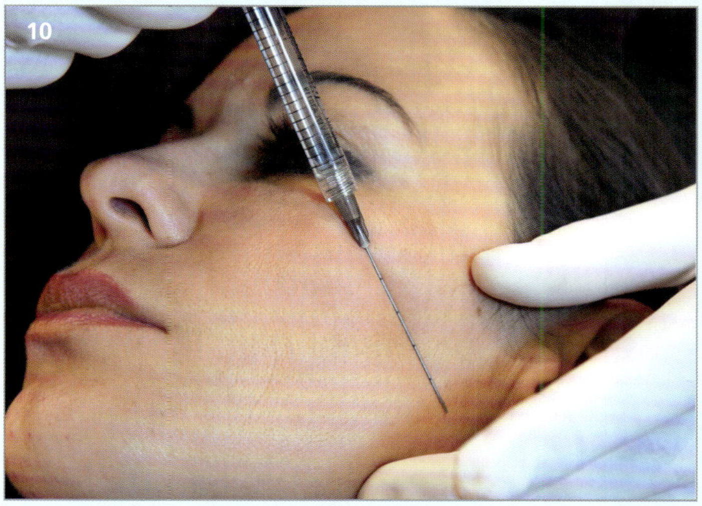

Fig. 7.41 The cannula is advanced towards the lateral aspect of the mandible. The volume injected depends on individual findings and varies from 0.3 to 1 ml. The cannula is then removed.

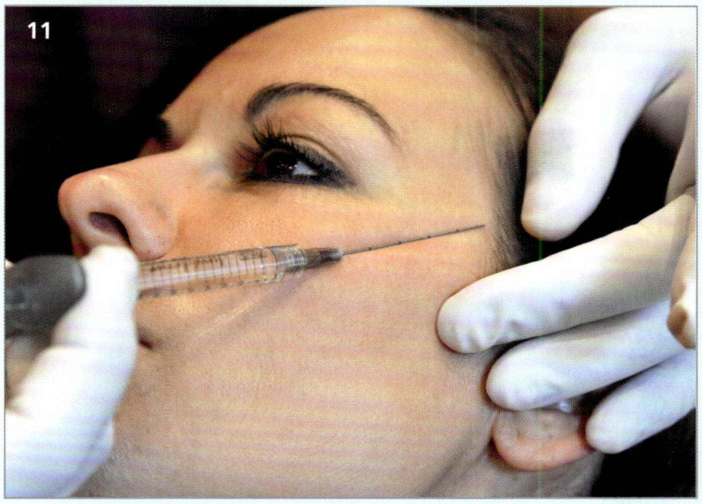

Fig. 7.42 The cannula is re-inserted via the same insertion site and advanced towards the temporo-auricular region. With low volumes (0.1–0.3 ml) of the filler injected, a harmonising augmentation is achieved while respecting the volumetric proportions of this area.

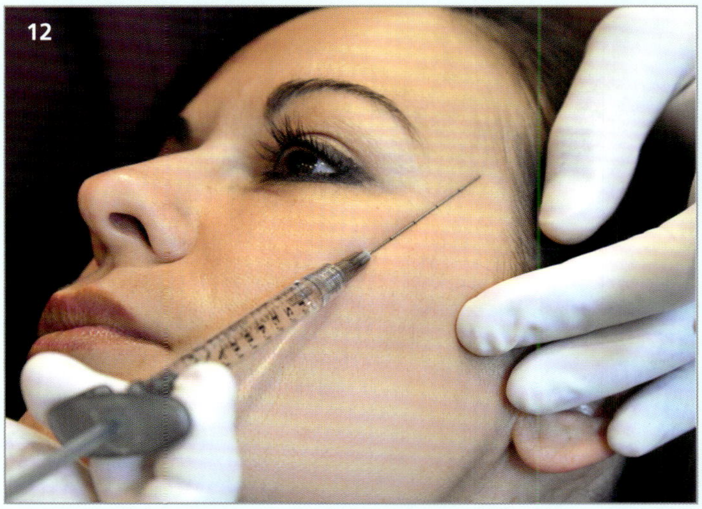

Fig. 7.43 After withdrawing the cannula, it is again advanced into the superior part of the temporal region close to the lateral border of the eyebrow. The augmentation here is also performed with the smallest volumes required (0.1–0.3 ml) in a retrograde thread.

⚠ Prior to injecting any filler, please refer to the latest manufacturer guidelines for specific instructions for use.

7.4.2 Zygomatic region (bucco-maxillary ligament and malar fat pad)

A prominent lateral cheekbone is considered an attractive and youthful feature of the face. With age-related loss of the soft tissues, the lateral cheek loses volume and the underlying bony structures become more prominent.

When the deep SOOF shrinks with ageing, the overlying superficial malar fat pad can look 'oedematous'. A visible grove also becomes prominent where the skin is retracted at the site of the bucco-maxillar ligament. Simultaneously, with ageing and mobilisation of the soft tissues, the nasolabial folds become more prominent.

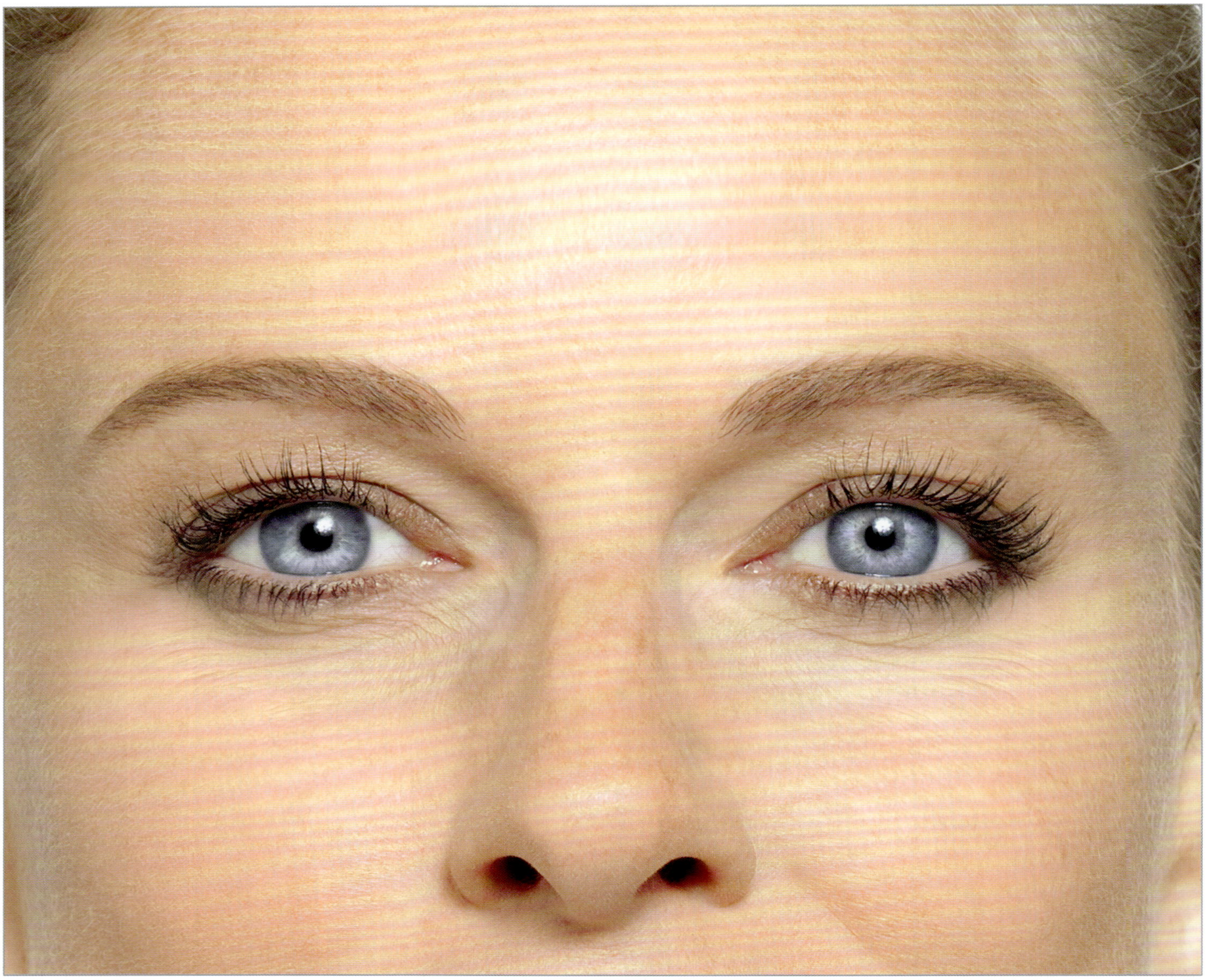

Patient selection

Patients presenting with advanced atrophy-related changes in the upper cheek region can benefit from filler injections into the malar fat pad or the bucco-maxillary ligaments. Focal augmentation of this region is an alternative to the more global augmentation of the midface described above, i.e. with the windmill technique. With focal vertical injections, the zygomatic region can be successfully augmented with minimal filler volume, by compensating the volume deficit of the atrophied soft tissue base.

Assessing the indication

Focal volume augmentation of the upper cheek, using a supraperiosteal approach to restore the deep soft tissue volume loss, allows for a causal and natural rejuvenation treatment approach. In fact, this treatment in some cases may negate the need for a surgical intervention, i.e. in cases when removal of the malar fat pad may be indicated.

Anatomy

The prominent zygomatic bone forms the most prominent element of the midface. It is covered with volumising fat layers, including the deep fat as well as the more superficial fat layer. With ageing, atrophy of the deeper fat layer (SOOF, 1) results in a perceived 'swelling' in the malar fat pad, which is situated more superficially. When the zygomaticus minor (2) and major (3) muscles contract with facial expressions, especially when smiling, the area is further elevated and projected. Anchoring onto the cheekbone, the real bucco-maxillary ligament (namely the maxillary portion) forms a columnar connection with the skin, running from the zygomatic region to the nasolabial fold (4). Age-related atrophy of the soft tissue base can provoke enhanced skin retraction where the ligament is located and as a result lead to a visible groove.

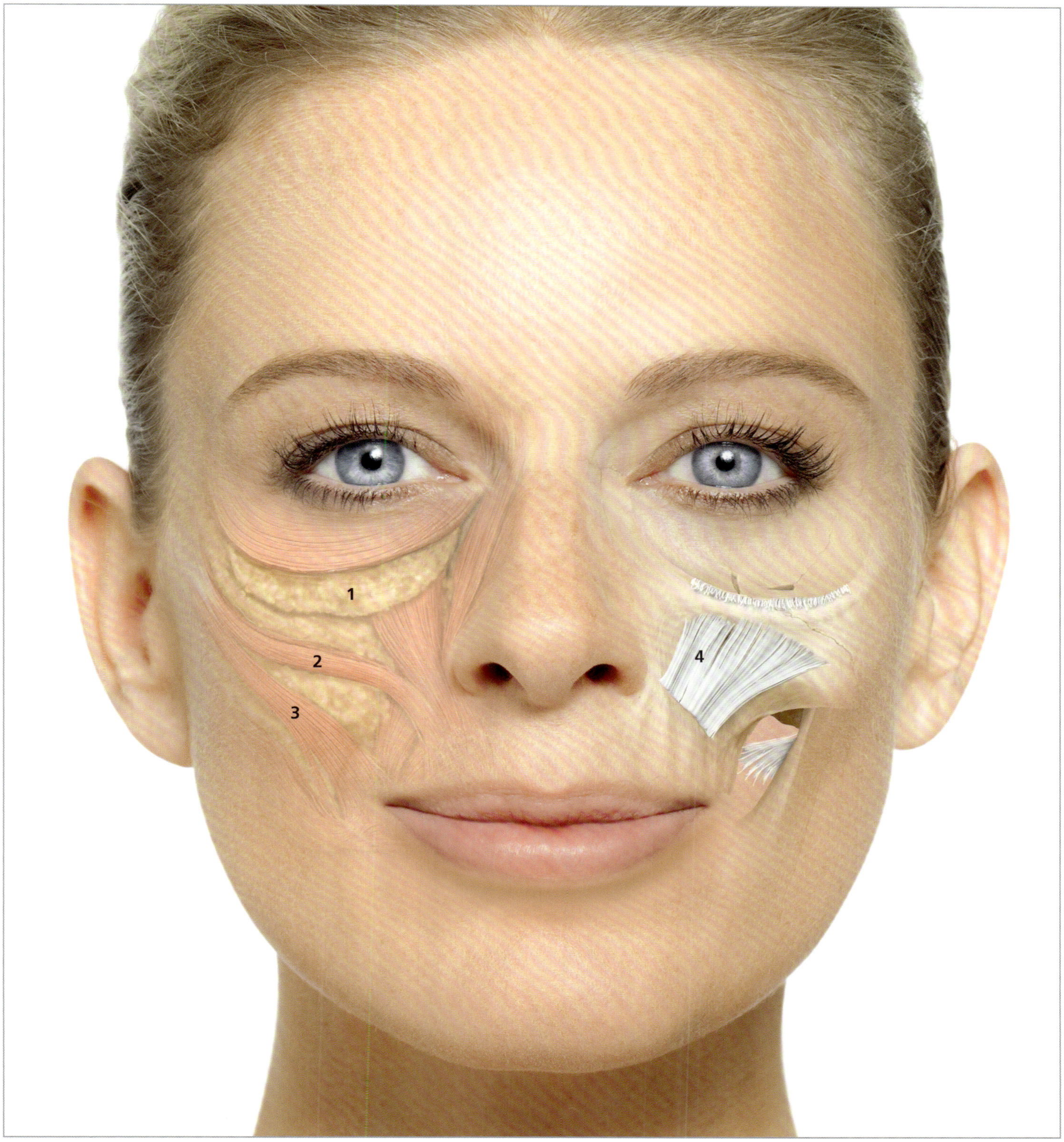

Treatment planning

Vertical, supraperiosteal injections with water-binding fillers can compensate for the atrophied conditions of the soft tissue base above the zygomatic bone. In addition, depending on the individual findings, the practitioner can administer vertical depots into the malar fat pad and/or the bucco-maxillary ligament. Importantly, upper midface augmentation allows for secondary improvement of the nasolabial fold.

Furthermore, minor amounts of supraperiosteally placed filler are sufficient to achieve the desired superficial harmonisation.

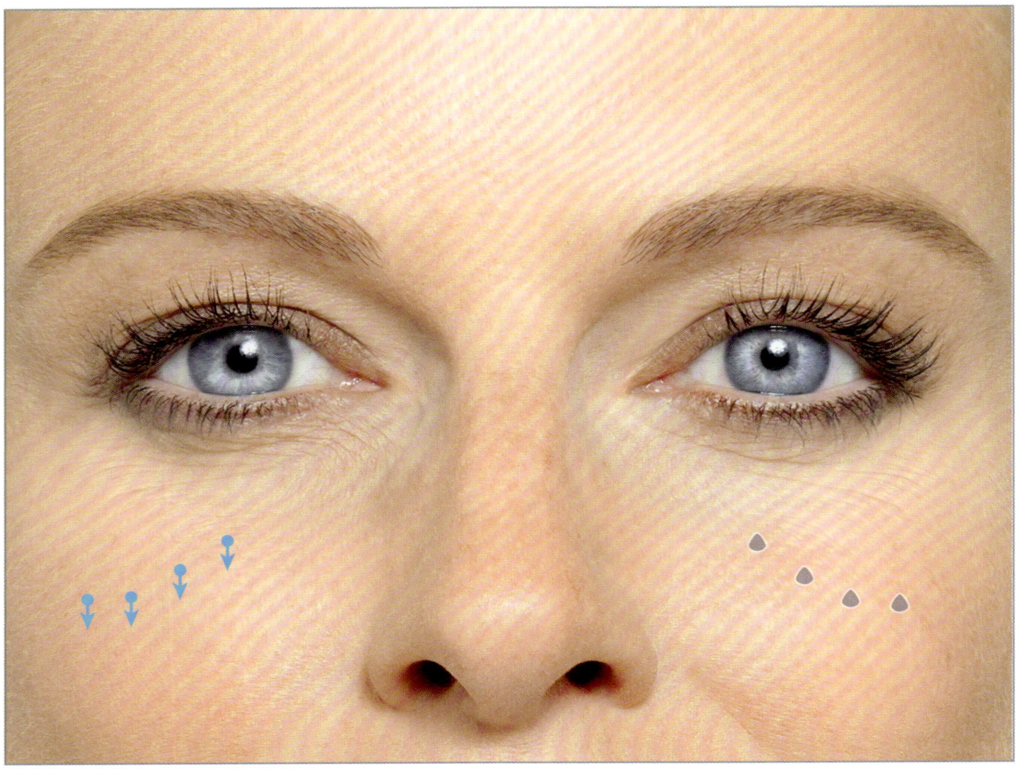

Technique: VSDT or tower technique (in case of pronounced volume atrophy)
Injection sites: three to four 'hot spots' into the groove created by the bucco-maxillary ligaments
Volume: 0.05–0.1 ml/injection point

Video: Bucco-maxillary ligament
http://www.kvm-tv.de/FIL/013.mp4

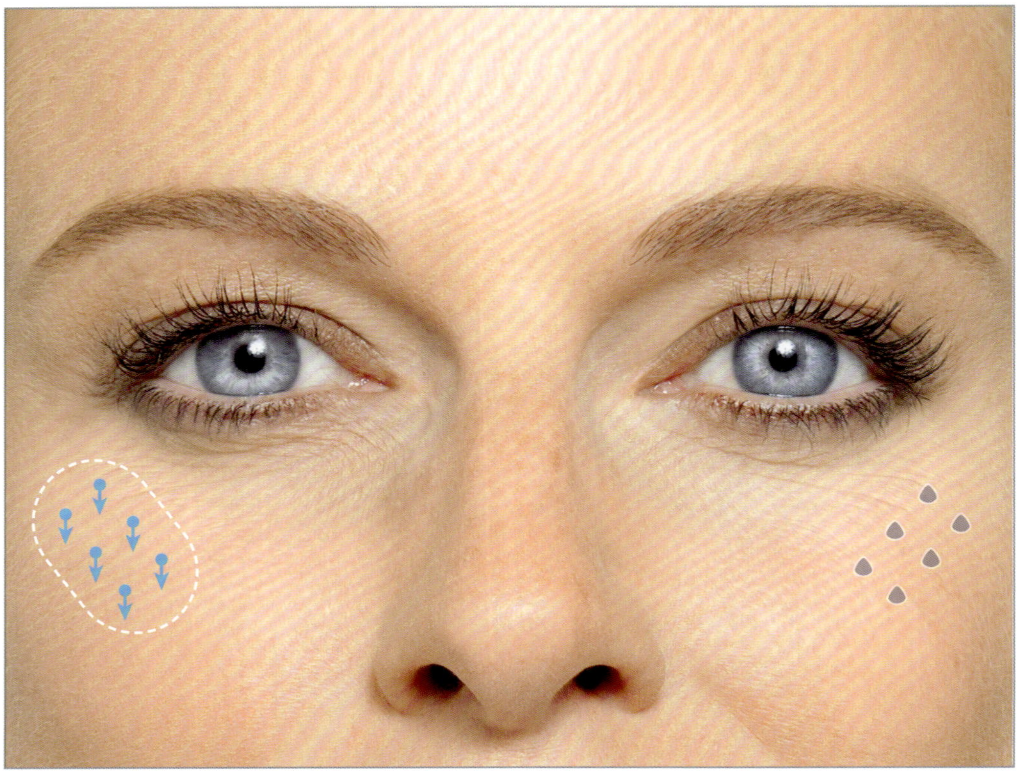

Technique: VSDT or tower technique (in case of pronounced volume atrophy)
Injection sites: six 'hot spots' into the malar fat pad
Volume: 0.02–0.03 ml/injection point

Video: Malar fat pad
http://www.kvm-tv.de/FIL/014.mp4

Treatment

VSDT

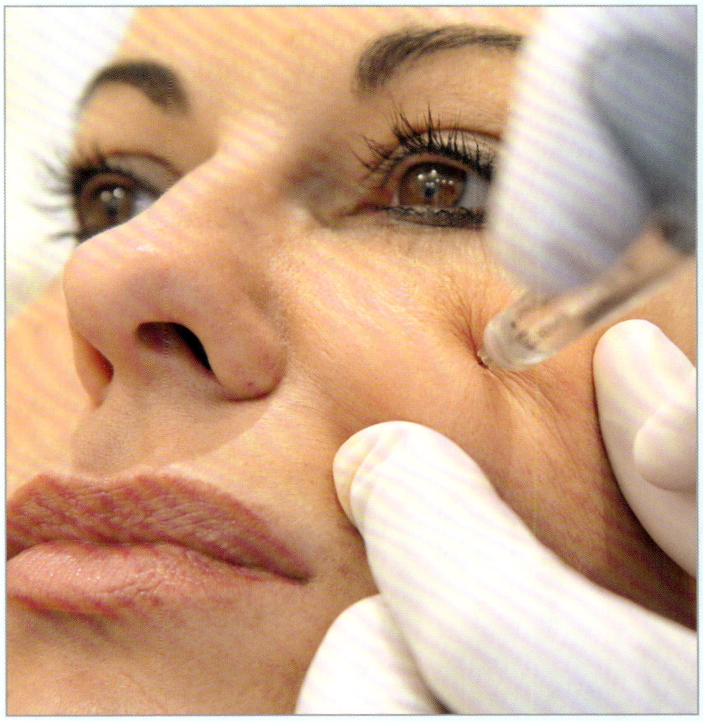

Fig. 7.44 The treatment area will get slightly compressed during vertical injections along the bucco-maxillary ligament.
The course of the groove where the bucco-maxillary ligament is located does vary between individuals.
Depending on the severity of the cheek atrophy, between 0.05 to 0.1 ml of the filler per depot can be injected.

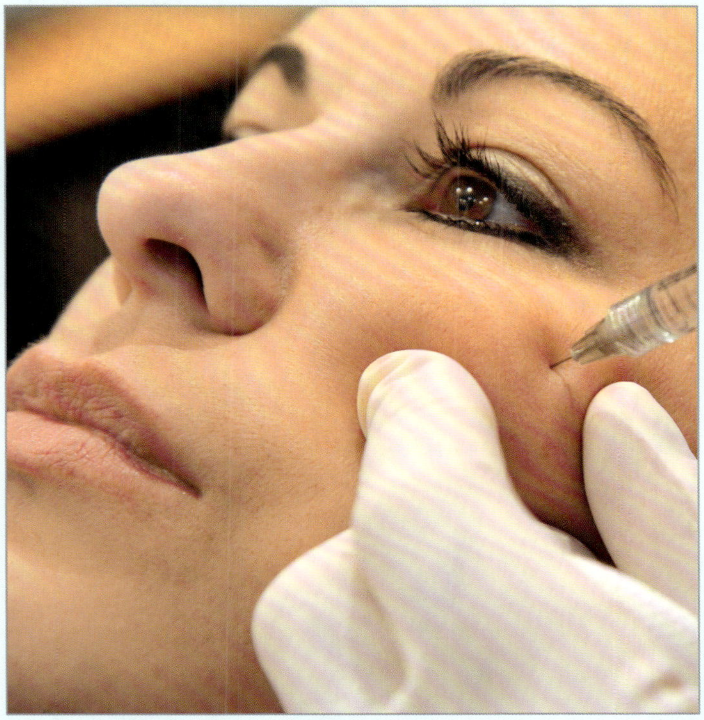

Fig. 7.45 While holding and stabilising the upper cheek, up to six vertical injections are delivered into the malar fat pad. In doing so, the atrophied soft tissue base (including the SOOF) is restored, leading to clinical harmonisation of the area, initially appearing as 'swollen'. Minimal amounts of the filler (0.02–0.03 ml per depot) are sufficient, provided that it is delivered ultra deep, i.e. supraperiosteally.

Treatment steps

- Remove makeup
- Disinfection
- Anaesthesia (optional)
- Injection: VSDT or TT
- Massage and mould (ensure appropriate distribution of the filler)
- Inform patient about post-treatment dos and don'ts
- Arrange a follow-up appointment

Filler selection

3 Deep injection (p. 66)
4 Ultra-deep injection (p. 67)

Combined treatment options

- Microdermabrasion
- Chemical peeling
- Medical needling
- Laser resurfacing

Complications/Managing complications

- Overcorrection should be avoided at all times, particularly with progressive long-term treatments, and hence progressive mild enhancement is recommended.
- Palpable nodules may form due to the aggregation of the filler. Thorough massage and moulding of the filler immediately after the injection ensures uniform distribution.

Practical tips

- In case of severe volume atrophy of the midface involving the superficial tissue layers, it may be necessary to attain additional stabilisation with the tower technique (TT) instead of the VSDT.
- Compensating for the lost volume in the upper midface will additionally achieve improvement of the nasolabial folds.

7.4.3 Nasolabial folds

The nasolabial fold exists in every human face and distinguishes it from primates. It is affected by numerous muscles and is thus involved in a variety of emotions. It is mostly pronounced during laughter. In general, the nasolabial fold is not a negative aesthetic attribute. However, with age, static nasolabial folds become more prominent in the context of soft tissue atrophy and the destabilisation of the facial anatomical units. The lines become deeper and cause unintended emotions to be expressed with greater intensity. The static lines in the transition zone between the fat-rich cheek region and the fat-poor oral region result as a consequence of the atrophy-related shrinking of the buccal fat and descent of the overlying tissues such as the skin, which are related to the bucco-maxillar retaining ligaments.

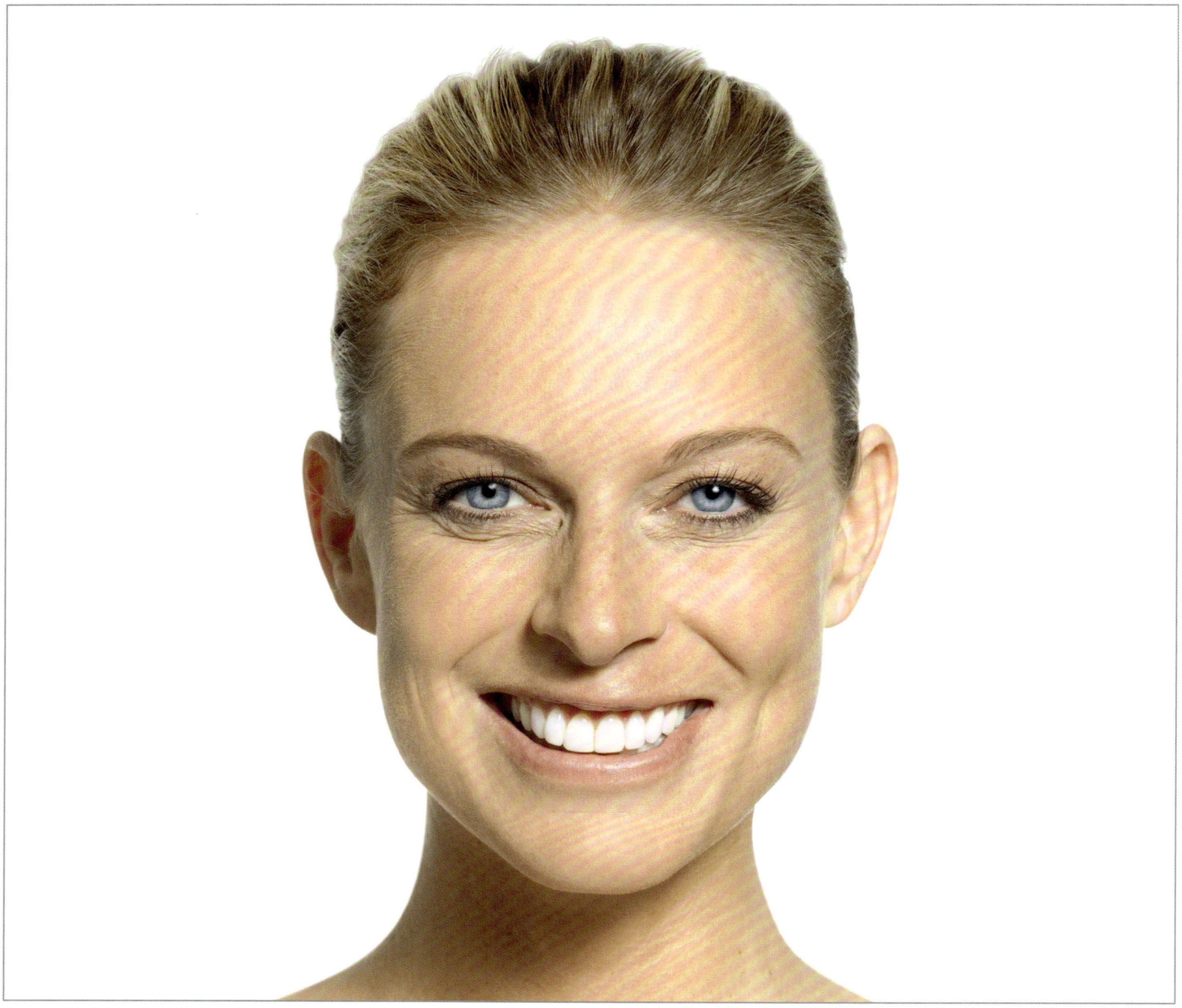

Patient selection
The presence of a natural nasolabial fold alone does not represent a negative aesthetic feature. However, if the natural, harmonious balance of the face becomes impaired by the prominence and depth of the nasolabial folds, filler augmentation treatments can restore this harmony. On the other hand, overcorrection of the nasolabial fold can also perceptibly impair the overall harmonious appearance of the face. It is important that the nasolabial fold remains soft and visible during natural facial expressions. In extreme cases, overcorrection can make the face look swollen.

Assessing the indication
Static nasolabial folds caused by loss of volume represent an excellent indication for filler augmentation. However, it is important not to try to fully obliterate the folds, but rather to soften them. Filler should ideally be placed below the musculature. The recommended technique is using a blunt cannula for deep supramucosal tissue mobilisation (i.e. mobilising the plane between the muscosa and the muscles).

Anatomy

The nasolabial fold extends from the upper lateral portion of the wing of the nose down to the corner of the mouth. Its depth can vary from individual to individual, ranging from minimally visible to very deep folds. It may extend down to the angle of the mouth, and in some cases join up with the marionette line and extend down towards the jawline.

The muscles that act on the nasolabial fold include:

- Levator labii superioris alaeque nasi muscle (1)
- Levator labii superioris muscle (2)
- Zygomaticus minor muscle (3)
- Zygomaticus major muscle (4)
- Levator anguli oris muscle (located deeper down) (5)

The dynamic creasing of the skin is most prominent where the zygomaticus major muscle (4) attaches to the skin. The levator labii superioris contributes to the formation and movement of the middle segment of the nasolabial folds. However, there are other causes for the development of nasolabial folds apart from the dynamic, muscle-related impacts, as discussed next.

With advanced skin ageing and soft tissue atrophy, the folds become visible at rest where the fat-rich buccal region adjoins the fat-deplete oral region. In the cranial aspect, the fold is the deepest where the maxillary part of the bucco-maxillary retaining ligaments (6) is acting with its retraction forces on the skin. In the inferior aspect, the buccal part of the bucco-maxillary retaining ligaments (7) attaches to the skin. That particularly weak ligament slackens early on in the ageing process and is not able to hold the required tension against the advancing ptosis of the buccal soft tissues. The manifestation of the fold at rest is therefore enhanced.

By mobilising the fixation point of the zygomaticus major muscle at the modiolus with a cannula, a harmonious augmentation of the nasolabial fold can be achieved.

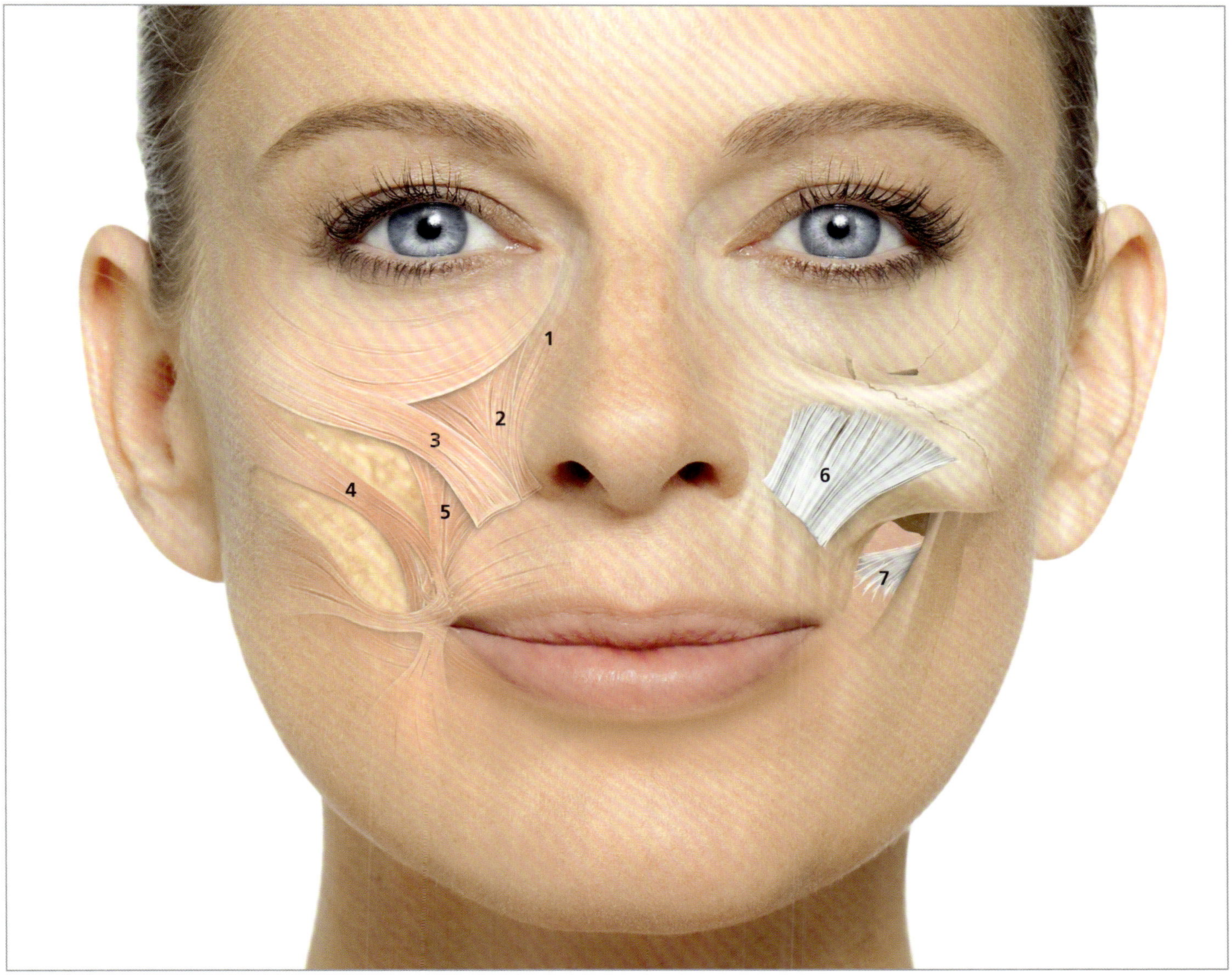

Treatment planning– Superficial correction

The aim of the superficial treatment is to achieve a decorative superficial covering, i.e. 'camouflage' of the persisting nasolabial fold. Hence, it should not be relied upon to remedy the causal volume deficit from below. Furthermore, superficial placement of the filler results in most of it being mobilised horizontally due to the constant muscular action.

Importantly, injecting too much filler in the superficial plane risks unnatural overcorrection of the fold; this in turn may disturb the facial harmony more so than the original manifestation of the fold itself.

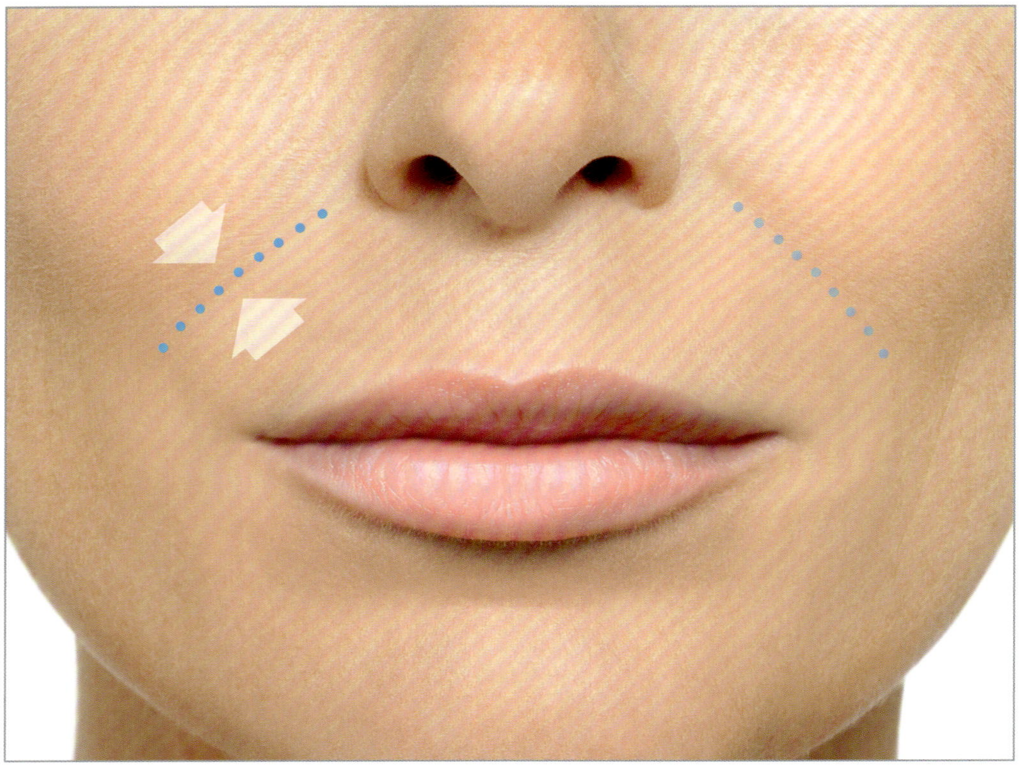

Technique: ● ● ● point technique with compression
Injection sites: ● serial injection points along the fold
Volume: 0.1–0.2 ml/side
Tool: 30 gauge needle

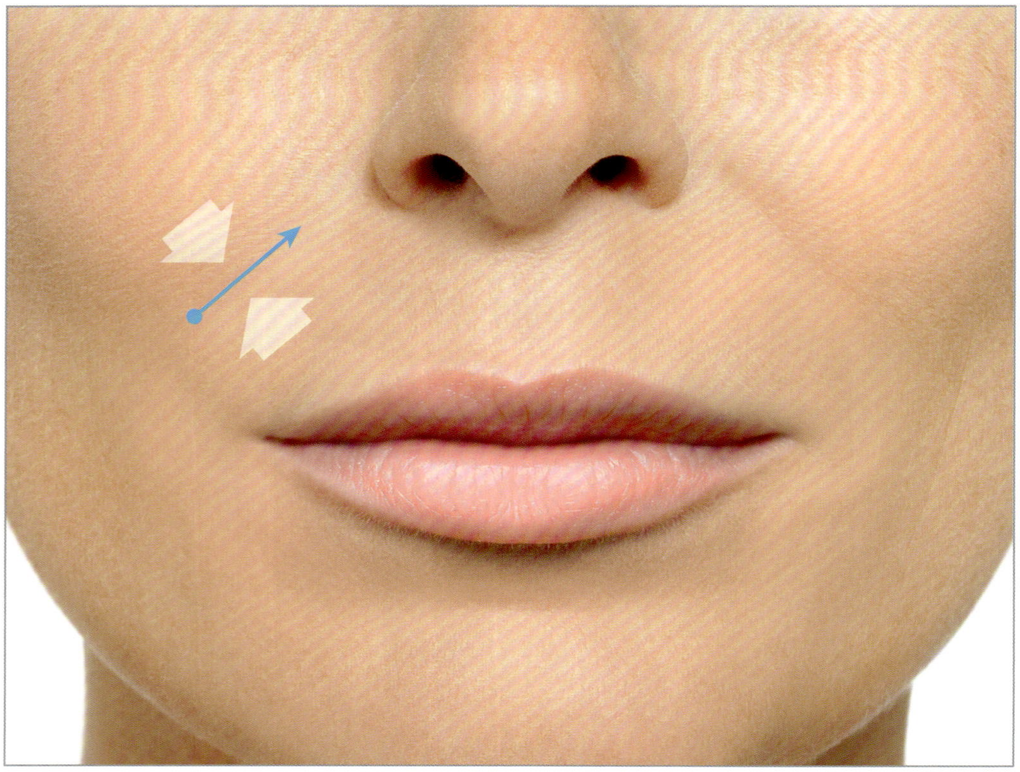

Technique: tunneling technique with compression
Injection sites: ● inferior end of the fold
Volume: 0.1–0.2 ml/side
Tool: 30 gauge needle

7

Treatment – Superficial correction

Tunneling technique

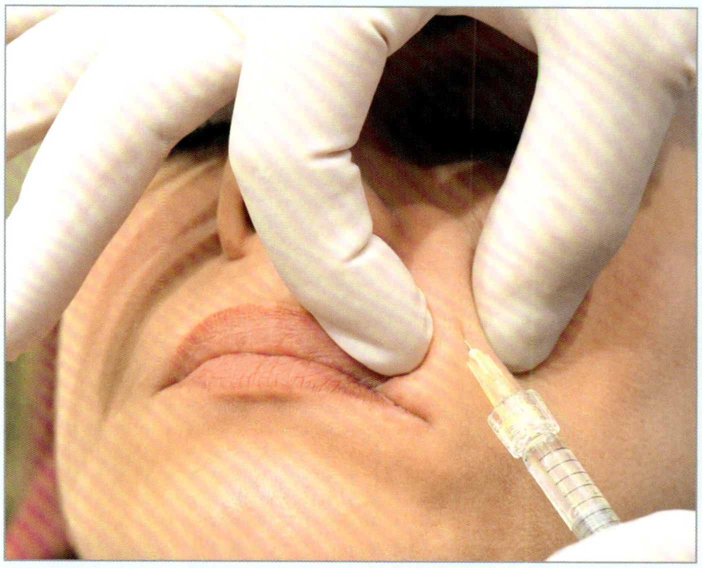

Fig. 7.46 The practitioner grasps the nasolabial fold in a gentle pinch grip with the non-injecting hand, compresses it gently and inserts the needle along the course of the line, starting at the inferior aspect and aiming superiorly. The filler is injected in a retrograde manner.

Point technique

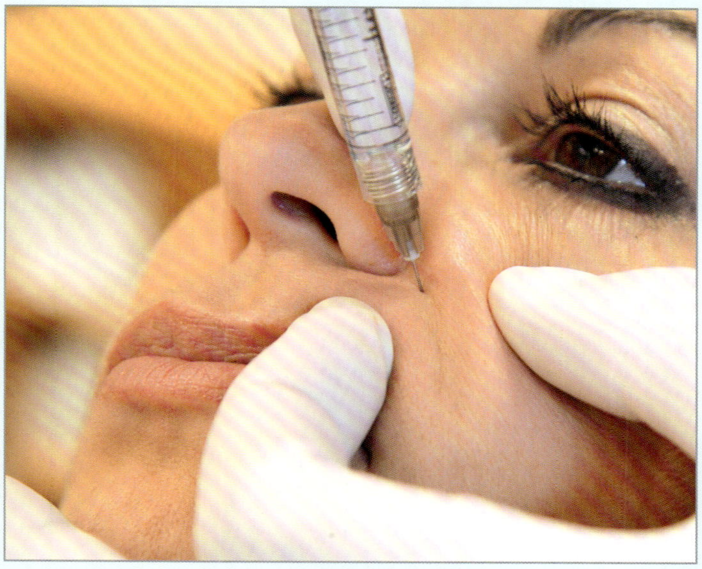

Fig. 7.47 When using the serial point technique, individual injection points are administered along the course of the fold with the needle inserted at a 90-degree angle.

Treatment steps

- Remove makeup
- Disinfection
- Anaesthesia (optional)
- Injection: compression technique (serial point or tunneling technique)
- Massage and mould (ensure appropriate distribution of the filler)
- Inform patient about post-treatment dos and don'ts
- Arrange a follow-up appointment

Filler selection

1 Superficial injection (p. 62)
2 Medium injection (p. 63)

Combined treatment options

- Microdermabrasion
- Chemical peeling
- Medical needling
- Laser resurfacing

Complications/Managing complications

- Optimal harmonisation and augmentation of the folds will be challenging to achieve with superficial techniques alone. Overfilling with superficial filler placement should be avoided. Supramucosal injections below the musculature are the target plane for this indication.
- Palpable nodules may form due to the aggregation of the filler. Thorough massage and moulding of the introduced filler immediately after the treatment ensures uniform distribution.

Practical tips

- For less pronounced nasolabial folds, satisfactory results can often be achieved just by filling the superior part of the fold using the sandwich technique.
- The distance between the origin (most proximal part) of the nasolabial fold and the tip of the nose in a profile view determines the subjective impression of facial ageing. The maximum elevation of the nasolabial fold at its origin is particularly significant in this respect. Several treatments may be necessary in deeper nasolabial folds.
- Superficial augmentation (above the muscles) is associated with significant horizontal distribution of the filler, due to the constant muscular activation, and as a result can only achieve a minimal lifting effect.
- Deep, supramucosal injection techniques can achieve natural and effective clinical outcomes.

Treatment planning – Volume compensation

The aim of a nasolabial fold treatment is to gently augment and create harmony within this part of the face. The treatment should allow for a reduction in the visibility of the fold when assessed at rest, but upon dynamic expression of the face – namely during smiling – the fold should still be visible. After all, it is not appropriate or possible to fully eradicate this anatomical feature. Supramucosal filler injections below the musculature are indicated here. Cannulas are useful when initiating this treatment, particularly as they allow for deep tissue mobilisation alongside augmentation. The resultant reduction in the mechanical forces, in combination with fluid-dependent tissue saturation alongside fibrogenesis, allow for optimal rejuvenation outcomes. Alternatively, in cases of deep nasolabial folds, additional stabilisation and augmentation can be achieved with the tower technique (TT).

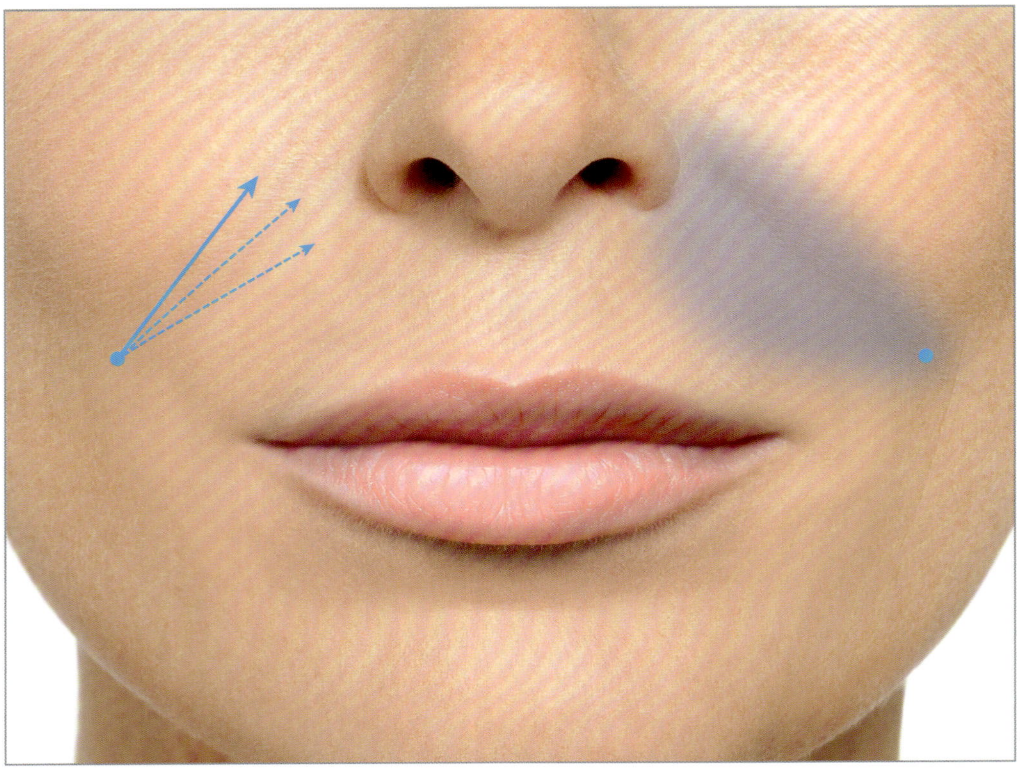

Technique: DHAC
Insertion site: at the insertion point of the zygomaticus muscle at the modiolus
Injection depth and direction: supramucosal, below the muscles
Volume: 0.2–0.3 ml/side
Tool: 22 gauge cannula

Video: Nasolabial fold DHAC http://www.kvm-tv.de/FIL/015.mp4

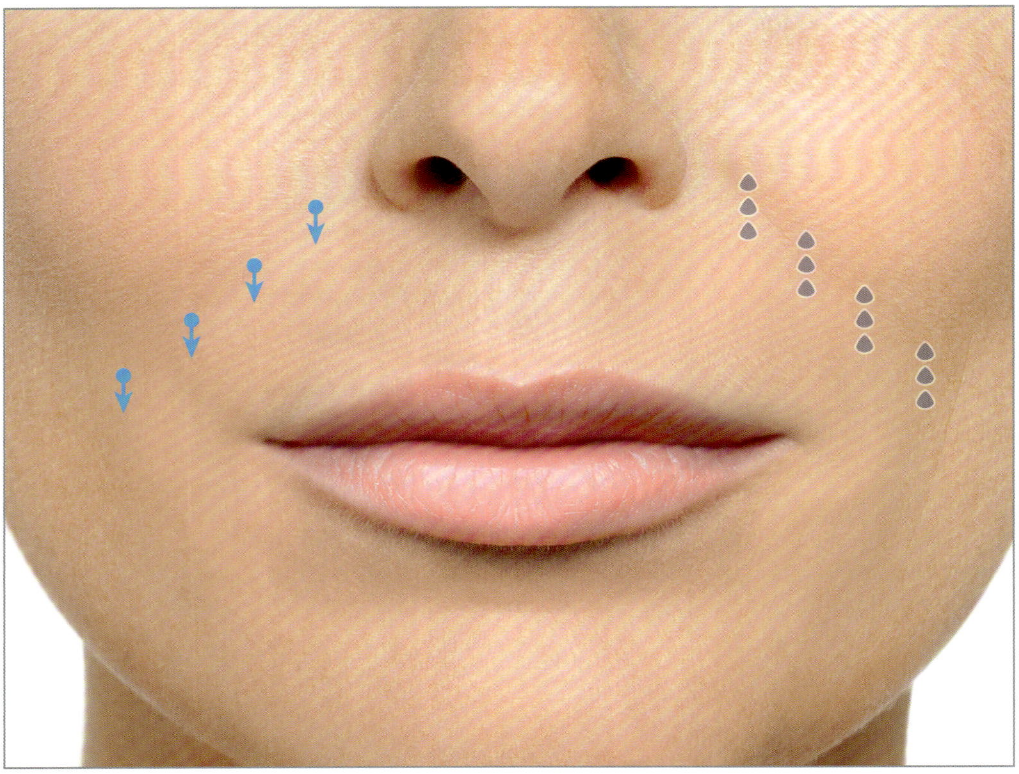

Technique: tower technique (TT)
Injection points: four to five 'hot spots' along the nasolabial fold
Volume: 0.5 ml/side
Tool: 27 gauge needle

Video: Nasolabial fold TT http://www.kvm-tv.de/FIL/016.mp4

7

Treatment – Volume compensation

DHAC

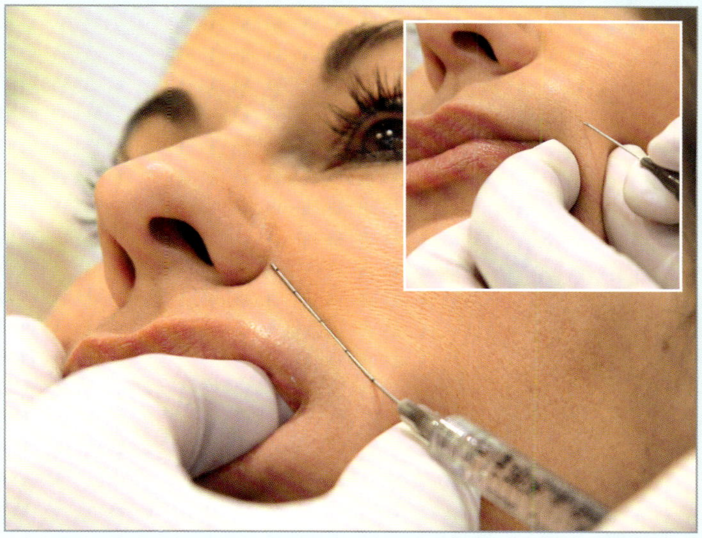

Fig. 7.48 The cannula is inserted below the modiolus (at the insertion site of the zygomaticus major muscle) and brought into the supramucosal plane. The tissue is then gently mobilised in a horizontal direction prior to small volumes of the filler being injected. The improved clinical outcome results from the anatomical release of the fixation elements together with a soft lifting effect of the filler.

Tower Technique

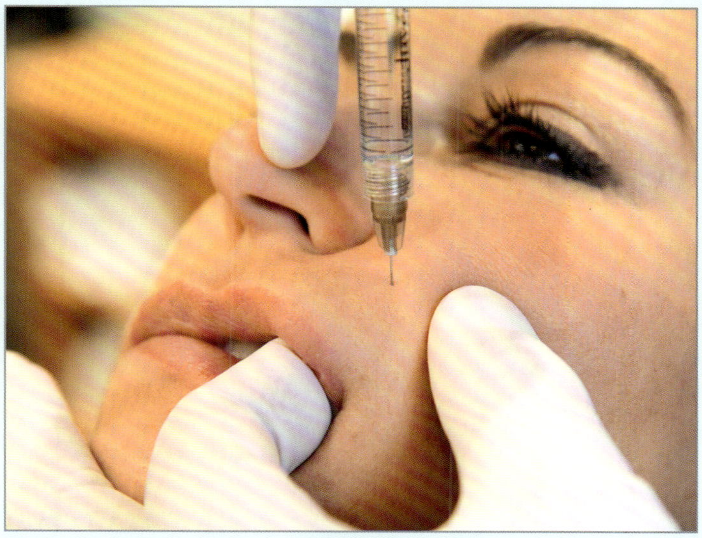

Fig. 7.49 When performing vertical injections above the smooth mucosa, it is advisable to closely monitor the penetration depth of the needle in order to gauge where the filler is deposited, by palpating intraorally with the non-injecting hand. (Caution should be exercised when doing this to avoid needlestick injuries.)
When the needle is vertically inserted into place, the first depot is then given directly above the mucosa. While slowly withdrawing the needle, further depots are given, one on top of each other in a 'stack of coins' formation, right up to the dermal plexus. Aspiration is recommended prior to injecting the filler to reduce the risk of intravascular injection. This is coupled with slow and minimal volume of filler injection techniques.

Treatment steps

- Remove makeup
- Disinfection
- Anaesthesia (optional)
- Injection: DHAC or TT
- Massage and mould (ensure appropriate distribution of the filler)
- Inform patient about post-treatment dos and don'ts
- Arrange a follow-up appointment

Filler selection

3 Deep injection (p. 66)

Alternative or combined (after a duration of 2 months) treatment options

Autologous fat transplantation

Complications/Managing complications

- Eradicating the nasolabial fold completely is not only aesthetically undesirable, but also physiologically impossible. Attempting to do this risks overfilling.
- Do not inject isolated strands of filler into the line; the deeper tissue around the line also needs to be supported and lifted.
- Be sure to inject below the musculature in order to avoid under- or overcorrection.
- Palpable nodules may form due to the aggregation of the filler. Thorough massage and moulding of the filler immediately after the injection allows ensures distribution.

Practical tips

- Make sure that you inject below the muscle (supramucosally) in order to achieve optimal clinical outcomes.
- Use a cannula for deep tissue mobilisation before injecting the filler itself. This will reduce the retraction forces acting on the skin, which increase the depth of the nasolabial fold. Additionally, this will induce fibrogenesis along with fluid-dependent tissue saturation.
- If the nasolabial folds are very deep and in association with advanced cheek atrophy, the tower technique (TT) can be used for enhanced stabilisation and saturation of the upper tissue layers.
- The distance between the origin (most proximal part) of the nasolabial fold and the tip of the nose in a profile view determines the subjective impression of facial ageing. The maximum elevation of the nasolabial fold at its origin is particularly significant in this respect. Several treatments may be necessary in deeper nasolabial folds.

7.5 Perioral Complex

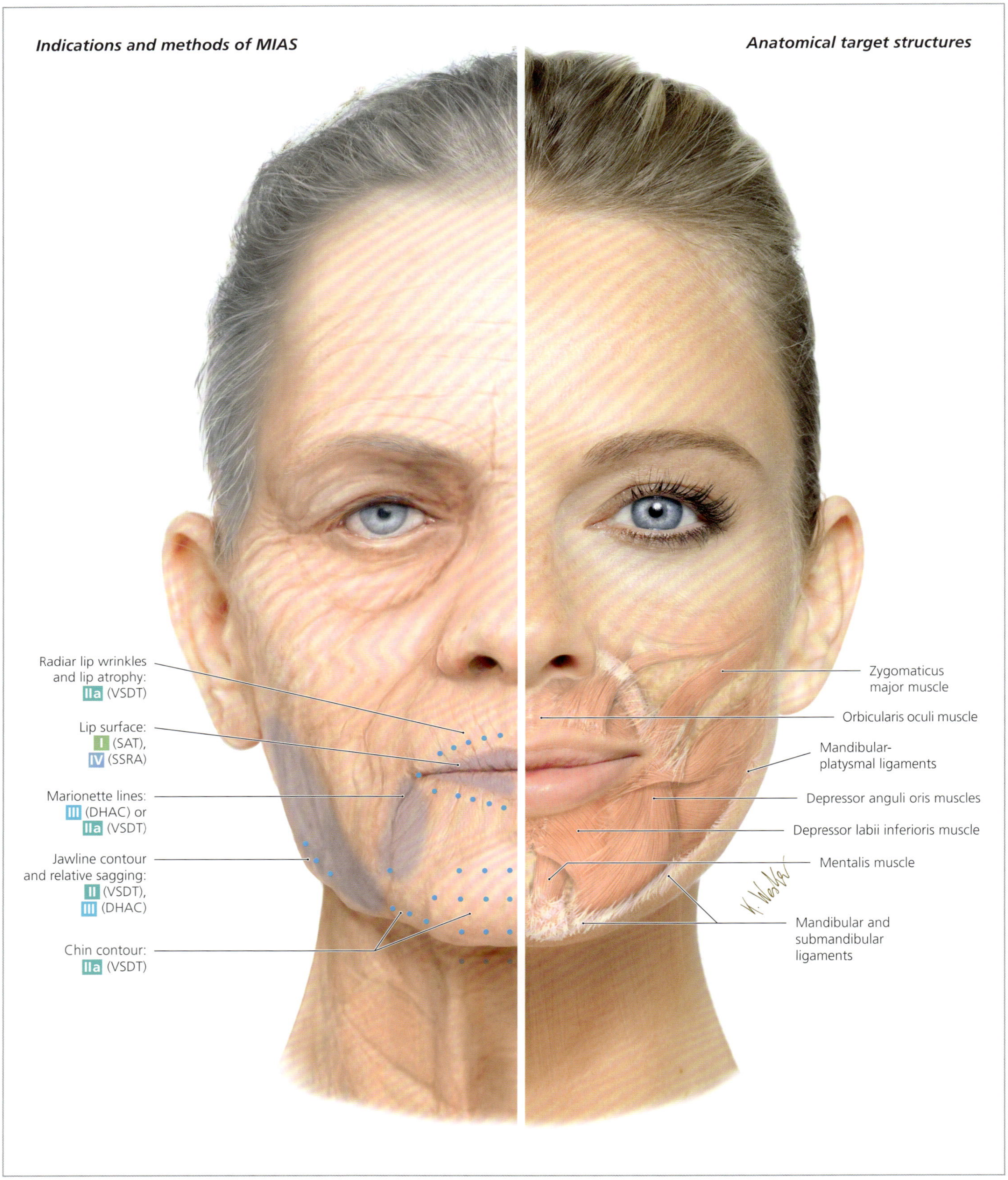

Fig. 7.50 Overview of the anatomy, target structures and cause-related augmentation techniques used in the perioral and chin region.
• VSDT (or, alternatively, superficial augmentation techniques [SAT] for camouflage purposes); DHAC.

A harmonious volumisation and augmentation of the perioral complex, including the lips, the marionette lines and the chin, elongates the face and achieves a more oval face shape.

Interestingly, as opposed to what was previously believed, it is not primarily the collapse and the disharmonious prolapse of the soft tissues, but rather an atrophy-related shrinkage that results in the visible signs of ageing of the face, particularly in this area.

Overall, it is the anterior projection achieved with fillers in the lower third of the face that is key to optimal facial rejuvenation of this region.

Facial rejuvenation with volume restoration in the perioral complex

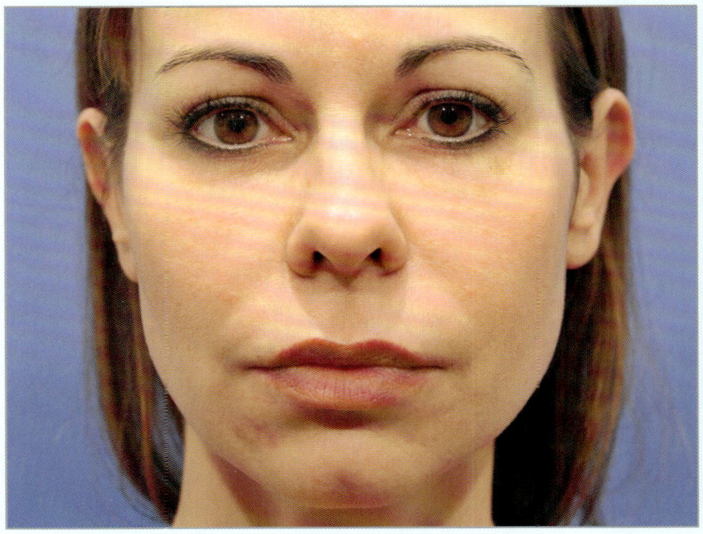

Fig. 7.51 Female patient with untreated chin, frontal view.

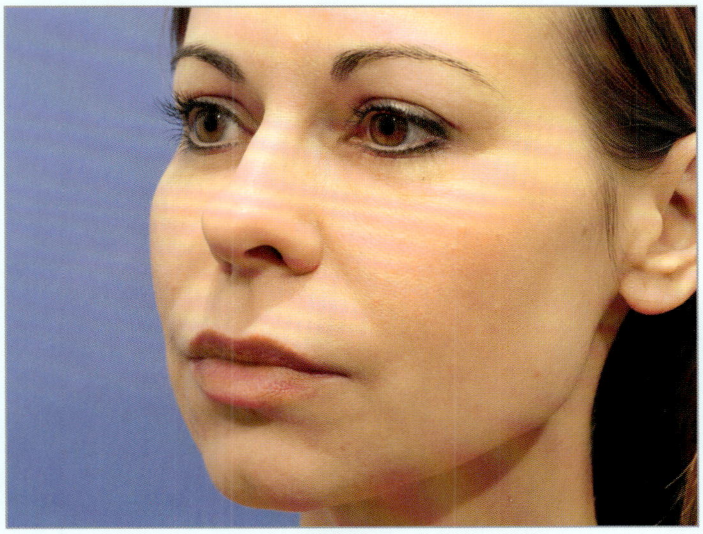

Fig. 7.52 Female patient with untreated chin, oblique view.

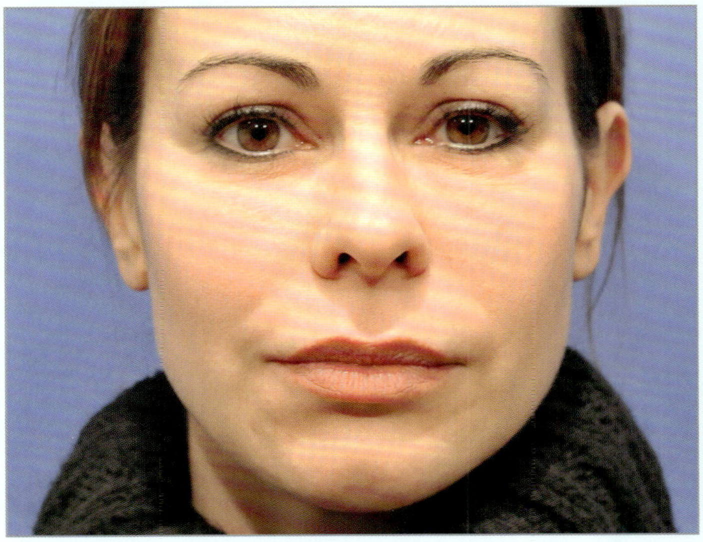

Fig. 7.53 Patient after volumisation of the chin with hyaluronic acid fillers, frontal view. The patient looks visibly younger and the effect is still natural.

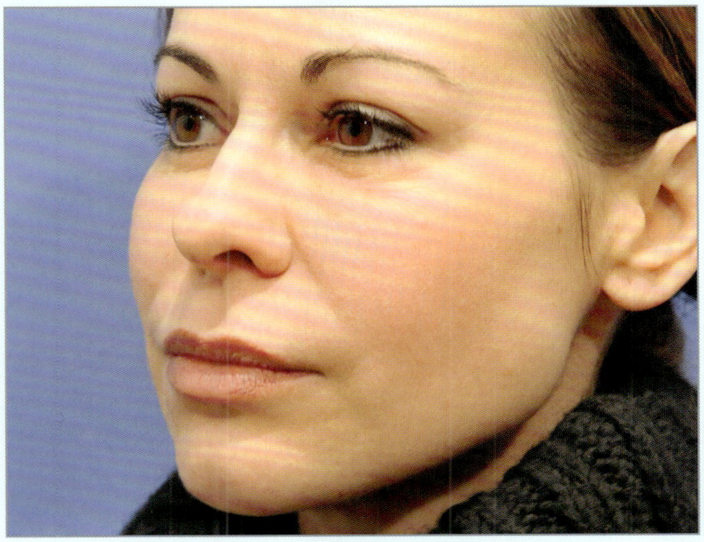

Fig. 7.54 Patient after volumisation of the chin, oblique profile. It becomes evident that the anterior projection of the chin achieves a harmonising elongation and rejuvenation of the face.

7.5.1 Perioral lines in the upper and lower lip

Perioral or radial lines on the upper and lower lip (i.e. radiating from the vermilion border into the white lip) constitute a significant concern in female patients in particular. The subcutaneous tissue of the upper lip is very thin. This fact, along with the pronounced activity of the orbicularis oris muscle, makes this area particularly prone to fine lines and wrinkles.

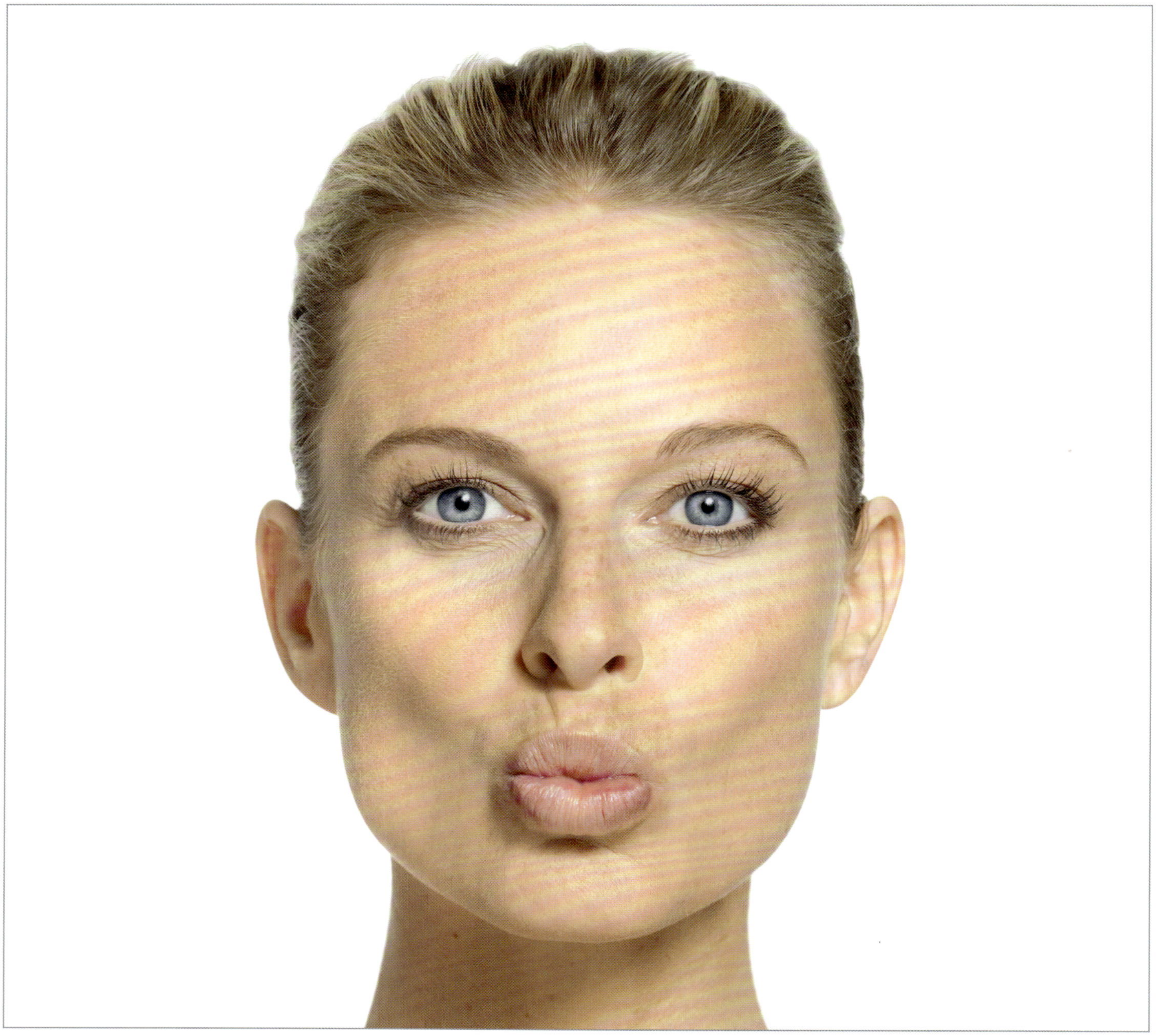

Patient selection
Patients with radial lines that are related to atrophy of the supramucosal soft tissue particularly benefit from filler augmentation. Preferably, the injection should be deep to compensate for the causal tissue deficit. Furthermore, lines arising from the dynamic effects of the underlying orbicularis oris are best treated with botulinum toxin type-A injections. Often a combination approach with both treatment modalities works best (i.e. initial treatment with botulinum toxin type-A, after which at 2 weeks or so, the filler augmentation with hyaluronic acid can be performed).

Assessing the indication
Perioral lines are a good indication for filler augmentation. Whereas previously filler treatment at a superficial level was the primary technique, today deep volumising techniques have been recognised as significant for this indication. By restoring the lost supramucosal volume with vertical filler injections, the practitioner is able to provide the lips with a new natural base to support the overlying structures. In doing so, the body of the lip (vermilion body or red lip) is also simultaneously enhanced.

Anatomy

Radial lines arise as a consequence of the atrophy-related shrinkage of the soft tissue base of the white lip. Additionally the contraction of the annular orbicular oris muscle (1) acts on the skin and contributes to wrinkle formation.

A link with frequent pursing of the lips, e.g. when smoking, has been associated with radial line formation, which is why these lines are also often referred to as 'smoker's lines'; however, this is mainly related to the general acceleration of extrinsic skin ageing caused by smoking itself.

The upper lip is supplied by the superior labial artery (A labialis superior, 2) and the lower lip by the inferior labial artery (A labialis inferior, 3).

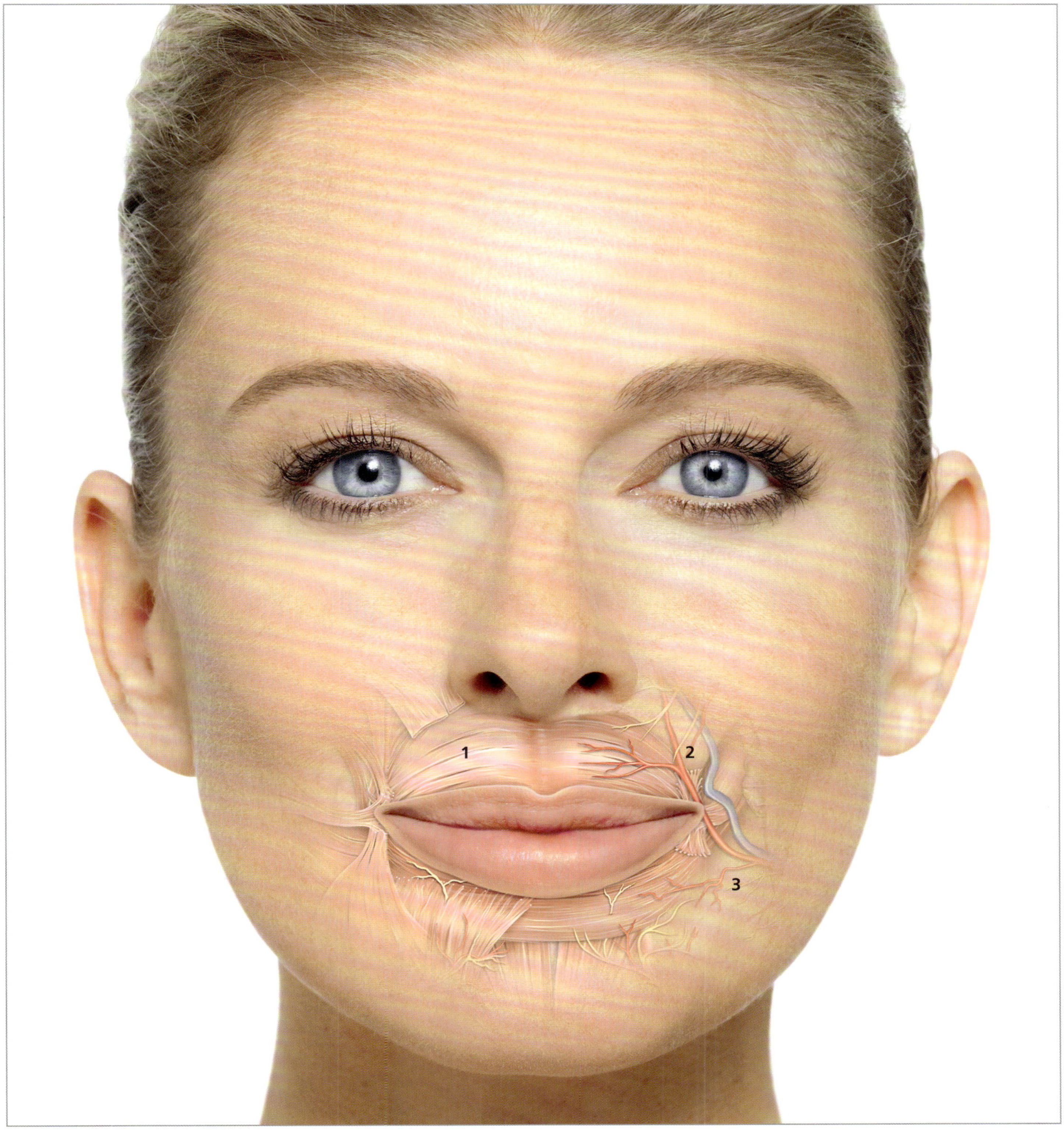

Treatment planning – Superficial correction
The treatment goal is a superficial correction of the radial lines on the upper and lower lip.

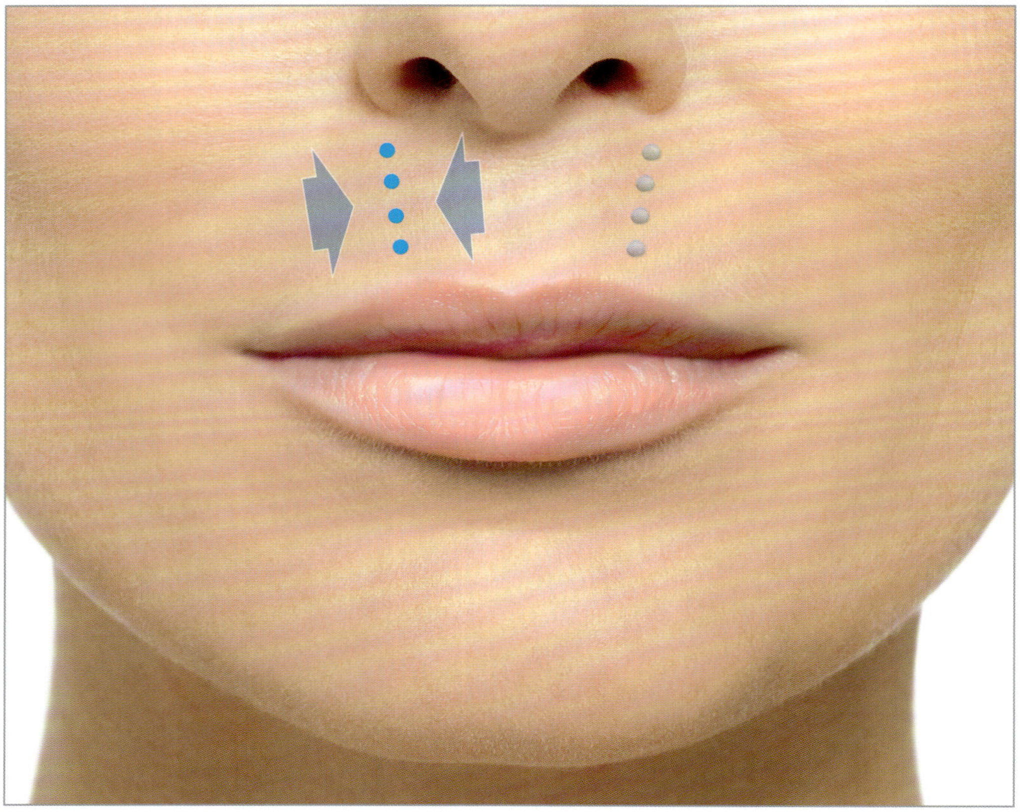

Technique: point technique with compression
Injection points: three to four points/line
Volume: minimal dose
Tool: 30–32 gauge needle

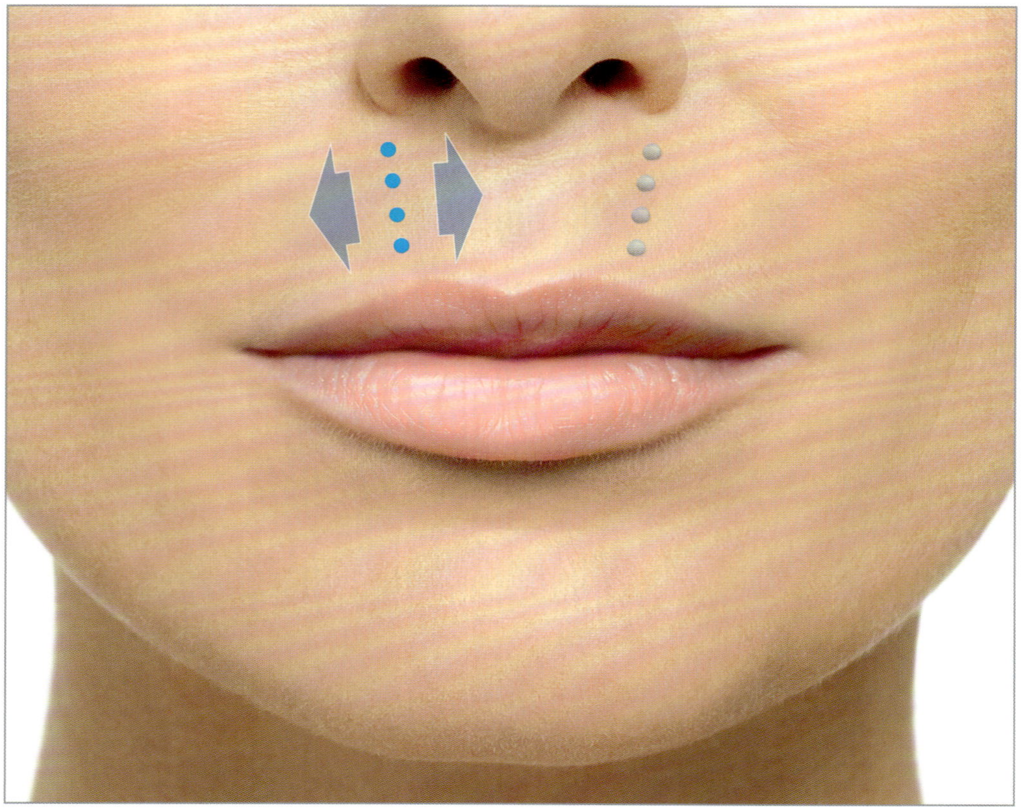

Technique: point technique with stretching, very superficially
Injection sites: three to four points/line
Volume: minimal dose
Tool: 30–32 gauge needle

Video: Radial lines – stretching
http://www.kvm-tv.de/FIL/017.mp4

Treatment – Superficial correction

Point technique with compression

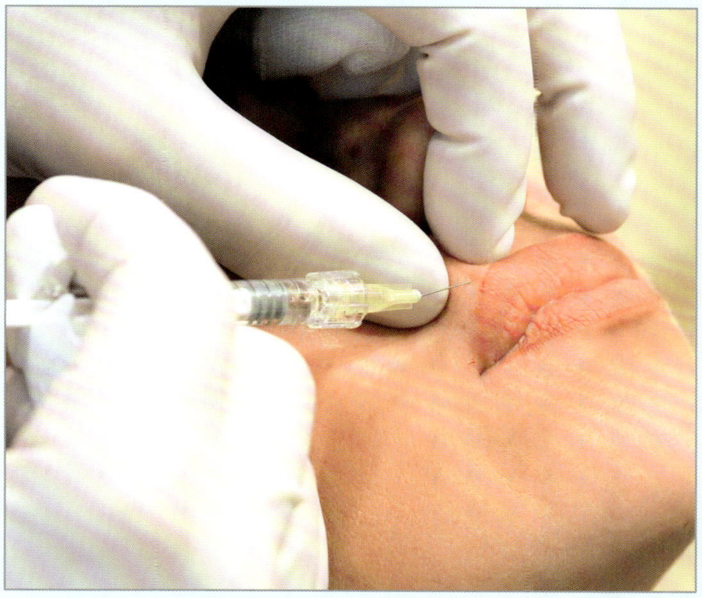

Fig. 7.55 The upper lip is grasped and compressed between the thumb and the index finger of the non-injecting hand. The injection is given at a right angle to the line. The point technique is performed, with individual injection points placed along the course of the line.

Point technique with stretching

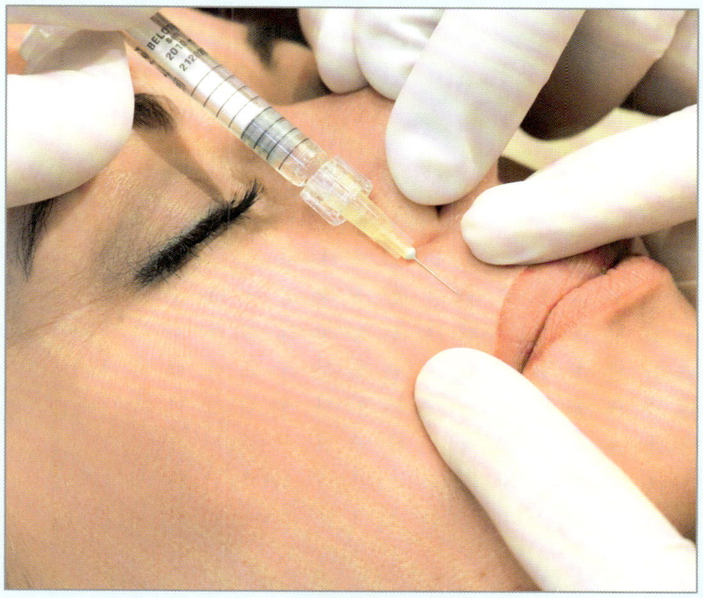

Fig. 7.56 The clinician or their assistant stretches the skin directly around the area to be injected (the upper lip in this case), while the needle is inserted into the skin of the upper lip towards its red margin. Multiple point injections are then made, as required.

Treatment steps

- Remove makeup
- Disinfection
- Anaesthesia
- Injection: point technique (with compression or stretching)
- Massage and mould (ensure appropriate distribution of the filler)
- Inform patient about post-treatment dos and don'ts
- Arrange a follow-up appointment

Filler selection

1 Superficial injection (p. 62)
2 Medium injection (p. 63)

Combined treatment options

Treatments inducing collagen synthesis without removing the epidermis:

- Non-ablative lasers
- Flash lamp
- Radiofrequency
- Dermal needling

Additional treatment options, depending on the skin findings:

- Ablative lasers
- Chemical peels
- Dermabrasion

Complications/Managing complications

Palpable nodules may form due to the aggregation of the filler used. Thorough massage and moulding of the injected filler directly after the injection ensures uniform distribution.

Practical tips

- The stretching technique can lead to complete smoothing of the deeper lines even when prominent elastotic skin changes are present. The key factor here is to use the technique correctly, with maximum stretching, to enable the filler to spread uniformly through the tissue and produce a smooth appearance. Consistent use of the stretching technique prevents overcorrection.
- Superficial filler augmentation of the radial lines achieves a camouflage of the radial wrinkles, rather than actually treating the causal deficit. The filler is applied into the soft tissue envelope and does not reach the 'hot spots' of the volume loss. For a complete treatment, vertical deep depots of filler placement are advised, as discussed below.

Treatment planning – Volume compensation
The treatment goal is to compensate for the lost volume in the deep supramucosal layer of the white lip region. This reduces the radial lines and simultaneously creates natural lip volume.

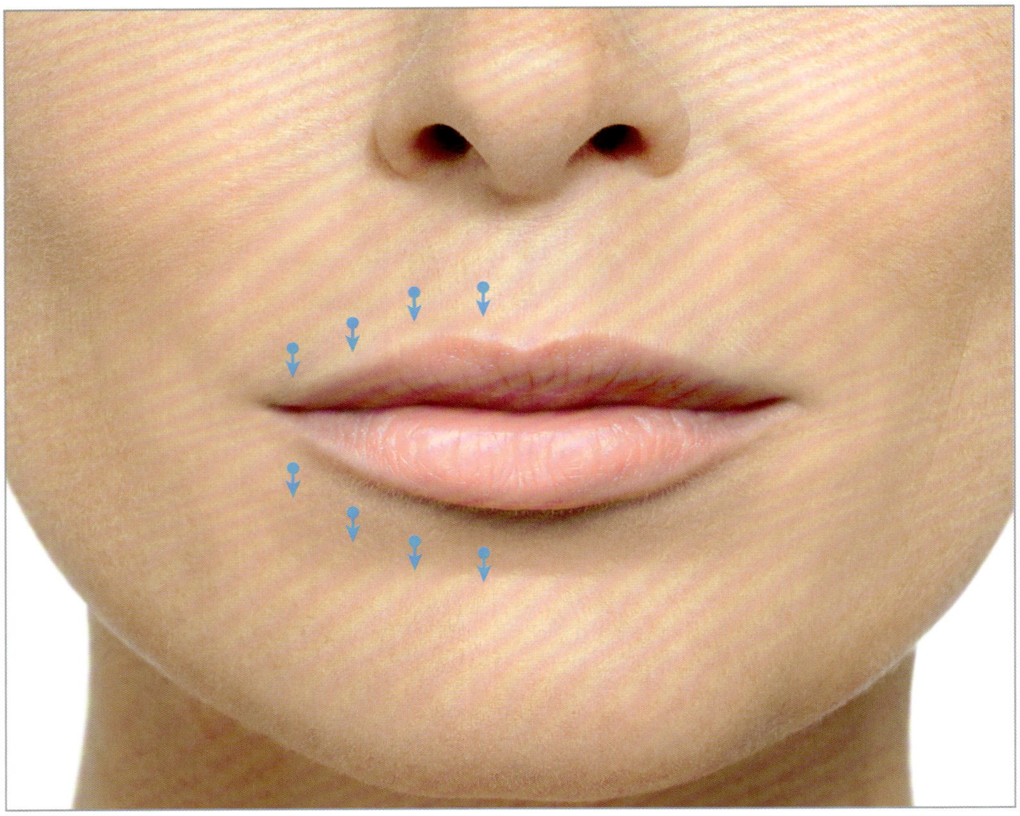

Technique: VSDT
Injection points: one 'hot spot'/line

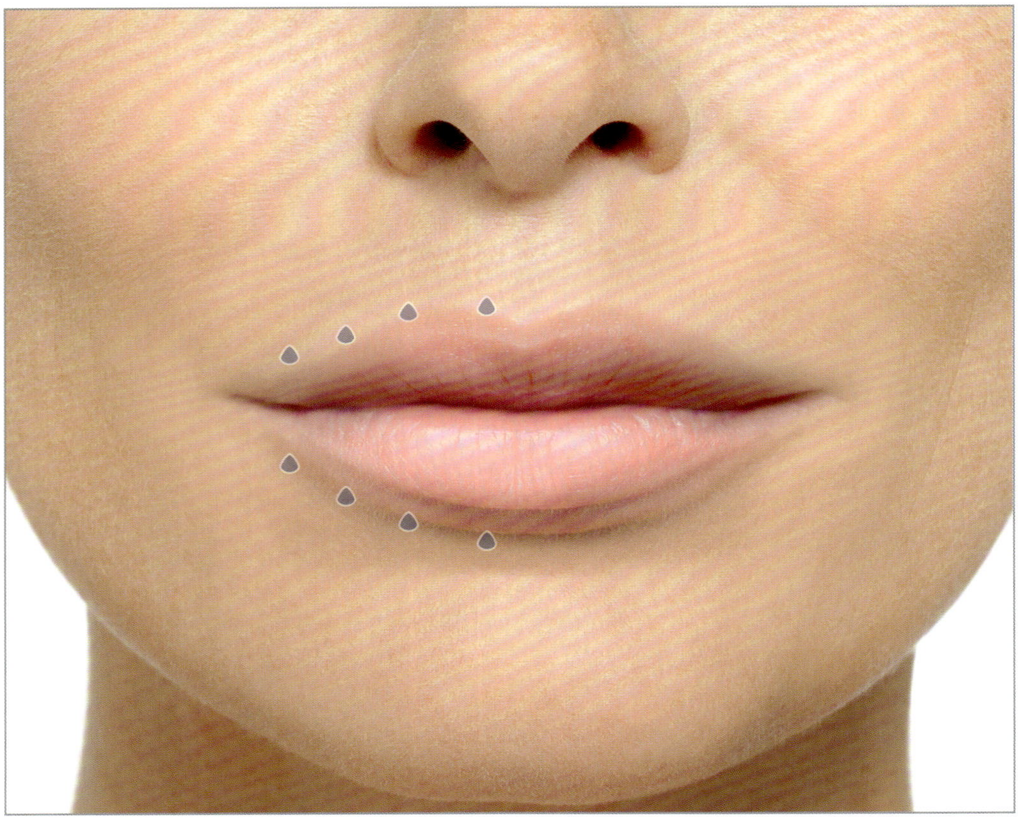

Volume: 0.2–0.3 ml per quadrant of the upper or lower lip
Tool: 27 gauge needle

Treatment – Volume compensation

VSDT upper white lip

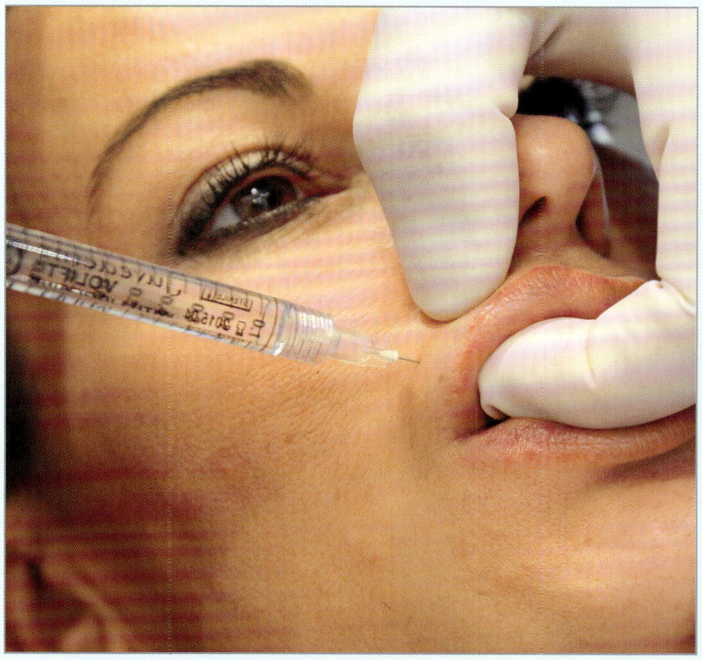

Fig. 7.57 The practitioner uses the non-injecting hand to create a stabilising counter bearing for the supramucosal injection. The needle is introduced in a vertical direction to the skin at the site of the deepest depression of each line and minimal doses of the filler are injected into the supramucosal plane. The volumes used amount to 0.1 to 0.3 ml of filler injected per quadrant of the upper or the lower lip.

VSDT lower white lip

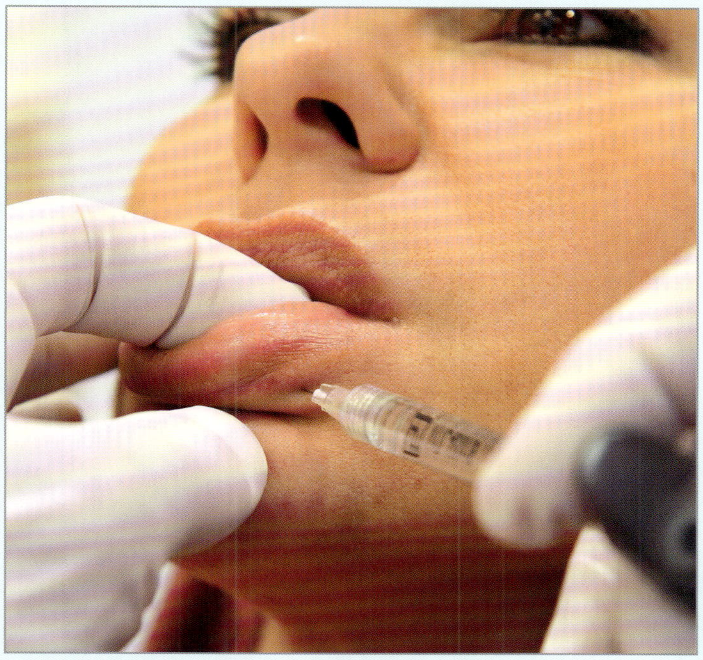

Fig. 7.58 The same procedure is applied to the lower lip. The vertical ultra-deep injection enables an optimal lifting effect, as the filler does not disperse into the overlying soft tissues. Simultaneously, lip volumisation is also achieved.

Treatment steps
- Remove makeup
- Disinfection
- Anaesthesia
- Injection: VSDT
- Massage and mould (ensure appropriate distribution of the filler)
- Inform patient about post-treatment dos and don'ts
- Arrange a follow-up appointment

Filler selection

3 Deep injection (p. 66)

B Special indication: lips (p. 70)

Combined treatment options
- Filler volumisation of the red lip
- Botulinum toxin type-A (for the dynamic perioral lines)

Complications/Managing complications
- Careful insertion of the needle down to the mucosa with slow penetration speed and aspiration reduces the risk of an intravascular injection.
- Palpable nodules may form due to the aggregation of the filler. Thorough massage and moulding of the filler directly after the injection ensures uniform distribution.

Practical tips
- Some practitioners use the index finger of the non-injecting hand as a counter bearing during the injection to facilitate the correct supramucosal placement of the filler; however, great care should be taken to avoid needlestick injuries.
- Supramucosal injections, unlike the superficial injections discussed above, ensure optimal augmentation as the filler does not displace and migrates into the superficial tissue layers.
- VSDT into the radial lines of the upper and lower white lip achieves a reduction or complete eradication of the lines and wrinkles, as well as achieving a natural enlargement of the lip base by restoring the ultra-deep volume. This in itself can eliminate the need for volume augmentation of the red lip.

7.5.2 Lips

Lips play a key functional role in facial expression, and furthermore, as a symbol of sensuality can influence an individual's level of attractiveness. Full, symmetrical lips, with upturned corners and a healthy colour are considered aesthetically appealing. With ageing, the corners tend to turn down, and the volume diminishes.

Lips are commonly augmented with fillers. However, it is also important to simultaneously consider treating the perioral complex to ensure overall harmony of the lower third of the face.

Importantly, lips are highly sensitive areas to treat given the high density of nerves, and hence anaesthesia is a key consideration in this treatment.

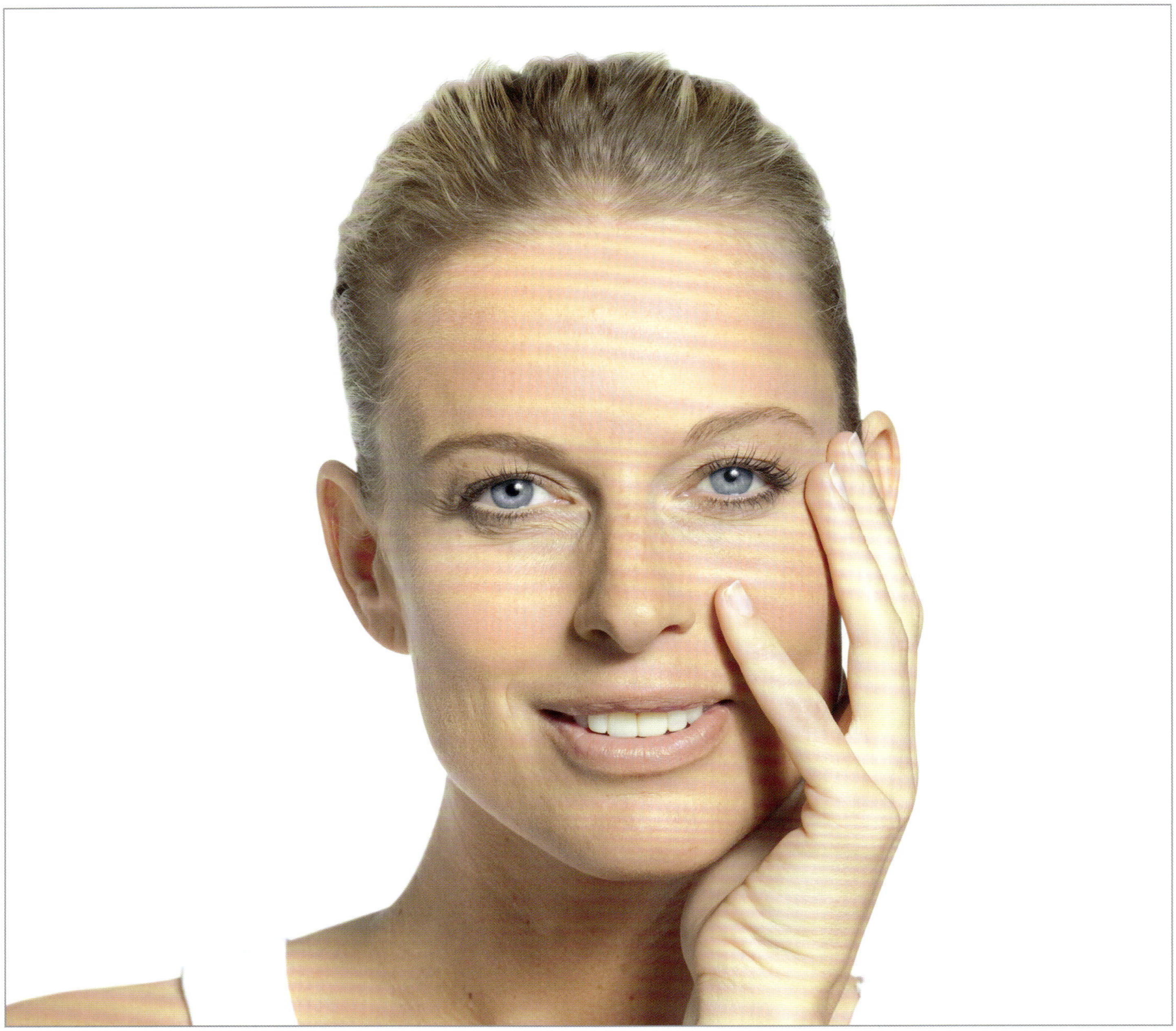

Patient selection

A thorough discussion regarding the desired treatment outcome is essential, as there are a number of treatment options available when considering lip and perioral rejuvenation and augmentation. Patients specifically seeking to enhance the volume of the lip should also be advised to assess the perioral complex, and if necessary, the surrounding structures (e.g. the marionette lines, corners of the lip, and the chin) should be treated simultaneously to achieve a harmonious clinical outcome to the lower third of the face.

Assessing the indication

A number of features can be treated when considering lip augmentation and rejuvenation, namely: the volume of the red lip (i.e. body of the lip); the vermilion border (i.e. the contour of the lip); the lip corners; Cupid's bow; the philtral columns, and the aforementioned radial lip lines.

Anatomy

The orbicularis oris muscle (1) plays a key role in the motor function of the lips. The section of the muscular ring that lies furthest from the oral aperture can reduce in size while protruding from the red margin of the lips, as in the case of whistling. When the part of the muscle that lies at the edge of the lips contracts in isolation, the red lip moves inwards towards the front teeth, so that less of it is visible.

The function of the orbicularis oris muscle is antagonised by the surrounding muscles of facial expression, which pull the lips or the corner of the mouth laterally, upwards or downwards, thus widening the oral aperture.

The skin of the red lip, which has three to five cell layers, is very thin compared to the cell layers of the skin covering the rest of the face. Light skin types have no melanocytes in the skin of their lips. The intense red colour of the lips comes from the superficial blood vessels. This colour is less pronounced in darker skin types, as their lips are pigmented. The blood supply of the lower lip is provided by the inferior labial artery (2) and that of the upper lip by the superior labial artery (3).

Since the skin of the lips has neither sweat glands nor sebaceous glands, it lacks the usual hydro-lipid film coating found in skin elsewhere. As a result, the skin of the lips dries faster and cracks more easily.

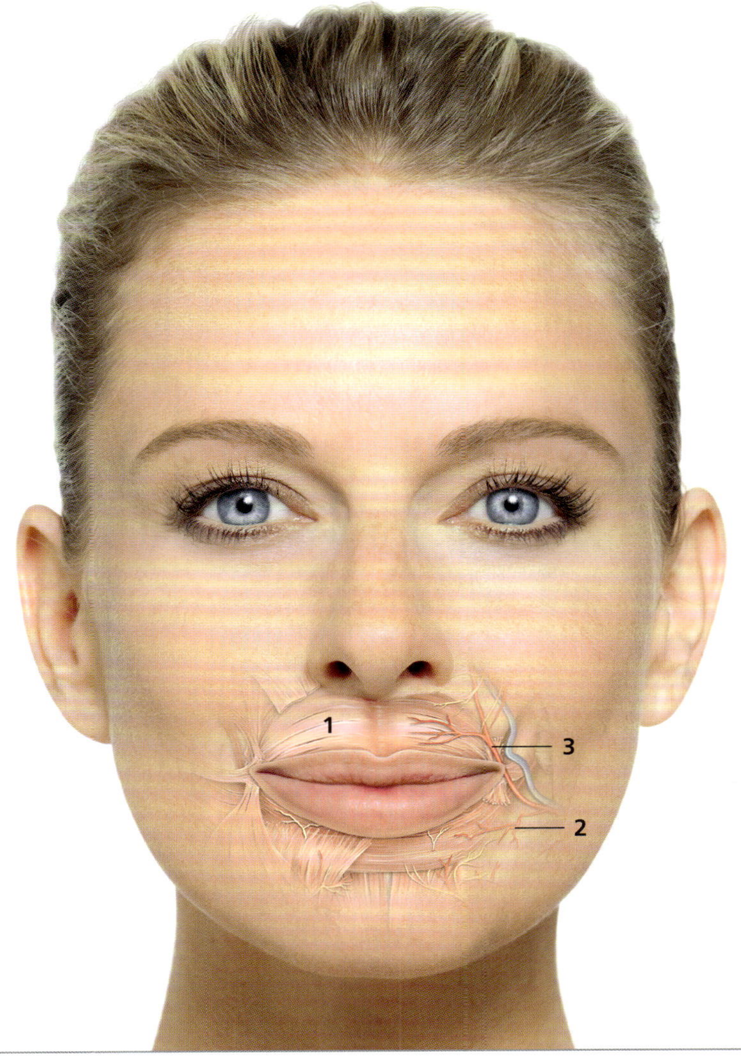

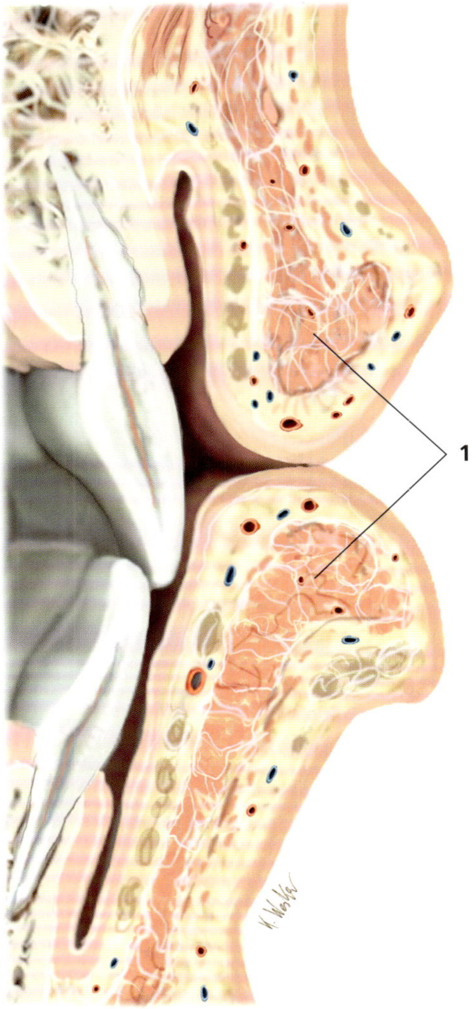

Orbicularis oris muscle

Origin	Insertion	Function	Innervation
• Mandible • Maxilla	• Upper and lower lip	• Closes the lips • Purses the lips during kissing or whistling	• Buccal branches and the marginal mandibular branch of the facial nerve (cranial nerve VII)

Treatment planning – Lip volume

The treatment goal is to create a homogeneous and harmonious volumisation of the lips, in line with the rest of the face.

Restoration of the atrophied deep soft tissue volume with vertical injections into the white lip, as discussed previously (see pp. 194 f.), rebuilds the natural base to lips that appear significant aged. Thereafter, the practitioner can correct the lip volume also by treating the red part of the lips, where the filler has sufficient space and structural support for a predictable distribution over the muscle.

Combining the white lip and red lip treatment can be useful, particularly in aged lips. Cannulas are a useful tool when treating the red lip, and achieve optimal results, although needles can also be used.

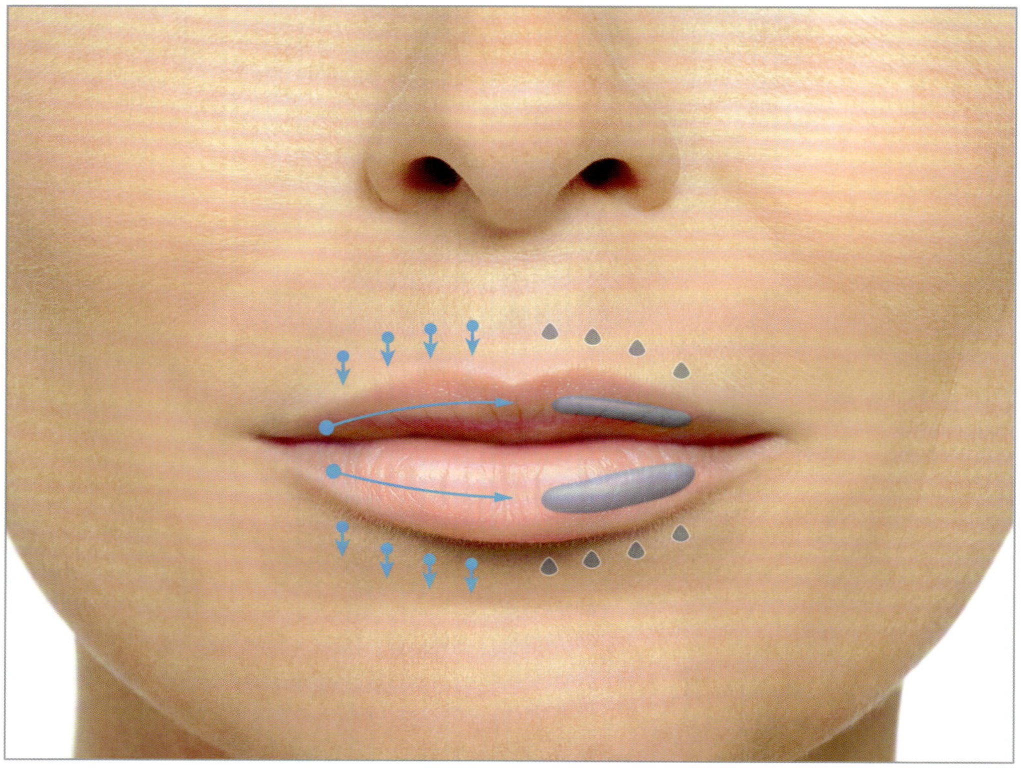

Technique: VSDT (white lip) and linear technique (red lip)
Injection points: white lip – three to four injection points into the radial wrinkles per quadrant of the lip (to build up the lip base); red lip – one injection site close to the corner of the mouth per quadrant of the lip
Injection depth and direction: white lip – supramucosal depots; red lip – above the muscle in the direction of the centre of the lips, parallel to their course
Volume: white lip –0.2–0.3 ml/quadrant of the lip; red lip – 0.1–0.25 ml/quadrant of the lip
Tool: 27–30 gauge needle

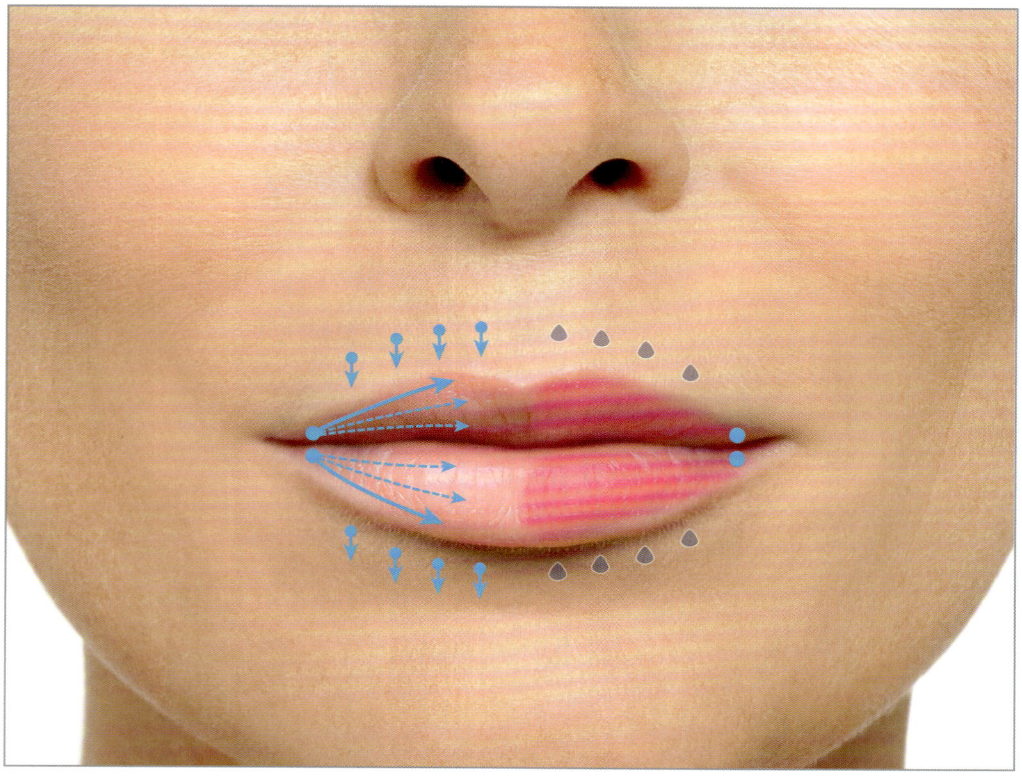

Technique: VSDT (white lip) and SHAC (red lip)
Injection points: white lip – see earlier; red lip – per quadrant of the lip, one insertion site close to the corner of the mouth
Injection depth and direction: white lip – supramucosal depots; red lip – above the muscle in the direction towards the centre of the lips, in a fan-like fashion while mobilising the tissues
Volume: white lip – see above; 0.2–0.3 ml/quadrant of the lip
Tool: needle for white lip (as per above), and 22–25 gauge cannula for the red lip

Treatment – Lip volume

Linear technique

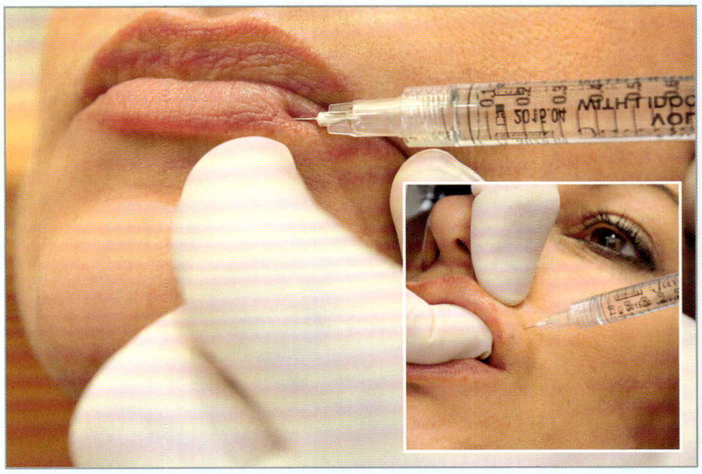

Fig. 7.59 Before augmentation of the red lip, volume restoration of the natural lip base should be accomplished with vertical injections into the white lip (small picture). The red lip is then treated above the orbicularis oris muscle. The filler can be carefully applied with a linear technique using a needle.

SHAC

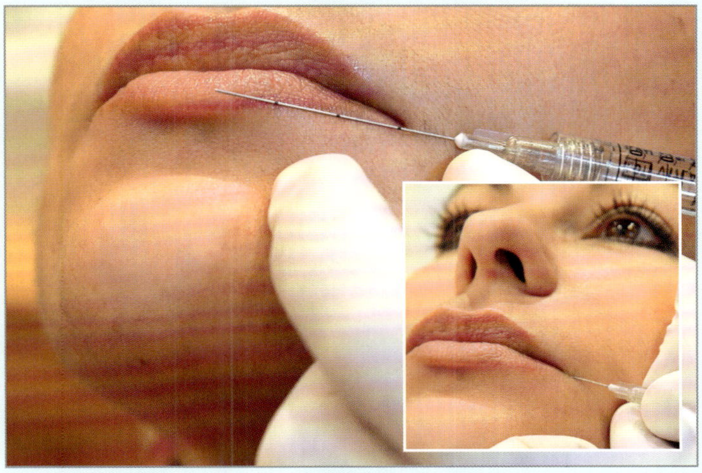

Fig. 7.60 Using cannulas to deposit the filler in a horizontal fashion is optimal for this region, and this practice reduces levels of discomfort and achieves the most uniform results. Gentle tissue mobilisation ensures this procedure also leads to fibrogenetic regeneration. Volumes of 0.2 to 0.3 ml per lip quadrant are delivered.

Treatment steps

- History: e.g. recurrent herpes infections (herpes prophylaxis with e.g. aciclovir may be necessary)
- Remove makeup
- Disinfection
- Anaesthesia
- Injection: VSDT/SHAC (or linear technique)
- Massage and mould (ensure appropriate distribution of the filler)
- Inform patient about post-treatment dos and don'ts
- Arrange a follow-up appointment

Filler selection

3 Deep injection (p. 66)
B Special indications: lips (p. 70)

Moderately cross-linked hyaluronic acid fillers are ideal for this indication due to their viscoelastic properties and longevity.

Complications/Managing complications

- Pain control is an important aspect to consider when treating lips, particularly when injecting with needles. Local anaesthesia (see section 6.8, p. 99) will need to be considered in most cases.
- When performing isolated augmentations on the red lip, the slim orbicularis oculi muscle forms the only underlying platform for the filler to distribute over. Too much filler volume in this plane can result in unpredictable and unsatisfactory results. This problem can be avoided by prior volume restoration of the natural lip base by vertical injections into the white lip.
- Palpable nodules may form due to the aggregation of the injected filler. Thorough massage and moulding of the injected filler immediately after the injection ensures uniform distribution.
- Swelling or small haematomas during the treatment can make the result look asymmetrical at first; monitor to ensure that equal volumes are administered on both the left and right side of the lip, unless correcting any existing asymmetry. To avoid overcorrection, a review and additional injections can be offered once the injection-related swelling has subsided (we recommend waiting at least a week post-treatment to do this).
- Avoid overfilling and creating overprojected 'duck lips'. This is unnatural and an off-putting example of a filler treatment gone wrong.
- Fillers should be injected towards the inner aspect of the red lip (i.e. close to the mouth opening), as more outward injections closer to the white lip tend to results in decreased red-lip show.
- Always build up lip volume over several sessions, to achieve a natural enhancement gradually.

Practical tips

- By volumising the shrunken soft tissue base of the lips with vertical injections into the white upper and lower lip, the lips recover their natural volume. In doing so, further volume-enhancing injections in the red lip may have a better clinical outcome.
- It is essential that filler injections do not impair the functionality of the lips (e.g. when speaking) or make them feel unnatural to touch (e.g. when kissing).
- Cannulas are optimal tools when delivering supramuscular augmentation of the red lip, as they allow for reduced levels of pain and discomfort. As such, local anaesthesia is not necessary in many cases. This technique also allows for uniform filler distribution, a natural clinical outcome along with fibrogenetic activation.

⚠ Prior to injecting any filler, please refer to the latest manufacturer guidelines for specific instructions for use.

Treatment – Lip contour

Contouring of the vermilion border is a popular treatment, as it enables better lip definition to be achieved, particularly for aged lips.

The treatment goal is to attain a uniform, precise, harmonious-looking enhancement of the vermilion border, as well as to avoid overinjection and a resultant overprojection.

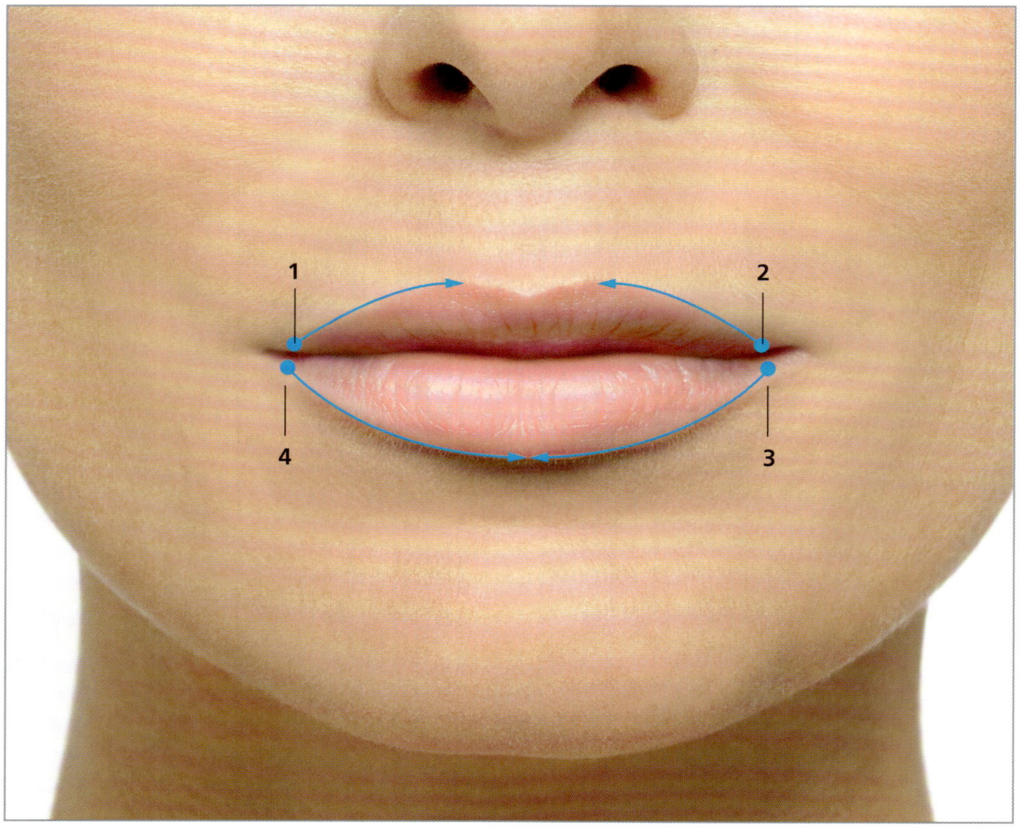

Technique: linear tunneling technique
Injection point: close to the angle of the mouth in the sequence shown above 1 to 4
Direction of injection: following the vermilion border, up to the apex of the Cupid's bow

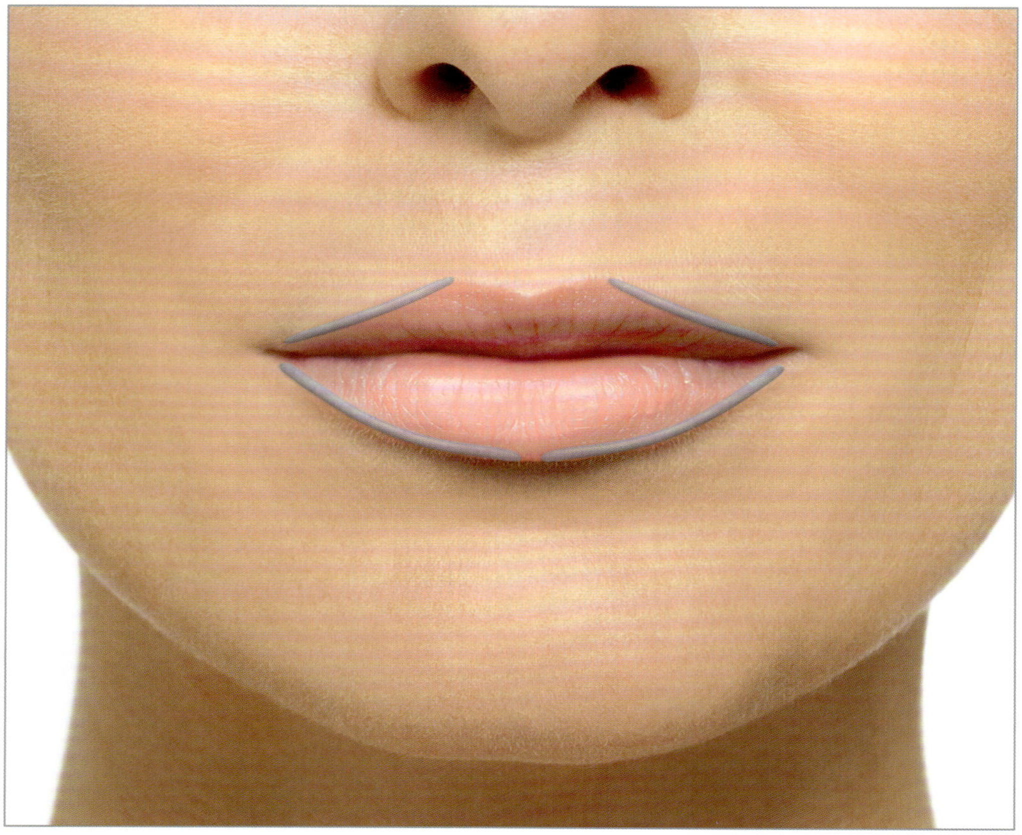

Volume: approximately 0.1 ml/quadrant of the lip
Tool: 30 gauge needle

7

Treatment – Lip contour

Tunneling technique

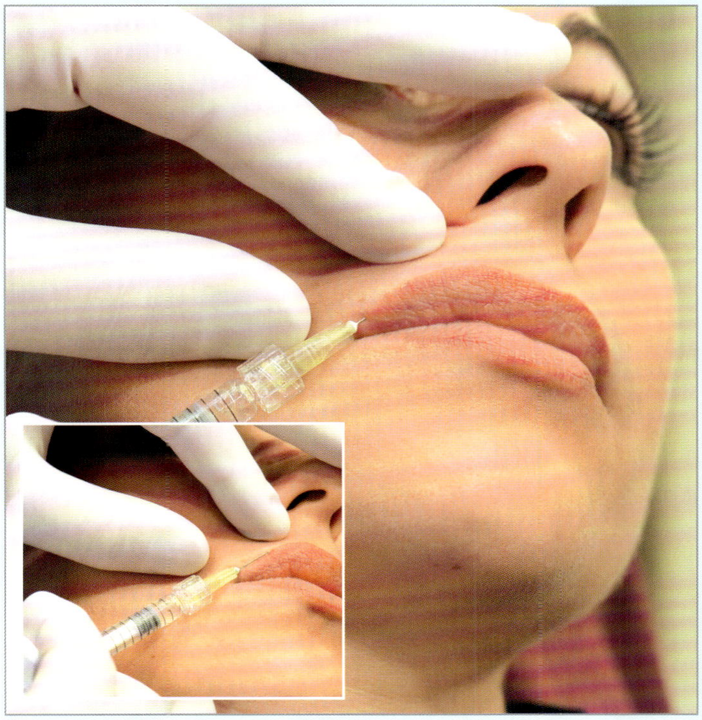

Fig. 7.61 The needle is inserted at the corner of the mouth within the vermilion border, and threaded towards the apex of the Cupid's bow. End-to-end linear threads are delivered with the needle. Once the needle is advanced as far as it will go, the filler is then injected as the needle is being withdrawn (i.e. in a retrograde fashion).

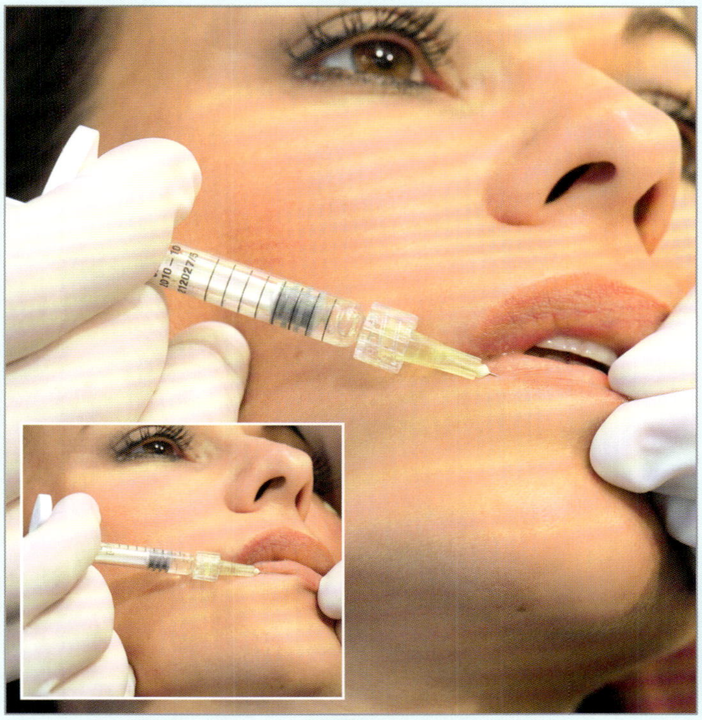

Fig. 7.62 The same procedure is used to contour the lower vermilion border.

Treatment steps

- History: e.g. recurrent herpes infections (herpes prophylaxis with e.g. aciclovir may be necessary)
- Remove makeup
- Disinfection
- Anaesthesia
- Injection: linear tunneling technique
- Massage and mould (ensure appropriate distribution of the filler)
- Inform patient about post-treatment dos and don'ts
- Arrange a follow-up appointment

Filler selection

2 Medium injection (p. 63)
B Special indications: lips (p. 70)

Moderately cross-linked hyaluronic acid fillers are ideal for this indication due to their viscoelastic properties and longevity.

Complications/Managing complications

- Palpable nodules may form due to the aggregation of the injected filler. Thorough massage and moulding of the filler immediately after the injection ensures uniform distribution.

Practical tips

- Not everyone will benefit from a contouring lip treatment, and hence it is worth discussing with the patient his or her desired treatment outcome, and assessing if filling the vermilion border will enhance and rejuvenate the overall aspect.
- It is essential that filler injections do not impair the functionality of the lips (e.g. when speaking) or feel unnatural to touch (e.g. when kissing).
- Pain control is an important aspect to consider when treating lips, and particularly when injecting with needles. Anaesthesia (see section 6.8, p. 99) will need to be considered in most cases.

Treatment planning – Cupid's bow and philtrum

The treatment goal is to accentuate or enhance the Cupid's bow and where necessary, adjunctive modification or reconstruction of the philtrum.

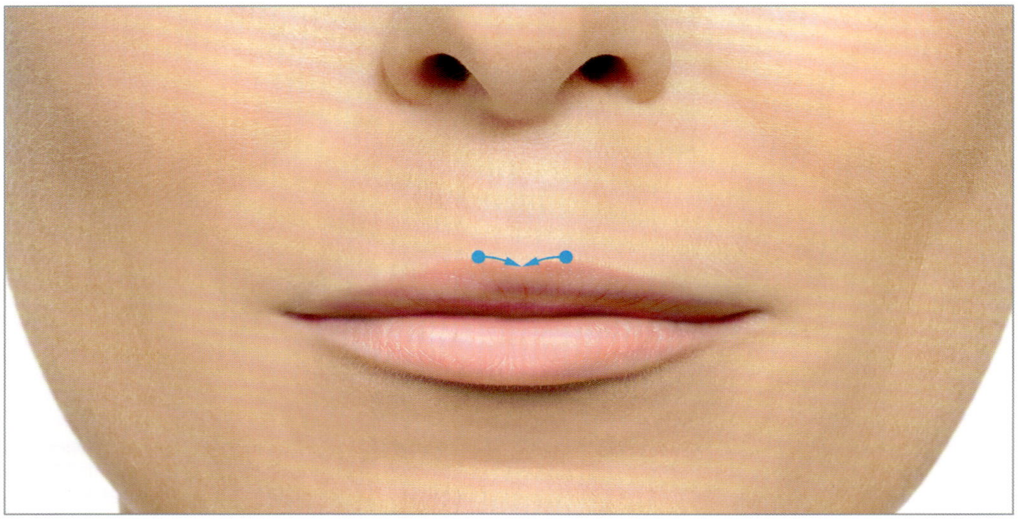

Technique: linear technique
Injection point: highest point of the Cupid's bow at the vermilion border
Direction of injection: towards the lowest point of the Cupid's bow at the vermilion border

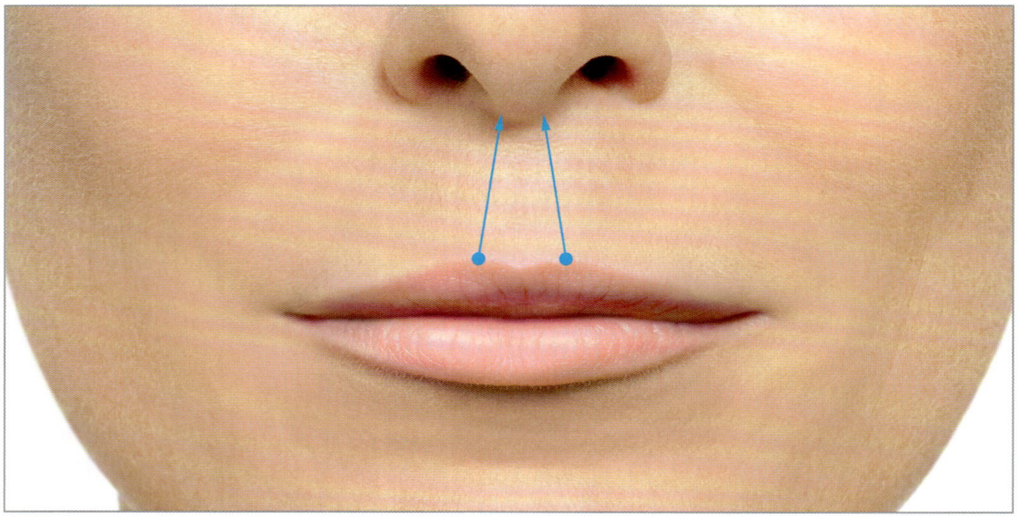

Technique: linear technique with compression
Injection point: highest point of the Cupid's bow
Direction of injection: following the philtral column up to the base of the nose

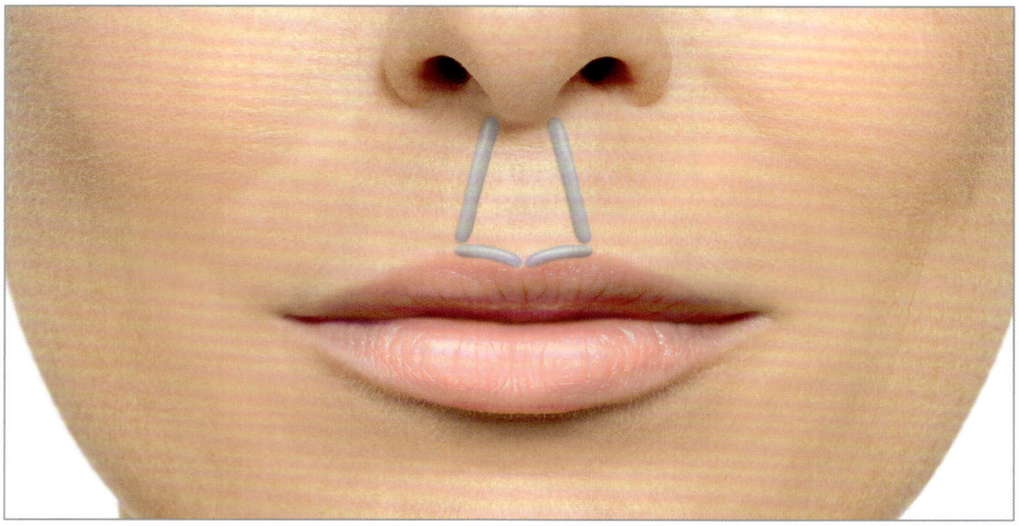

Volume: Cupid's bow – the minimum amount possible; philtrum – approximately 0.1 ml per column
Tool: 30 gauge needle

Treatment – Cupid's bow and philtrum

Tunneling technique / Compression technique

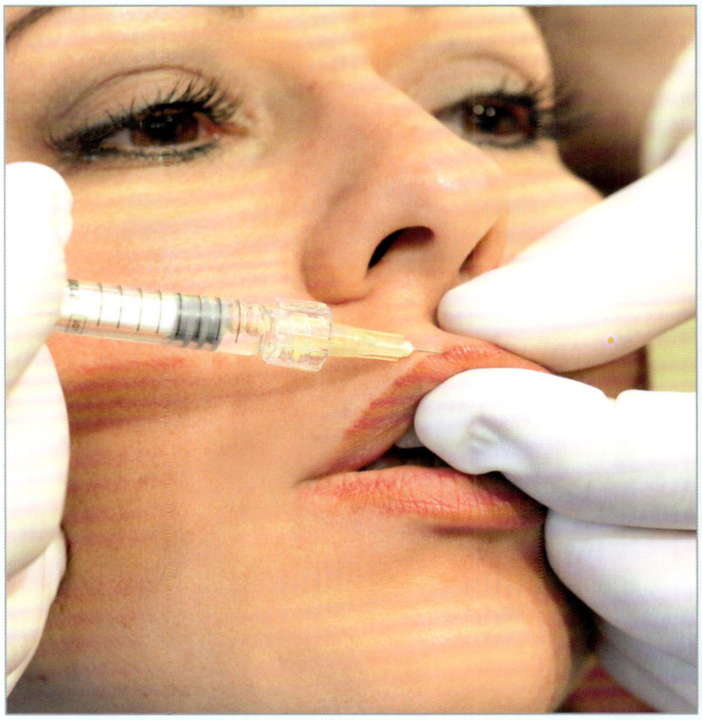

Fig. 7.63 The needle is inserted at the vermilion border, at the highest point of the Cupid's bow. The needle is advanced up to the lowest point of the Cupid's bow. The filler is injected as the needle is being withdrawn (i.e. in a retrograde fashion).

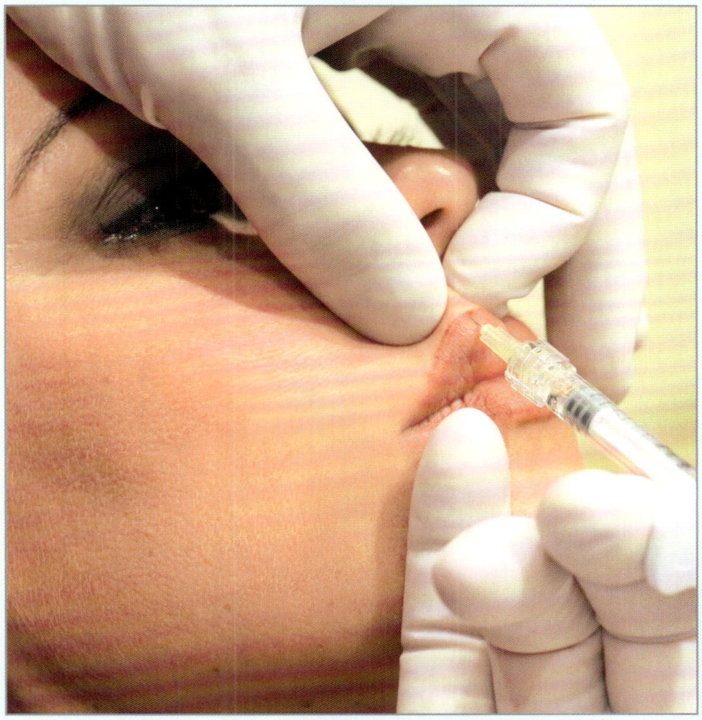

Fig. 7.64 The practitioner grasps the upper lip between the thumb and the index finger of the non-injecting hand. The needle is inserted at the vermilion border at the apex of the Cupid's bow. Using the linear technique with compression, the needle is advanced as far as is necessary, and the filler injected as the needle is being withdrawn.

Treatment steps

- History: e.g. recurrent herpes infections (herpes prophylaxis with e.g. aciclovir may be necessary)
- Remove makeup
- Disinfection
- Anaesthesia
- Injection: linear technique with compression
- Massage and mould (ensure appropriate distribution of the filler)
- Inform patient about post-treatment dos and don'ts
- Arrange a follow-up appointment

Filler selection

2 Medium injection (p. 63)
B Special indications: lips (p. 70)

Complications/Managing complications

Palpable nodules or threads may form due to the aggregation of the filler used. Thorough massage and moulding of the filler directly after the injection ensures uniform distribution.

Practical tips

- Not everyone will benefit from a Cupid's bow or philtral column injections. A thorough assessment and discussion with the patient should help to determine the desired treatment goal. Importantly, it is useful to understand what the patient looked like in their youth, with regard to the prominence of these features. If not present in the first place, performing these treatments may not be appropriate or desirable.
- Use the filler sparingly; avoid overcorrection as this produces an unnatural and overprojected appearance.

Treatment planning – Mouth corners
The treatment goal is to achieve a gentle and symmetrical elevation of the mouth corners (i.e. the labial angles). Supporting drooping mouth corners by placing small filler depots into this region often leads to marked improvement in the appearance of the mouth and gives the whole face a friendlier and more positive outlook.

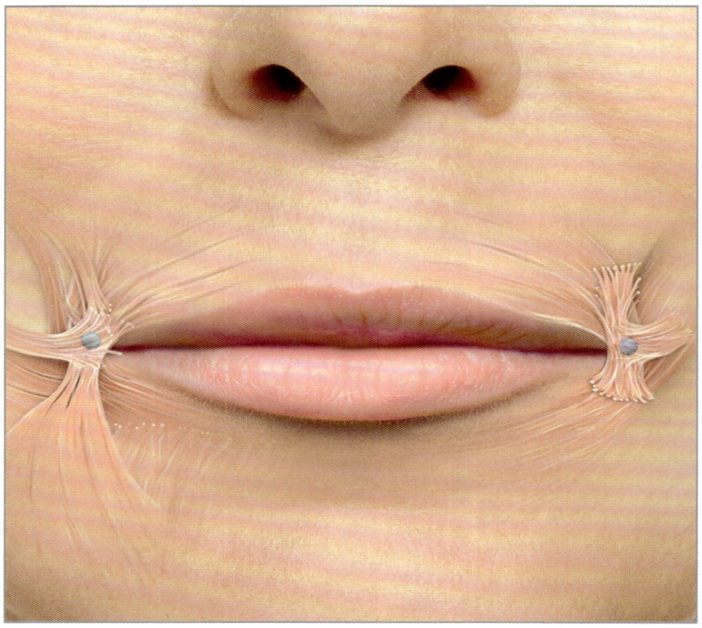

Injection site: (●) The first injection is made at the apex of the angle of the mouth. The depth of the injection is about 1 mm and the filler should be spread centrifugally to the upper and lower lip.

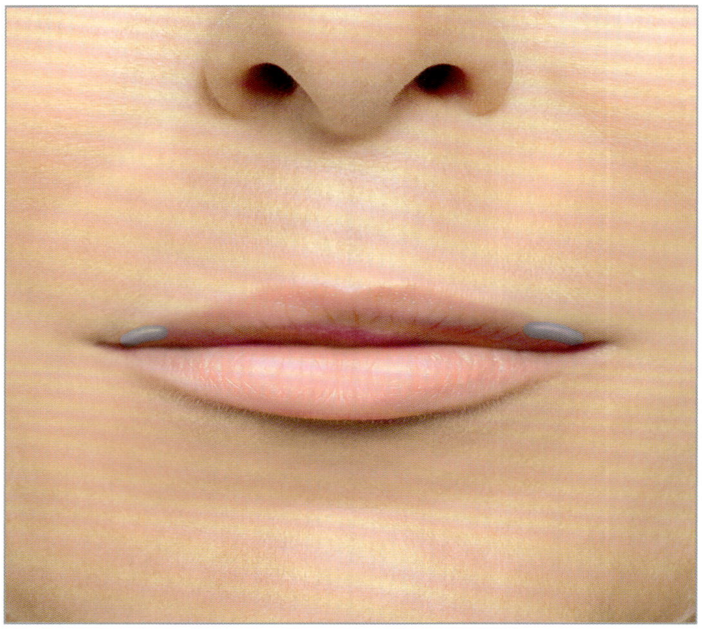

Injection site: (●) The second injection is given slightly above the first, at the vermilion border. The injection is given in the red lip but above the muscle into a depth of about 1 mm, in a retrograde direction after advancement of the needle 5 mm towards the middle of the lip.

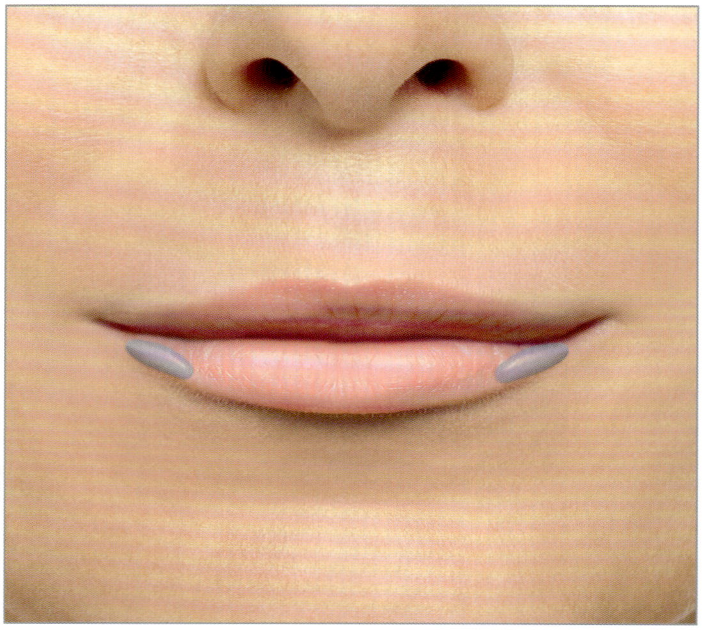

Injection site: (●) The third injection is placed slightly below the first point. The needle is inserted at the vermilion border in the subdermal plane. The direction of the injection is along the body of the muscle but above the muscle, at a depth of approx. 1 mm. The filler is injected as the needle is being withdrawn. This injection pads out the angle of the mouth in the lateral region.

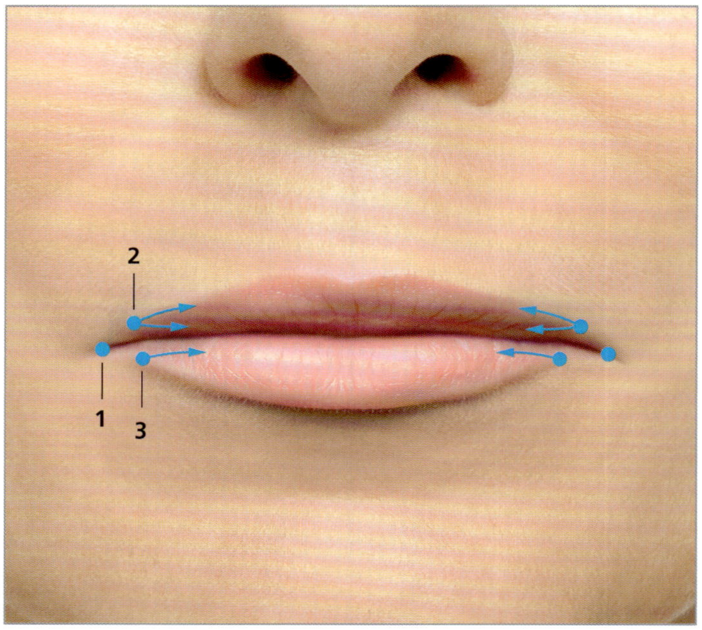

Volumes: (1) 0.05–0.1 ml; (2) 0.1–0.2 ml; (3) 0.1–0.2 ml
Tool: 30–32 gauge needle

Video: Mouth corners
http://www.kvm-tv.de/FIL/018.mp4

Treatment – Mouth corners

Point technique

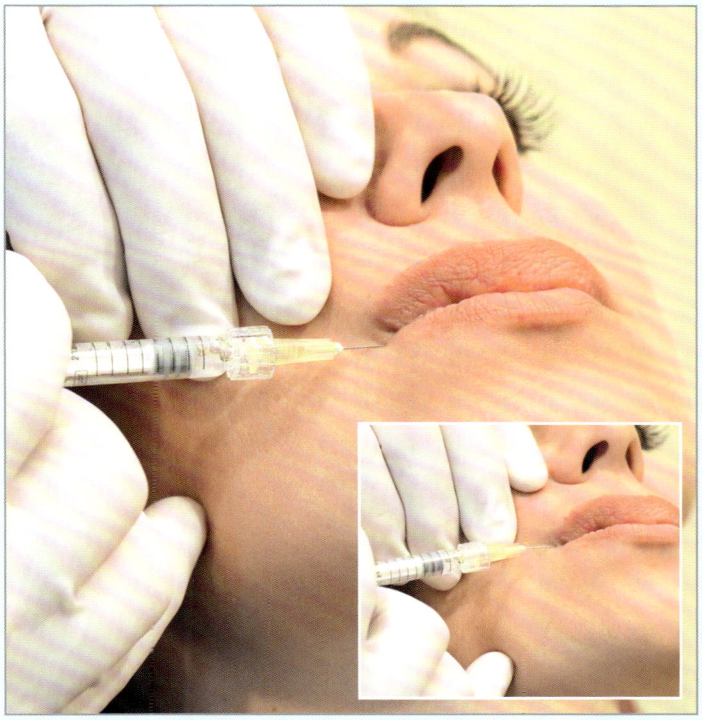

Fig. 7.65 The needle is inserted at the apex of the angle of the mouth, directly into the modiolus. The depth of the injection is about 1 mm.

Linear technique

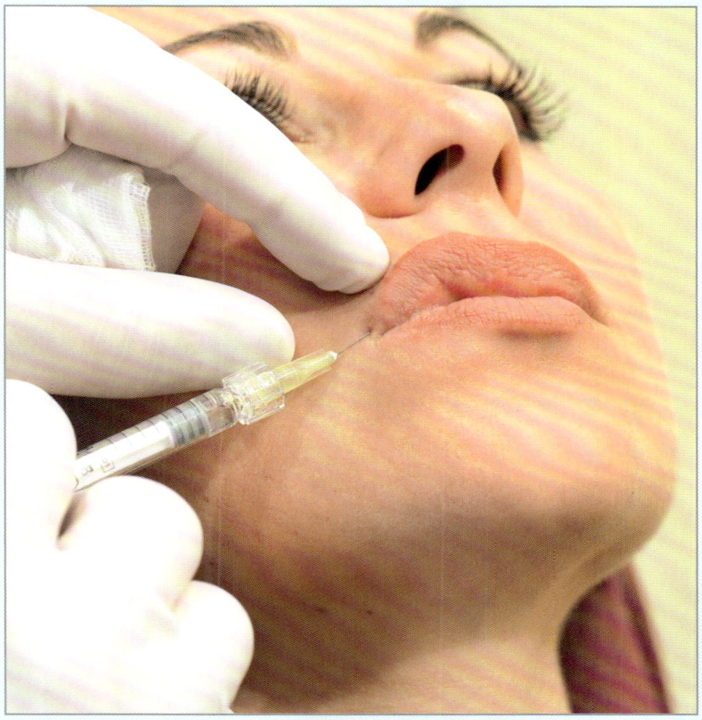

Fig. 7.66 The second injection is placed slightly above the first, to a depth of about 1 mm, advancing the needle 5 mm above and within the subdermal plane above the orbicularis oris muscle. The filler is injected as the needle is being withdrawn. The third injection point is placed slightly below the first one. The direction of injection follows the course of the orbicularis oris muscle, but above the muscle, and the filler is injected as the needle is being withdrawn (see small image, left).

Treatment steps

- History: e.g. recurrent herpes infections (herpes prophylaxis with e.g. aciclovir may be necessary)
- Remove makeup
- Disinfection
- Anaesthesia
- Injection: point technique, linear technique
- Massage and mould (ensure appropriate distribution of the filler)
- Inform patient about post-treatment dos and don'ts
- Arrange a follow-up appointment

Filler selection

2 Medium injection (p. 63)
B Special indications: lips (p. 70)

Combined treatment options

If the mouth corners are affected by excessive facial movements, i.e. by increased activity of the depressor anguli oris muscle, bilateral botulinum toxin type-A injections into this muscle can also be considered.

Complications/Managing complications

- Palpable nodules may form due to the aggregation of the filler used. Thorough massage and moulding of the injected filler directly after the treatment ensures uniform distribution.
- Hyaluronic acid augmentation at the angles of the mouth is prone to the Tyndall effect, and hence care should be taken to ensure appropriate injections are delivered (see p. 103).

Practical tips

- In cases where the droop at the corners of the mouth is pronounced, several augmentation treatments may be required to achieve a satisfactory result.
- Treating the marionette lines simultaneously also enhances the lifting effect of the corners of the mouth, and hence is often recommended as an adjunctive treatment.

Treatment planning – Surface regeneration of the lips
The goal of the treatment is to rehydrate and revitalise the lip surface. Given the absence of sebaceous glands, the skin of the lips is prone to being dry and chapped. Improving the lip surface and hydration by providing new water-binding capacity with hyaluronic acid fillers will achieve softer looking and more youthful lips.

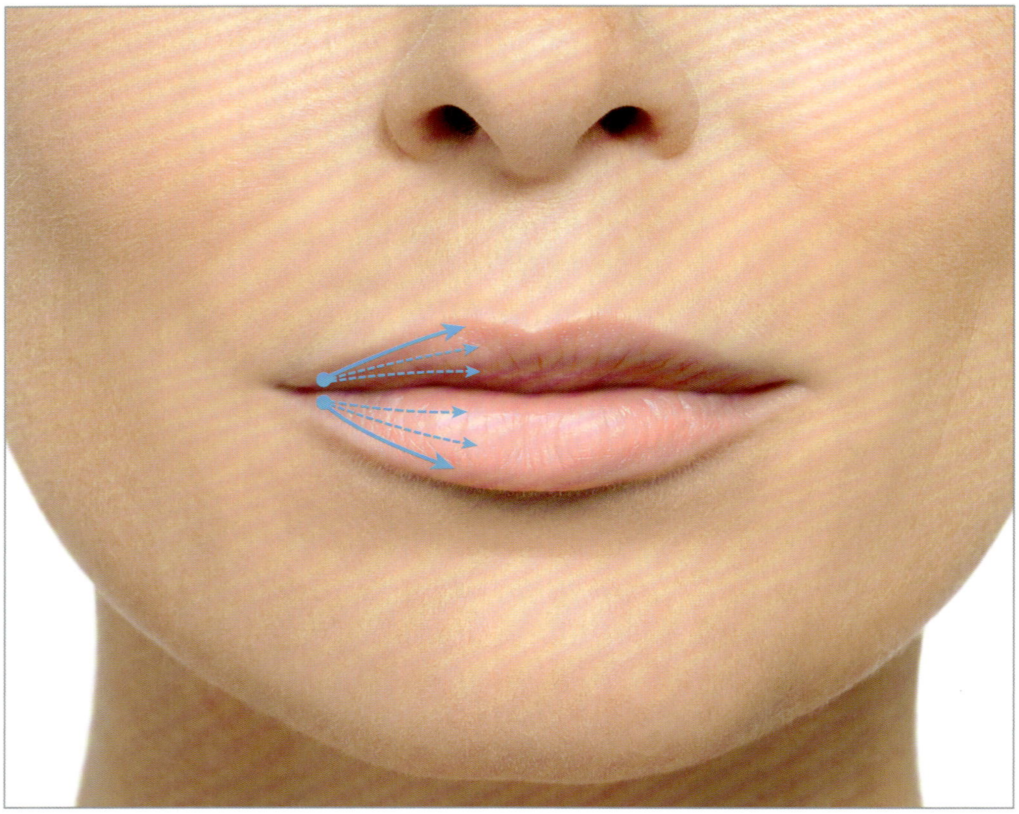

Technique: very superficial SHAC
Injection point: close to the labial angle of each lip quadrant
Injection depth and direction: intradermal or directly subdermal, advancing the needle in a fan-like fashion from lateral to medial

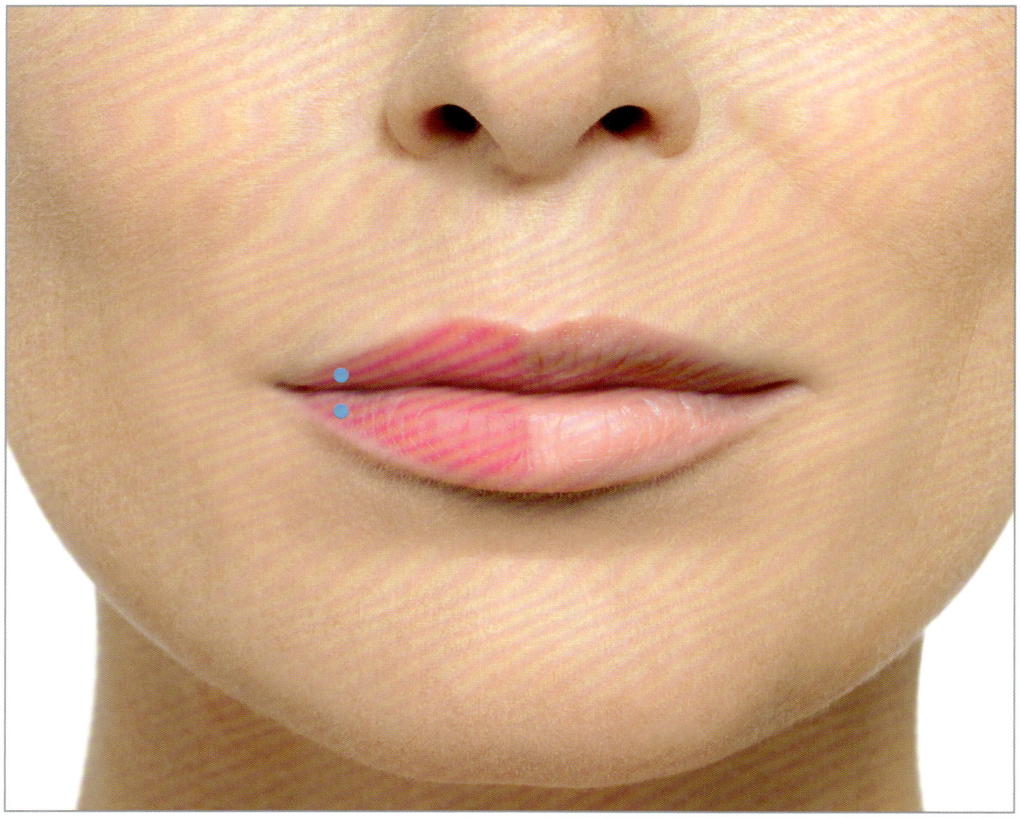

Volume: 0.1–0.2ml / lip quadrant
Tool: 27 gauge cannula

Treatment – Surface regeneration of the lips

SHAC lower lip

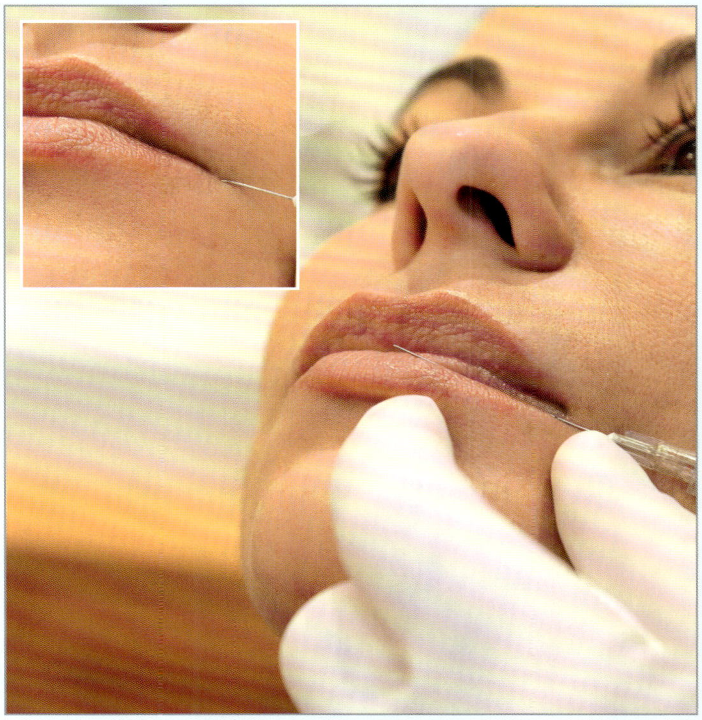

Fig. 7.67 The microcannula is inserted below the thin skin of the lower lip from a lateral point of insertion, close to the mouth corner. Under gentle and smooth mobilisation of the dermal or subdermal layer, the practitioner injects 0.1 to 0.2 ml of the hyaluronic acid filler per lip quadrant.

SHAC upper lip

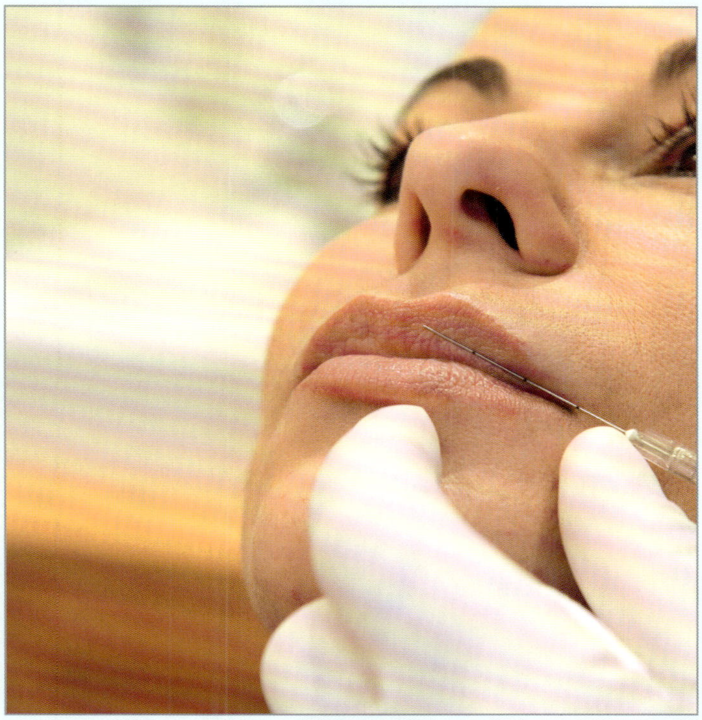

Fig. 7.68 The same procedure is repeated on both halves of the upper lip. The aim of the treatment is to provide a homogenously spread thin layer of a water-binding filler, and to simultaneously stimulate fibrogenetic tissue regeneration through tissue mobilisation.

Treatment steps

- History: e.g. recurrent herpes infections (herpes prophylaxis with e.g. aciclovir may be necessary)
- Remove makeup
- Disinfection
- Anaesthesia
- Injection: SHAC (or multi-injection systems)
- Massage and mould (ensure appropriate distribution of the filler)
- Inform patient about post-treatment dos and don'ts
- Arrange a follow-up appointment

Filler selection

A Special indications: skin surface regeneration (p. 69)
B Special indications: lips (p. 70)

Combined treatment options

Topical cosmetic preparations

Complications/Managing complications

Palpable nodules may form due to the aggregation of the filler used. Thorough massage and moulding of the injected filler directly after the treatment ensures uniform distribution.

Practical tips

- The SHAC offers an ideal treatment approach for lip surface regeneration, as it enables a painless and homogenous augmentation along with fluid-dependent and fibrogenetic tissue regeneration.
- Alternatively, multi-injection systems can be used for skin regeneration or mesotherapy of the lips with hyaluronic acid fillers.
- Pain control is an important aspect to consider when treating lips, and particularly when injecting with needles. Anaesthesia (see section 6.8, p. 99) will need to be considered in most cases.

⚠ Prior to injecting any filler, please refer to the latest manufacturer guidelines for specific instructions for use.

7.5.3 Marionette lines

Marionette lines arise from the angles of the mouth and continue down towards the chin. Prominent marionette lines give the face a frustrated, disappointed and a dissatisfied expression. Drooping mouth corners alongside marionettes are one of the most powerful negative messages communicated by the face, second only to the frown lines in the glabella. The key factors associated with the intensity of these lines include the atrophy-related shrinkage of the soft tissue base, alongside the adherent depressor muscles (depressor anguli oris and depressor labii inferiors) anchoring at the base and thus pulling the skin downwards.

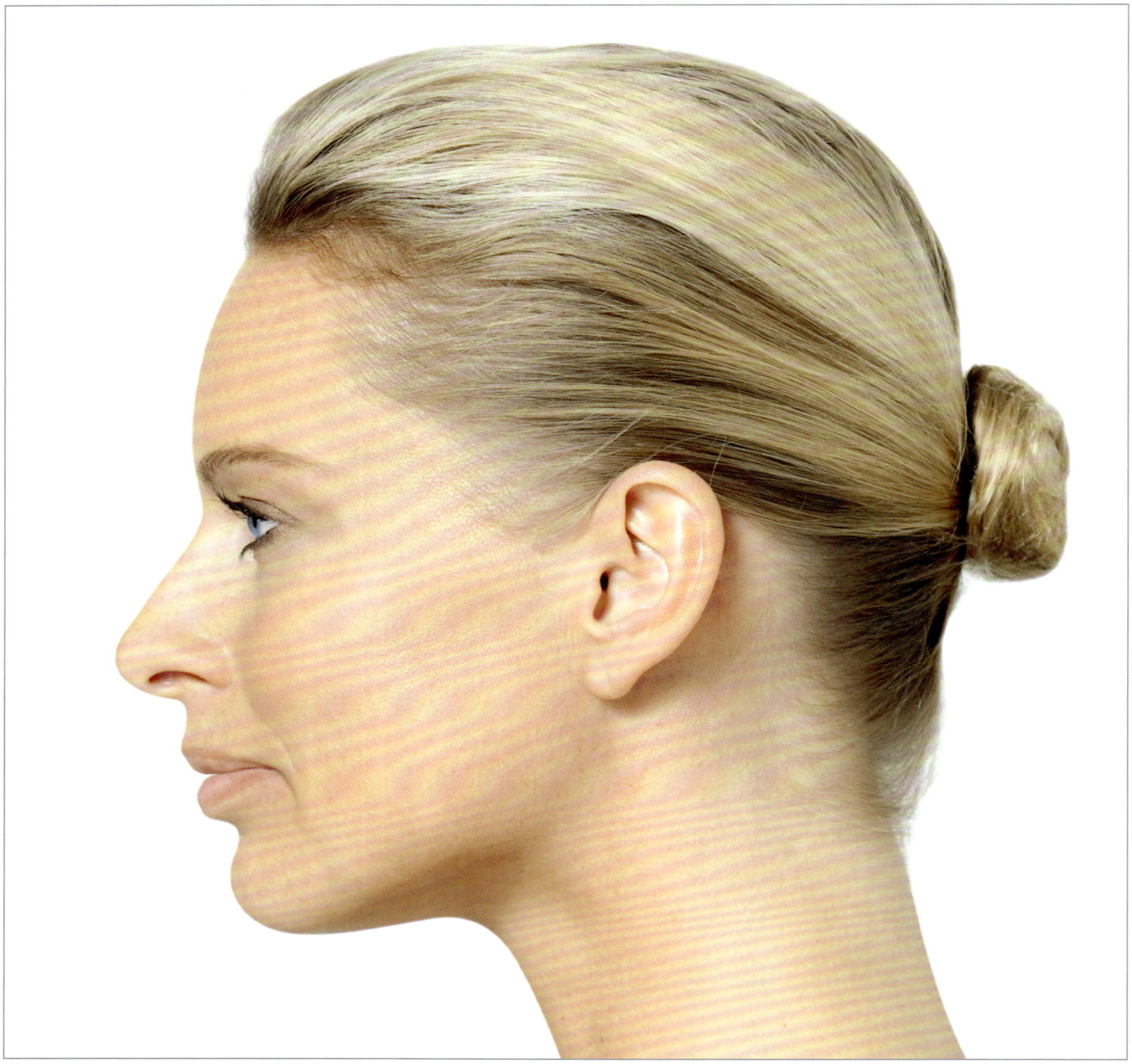

Patient selection
Patients who present with subcutaneous tissues showing age-related laxity and involutional changes can benefit from augmentation with hyaluronic acid fillers. In contrast, patients who produce or intensify these lines dynamically and voluntarily benefit from botulinum toxin type-A treatment. However, in many cases both treatments can be used to achieve an optimal clinical outcome.

Anatomy

The perioral muscles are built up into several layers. The depressor anguli oris muscle (1) is the most superficial muscle in the chin region. When it contracts, this muscle together with the platysma pulls down the angles of the mouth, giving the face a frustrated, disappointed and dissatisfied expression. Below the depressor anguli oris muscle lies the depressor labii inferioris muscle (2), which directly connects with the mucosa. Following atrophy of the soft tissue base, it is possible that these muscles have a stronger retracting effect on the skin. This leads, together with hyperactivity of the muscles, to deepening of the marionette lines. Anatomical release of the muscles via supramucosal cannula mobilisation can reduce the severity of these lines.

Close to the mouth corners, a fibrous structure called the modiolus (3) forms an actinoid connection with numerous perioral muscles. Using this structure as the insertion point for the cannula enables it to reach the supramucosal mobilisation plane below the muscles.

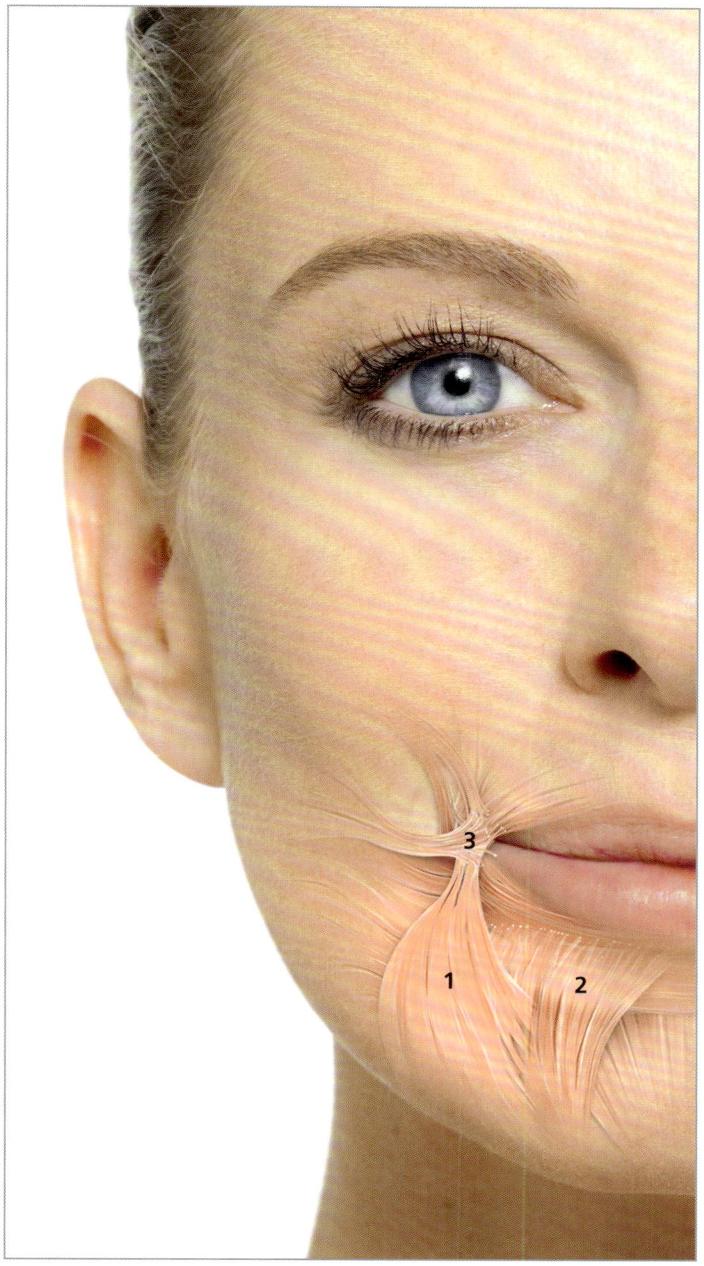

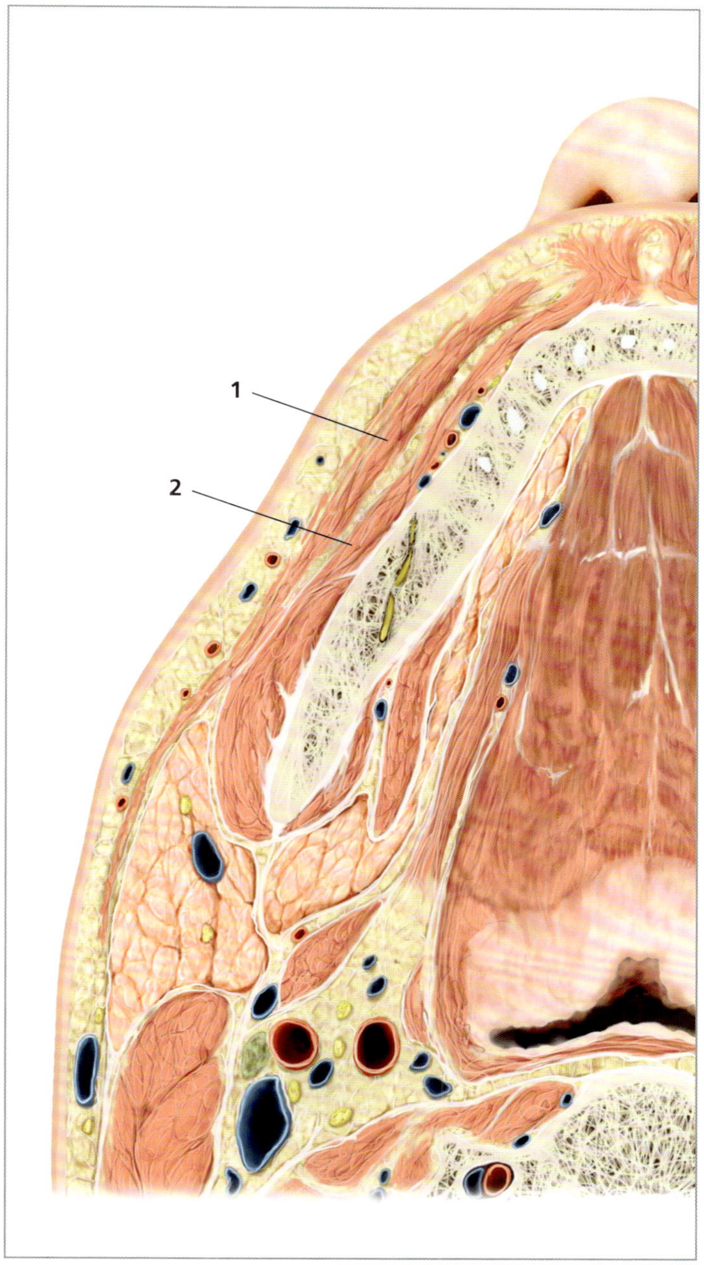

Depressor anguli oris muscle

Origin	Insertion	Function	Synergists	Antagonists	Innervation
Lower edge of the mandible, inferior to the mental foramen	Angle of the mouth (modiolus)	Pulls the corner of the mouth downwards	• Platysma • Depressor labii inferioris muscle	• Zygomaticus major muscle • Levator anguli oris muscle	Marginal mandibular branch of the facial nerve (cranial nerve VII)

Treatment planning – Marionette lines
The aim of the treatment is to achieve a harmonious and causal correction of the marionette lines. This can be best achieved by using cannulas for deep horizontal tissue mobilisation and augmentation techniques below the muscles. If the result is not sufficient, the marionette lines can also be elevated with vertical supramucosal depot injections using needles.

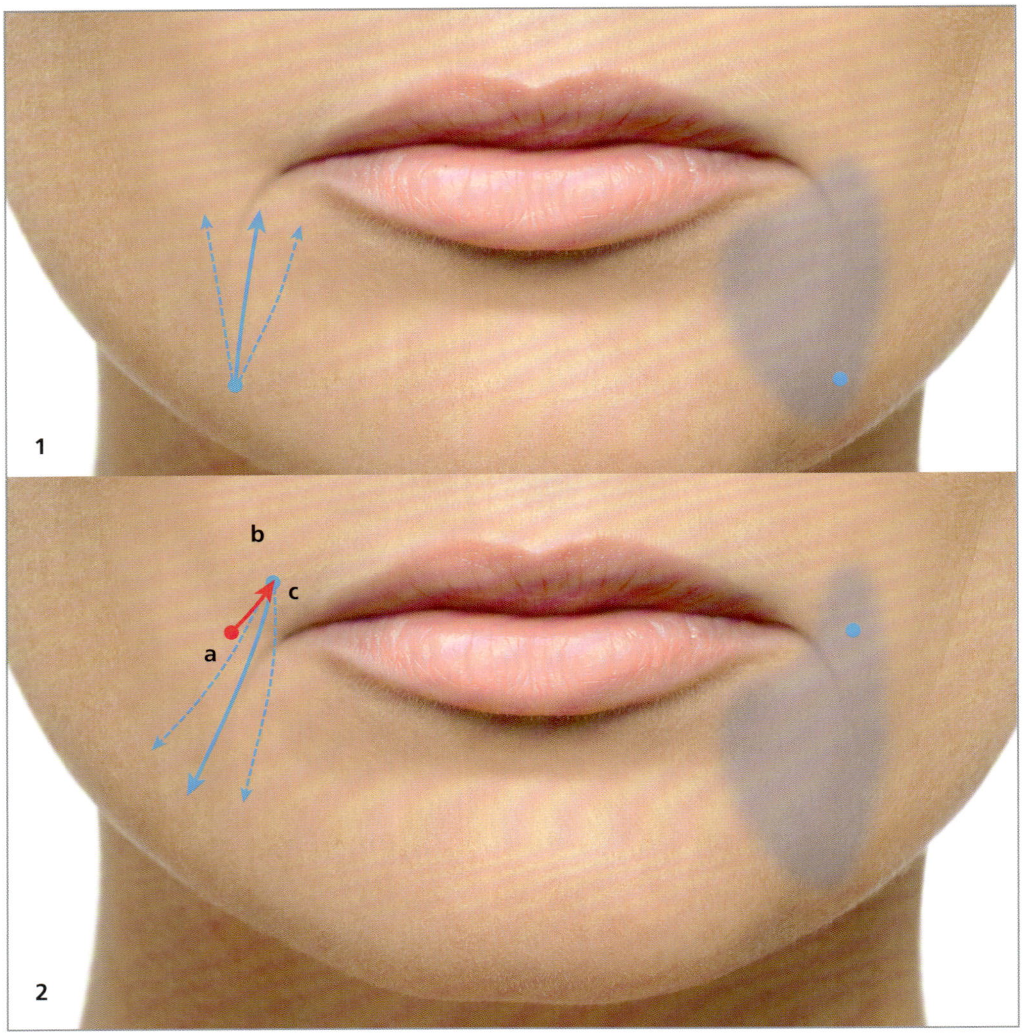

Technique: DHAC
Insertion sites: (1) • Caudal endpoint of the marionette line on the chin or (2) • above the modiolus (thick connective tissue zone)
Injection depth and direction: Supramucosal tissue mobilisation (1) injecting the filler in a fanning technique from the chin in the direction towards the mouth corner, or alternatively (2) (**a**) a short length of the cannula is insersted deep into the supramucosal plane, in the direction of the nasolabial fold (diagonal direction, see red arrow). The forefinger of the non-injecting hand is placed intraorally to help monitor the cannula to ensure it is within the supramucosal plane. Importantly, the cannula is only inserted a short distance, and no filler is deposited at this stage unless treating the nasolabial fold also is desired. (**b**) The cannula is now rotated in a 170 degrees in an anti-clockwise direction while still in the supramucosal plane and under the guidance of the intraorally placed forefinger of the non-injecting hand. Finally, the filler is injected in a fanning fashion while mobilising the cannula in the supramucosal plane (see blue arrow) (**c**).
Volume: 0.2–0.3 ml/side
Tool: 22 gauge cannula

Video: Marionette lines DHAC 2
http://www.kvm-tv.de/FIL/019.mp4

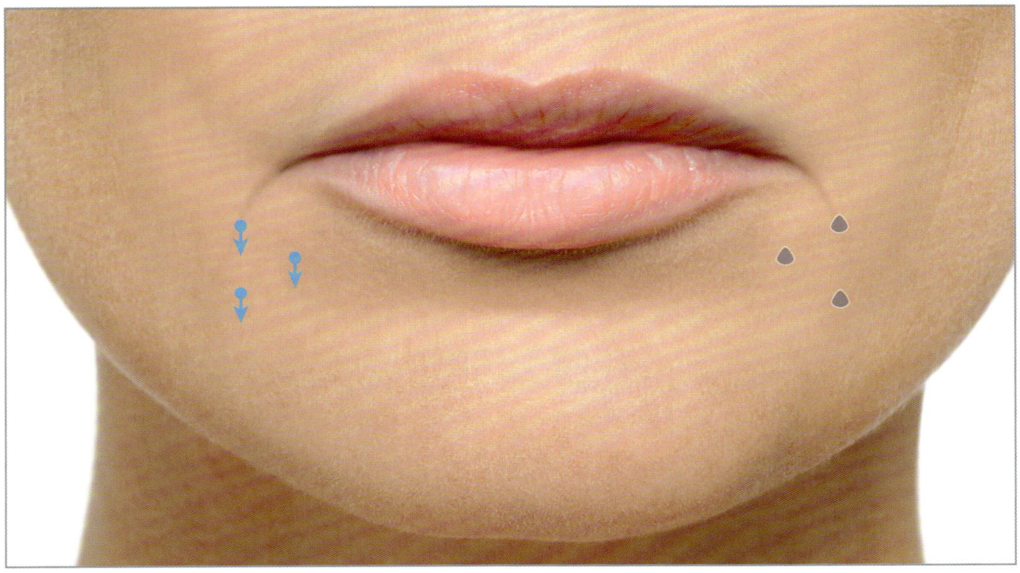

Technique: VSDT
Injection points: • depending on individual findings, two to three 'hot spots' along and medial to the marionette line
Volume: 0.05–0.1 ml/injection point

Video: Marionette lines VSDT
http://www.kvm-tv.de/FIL/020.mp4

Treatment – Marionette lines

DHAC

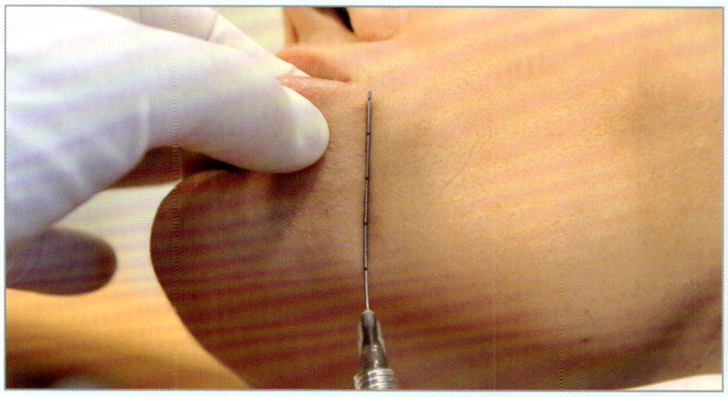

Fig. 7.69 The cannula is inserted and brought into the supramucosal plane below the perioral muscles. This can be done by starting from the inferior aspect of the marionette (as shown), advancing the cannula with gentle, mobilising movements to the superior portion close to the corners of the mouth. In doing so, the muscles are anatomically released and the retraction forces acting on the skin that deepen the line are reduced. Along with the mechanical mobilisation technique, the practitioner injects 0.2 to 0.3 ml of the water-binding hyaluronic acid filler into the supramucosal anchoring layer. This technique enables a harmonious and natural augmentation of the marionette lines. It is possible to use a finger of the non-injecting hand as a counter bearing during the supramucosal mobilisation and injection.

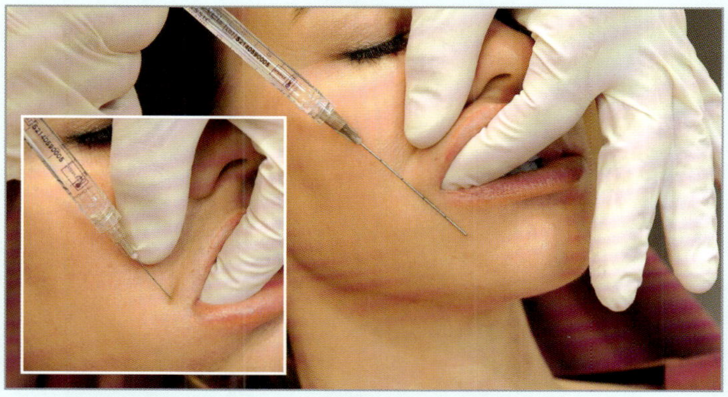

Fig. 7.70 Alternatively, the cannula can be inserted directly above the modiolus. This technique aims at reaching the supramucosal, submuscular plane, without getting the cannula embedded within the modiolus (thick connective tissue zone). To do so, an insertion point for the cannula is made with an introducer needle directly above the modiolus. A short length of the cannula is then inserted deep into the supramucosal plane, in the direction of the nasolabial fold. The forefinger of the non-injecting hand is placed intraorally to help monitor the cannula to ensure it is within the supramucosal plane. The cannula is now rotated in a 170 degrees in an anti-clockwise direction while still in the supramucosal plane and under the guidance of the intraorally placed forefinger of the non-injecting hand. Finally, the filler is injected in a fanning fashion while mobilising the cannula in the supramucosal plane to treat the marionette line.

Treatment steps

- History: e.g. recurrent herpes infections (herpes prophylaxis with e.g. aciclovir may be necessary)
- Remove makeup
- Disinfection
- Anaesthesia
- Injection: DHAC, possibly with VSDT
- Massage and mould (ensure appropriate distribution of the filler)
- Inform patient about post-treatment dos and don'ts
- Arrange a follow-up appointment

Filler selection

2 Medium injection (p. 63)
3 Deep injection (p. 66)
4 Ultra-deep injection (p. 67)

Combined treatment options

Superficial, very fine lines can be additionally treated with:

- Microdermabrasion
- Dermabrasion
- Chemical peeling
- Laser resurfacing
- Medical needling

Deeper lines can additionally be treated with:

- Botulinum toxin type-A
- Autologous fat augmentation (as an alternative or additionally after some weeks)

Complications/Managing complications

Palpable nodules may form due to the aggregation of the filler used. Thorough massage and moulding of the injected filler directly after the treatment ensures uniform distribution.

Practical tips

- Marionette lines are a significant facial ageing feature that benefit considerably from filler augmentation. Blunt tissue mobilisation in combination with the VSDT is a useful method for significantly reducing deep marionette lines. However, several treatments are often required to achieve optimal results, and hence patients should be made aware of this from the outset.
- The cannula technique allows for the mechanical tissue release and fibrogenetic regeneration along with immediate augmentation, and hence is an ideal tool for this indication.
- It is easy to penetrate into the supramucosal anchoring layer by inserting the cannula from the fibrous modiolus, and perhaps even more so than trying to reach it from the inferior aspect of the marionette line.
- Forming a mechanical counter bearing for the mobilisation and injection using a finger of the non-injecting hand can facilitate the treatment.
- Superficial, fine lines can be injected using the stretching or compression technique.

7.5.4 Chin and jawline

A well projected, smooth and volumised chin is often taken for granted, and yet is a key feature of a rejuvenated and a harmonious face. With ageing, progressive tissue atrophy leads to volume loss and regression of the mental nerve and the mandibular base. As a result, irregularities in the chin relief and the contour of the jawline become visible. These irregularities, seen as depressions and swellings, particularly emerge where the retaining ligaments connect the base with the skin and as a result retract it. It is now accepted that the sagging seen in the jawline is attributed to the atrophy-related shrinkage of the surrounding soft tissues, rather than the previously assumed simple descent and drooping of the soft tissues.

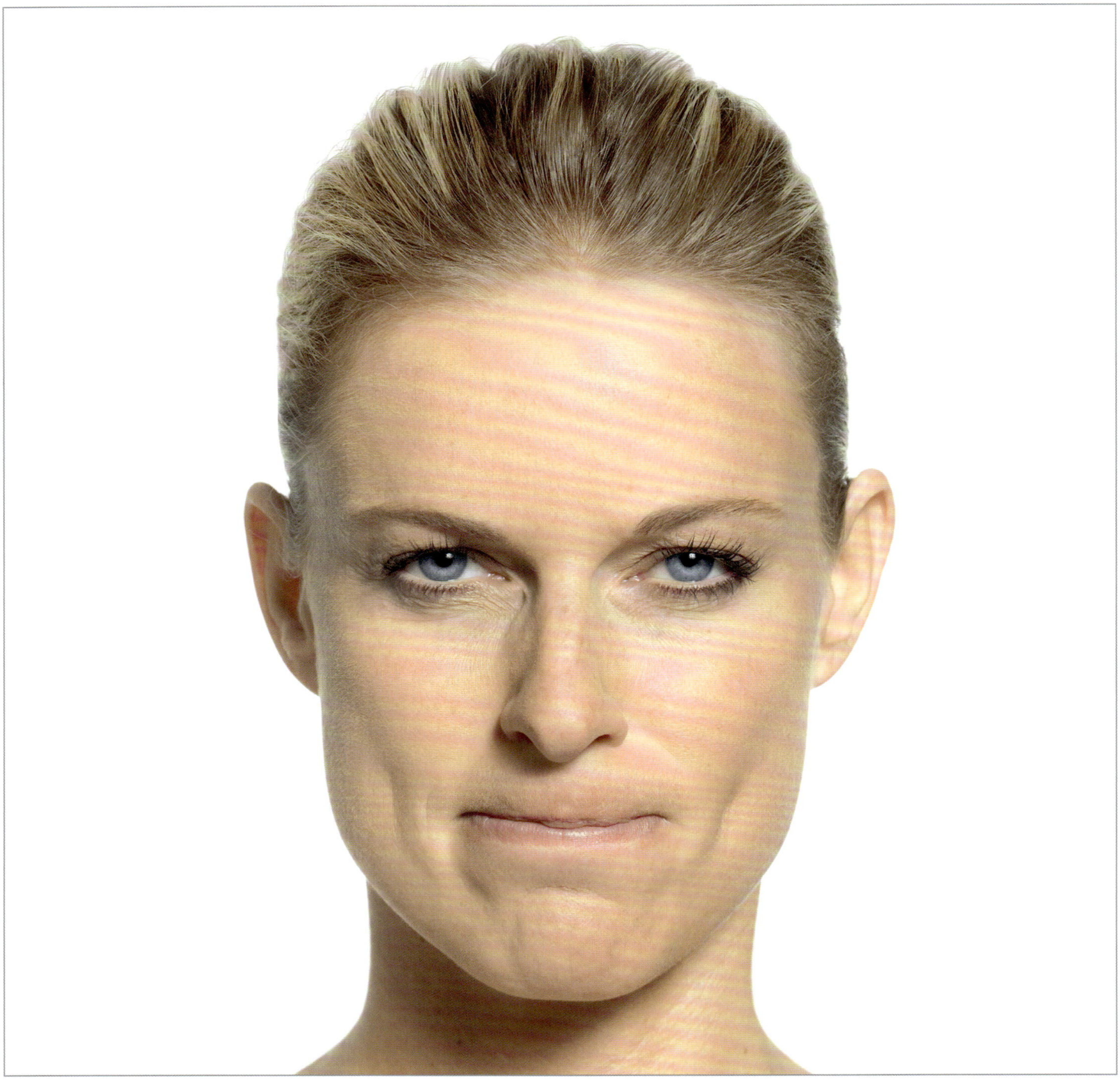

Patient selection/Assessing the indication
Volume augmentation in this region should be seen as the key and foremost treatment option to harmonise the age-related changes. In many cases, botulinum toxin type-A treatments may no longer be required after filler augmentation. Furthermore, by volumising the chin complex, the marionette lines also improve.

Anatomy

The mental complex is influenced by the actions of the perioral depressor muscles: ([1] depressor anguli oris, [2] depressor labii inferioris) and [3] mentalis muscle. Contraction of the mentalis muscle in combination with the anchoring system of the ligament leads to an uneven, irregular, and a cobblestone-like wrinkling on the skin surface of the chin.

The significance of the retaining ligaments needs to be particularly highlighted when considering chin anatomy, alongside the associated age-related changes. Mental, submental and mandibular ligaments provide the static retaining elements of the lower part of the face. Over areas where the soft tissue base is atrophied, the skin is more retracted by the ligaments than in younger individuals. Depressions on the surface of the skin are the consequence of this, and are initially seen as shadows and later progress to surface irregularities and relative swellings, i.e. the sagging between the mandibular and the mandibular–platysmal ligaments on the jawline.

> Around the sites where the ligamentous attachments connect to the skin, with ageing and progressive fat atrophy, the skin begins to sag. The bone also becomes palpable where the fat has atrophied. Harmonisation of the chin and jawline contours can be achieved by focal volume-compensating injections at the sites where the ligaments are located.

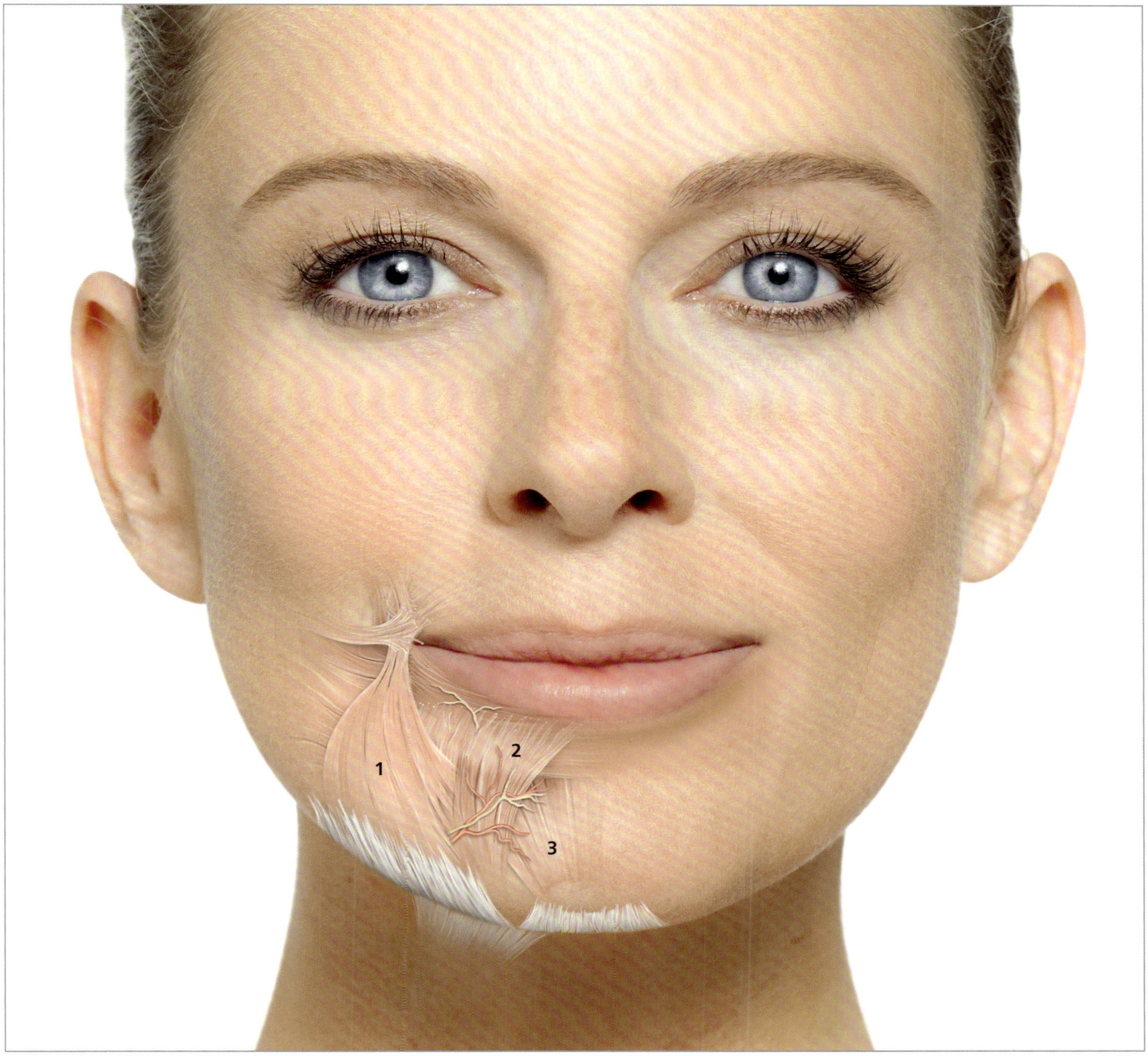

Treatment planning – Chin contouring

The aim of the treatment is to volumise, recontour the chin back to its more youthful state and improve the surface by compensating for the atrophy-related deficits at the soft tissue anchoring base. In some cases, however, the aim is to augment a chin that has been always retracted, and hence restructure the anatomical position completely.

This treatment also creates a globally rejuvenating oval shape to the face, as well as improving the adjacent marionette lines.

The vertical depot injections aim at refilling the base of the skin-retracting mental and submental ligaments. It is important to manage all the ligaments involved.

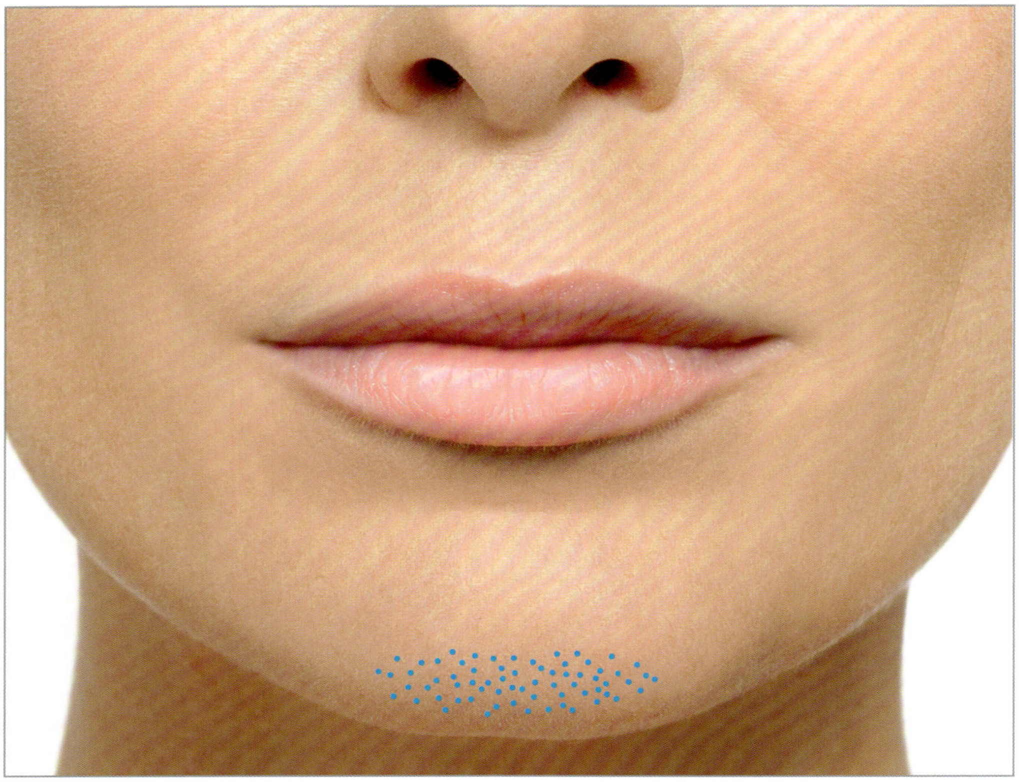

Technique: point technique with compression, suitable for superficial defects in the contour of the chin
Injection points: serial point injections at the site of the deficit
Volume: minimal amount < 0.05 ml/injection point
Tool: 30 gauge needle

Video: Chin superficial injections http://www.kvm-tv.de/FIL/021.mp4

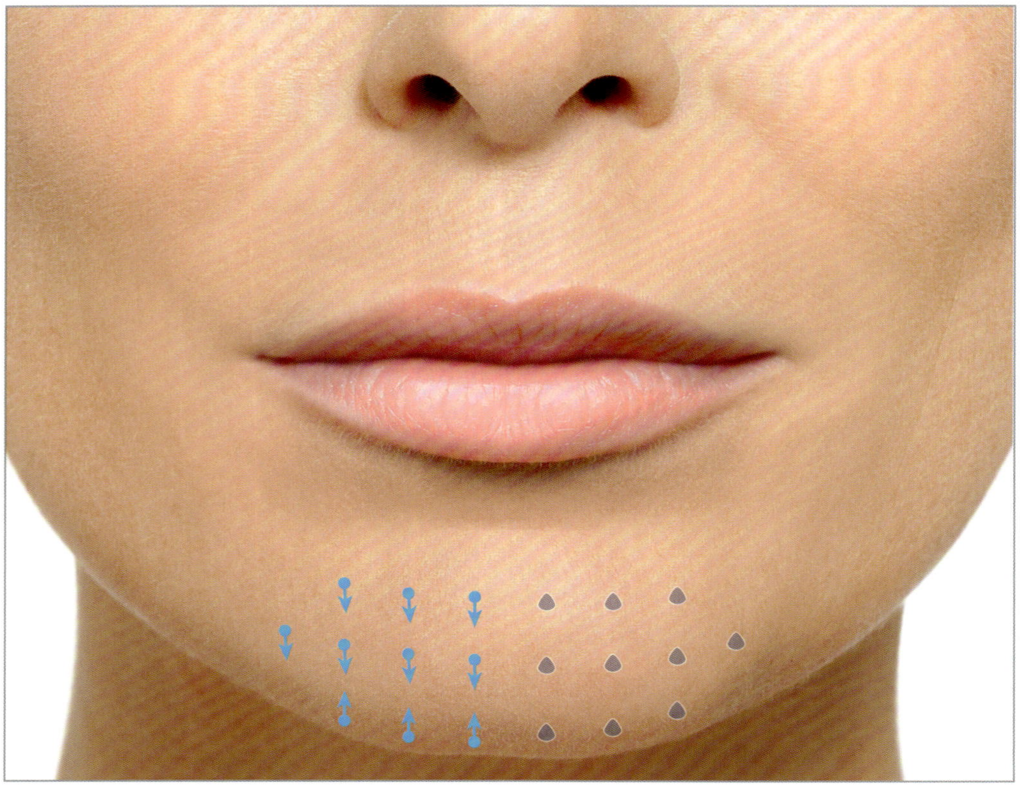

Technique: VSDT
Injection points: depending on individual requirements, into the 'hot spots' of the involved mandibular and submandibular ligaments
Volume: 0.05–0.1 ml/injection point
Tool: 27 gauge needle

Video: Chin VSDT http://www.kvm-tv.de/FIL/022.mp4

Treatment – Chin contouring

Point technique

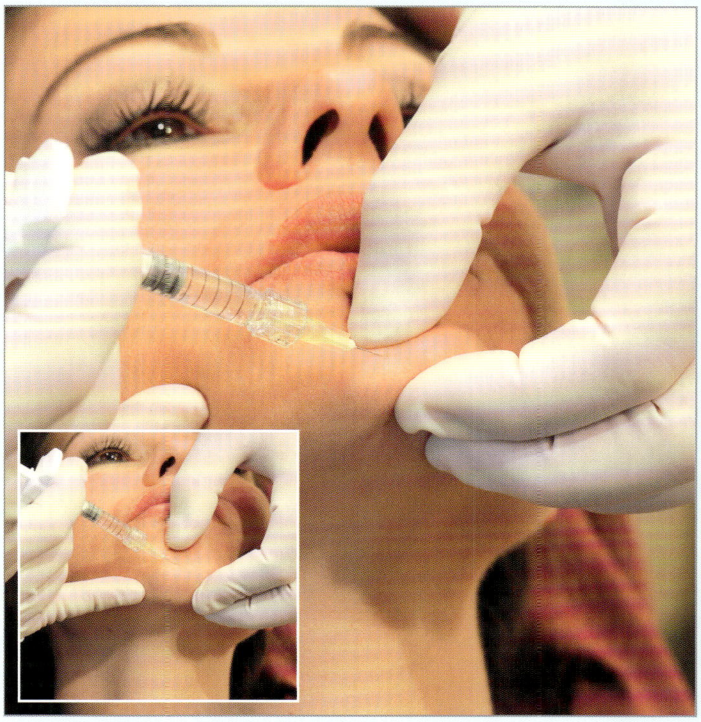

Fig. 7.71 The injections are given using the serial point technique. The needle is inserted at a 45-degree angle and the injection is given superficially, assisted by compression or stretching (see small image).

VSDT

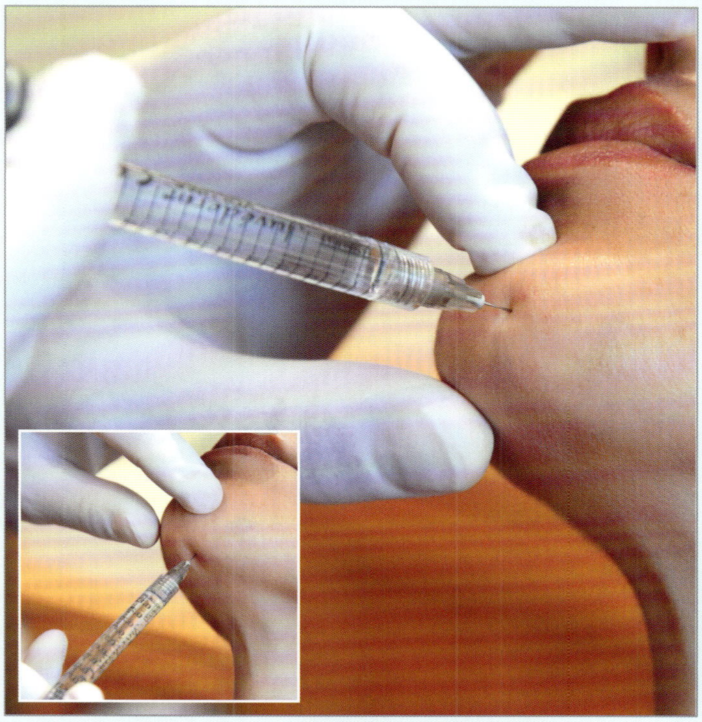

Fig. 7.72 The practitioner delivers tangential depots into the 'hot spots' of the mental ligaments in order to compensate for the causal-atrophy. Depending on individual findings, the submandibular ligaments are injected with vertical injections (see small picture).

Treatment steps

- Remove makeup
- Disinfection
- Anaesthesia (optional)
- Injection: serial point technique, superficially/vertical depots for contouring
- Massage and mould (ensure appropriate distribution of the filler)
- Inform patient about post-treatment dos and don'ts
- Arrange a follow-up appointment

Filler selection

Superficial lines:

1 Superficial injection (p. 62)

2 Medium injection (p. 63)

Deeply retracted chin:

3 Deep injection (p. 66)

4 Ultra-deep injection (p. 67)

Combined treatment options

- In patients presenting with an overactive mentalis muscle: botulinum toxin type-A
- In cases of elastosis/sun damage: chemical peeling; laser resurfacing; medical needling

Complications/Managing complications

Palpable nodules may form due to the aggregation of the filler used. Thorough massage and moulding of the injected filler directly after the treatment ensures uniform distribution.

Practical tips

- Compensating the soft tissue atrophy with vertical depot injections into the ligaments sometimes eliminates the need for further treatment with botulinum toxin type-A .
- Augmentation achieving anterior projection of the chin allows to correct the ageing in this region.

⚠ Prior to injecting any filler, please refer to the latest manufacturer guidelines for specific instructions for use.

Treatment Planning – Jawline

The aim of the treatment is to harmonise the jawline contour, and mask some of the jowling and sagging. The main target structures are the mandibular and mandibular–platysmal ligaments, which exert their forces onto the skin, causing it to retract. By restoring the fatty tissue in which the ligaments are embedded, the soft tissue envelope can be naturally enhanced and the surface irregularities minimised. Besides vertical injections into the 'hot spots' (i.e. referring to the sites of the deepest skin retractions of the ligaments), horizontal mobilising treatments using cannulas are also viable here.

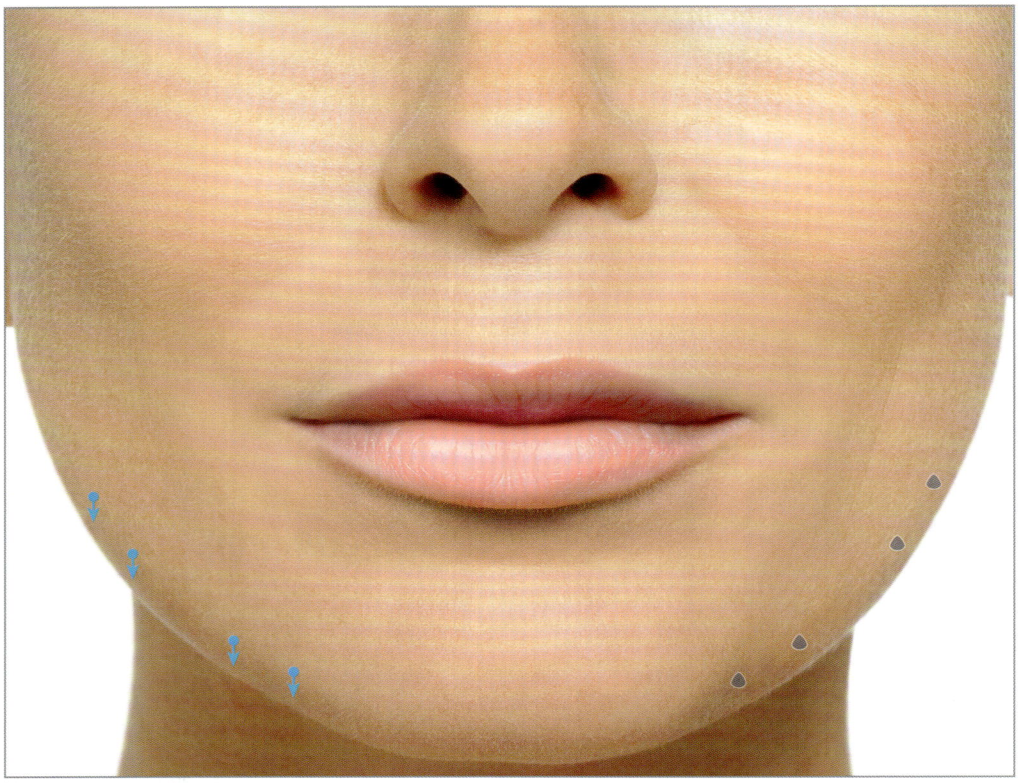

Technique: VSDT
Injection points: into the 'hot spots' of the mandibular and mandibular–platysmal ligaments (causing the relative sagging)
Volume: 0.05–0.1 ml/injection point
Tool: 27 gauge needle

Video: Jawline VSDT http://www.kvm-tv.de/FIL/023.mp4

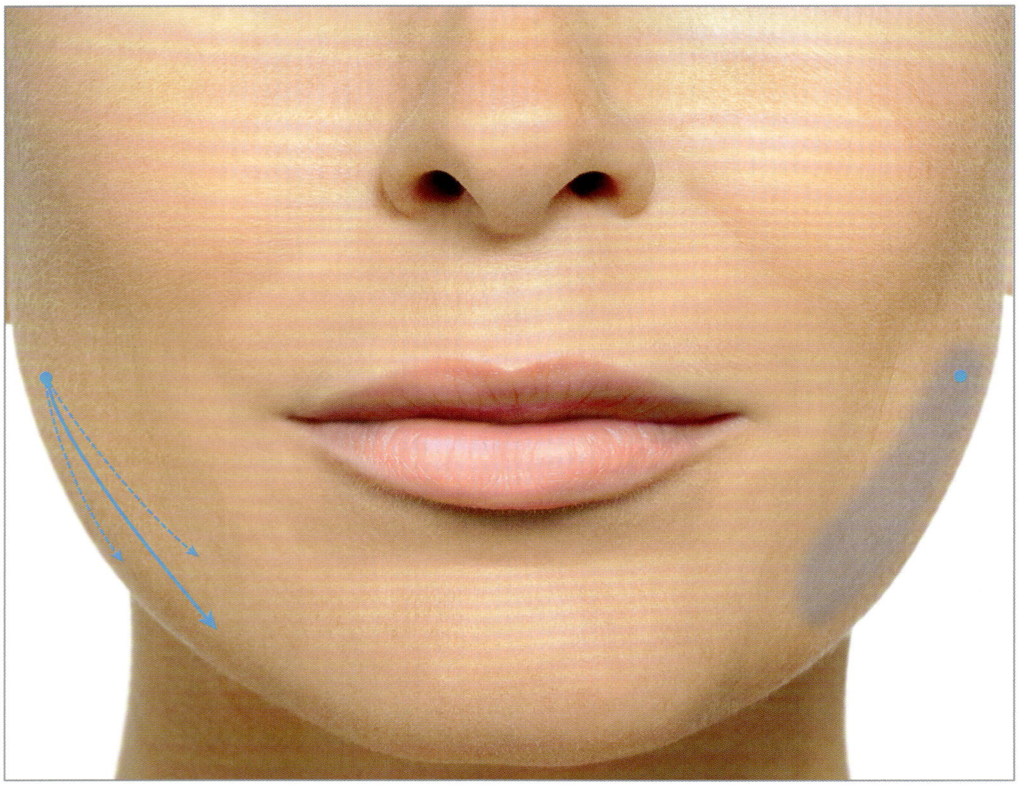

Technique: DHAC
Insertion site: auricular border of the mandible
Injection depth and direction: subcutaneous, direction of the injections is towards the chin
Volume: 0.1 ml/side
Tool: 22–25 gauge cannula

Video: Jawline and inferior cheek HAC http://www.kvm-tv.de/FIL/024.mp4

7

Treatment – Jawline

VSDT

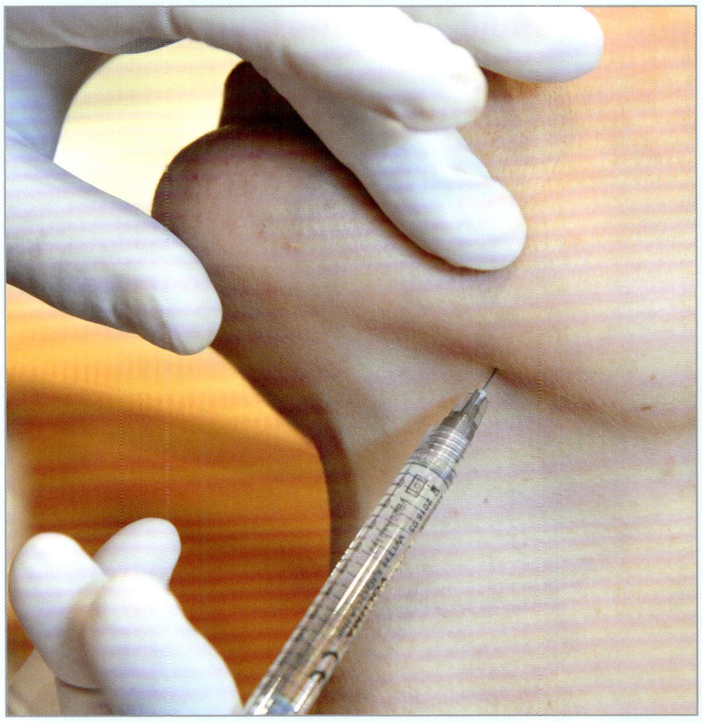

Fig. 7.73 The injection is given vertically down onto the supraperiosteal base of the mandibular ligaments. The injected volume is between 0.05 and 0.1 ml per 'hot spot'. Where the focal lifting has been achieved, the mandibular soft tissue envelope will reach its original level, resulting in harmonisation of the jawline contour.

DHAC

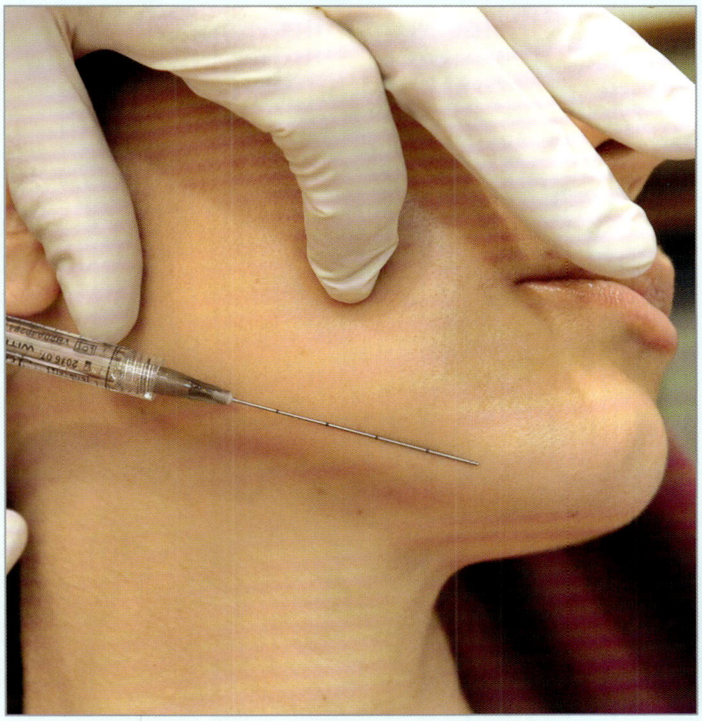

Fig. 7.74 To achieve mechanical release of the ligaments, and a more global, harmonised augmentation, a cannula is the ideal tool within the supraperiosteal soft tissue plane. The injection is made from the lateral aspect of the jawline towards the chin, advancing the cannula back and forth while mobilising the tissues gently. Approximately 0.1 ml of the filler is injected per thread.

Treatment steps
- Remove makeup
- Disinfection
- Anaesthesia (optional)
- Injection: VSDT/DHAC
- Massage and mould (ensure appropriate distribution of the filler)
- Inform patient about post-treatment dos and don'ts
- Arrange a follow-up appointment

Filler selection

3 Deep injection (p. 66)

4 Ultra-deep injection (p. 67)

Combined treatment options

In cases of elastosis/sun damage: chemical peeling; laser resurfacing; medical needling

Complications/Managing complications

Palpable nodules may form due to the aggregation of the filler used. Thorough massage and moulding of the injected filler directly after the treatment ensures uniform distribution.

Practical tips
- With vertical lifting of the atrophied mandibular base, deep depressions and irregularities along the jawline, including some of the visible sagging, can be satisfactorily improved.
- Horizontal augmentation techniques using cannulas have the advantage of activating fibrogenetic tissue regeneration along with the instant visible augmentation. However, the lifting effect is perhaps less significant with cannulas.
- Anaesthesia is advisable given the sensitivity of the perioral region.

⚠ Prior to injecting any filler, please refer to the latest manufacturer guidelines for specific instructions for use.

7.6 Special Indications

7.6.1 Neck and décolleté

In the neck region, the elastotic skin changes that occur with progressive ageing become apparent and manifest as a loss of resilience alongside the onset of fine, horizontal wrinkling. These findings are intensified by the atrophy-related regression of the volumising soft tissue base of the neck and the décolletage. Furthermore, age-related changes of the platysma manifest in the form of vertical platysmal cords or bands. They stand out prominently when the muscles of facial expression are used, i.e. when speaking, and may impair a person's overall aesthetic appearance.

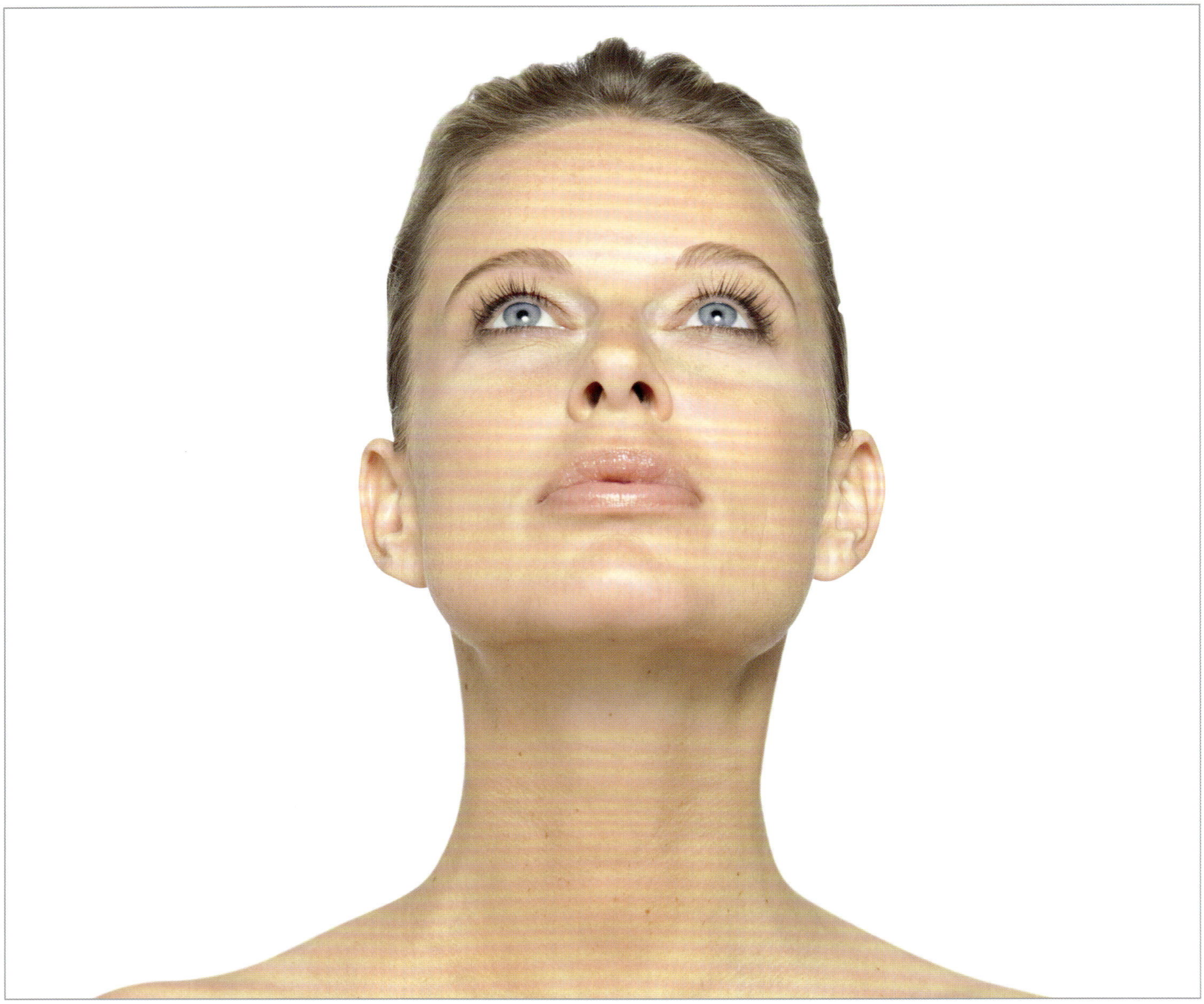

Patient selection
During the consultation and examination process, it is important to note any previous non-surgical and surgical treatments carried out in this region.

The extent of the fine horizontal lines as well as the atrophy-related skin laxity should be assessed to determine the extent of improvement that can be achieved with filler augmentation. Presence of severe elastotic changes can be further addressed with skin surface regenerating methods using hyaluronic acid injections, medical needling, chemical peeling or laser resurfacing modalities, in addition to filler augmentation.

Platysmal cords or bands are better treated with chemical denervation using botulinum toxin type-A.

Assessing the indication
To achieve optimal, long-term results, treatment of the neck region generally requires a multi-modal approach.

Anatomy

The platysma is a large and flat muscle, extending down to the décolletage region. When contracted voluntarily, it can tighten the skin of the anterior aspect of the neck from the lower jaw to below the clavicles. When this happens, its individual muscle cords or bands often become visible.

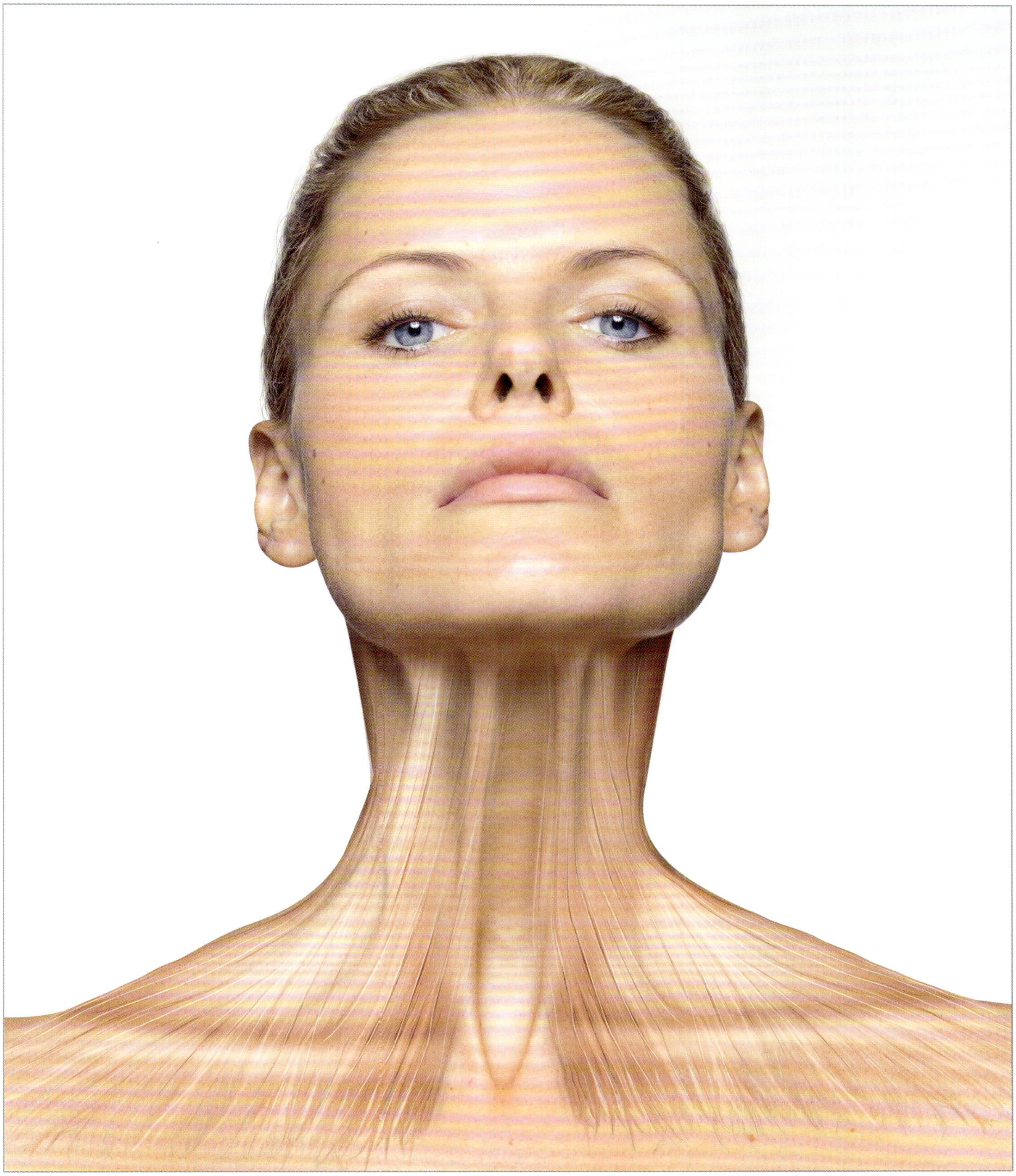

Treatment planning – Horizontal neck lines

The aim of the treatment is to smooth the fine, horizontal lines on the neck. The treatment can be accomplished by either: superficial intradermal injections; immediately subdermal linear injections; or by deeper subcutaneous, supramuscular volume compensation at the sites of the horizontal lines. It is important that only the smallest possible volumes of the filler are injected below the thin skin, and accompanied by mechanical stretching of the skin, in order to achieve natural clinical results.

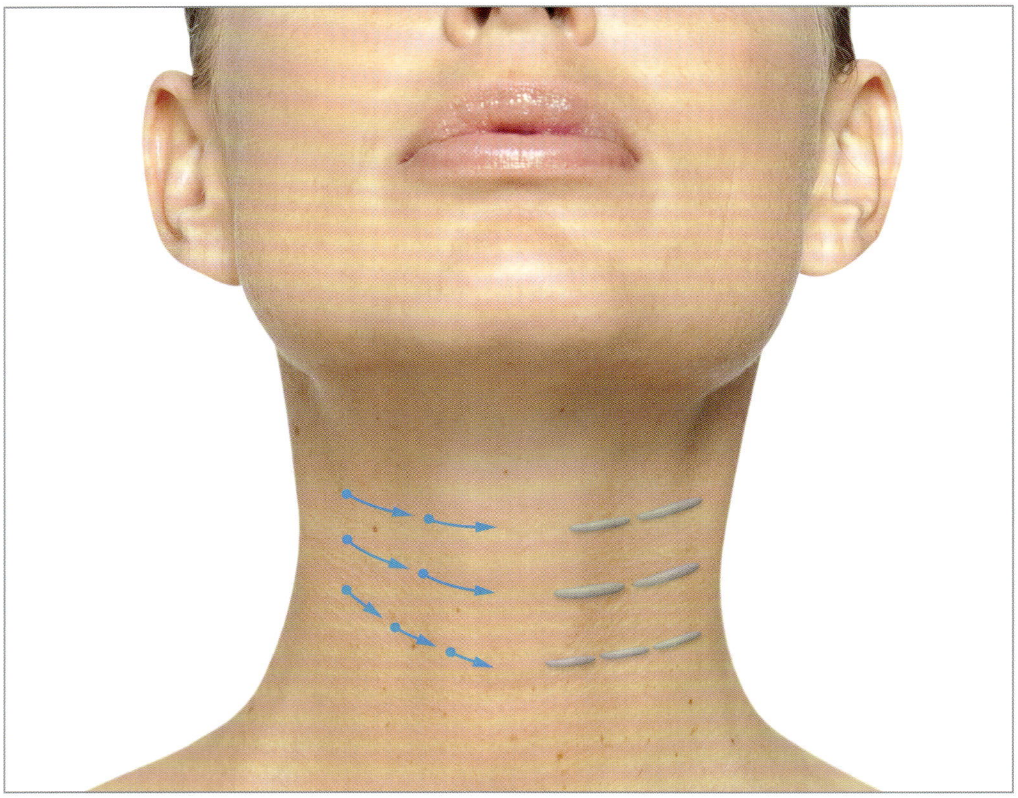

Technique: superficial linear technique alongside skin stretching
Injection points: two to three injections/line, or as required
Injection depth and direction: superficial (intradermal or immediately subdermal). Insert the needle in a tangential direction to the skin surface from lateral to medial, injecting the filler as the needle is withdrawn
Volume: 0.05 ml/thread
Tool: 30–32 gauge needle

Video: Neck lines tunneling http://www.kvm-tv.de/FIL/025.mp4

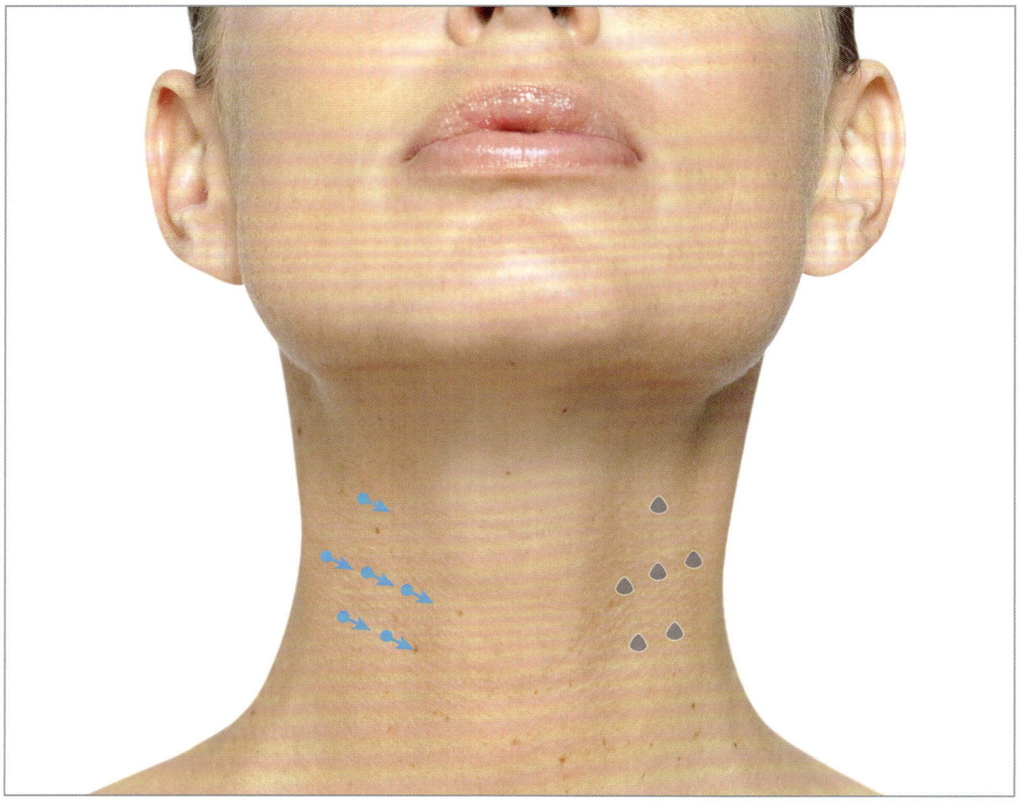

Technique: deep linear technique with skin stretching
Injection points: two to three thread/line, or as required
Injection depth and direction: supramuscular, from lateral to medial along the horizontal lines
Volume: 0.01–0.03 ml/thread
Tool: 27–30 gauge needle

Video: Neck lines deep http://www.kvm-tv.de/FIL/026.mp4

7

Treatment – Horizontal neck lines

Stretching

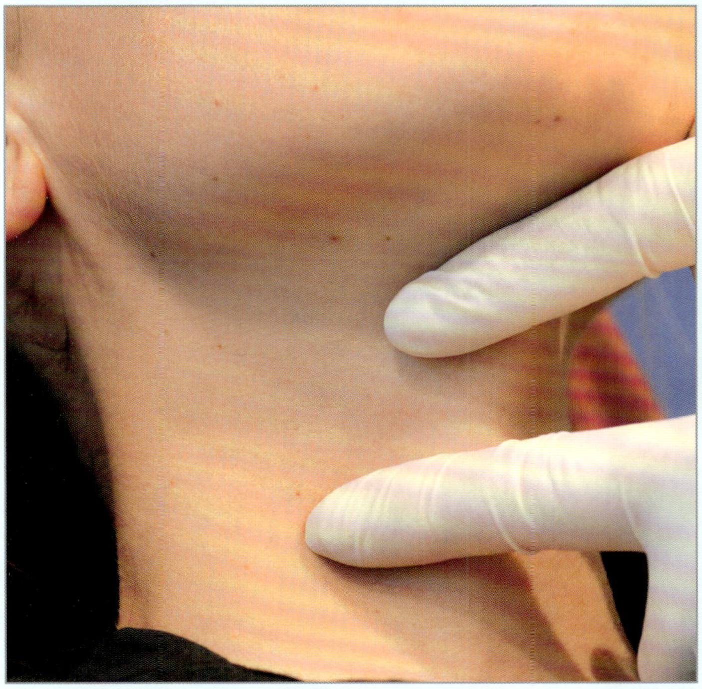

Fig. 7.75 It can be beneficial to have an assistant manage the continuous stretching of the skin during treatment. The assistant tightens the skin gently so that the lines remain only just visible, while the skin is held in place.

Linear technique

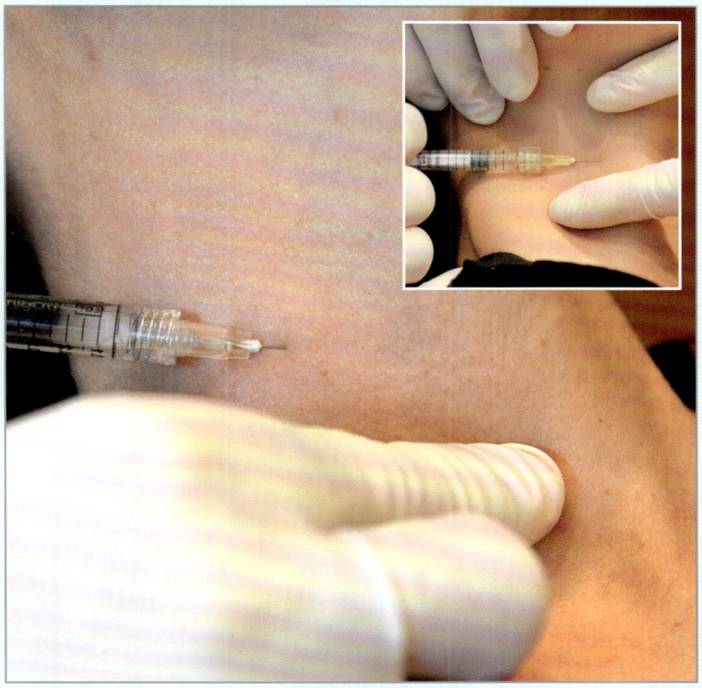

Fig. 7.76 The needle is inserted superficially from the lateral side, following the course of the line. It can be brought into the dermal or subdermal plane for superficial correction (see small image) or into the subcutaneous tissue above the muscle (see large image) where the retaining ligaments (between the skin and the muscle) are located. The filler is injected as the needle is being withdrawn in a retrograde fashion.

Treatment steps

- Remove makeup
- Disinfection
- Anaesthesia (optional)
- Injection: linear retrograde technique (superficial or deep)
- Massage and mould (ensure appropriate distribution of the filler)
- Inform patient about post-treatment dos and don'ts
- Arrange a follow-up appointment

Filler selection

1 Superficial injection (p. 62)
2 Medium injection (p. 63)
3 Deep injection (p. 66)

Combined treatment options

In the case of superficial lines:

- Microdermabrasion
- Chemical peeling
- Medical needling
- Laser resurfacing

In the case of prominent platysmal bands:

- Botulinum toxin type-A

Complications/Managing complications

Palpable nodules may form due to the aggregation of the filler used. Thorough massage and moulding of the injected filler immediately after the treatment ensures uniform distribution.

Practical tips

- Overcorrection must be avoided at all times when using the linear technique to treat the horizontal lines on the neck.
- The most optimal augmentation can be achieved by injecting small amounts of the filler deep into the subcutaneous tissue above the muscle accompanied with skin stretching.

Treatment planning – Neck elastosis
Filler augmentation aims at improving the elastosis of the skin, i.e. drooping, reduced laxity and wrinkling. In particular, tightening of the skin envelope can be achieved by volume compensation of the atrophied static base of the neck, leading to an increase in the stabilising tensions. Vertical depots can be injected along the course of the horizontal lines, as it is here where the ligamentous attachments are located (connecting the skin to the muscles). Furthermore, the quality of the skin can be improved with superficial serial injections with rehydrating filler agents or mesofillers. If the elastosis is very advanced, adjuvant treatments with chemical peeling, dermal needling or laser resurfacing should also be considered.

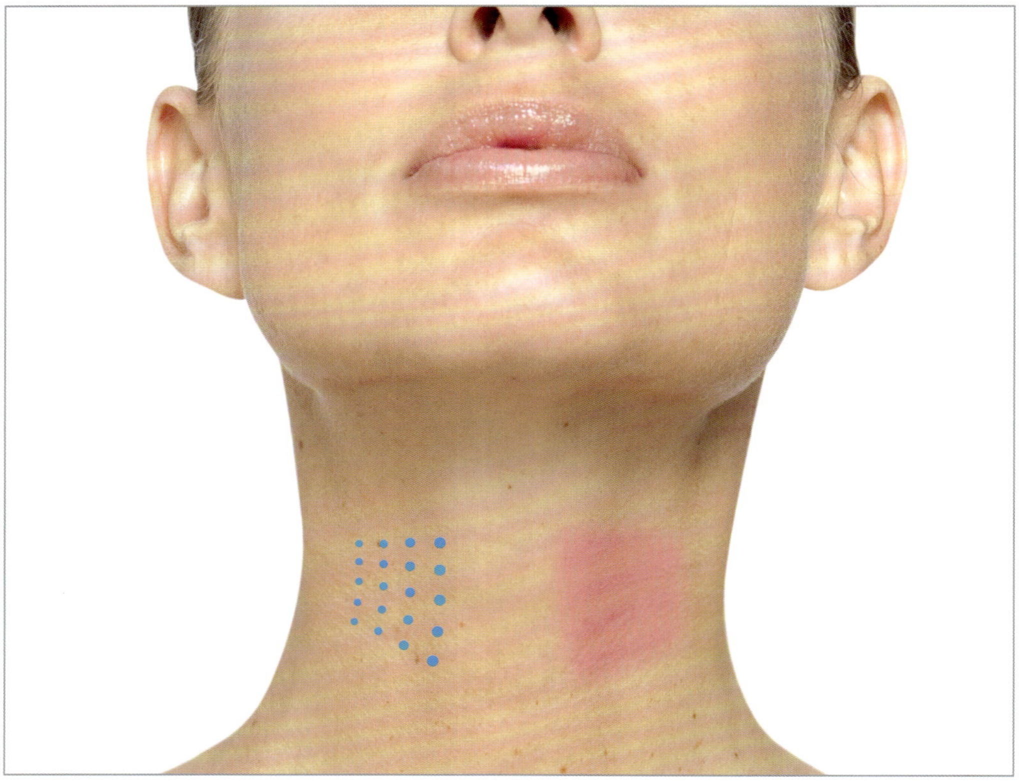

Technique: serial point technique with skin stretching
Injection points: serial micro-boluses spread out over the elastotic area (assisted injection systems [AIS] can be useful in this treatment)
Volume: smallest possible volume: 0.01 ml/injection point
Tool: 30–32 gauge needle

Video: Neck elastosis point
http://www.kvm-tv.de/FIL/027.mp4

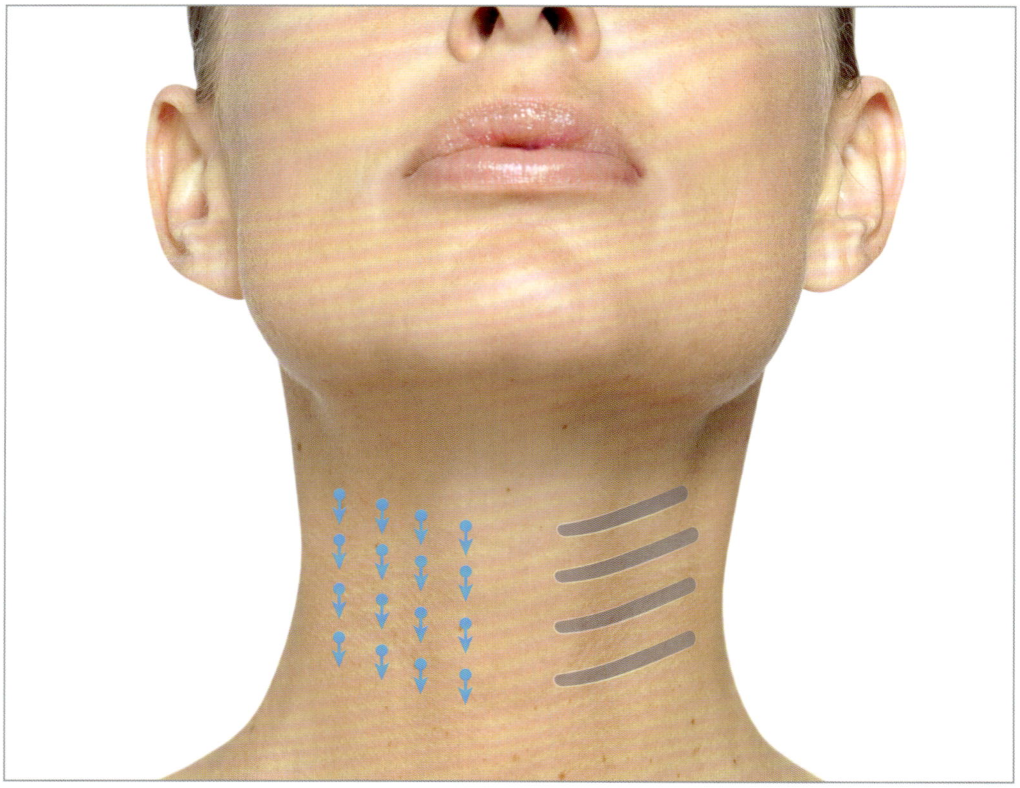

Technique: VSDT alongside skin elevation
Injection points: depending on individual needs, several 'hot spots' can be treated along the course of the horizontal lines
Volume: 0.1 ml/depot
Tool: 27 gauge needle

Video: Neck elastosis deep
http://www.kvm-tv.de/FIL/028.mp4

7

Treatment – Neck elastosis

Neck volumisation

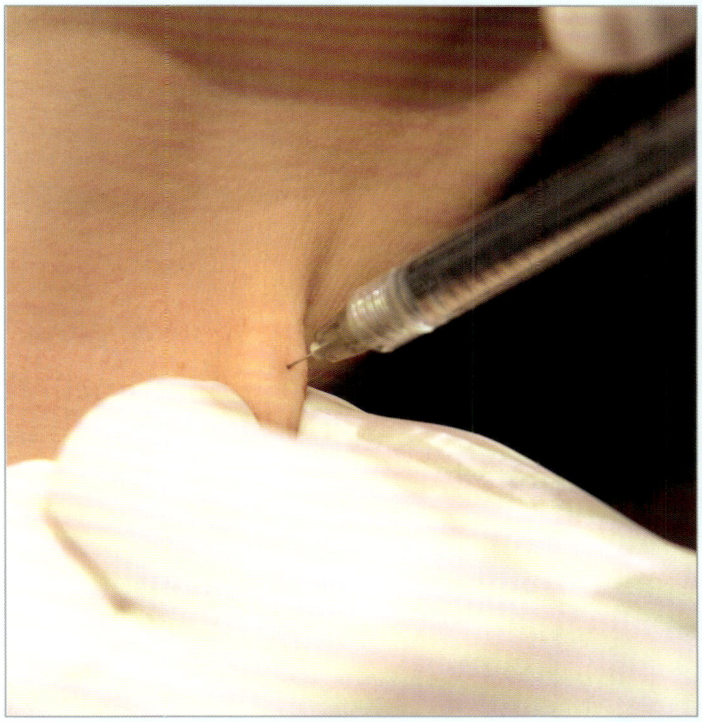

Fig. 7.77 The volumisation is achieved by depositing several vertical depots on the static base of the neck above the muscle. Before injecting the filler, the skin is grasped with two fingers of the non-injecting hand where the horizontal lines are located and is maximally elevated.

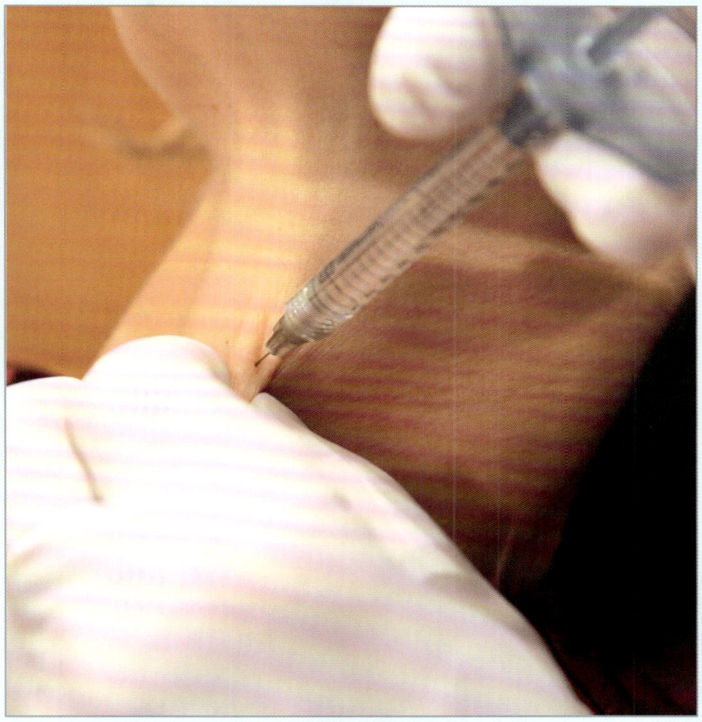

Fig. 7.78 Injecting with skin elevation avoids an intramuscular deposition of the filler. Target volumes per injection should amount to 0.1 ml per depot.

Treatment steps
- Remove makeup
- Disinfection
- Anaesthesia (optional)
- Injection: VSDT for volume build-up; serial point technique for surface improvement
- Massage and mould (ensure appropriate distribution of the filler)
- Inform patient about post-treatment dos and don'ts
- Arrange a follow-up appointment

Filler selection

Point technique (surface improvement):

1 Superficial injection (p. 62)

A Special indications: skin surface regeneration and mesotherapy (p. 69)

VSDT (volume build-up):

3 Deep injection (p. 66)

Combined treatment options
- Microdermabrasion
- Chemical peeling
- Medical needling
- Laser resurfacing

Complications/Managing complications
- To avoid an accidental intramuscular injection of the filler, it is important to perform the vertical injections under maximum elevation of the skin. This ensures correct placement of the filler on the static supramuscular neck base.
- Palpable nodules may form due to the aggregation of the filler used. Thorough massage and moulding of the filler immediately after the injection ensures uniform distribution.

Practical tip

Given the very thin skin alongside the minimal fat padding of the neck, the subcutaneously injected filler should be mouldable and smooth, on the one hand, and at the same time obtain good stabilising properties. Suitable filler products include Juvéderm® VOLIFT, Emervel® Deep, Restylane®, and BELOTERO® Volume Lidocaine.

7.6.2 Nose

Treatment planning

The indentation at the root of the nose becomes more pronounced with age. Modification of this indentation with volume replacement leads to a more harmonious and youthful appearance. Any unsightly nasal lumps and protuberances can also be smoothed out in this fashion. The marks caused by the nose pads in spectacle wearers can also be accurately filled. Furthermore, a sunken tip of the nose can be elevated without the need for a surgical intervention.

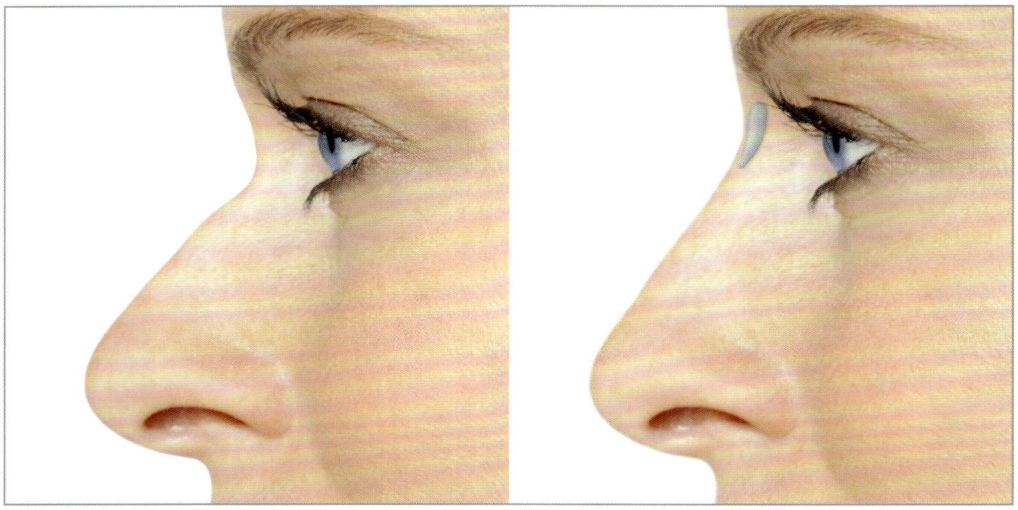

Augmentation of the indentation at the root of the nose
Technique: VSDT – bolus injection
Injection site: root of the nose
Volume: 0.2–0.5 ml total
Tool: 30 gauge needle

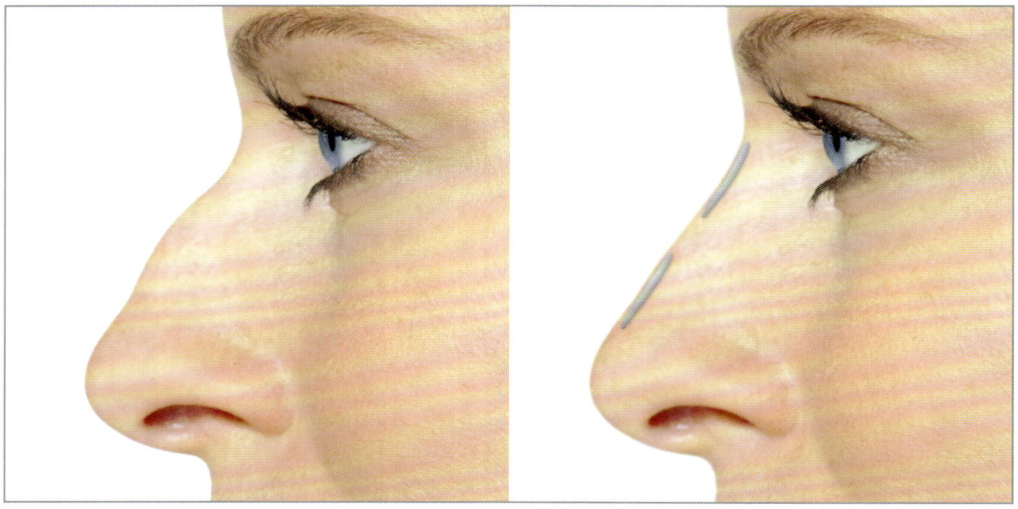

Straightening the bridge of the nose
Technique: VSDT/tunneling technique (depending on the anatomical findings)
Depth: supraperiosteal
Injection site: bridge of the nose
Volume: 0.3–0.8 ml total
Tool: 30 gauge needle

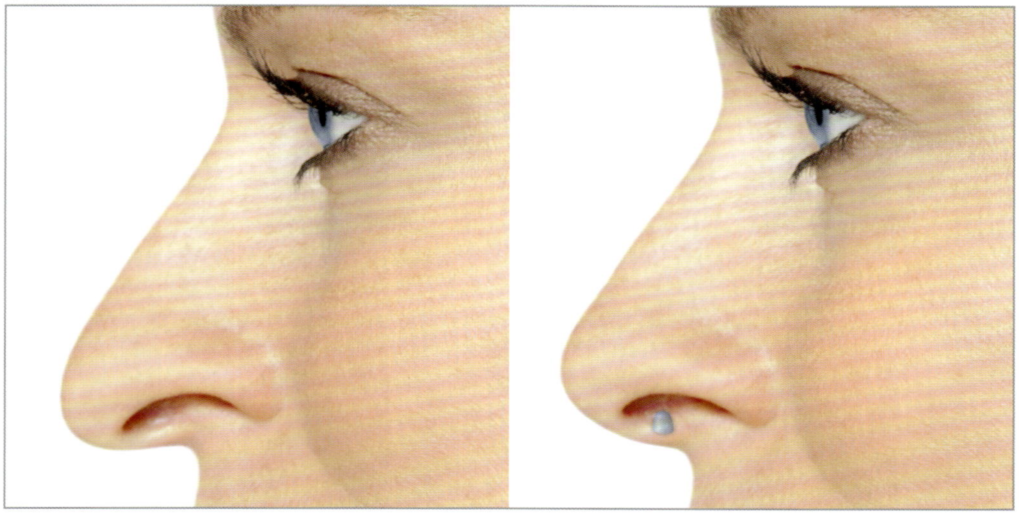

Elevation of the tip of the nose
Technique: VSDT
Depth: above the bone directly beneath the nasal septum
Injection site: proximal part of the nasal septum
Volume: 0.1–0.3 ml total
Tool: 30 gauge needle

Treatment

Straightening the root and dorsum of the nose

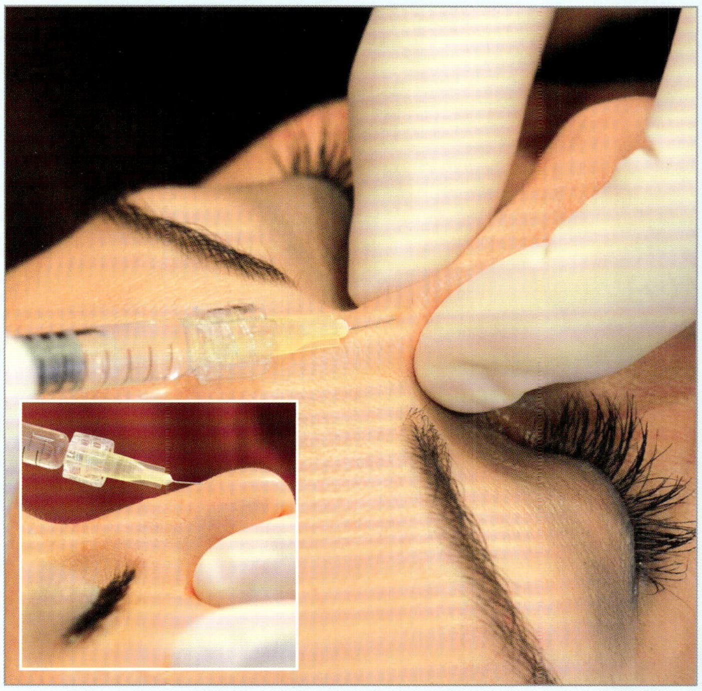

Fig. 7.79 Indentation at the root of the nose: The skin over the root of the nose is grasped and held in place with the thumb and the index finger of the non-injecting hand. The needle is inserted from the cranial end of the nose and directed downwards. The filler is injected at the deepest point at the supraperiosteum. Strict supraperiosteal injections are advocated here.
Along the dorsum/bridge of the nose: Several depots are injected along the dorsum/bridge of the nose, until the nasal profile is straightened. The tunneling or point technique can be used, depending on the clinical presentation.
Level of injection: On the bone or cartilage.

Elevating the tip of the nose

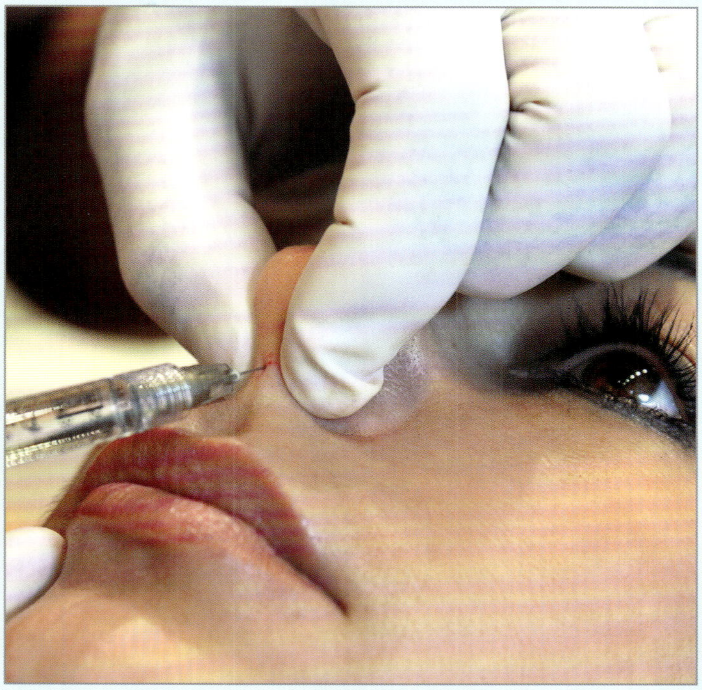

Fig. 7.80 The practitioner uses two fingers of the non-injecting hand to gently compress the nostrils, whilst asking the patient to breathe through their mouth. The injection is given above the bone directly beneath the nasal septum. Injection depth and augmentation are controlled with palpation.

Treatment steps
- Remove makeup
- Disinfection
- Anaesthesia (optional)
- Injection: VSDT (or tunneling technique)
- Massage and mould (ensure appropriate distribution of the filler)
- Inform patient about post-treatment dos and don'ts
- Arrange a follow-up appointment

Filler selection

2 Medium injection (p. 63)
3 Deep injection (p. 66)
4 Ultra-deep injection (p. 67)

Combined treatment options
- Chemical peeling
- Medical needling
- Laser resurfacing

Complications/Managing complications

Palpable nodules may form due to the aggregation of the filler used. Thorough massage and moulding of the filler immediately after the injection ensures uniform distribution.

Practical tips
- Augmentation of the bridge of the nose should really be considered a surgical indication on the whole, but in some cases non-surgical correction with injectable fillers can be effective, particularly in patients who have undergone previous surgery.
- In principle, filler augmentation can simulate the results of surgery. As long as optimal anatomical relationships (straight septum) are intact and nasal breathing is not impaired in a patient seeking aesthetic correction or enhancement, augmentation with fillers is indicated as the initial treatment, since this method is associated with a significantly lower risk compared to a surgical intervention.

⚠ Prior to injecting any filler, please refer to the latest manufacturer guidelines for specific instructions for use.

7.6.3 Ear

Treatment planning
The signs of ageing show distinctly on and around the ear. Consequently, the ear needs to be considered as part of an overall facial rejuvenation strategy.

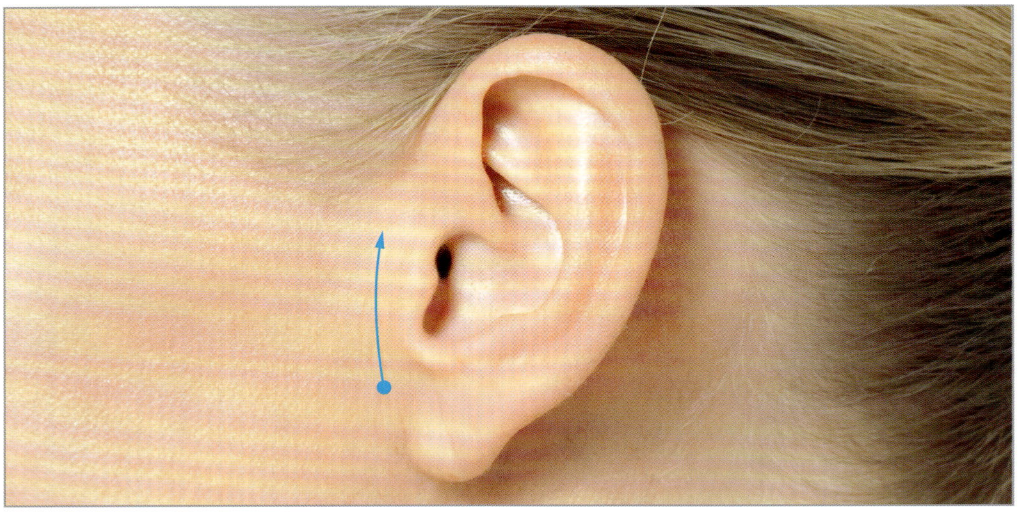

Pre-auricular lines/wrinkles
Technique: linear technique
Depth: intradermal or immediately subdermal
Volume: 0.1–0.2 ml/injection point
Tool: 30 gauge needle

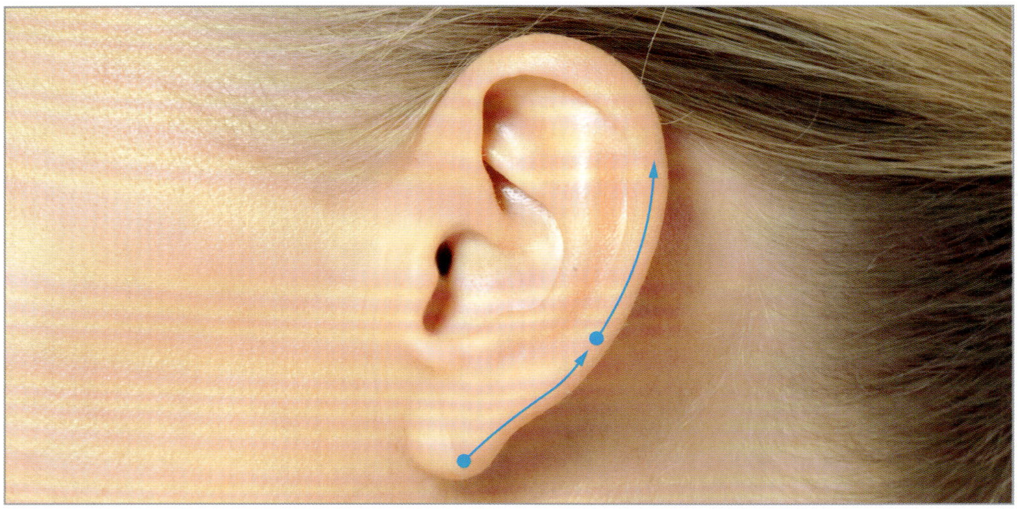

Contouring of the helix
Technique: linear technique
Depth: intradermal or immediately subdermal
Volume: 0.1–0.2 ml/thread
Tool: 30 gauge needle

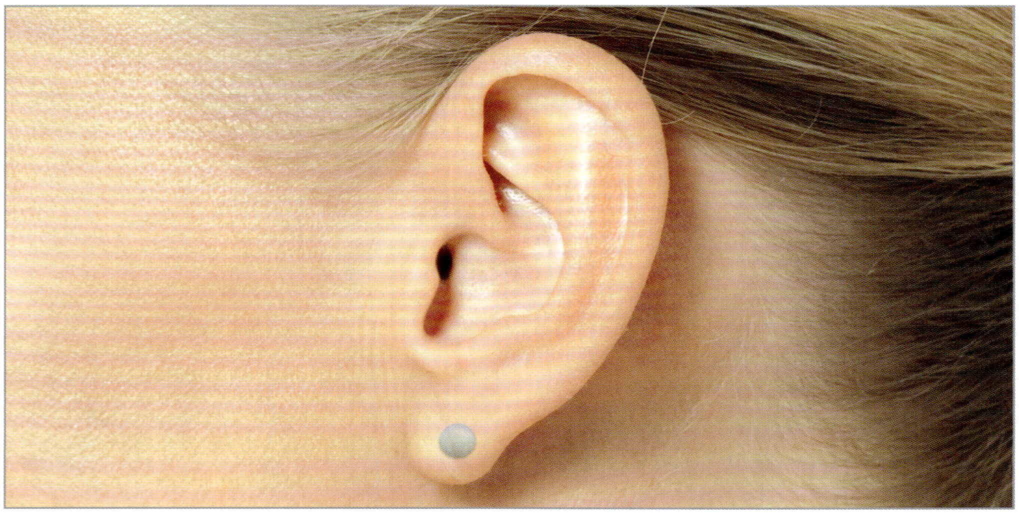

Earlobe augmentation
Technique: point technique – bolus injection
Depth: intradermal or immediately subdermal
Volume: 0.2–0.4 ml/side
Tool: 30 gauge needle

7

Treatment

Pre-auricular lines/wrinkles

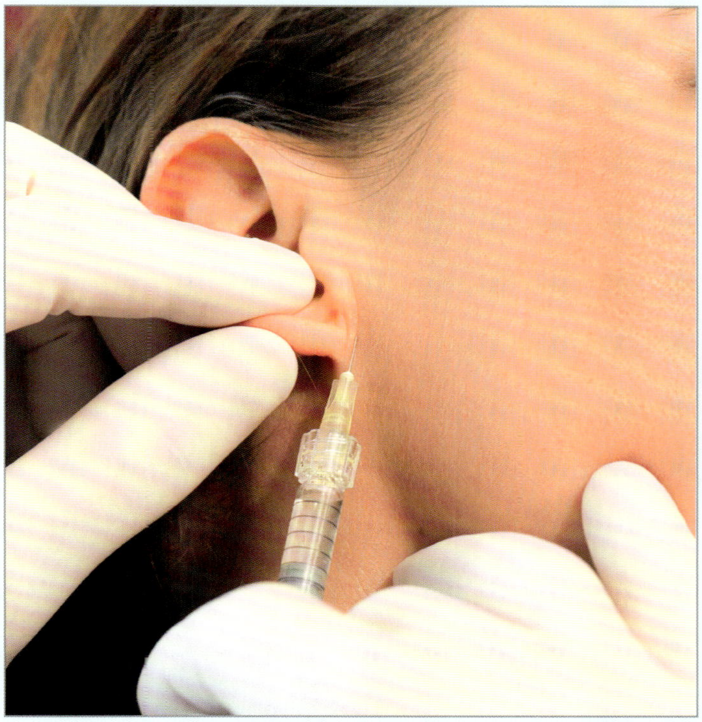

Fig. 7.81 The linear technique is suited for both the pre-auricular lines and wrinkles, as well as when contouring the helix. The injection is given at the base of the wrinkle using the linear technique, injecting the filler as the needle is being withdrawn.

Earlobe augmentation

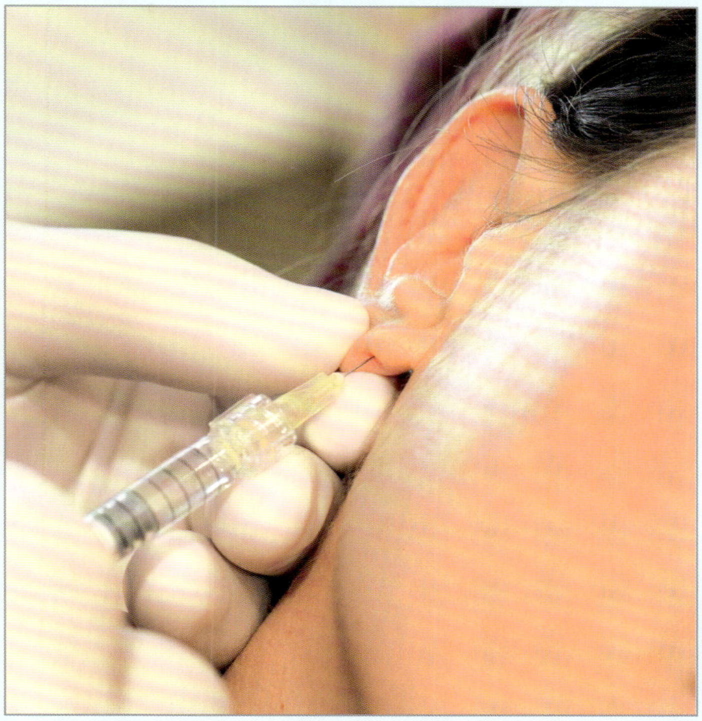

Fig. 7.82 The point technique is best suited to earlobe augmentation. The needle is inserted into the tip of the earlobe and a bolus of 0.2–0.4 ml is administered into the centre of the earlobe.

Treatment steps
- Remove makeup
- Disinfection
- Anaesthesia (optional)
- Injection: linear technique/point technique
- Massage and mould (ensure appropriate distribution of the filler)
- Inform patient about post-treatment dos and don'ts
- Arrange a follow-up appointment

Filler selection

Pre-auricular lines/wrinkles:

1 Superficial injection (p. 62)

2 Medium injection (p. 63)

Contouring of the helix and earlobes augmentation:

3 Deep injection (p. 66)

4 Ultra-deep injection (p. 67)

Combined treatment options
- Chemical peeling
- Medical needling
- Laser resurfacing

Complications/Managing complications

Palpable nodules may form due to the aggregation of the filler used. Thorough massage and moulding of the filler immediately after the injection allows for uniform distribution.

7.6.4 Hands

Treatment planning

External environmental ageing factors do not only affect the face and the neck. UV radiation exposure on the dorsal aspect of the hands that are not adequately protected leads to actinic elastosis. Furthermore, natural ageing processes affect the dorsal fat pads, which diminish with age. Fillers can be used to augment and build-up the atrophied base that leads to skin laxity, as well as to revitalise the surface of the skin.

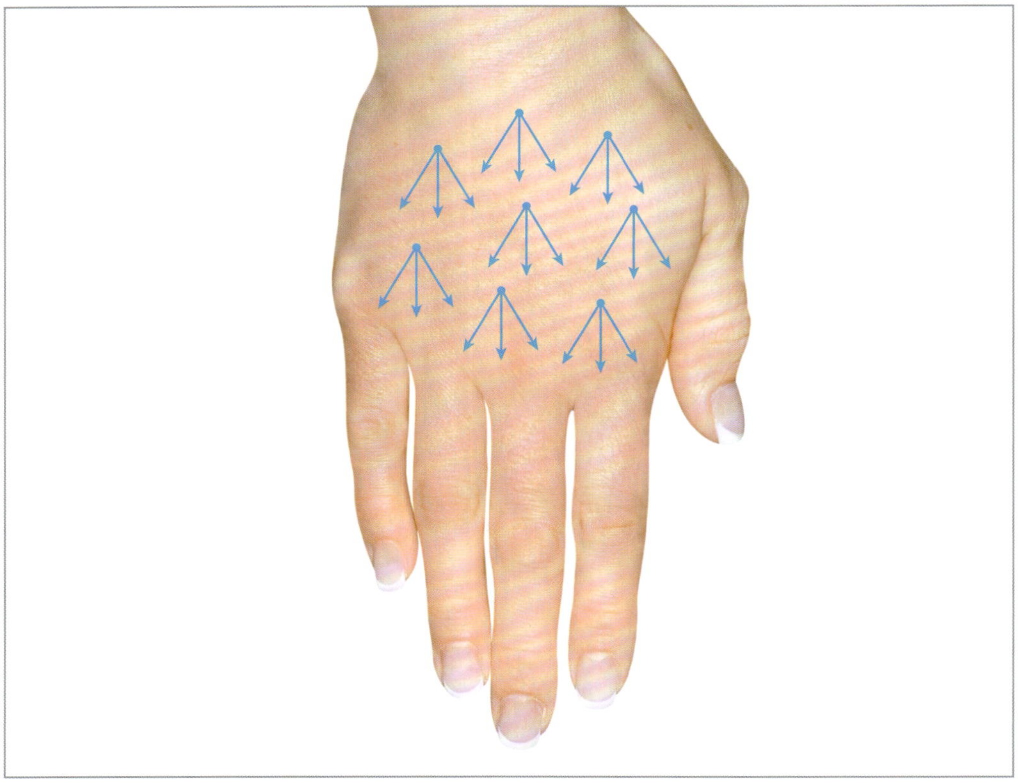

Technique: fanning technique
Depth: immediately subdermal
Injection sites: multiple fanning injections to augment the back of the hand
Volume: 0.1–0.2 ml/thread
Tool: 30 gauge needle

Video: Hands point http://www.kvm-tv.de/FIL/029.mp4

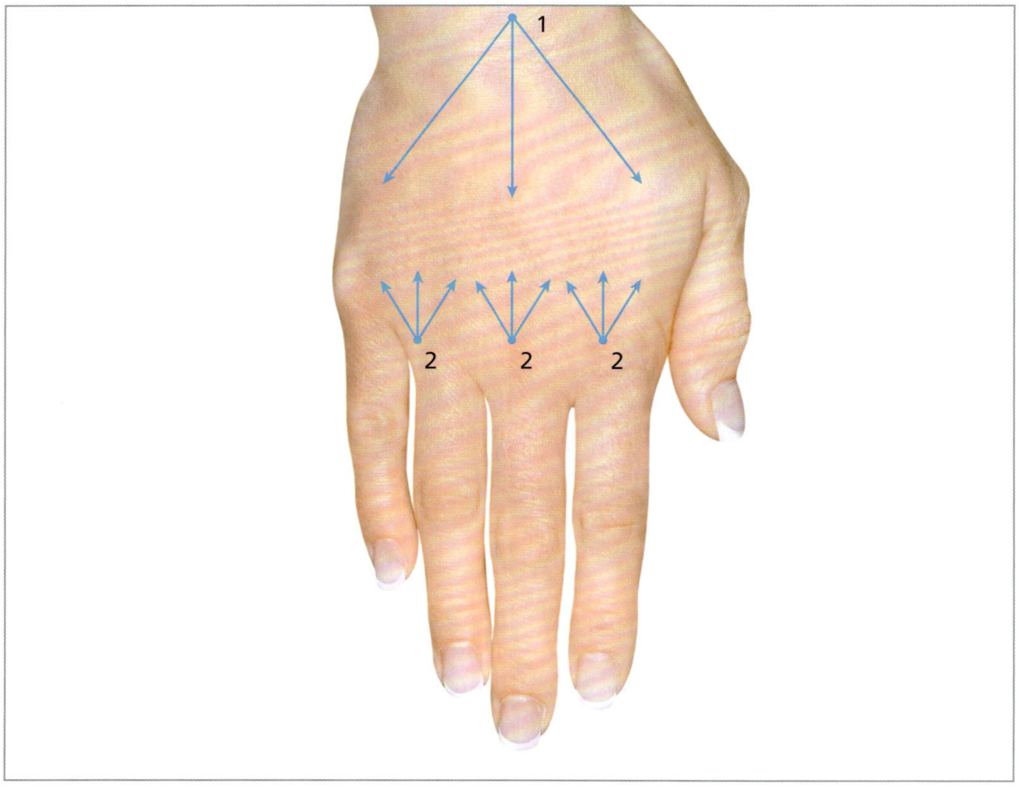

Technique: horizontal augmentation technique using a cannula (HAC) in a fanning fashion
Insertions sites: (1) at the proximal aspect of the metacarpal bones, and between the tendons (2) at the distal aspect of the metacarpal bones and between the knuckles
Injection depth and direction: subcutaneous, (1) starting from the proximal aspect, and then (2) injecting from the distal end (delivering multiple fans between the knuckles) to fill out the intertendinous volume loss, as well as to provide a smooth plane of filler to the whole dorsal aspect of the hand
Volume: depending on findings – 1.5–3.0 ml total for both hands
Tool: 22–25 gauge cannula

Video: Hands DHAC http://www.kvm-tv.de/FIL/030.mp4

Treatment

HAC

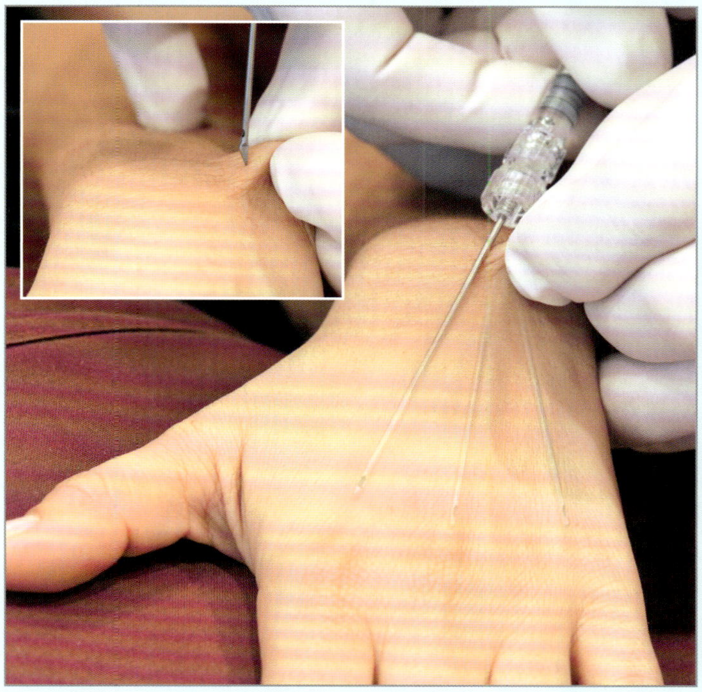

Fig. 7.83 At the insertion site at the base of the metacarpal bones, the skin is tented and a point incision (see small image) is made before a blunt cannula is advanced into the immediate subdermal space. The tissue is gently mobilised and filled in a fanning fashion. The same procedure is repeated from the distal aspect between the knuckles, this time in the opposite direction. In doing so, the overall dorsum of the hand can be augmented. A total of 1.5 to 3 ml of the filler can be injected in both hands.

Fanning technique

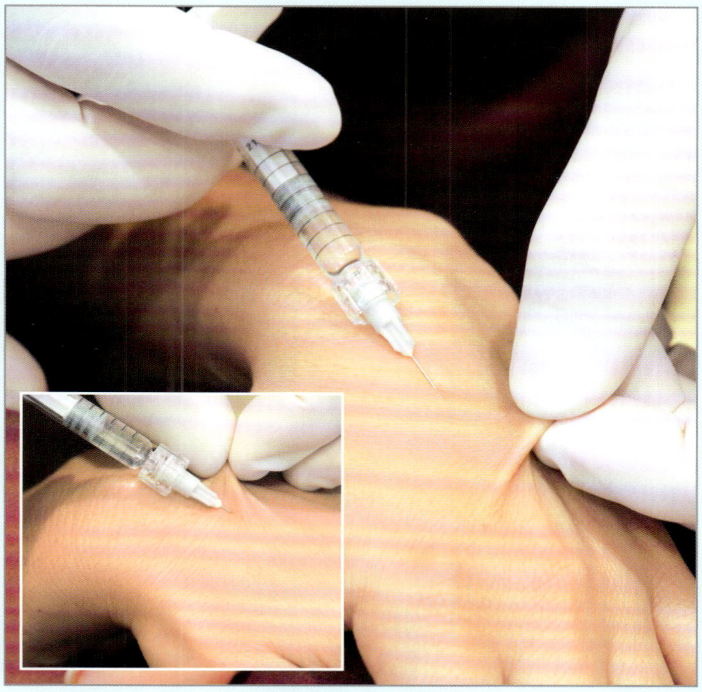

Fig. 7.84 A fold of skin is raised with the thumb and forefinger of the non-injecting hand. The needle is inserted into this fold (avoiding prominent vessels) placing the needle immediately subdermally (see small image). Fanned injections of 0.1–0.2 ml/line are delivered from this point.

Treatment steps
- Disinfection
- Anaesthesia (optional)
- Injection: fanning technique / HAC
- Massage and mould (ensure appropriate distribution of the filler)
- Inform patient about post-treatment dos and don'ts
- Arrange a follow-up appointment if necessary

Filler selection

2 Medium injection (p. 63)

3 Deep injection (p. 66)

Hyaluronic acid fillers, which are easy to massage and mould, are most suitable for application below the thin skin of the dorsal aspect of the hands. Calcium hydroxylapatite is also a commonly used filler for this indication, particularly as its opaque colour masks the bluishness of the dorsal veins, which are considered one of the key features of concern for many patients.

Combined treatment options

Superficial treatments including:
- Microdermabrasion
- Chemical peeling
- Medical needling
- Laser resurfacing

Complications/Managing complications
- It is vital not to damage the hyperplastic veins on the backs of the hands, if one is to avoid an extensive haematoma, and so a gentle technique is advocated.
- Palpable nodules may form due to the aggregation of the filler used. Thorough massage and moulding of the filler immediately after the injection ensures uniform distribution.

Practical tips
- Occasionally, several proximal and distal fans can be delivered to cover a larger dorsal surface area and to volumise the focal intertendinous spaces and immediately around the prominent veins. However, in smaller hands with minimal volumes loss, one fan delivered in the middle from the proximal aspect can be sufficient with the use of a long cannula.
- Thorough manual massage is needed after the treatment to distribute the filler (up to 5 minutes per hand).

8 Case Studies

8 Case Studies

Case 1 – Lip augmentation

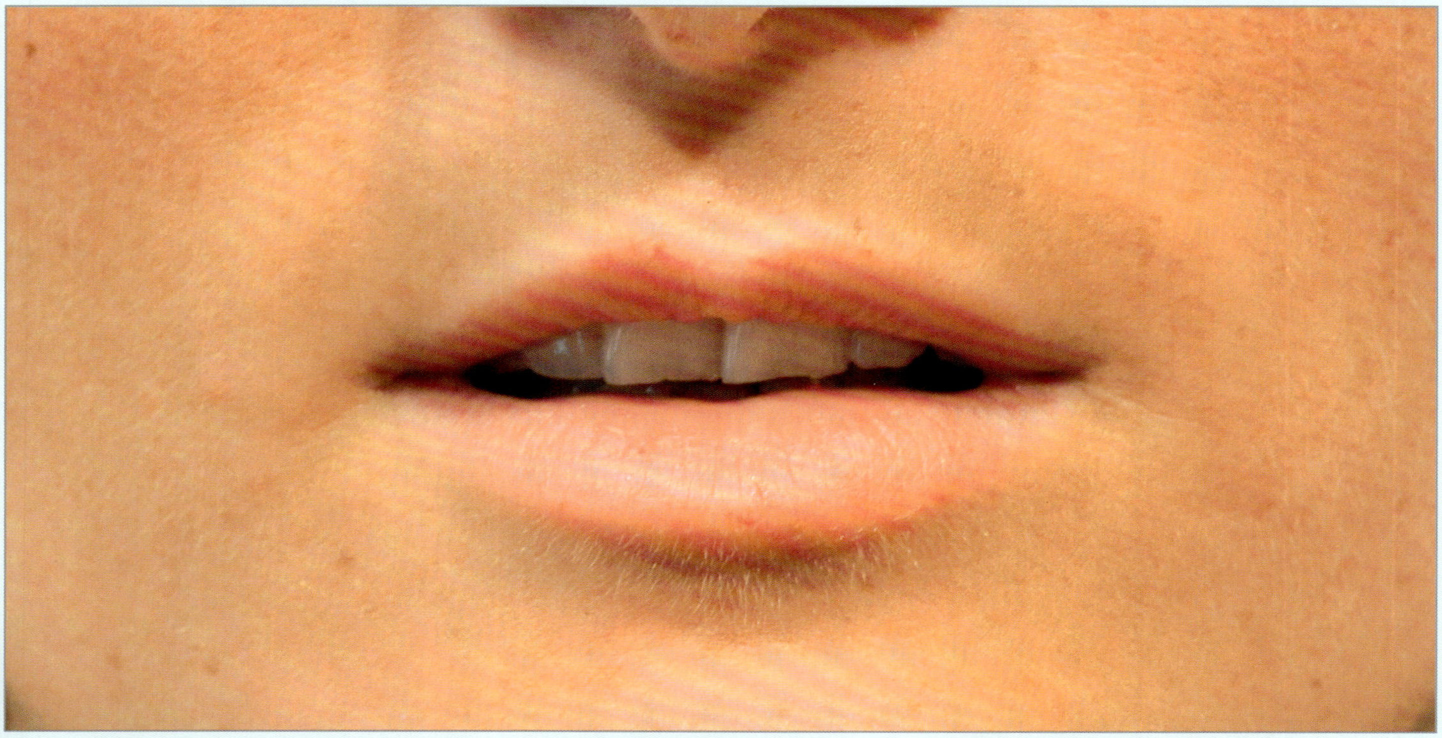

Baseline: 24-year-old female with narrow and somewhat asymmetrical lips.

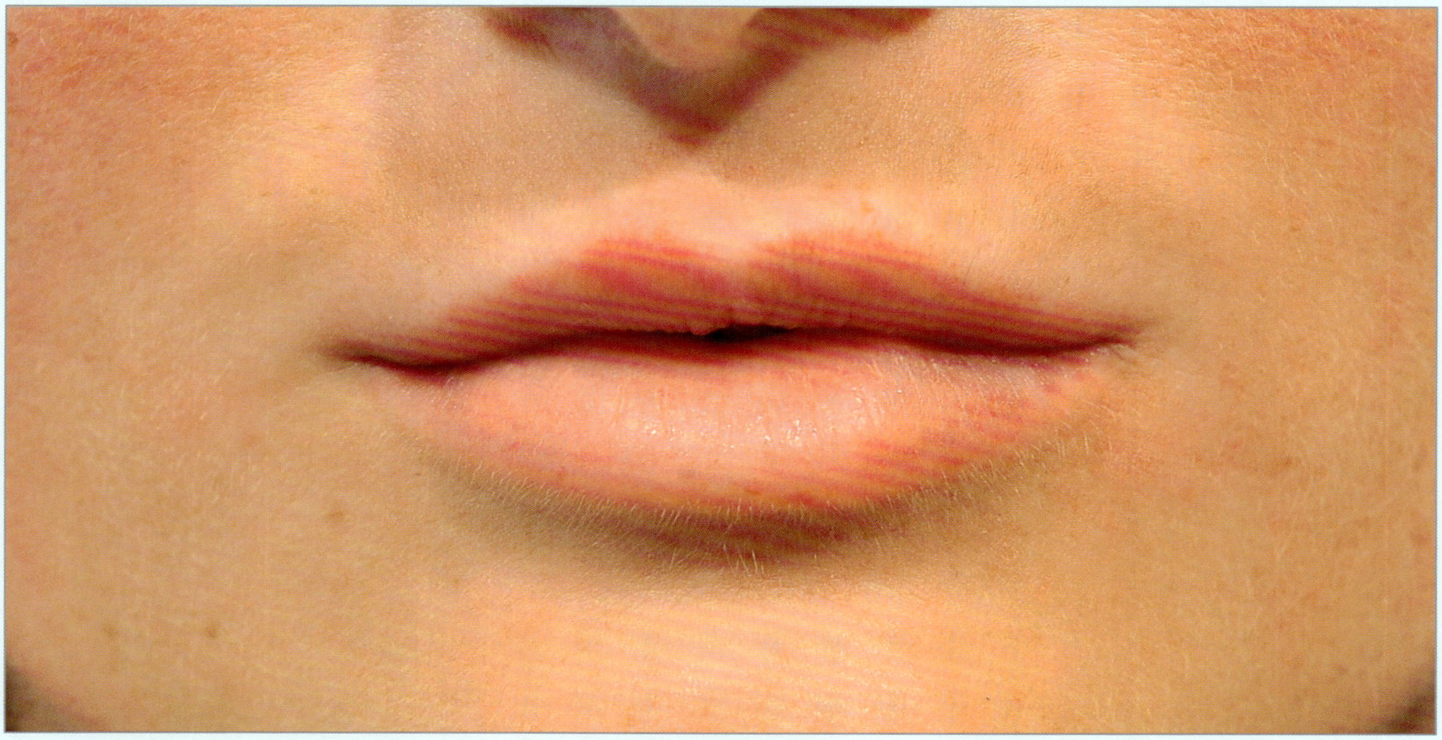

Result: 4 weeks after augmentation of the upper and lower lip with a total of 0.8 ml of a hyaluronic acid filler injected.

Case 2 – Lip augmentation

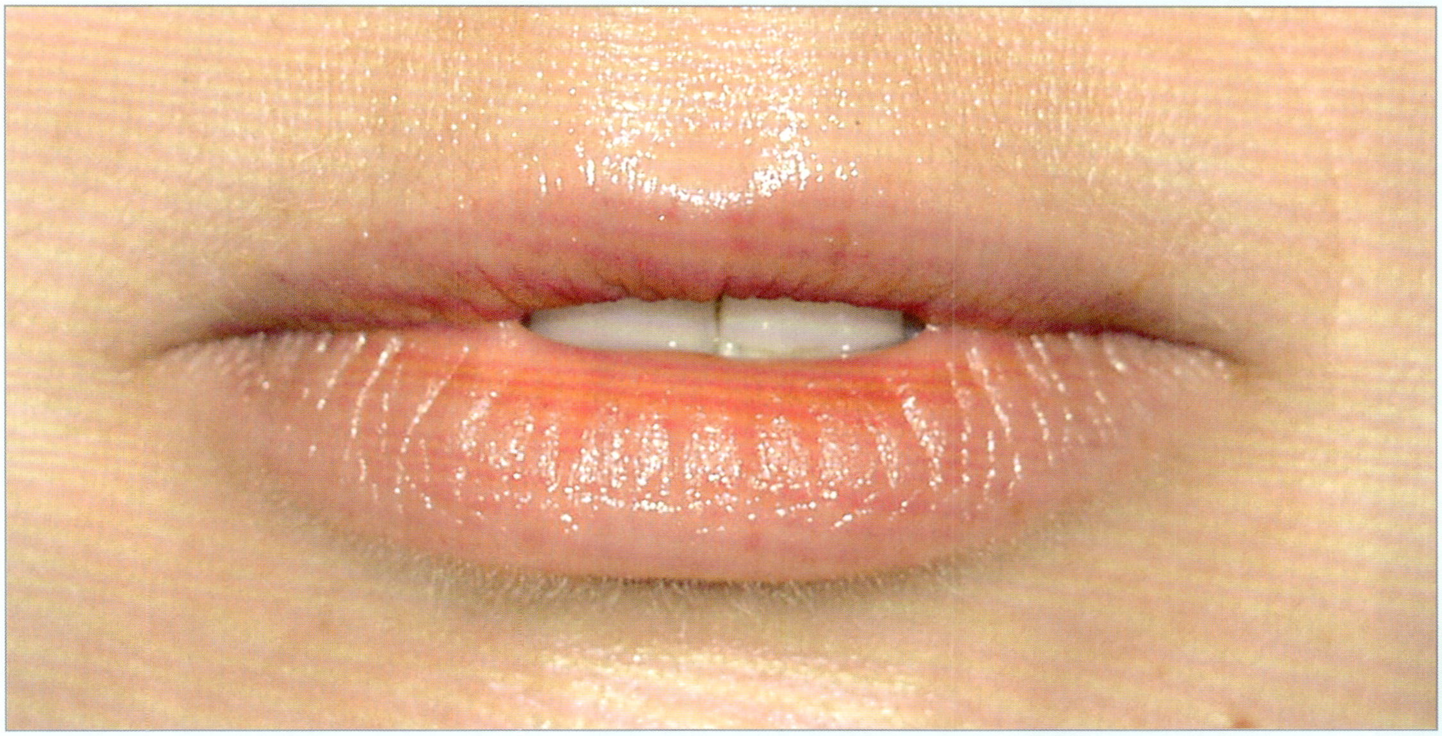

Baseline: 28-year-old female with mild lip asymmetry and volume deficit in the left lower lip.

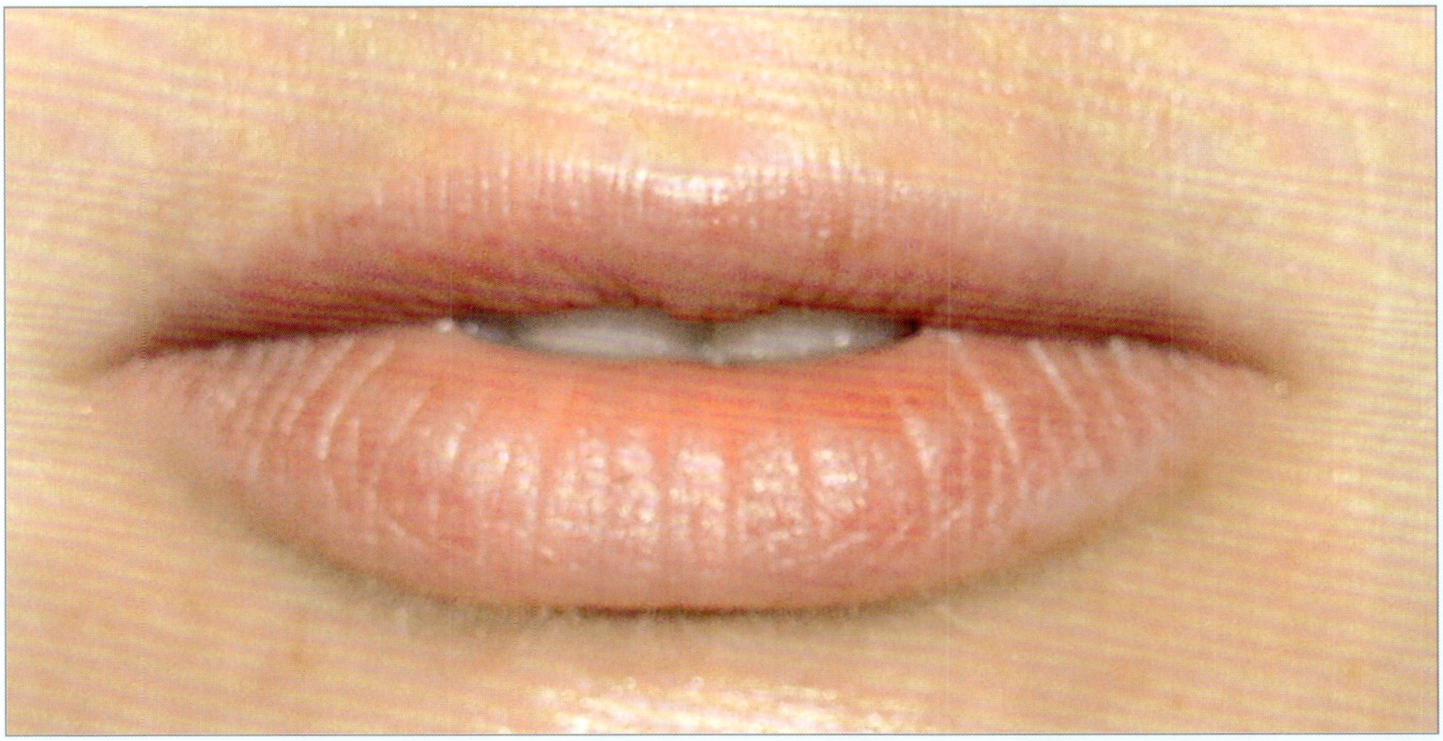

Result: 8 weeks after volume augmentation in the red margin of the lips, taking into account the prior asymmetry.

Case 3 – Severe volume loss in the midface

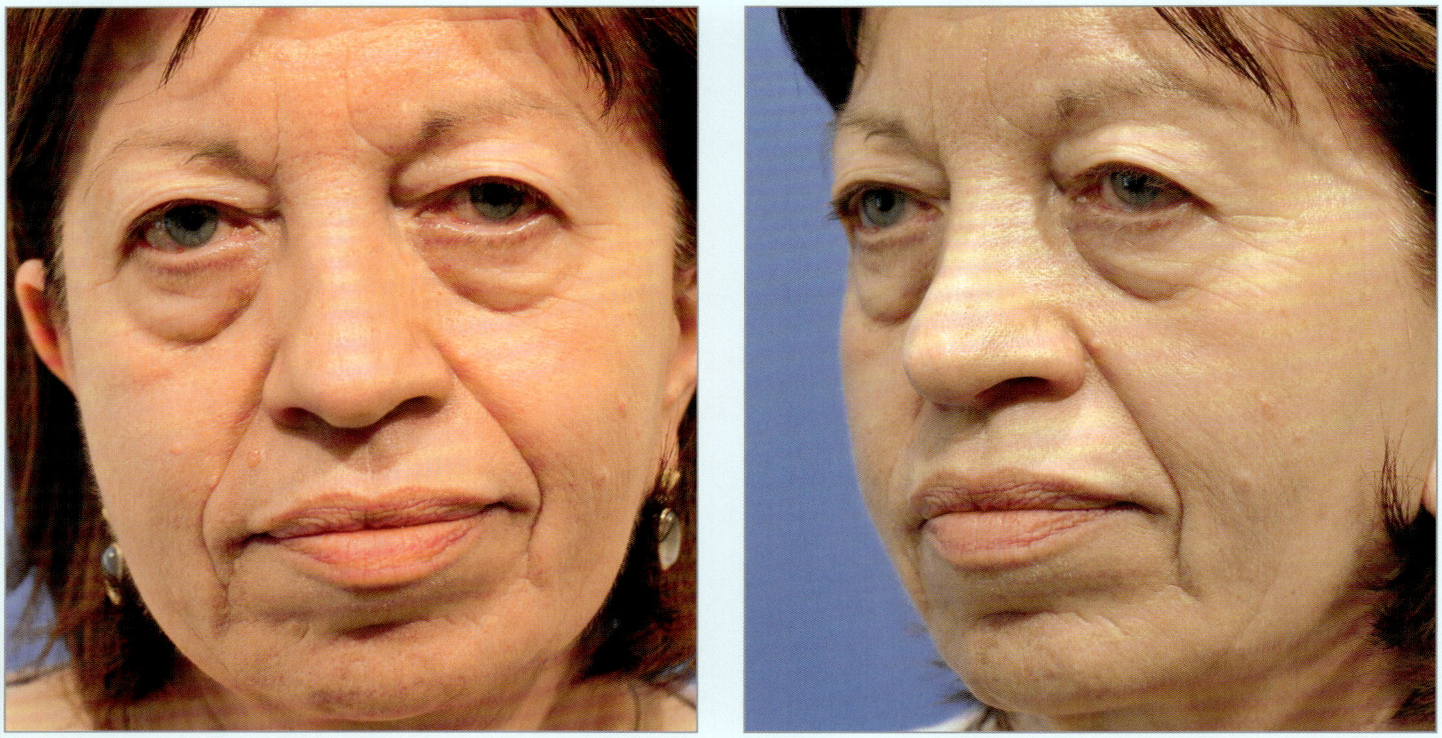

Baseline: 60-year-old female with extensive elastosis and considerable loss of volume in the midface.

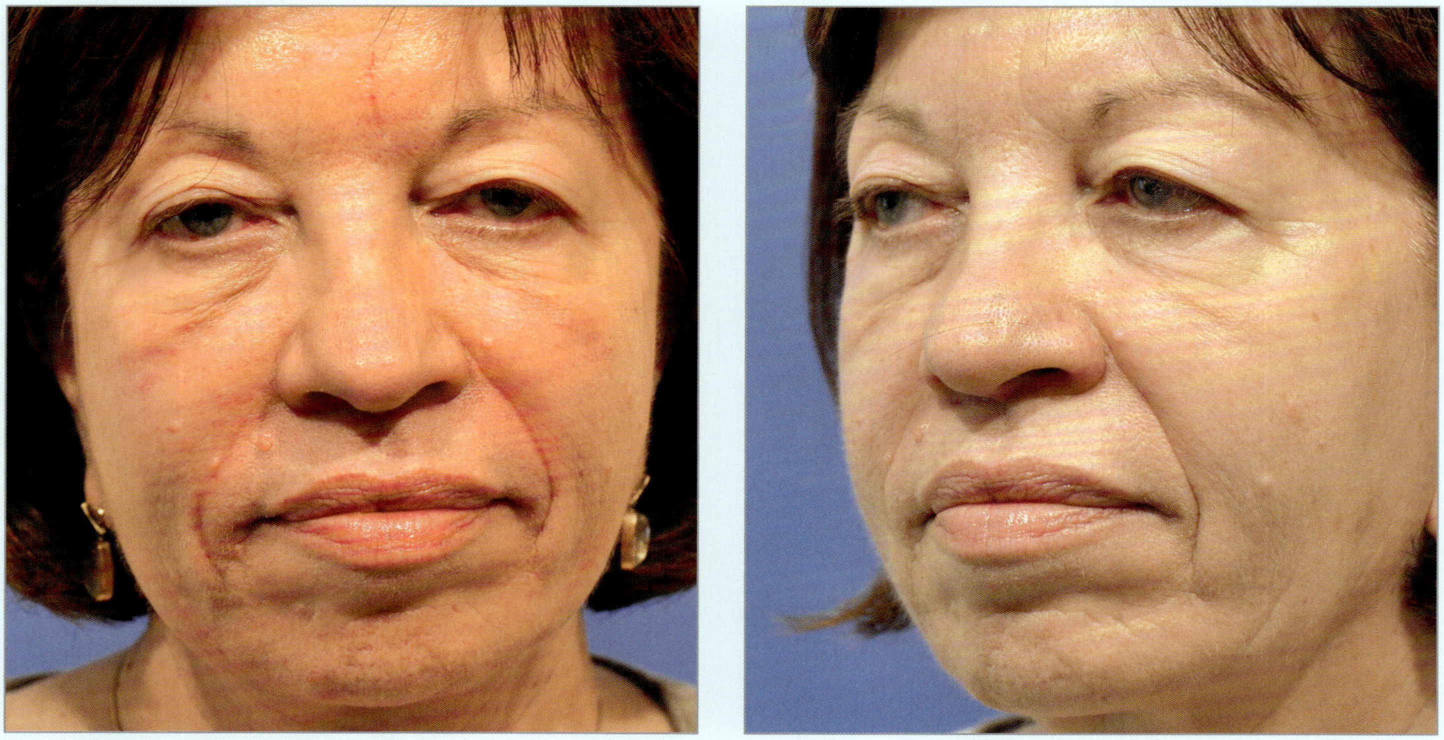

Result: 17 days after the initial treatment with a hyaluronic acid filler, using a total of 8 ml. Vertical injections were made into the SOOF, the lower lid region, the nasolabial folds, and the marionette lines. Superficial injections were made using the stretching technique into the lines in the lower cheeks, the lateral canthal lines around the eyes, and the glabella. Adjuvant injections of botulinum toxin type-A were also performed in the upper third of the face. Image taken prior to performing a blepharoplasty.

Case 3 – Long-term results

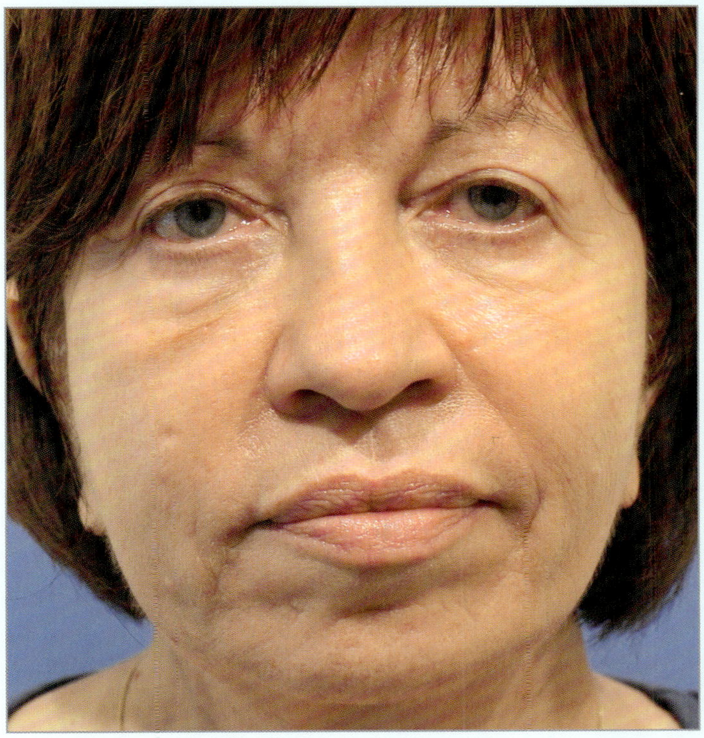

At 2.5 months after initial filler augmentation. A further 1.5 ml is planned to be injected.

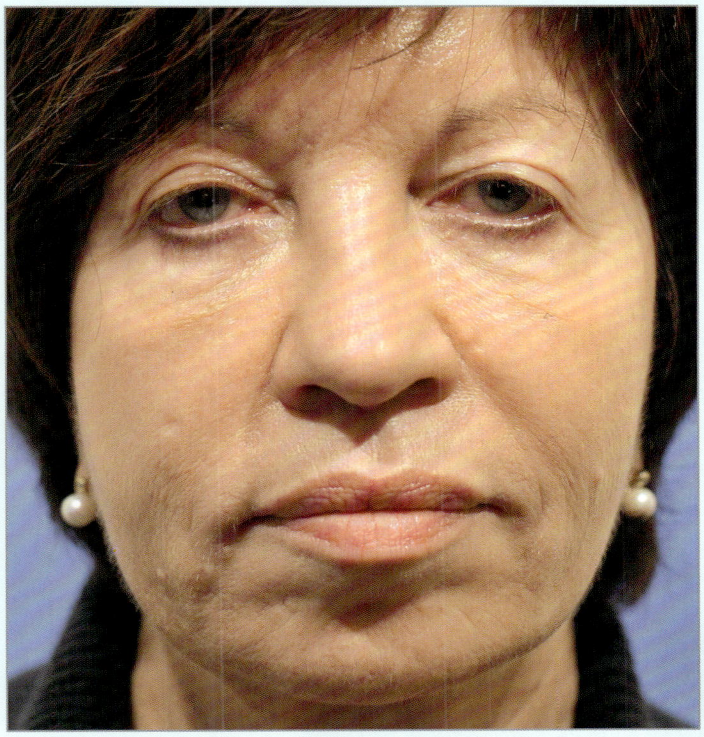

At 5 months after initial treatment. It is agreed that the patient will come back for long-term follow-up after 1 year.

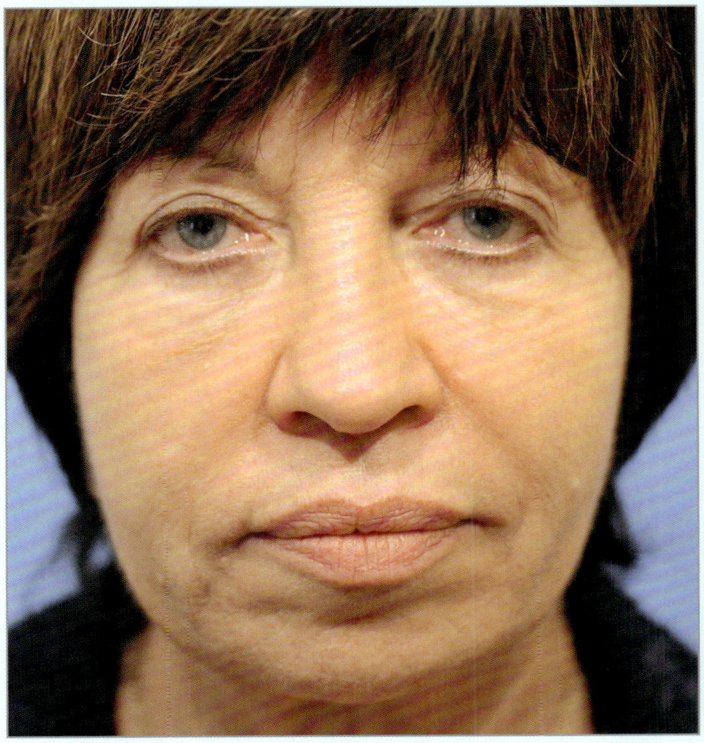

Status at 1 year after last treatment, with no further treatments performed in between.

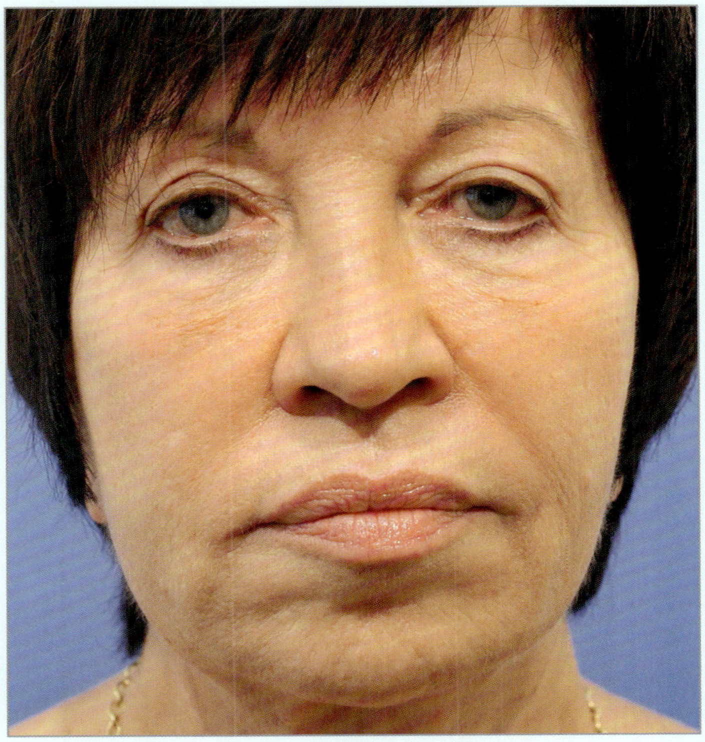

At 3 years after starting the long-term treatment. Status after four further treatments with hyaluronic acid using doses of 1.5/1/1/2 ml injected at intervals of between half to 1 year, alongside two adjuvant treatments with botulinum toxin type-A in the upper third of the face.

Case 4 – Facial elastosis

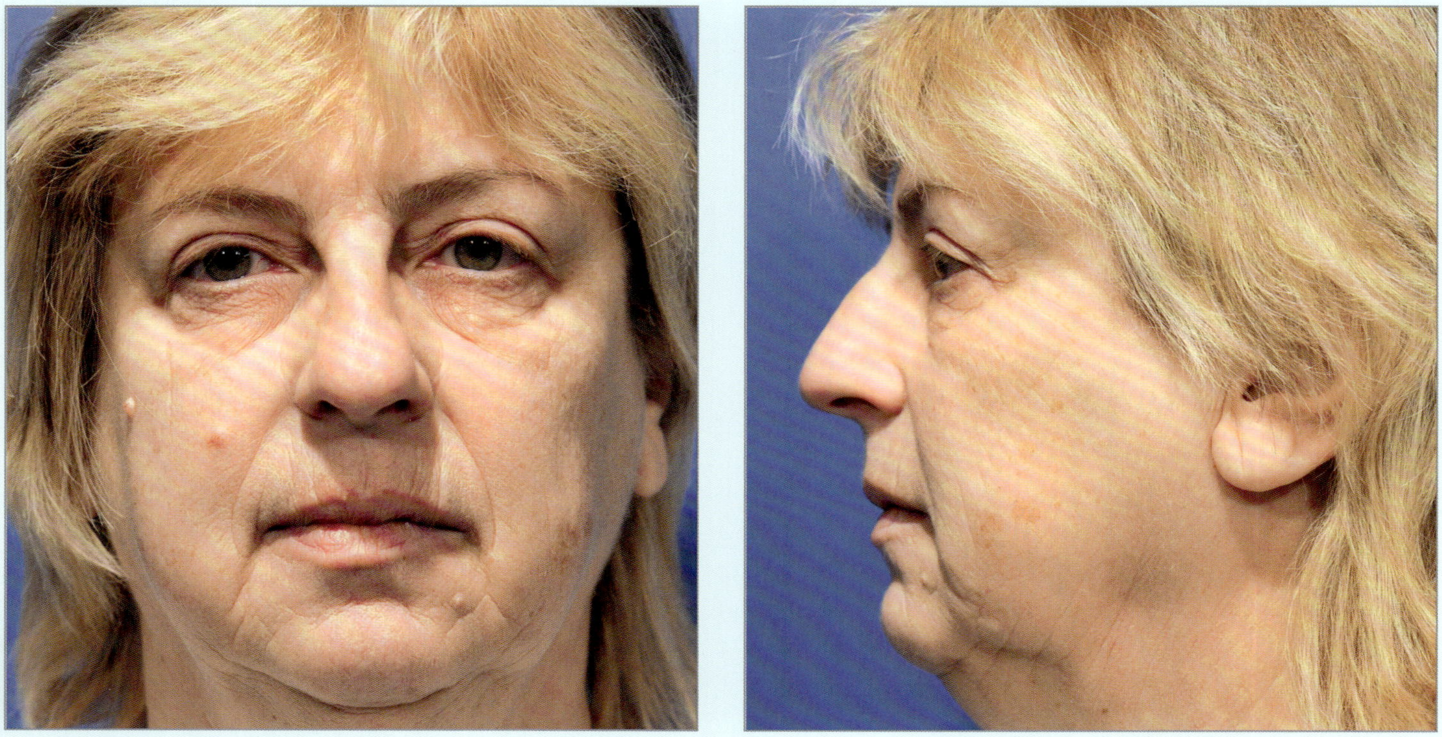

Baseline: 58-year-old female with marked facial elastosis particularly affecting the lower eyelids, perioral region and cheeks. Lipomatosis and several exophytic fibromas present on the cheeks and chin. Midface and lower eyelid volume deficit, as well as pronounced nasolabial and marionette lines are also noted.

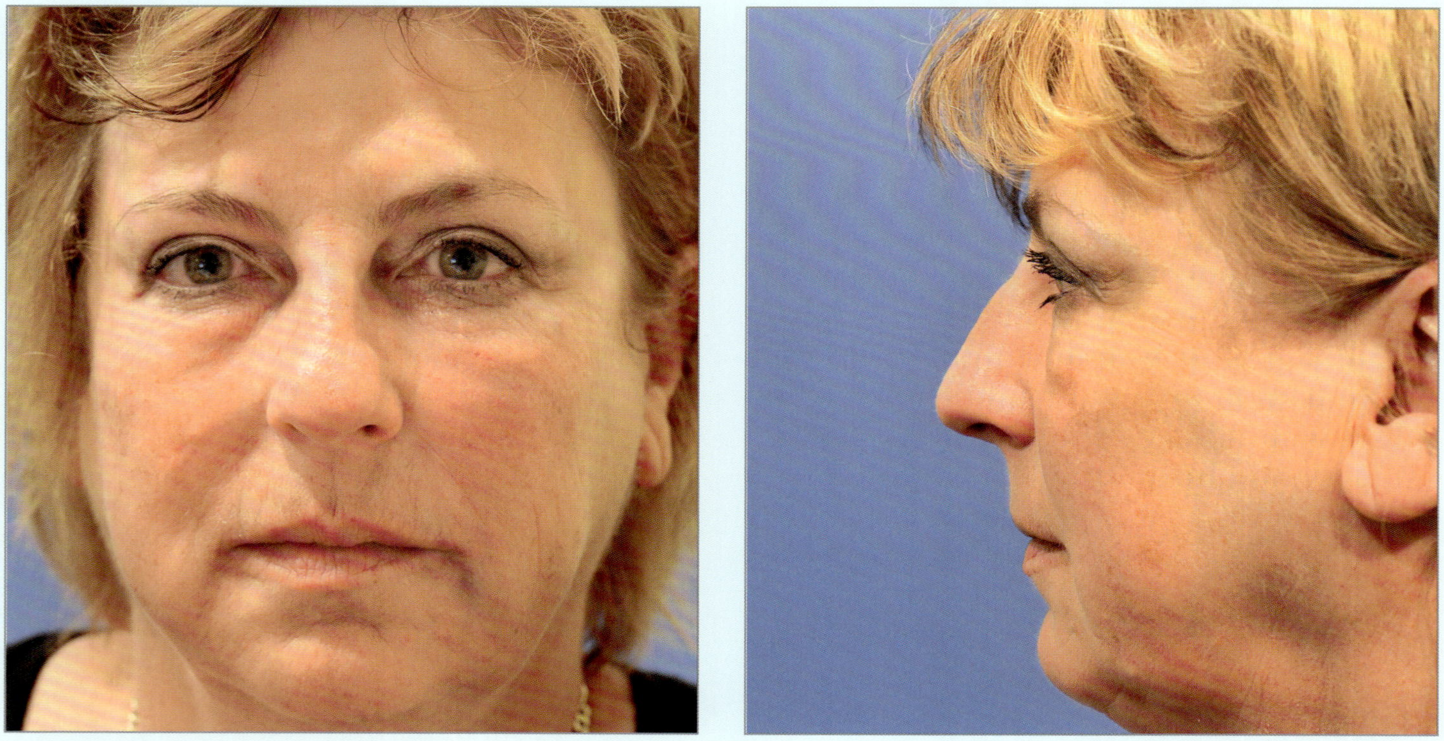

Result: 5 months after combination treatment, including: volume augmentation with a hyaluronic acid filler in the midface and lower eyelid region using the criss-cross technique, alongside fine line augmentation; botulinum toxin type-A injections into the upper half of the face; liposuction of the neck; and surgical excision of the papillomatous fibromas.

Case 5 – Incipient volume loss in the midface

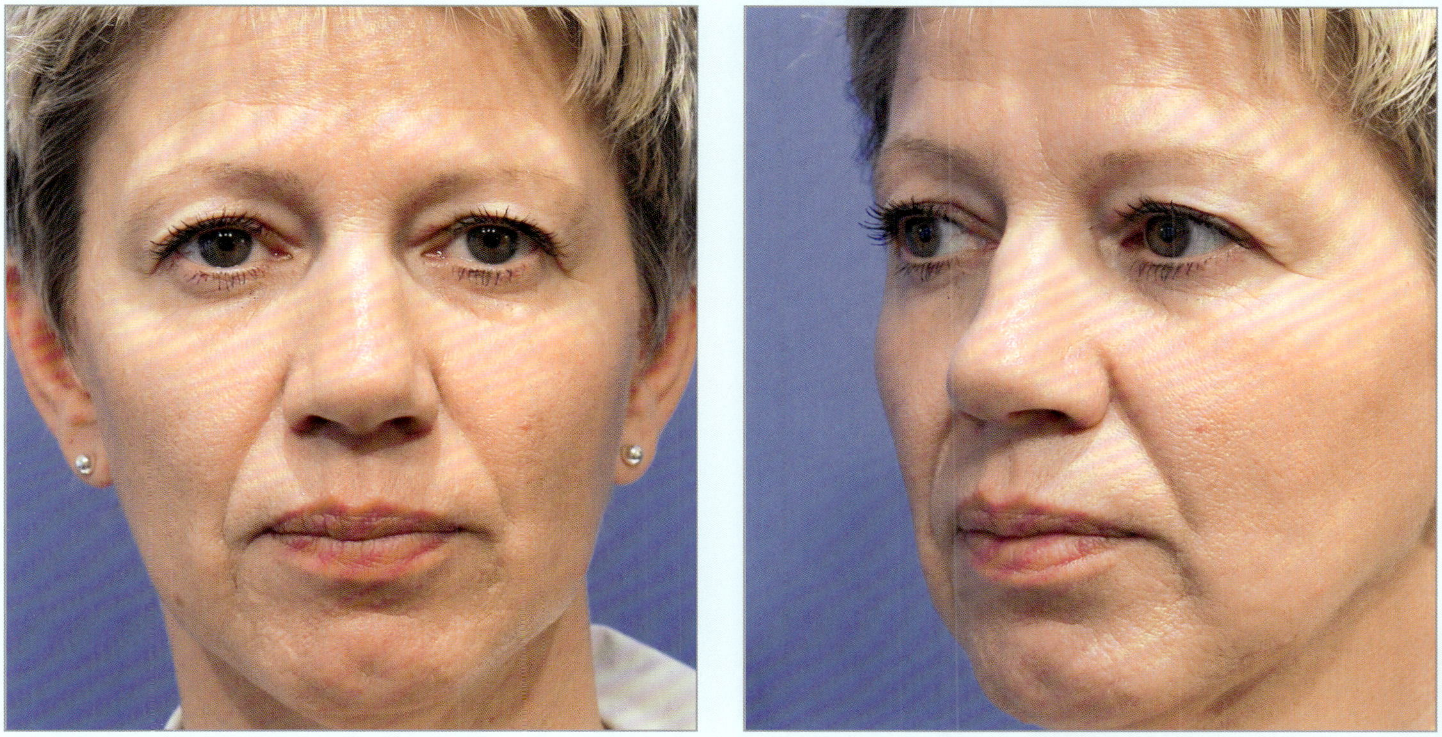

Baseline: 48-year-old female with incipient volume loss in the midface and the lower eyelid region, alongside the emergence of nasolabial folds and marionette lines.

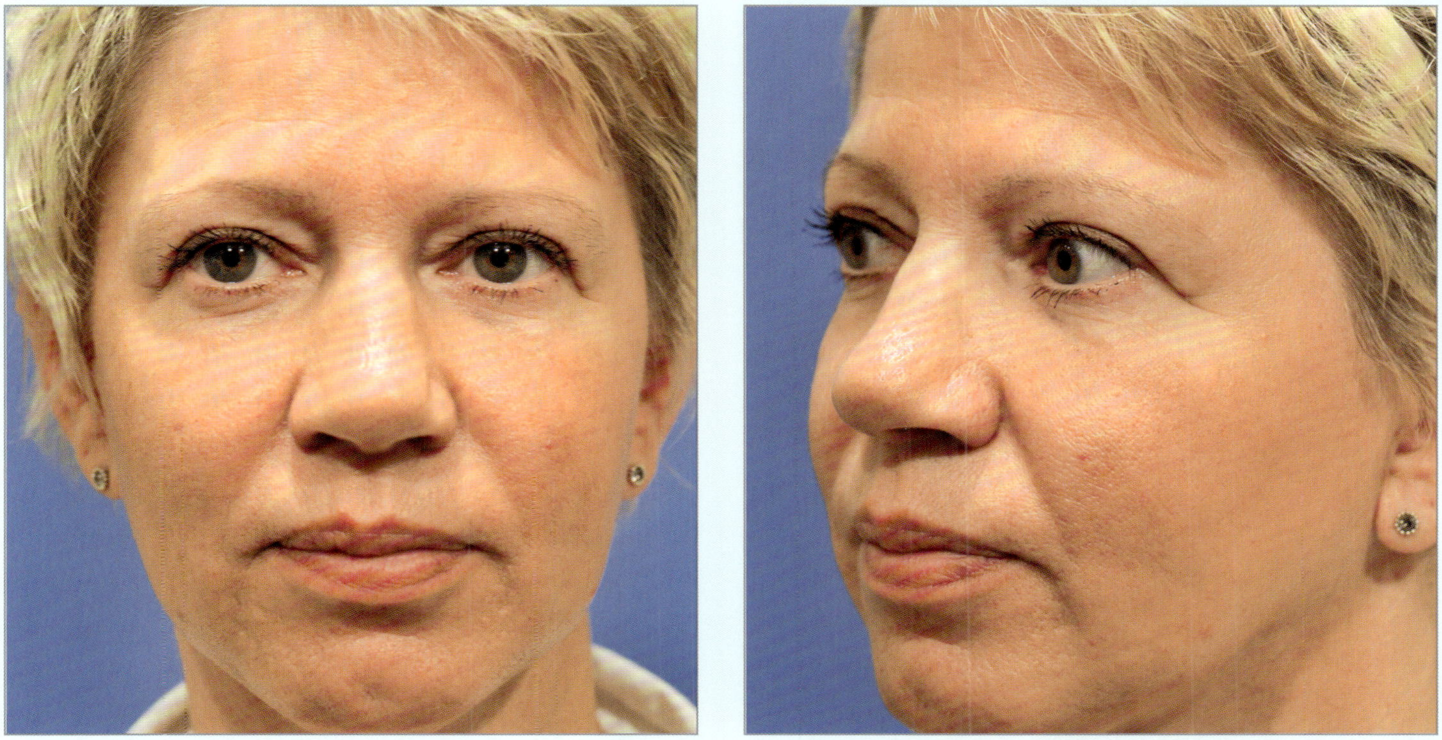

Result: 6 months after combination treatment, including: volume augmentation with a hyaluronic acid filler using the windmill technique in the cheeks, lower eyelids, nasolabial folds and marionette lines; alongside botulinum toxin type-A and Thermage® treatment in the forehead and chin.

Case 6 – Pronounced volume loss in the midface

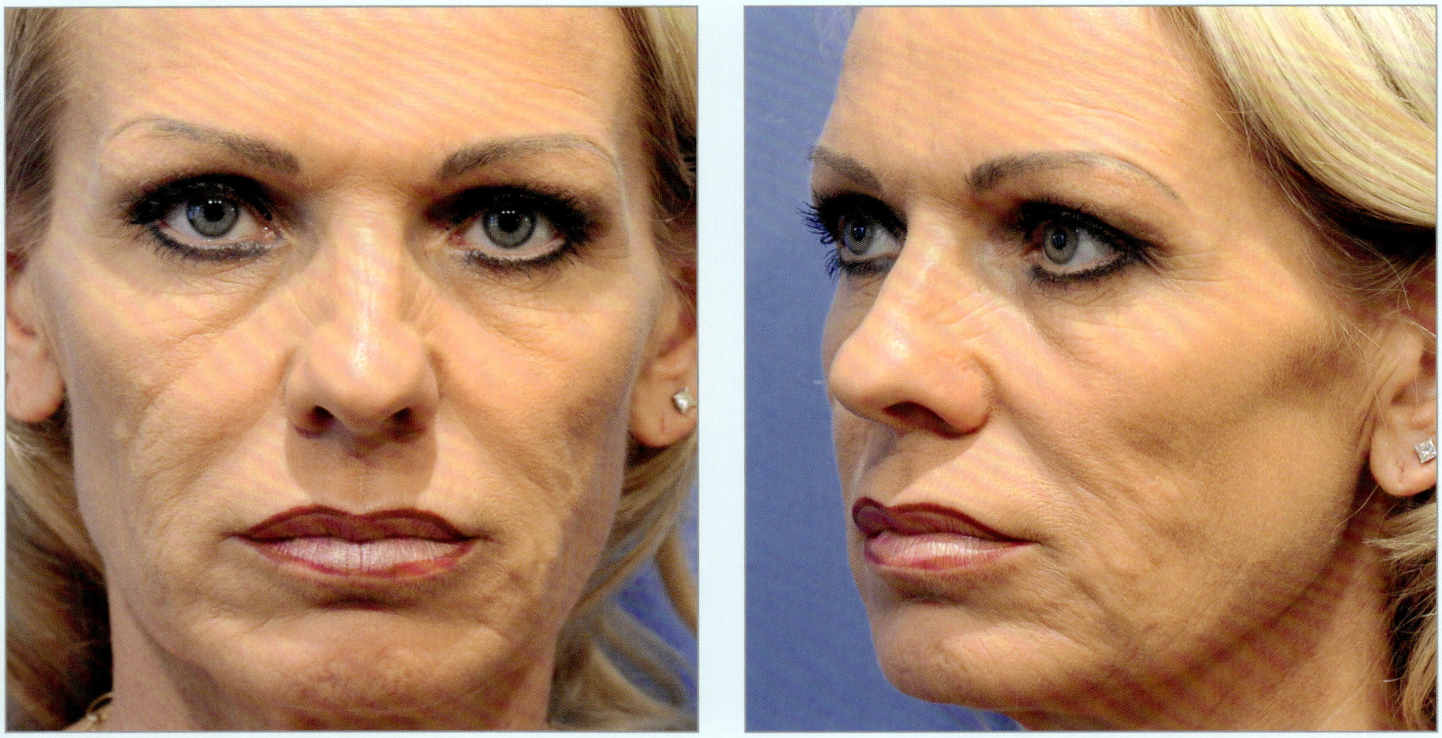

Baseline: 46-year-old female with pronounced loss of the midface volume alongside superficial elastosis in the cheek region.

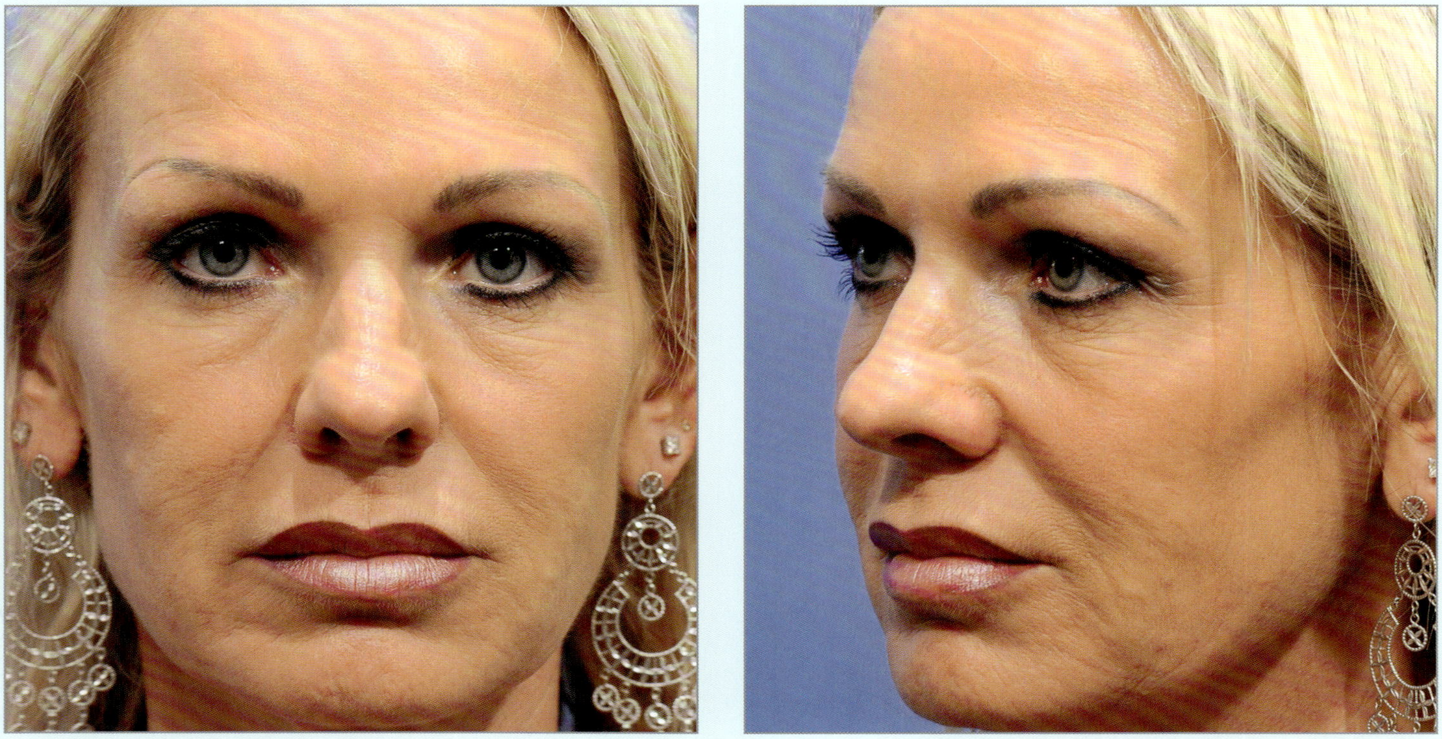

Result: 4 months after a single augmentation treatment using the windmill technique with a total of 8 ml of a hyaluronic acid filler injected.
Note: several treatments with botulinum toxin type-A have been performed prior to the filler augmentation.

Case 7 – Volume loss in the midface

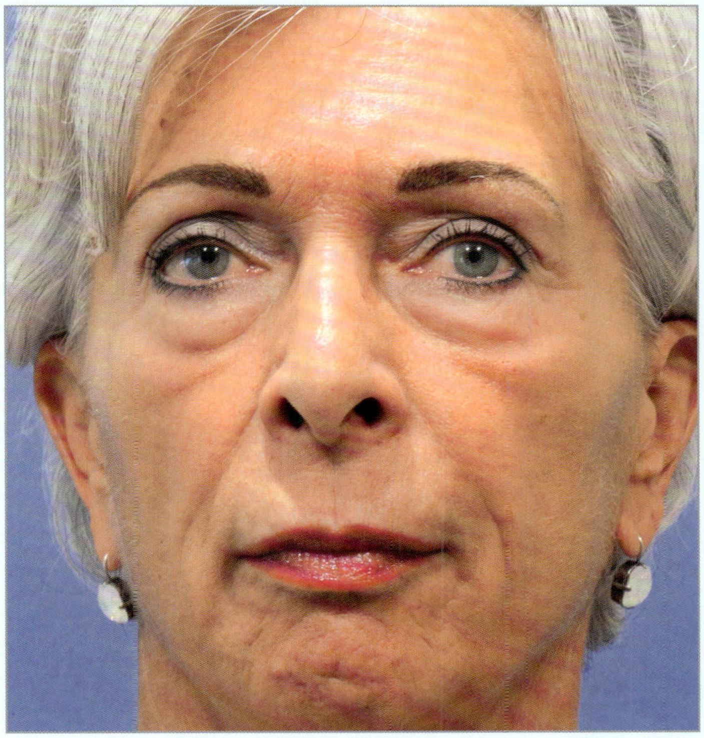

Baseline: 70-year-old female presenting with loss of volume in the midface despite a satisfactory facelift 3 years previously.

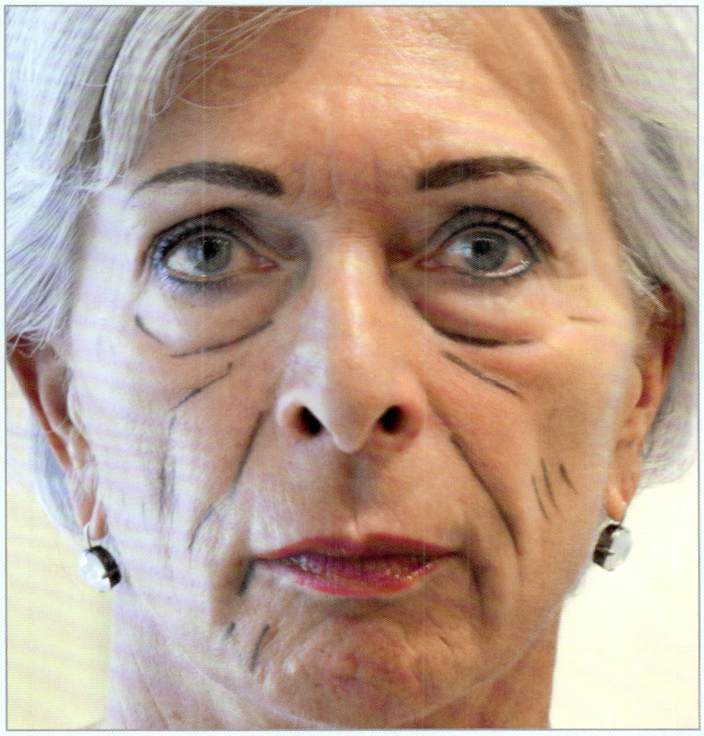

Skin markings highlight the focal areas of volume loss.

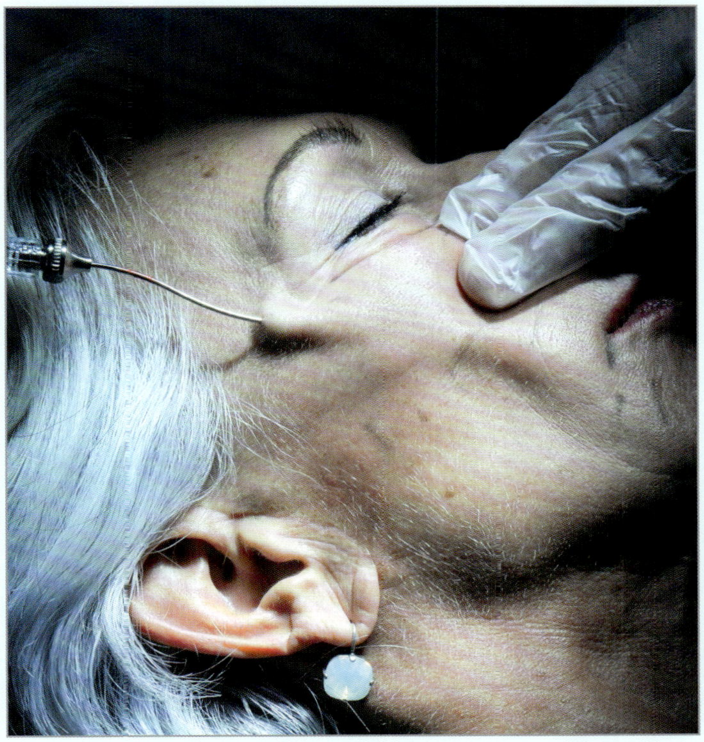

Light and shade contrast photograph highlighting the volume deficit and insertion of the cannula.

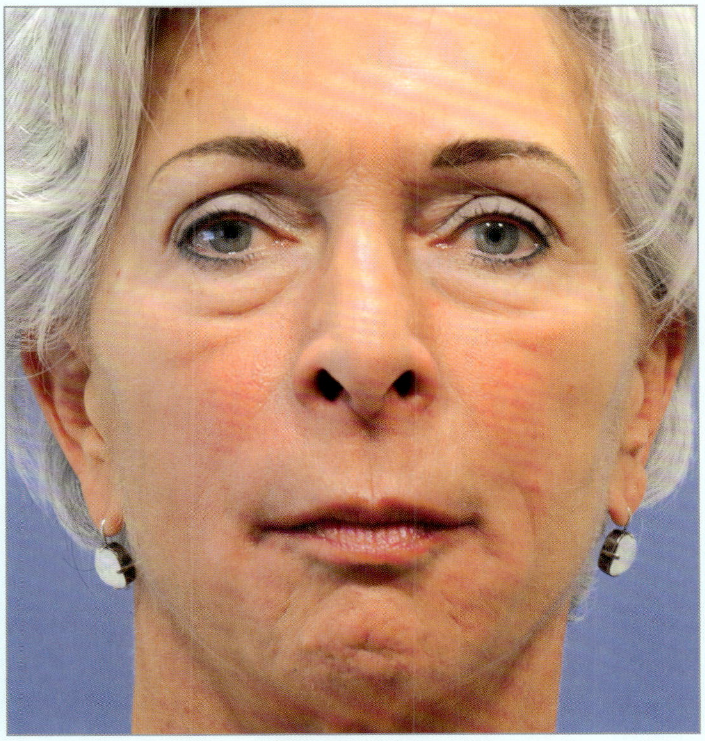

Result: Following 5 ml of hyaluronic acid filler injected into each cheek using the windmill technique.

Case 8 – Facial elastosis with volume loss

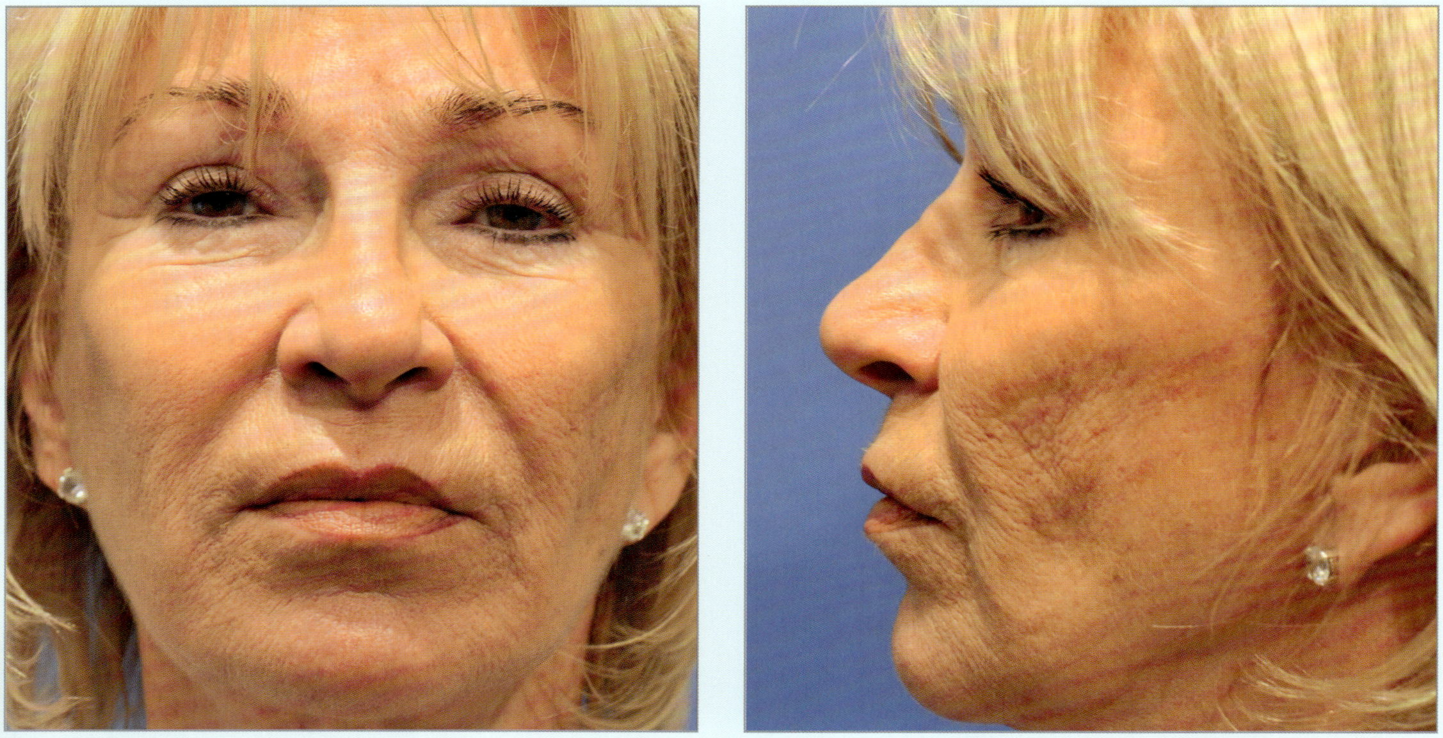

Baseline: 62-year-old female with senile elastosis and volume loss alongside prominent nasolabial folds.

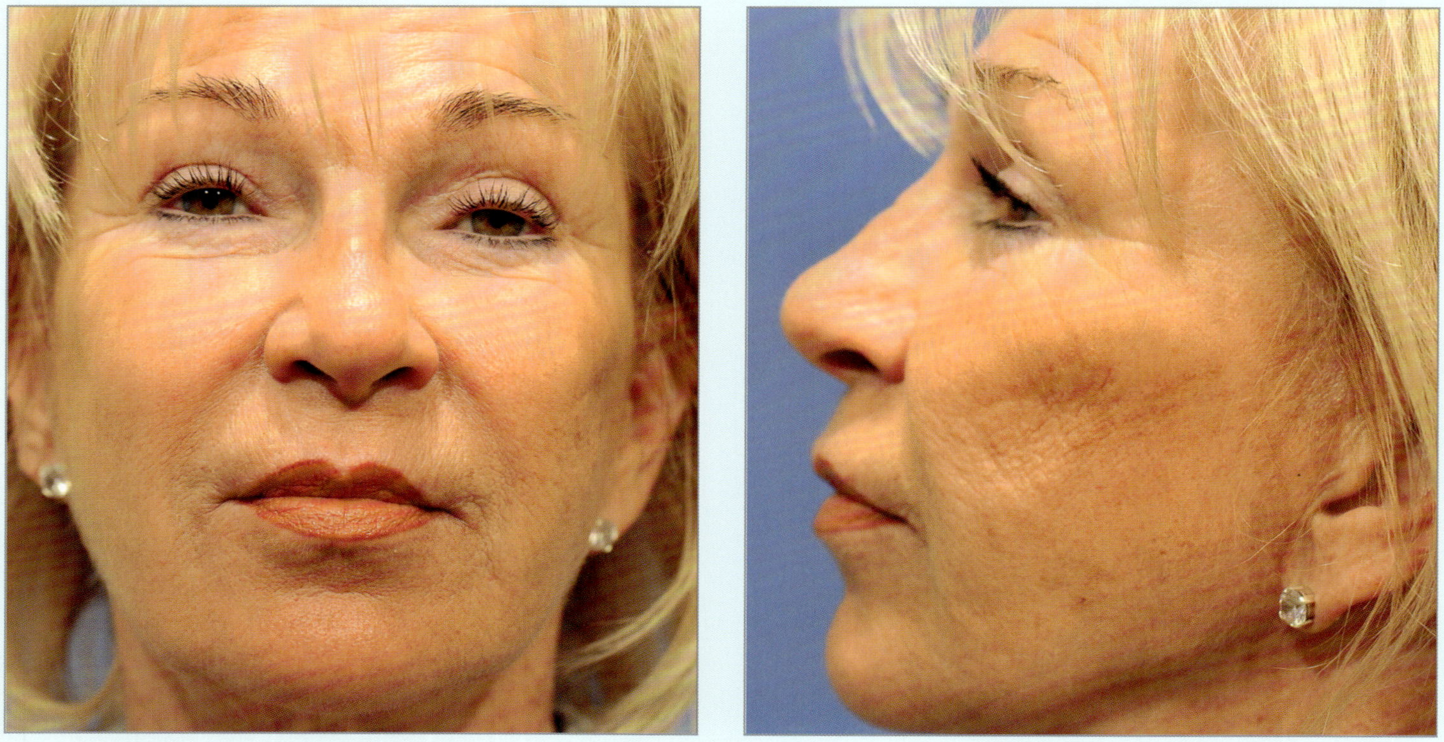

Result: 2 months after hyaluronic acid filler augmentation of the cheeks using the tower technique. The fine superficial wrinkles of the lower eyelid, the nasolabial folds and perioral region were treated with a total of 9 ml of a hyaluronic acid filler. No additional superficial augmentation or botulinum toxin type-A therapy was performed.

Case 9 – Pronounced nasolabial folds and marionette lines

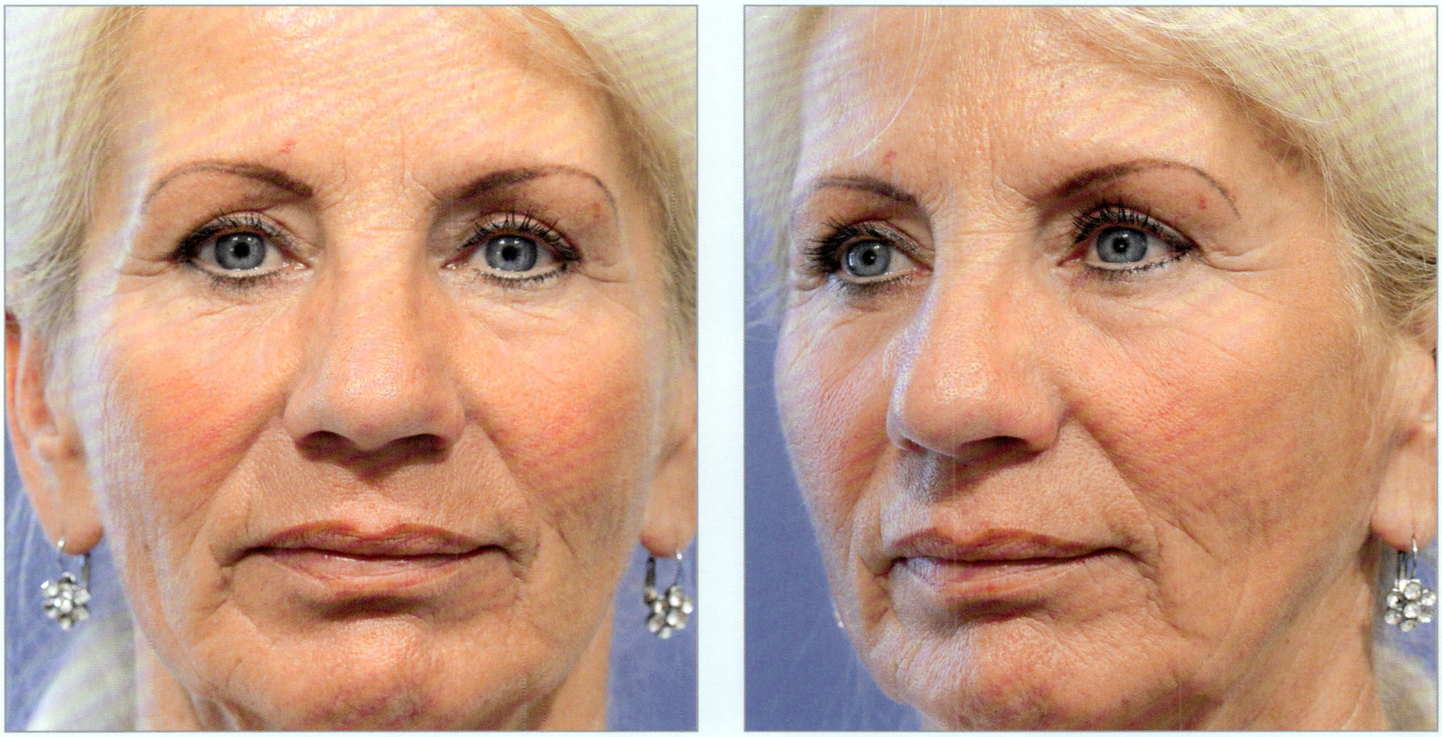

Baseline: 60-year-old female with pronounced nasolabial folds, marionette lines and incipient midface volume loss alongside moderate superficial elastosis.

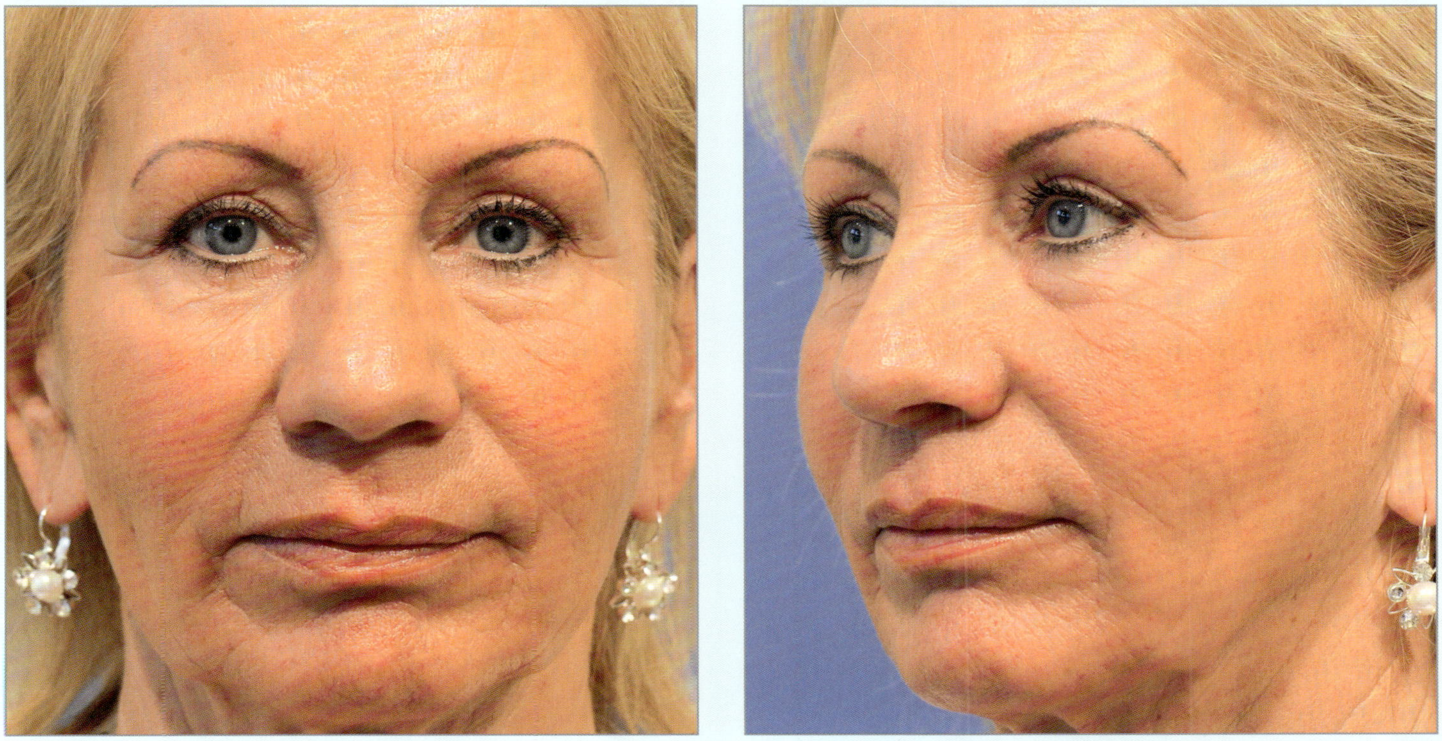

Result: 6 months after volume augmentation of the nasolabial folds, marionette lines and the cheek region using the tower technique. Additional superficial wrinkle augmentation using the stretching technique with linear injections around the mouth and the cheek region was also performed.

Case 10 – Perioral lines

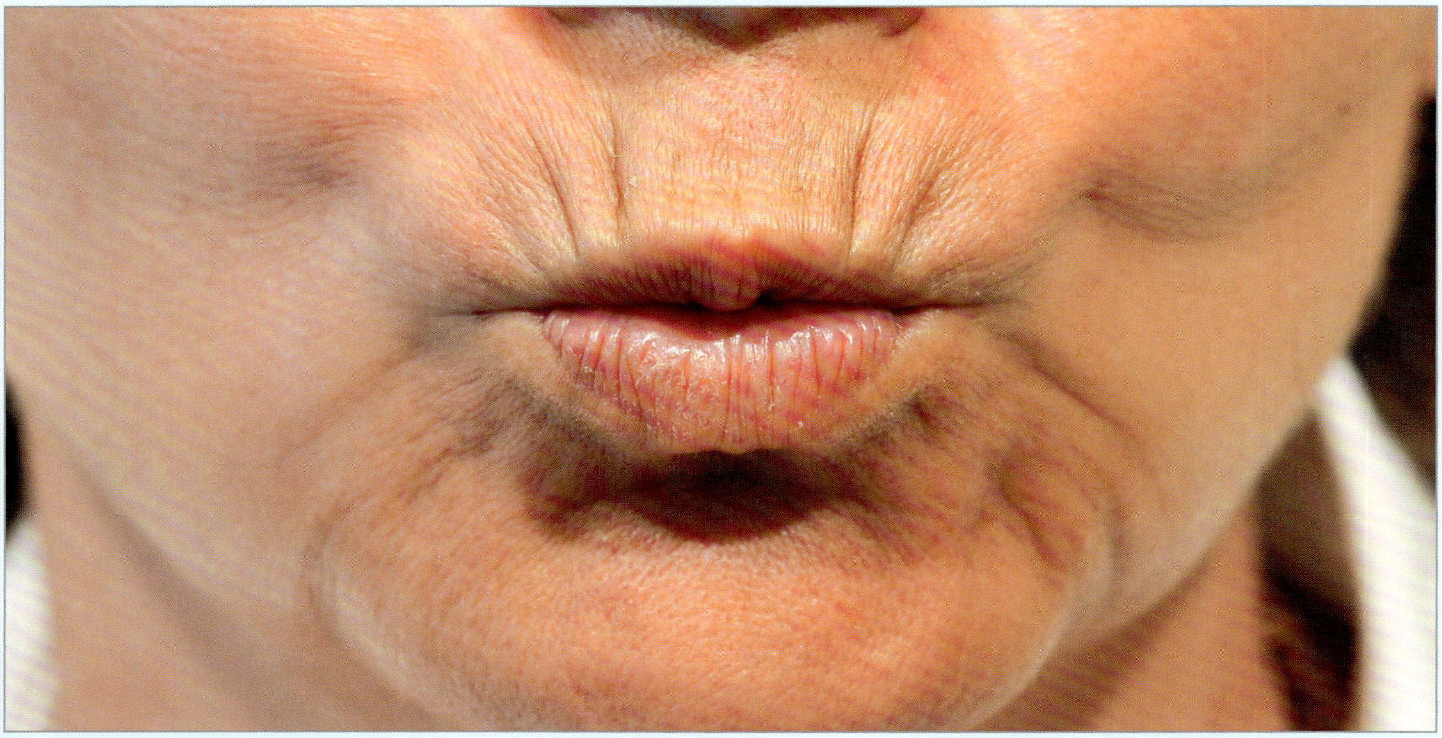

Baseline: 57-year-old female with pronounced perioral lines.

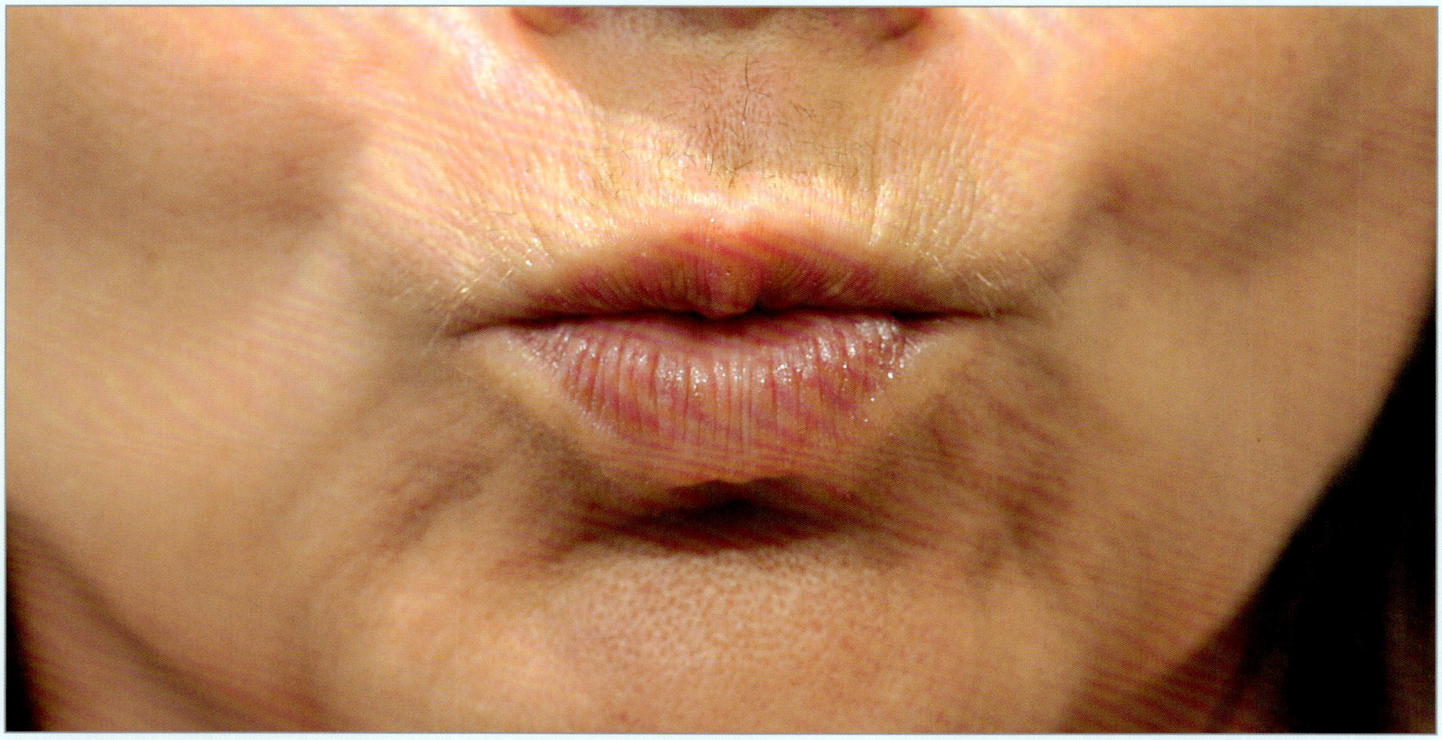

Result: 8 weeks after hyaluronic acid augmentation (total volume of 0.6 ml) used to smooth the skin relief with the forced stretching and linear injection techniques. Result obtained without the use of botulinum toxin type-A therapy.

Case 11 – Perioral lines

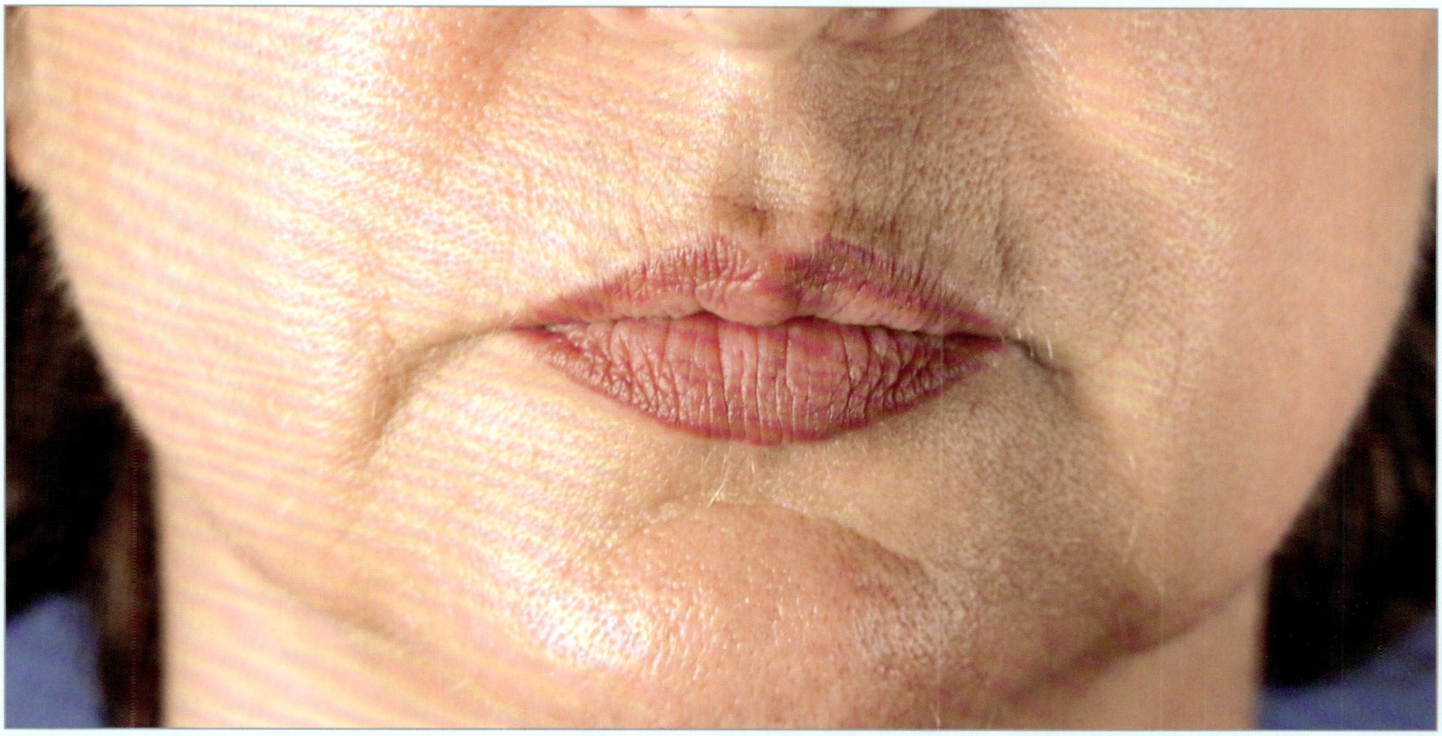

Baseline: 54-year-old female with perioral lines, marionette lines and incipient lip volume deficit.

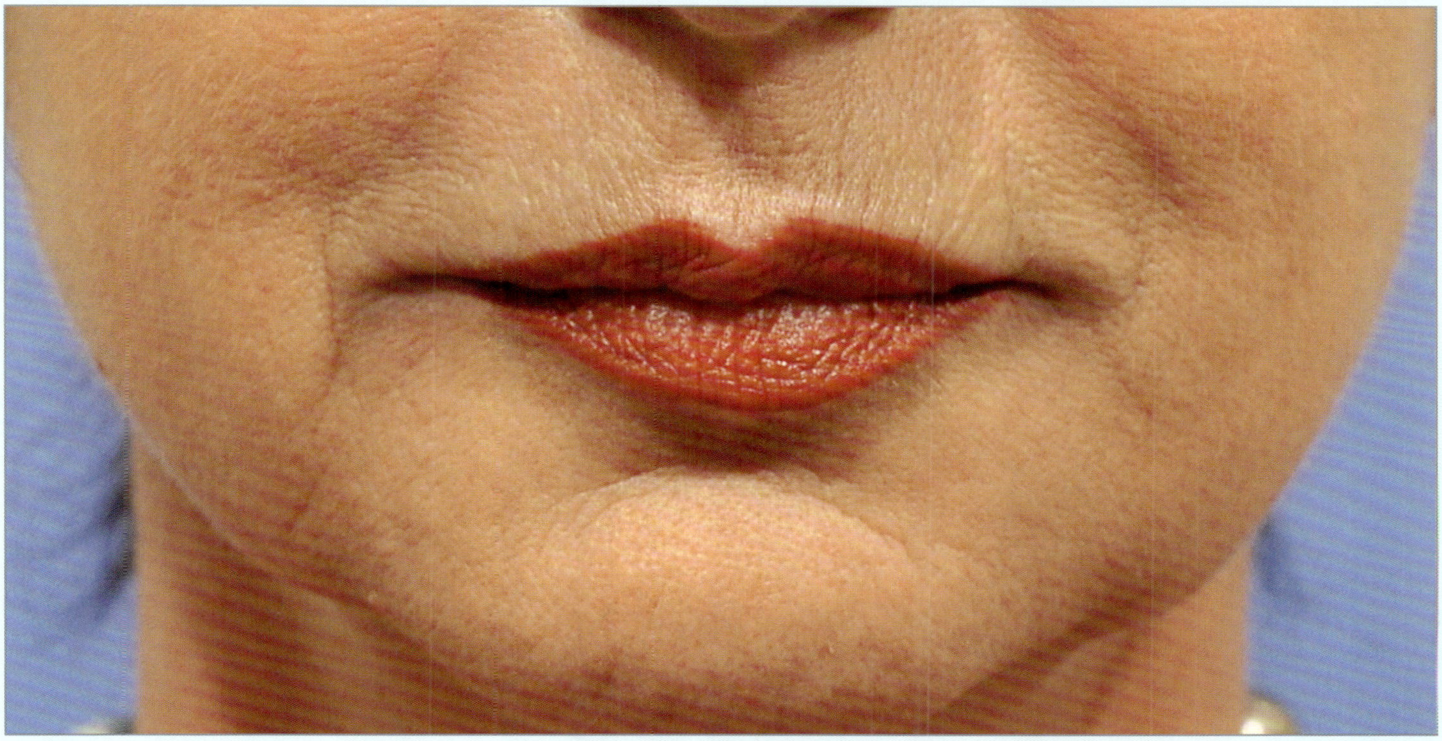

Result: 6 months after treatment with: poly-l-lactic acid (extensively) in the perioral area; augmentation of the radial lines with a hyaluronic acid filler using the stretching technique; volume replacement in the marionette line region with a hyaluronic acid filler; and augmentation of the lip margins with a hyaluronic acid filler.

Case 12 – Senile elastosis on the dorsal aspect of the hand

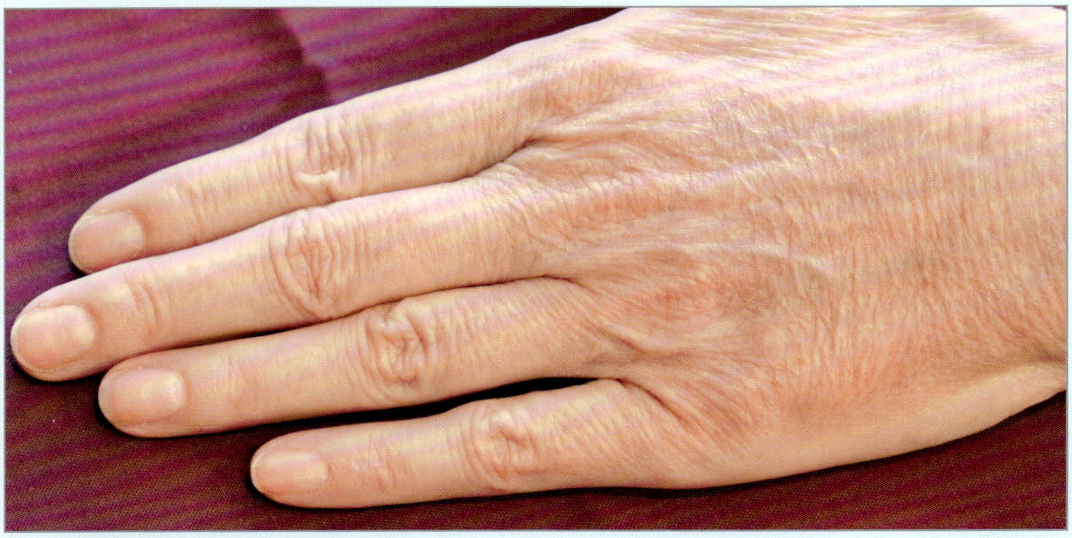

Baseline: 58-year-old female with pronounced senile elastosis on the back of the hand.

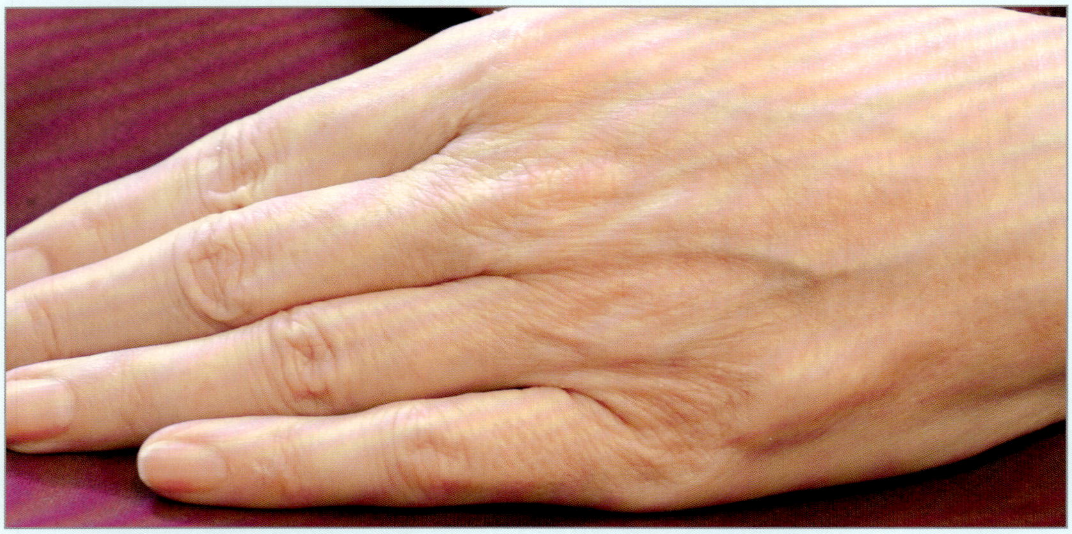

Result: following an injection of 5 ml of a hyaluronic acid filler using a cannula with the fanning technique in the dorsal aspect of the hands. Adjuvant treatment consisted of fractionated CO_2 laser therapy with FRAXEL REPAIR® at a total energy of 0.3 kJ.

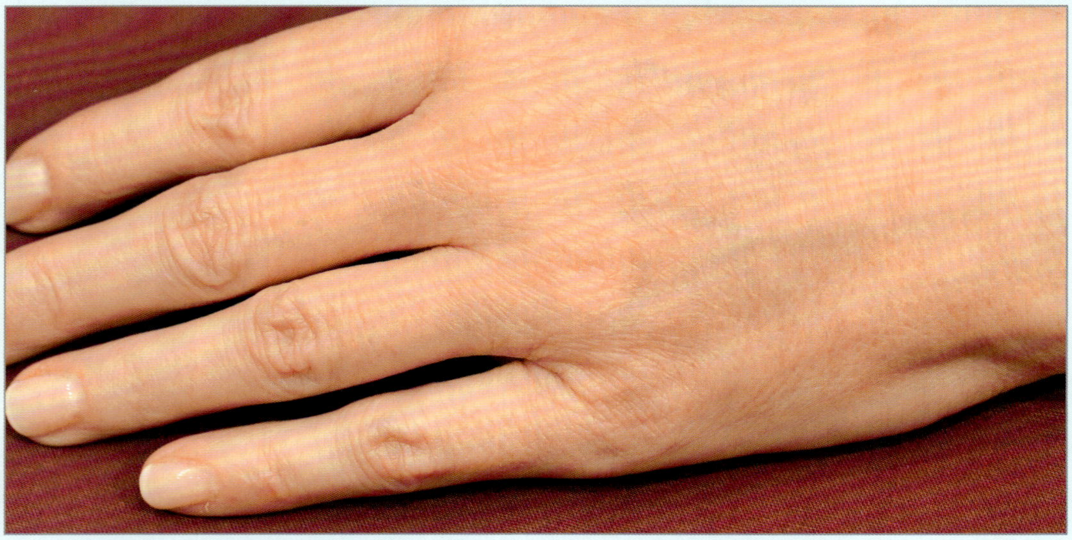

Clinical outcome 2 months post-treatment.

Case 13 – Incipient senile elastosis of the face

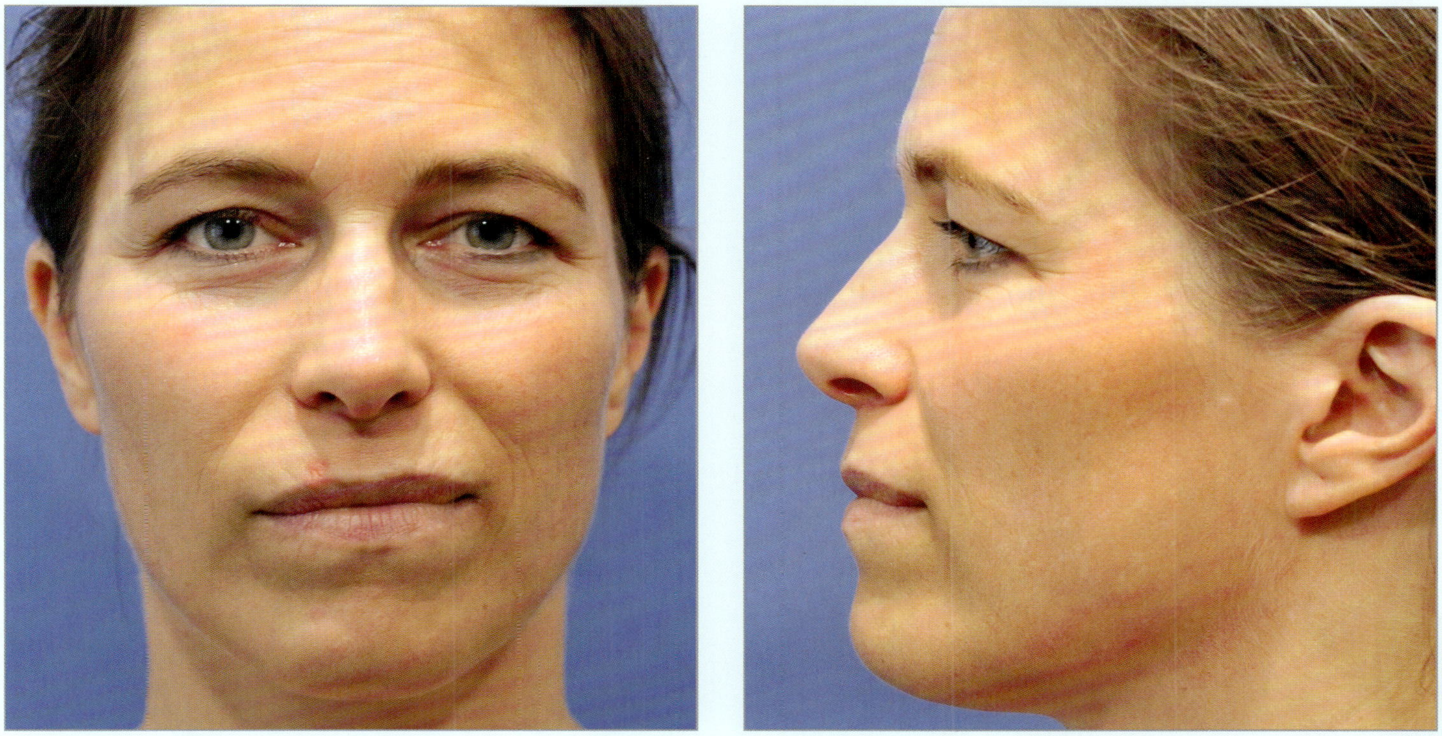

Baseline: 38-year-old female showing the initial signs of elastosis and volume loss in the periorbital, perioral and cheek region.

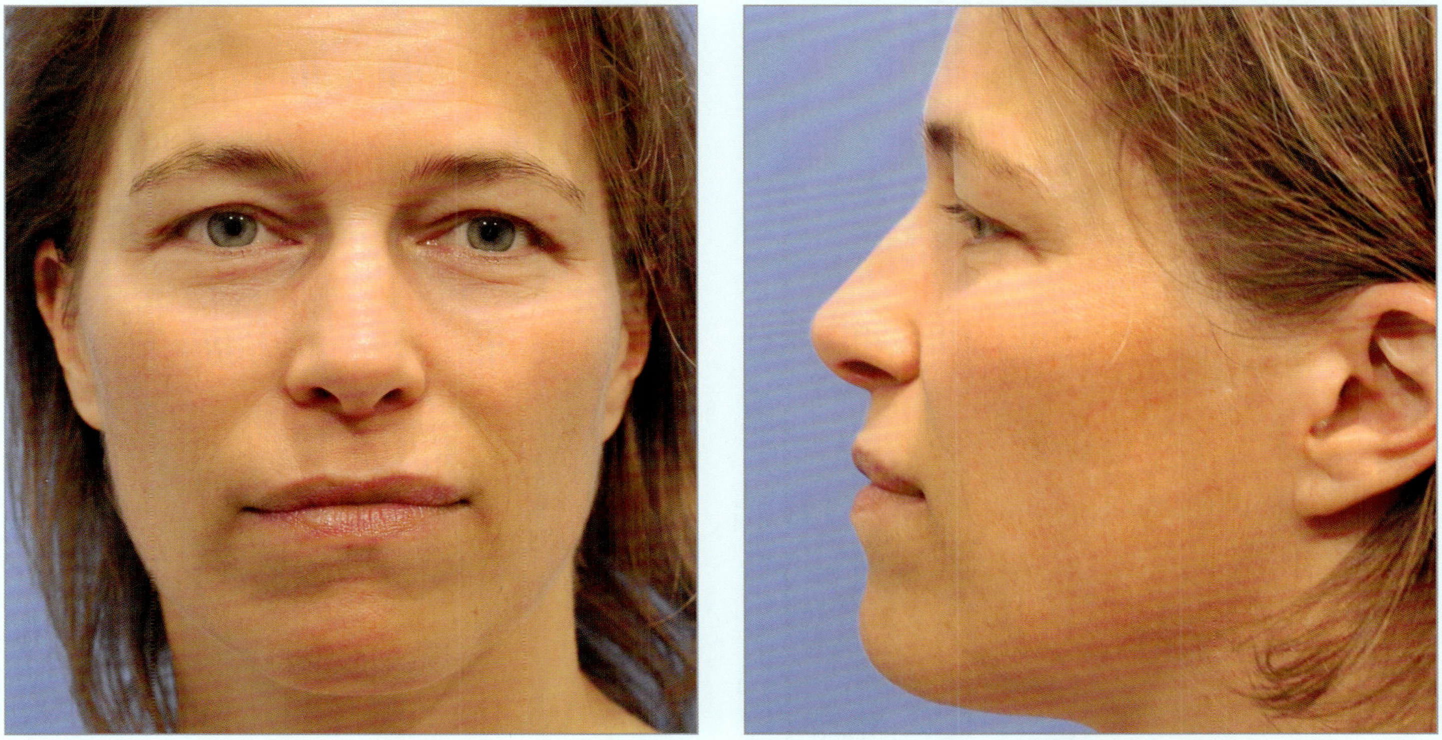

Result: 4 months after a single augmentation treatment with a hyaluronic acid filler injected vertically into the infraorbital hollow, cheeks and around the mouth. Harmonisation of the lips has been achieved with vertical injections in the white upper and lower lip (compare with Ch. 7, p. 192 and 193). Adjuvant treatment with botulinum toxin type-A in the upper third of the face was also performed.

Case 14 – Incipient volume loss in the perioral and periorbital regions

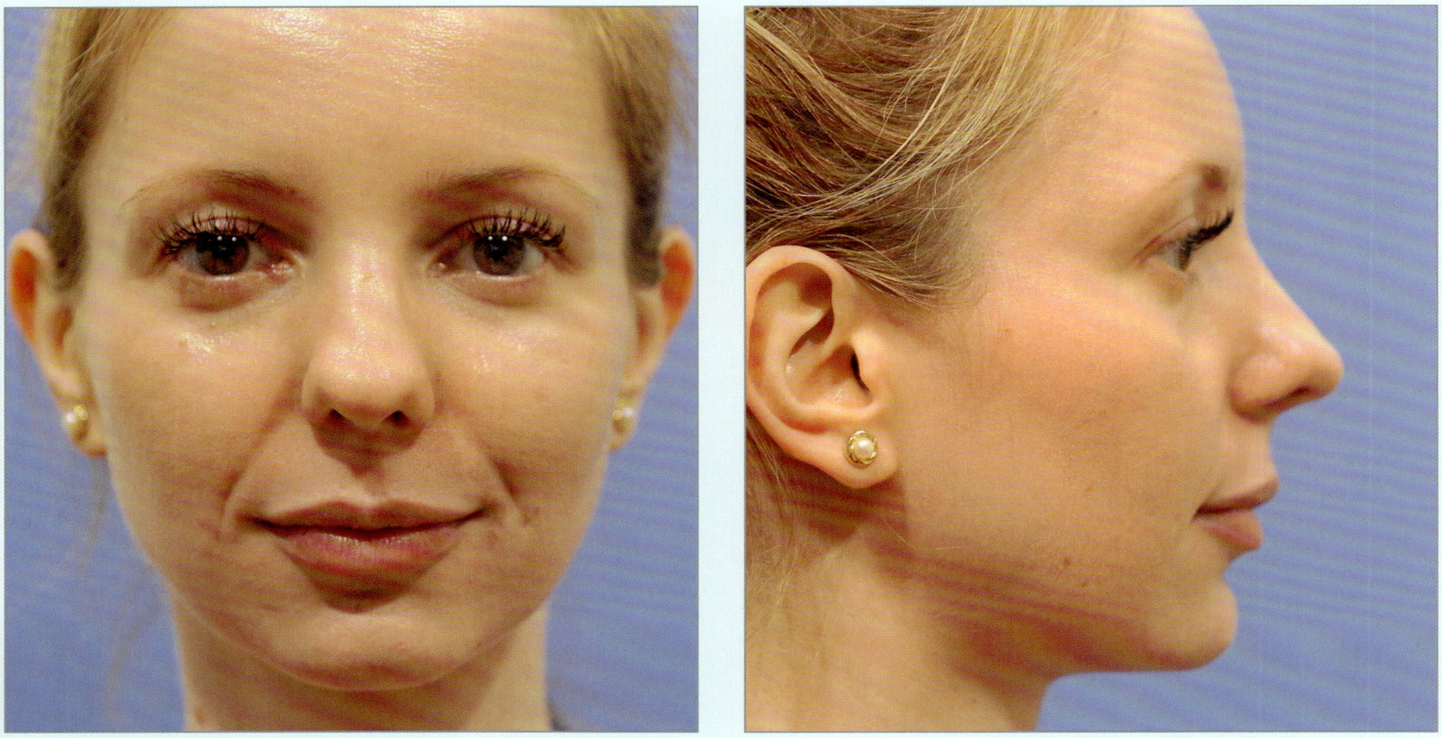

Baseline: 36-year-old female with incipient volume loss in the periorbital and perioral regions.

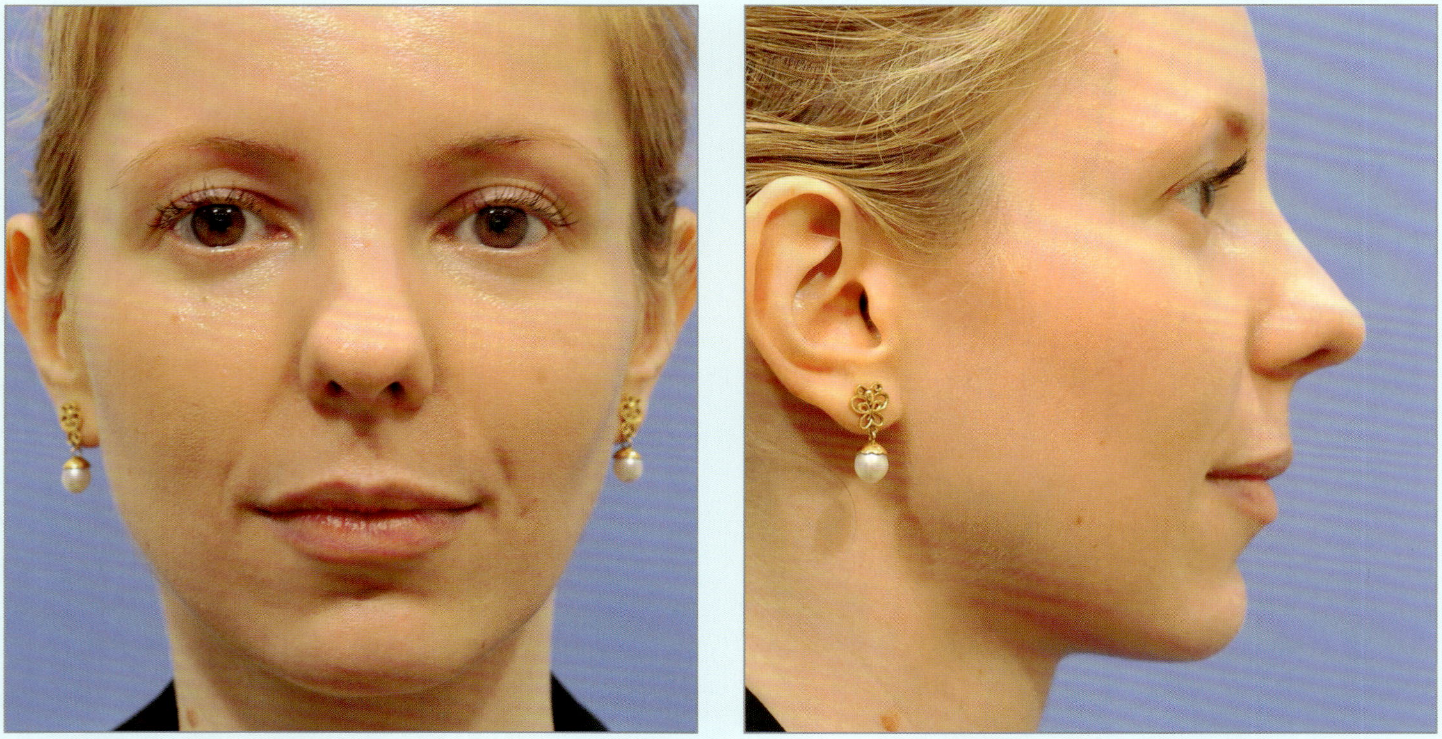

Result: 3 months after a single augmentation treatment using a total volume of 3 ml of a hyaluronic acid filler injected vertically into the infraorbital hollow and around the mouth. Harmonisation of the lips has been achieved with vertical injections in the white upper and lower lip (compare with Ch. 7, p. 192 and 193).

Case 15 – Asymmetrical lips and a prominent tear trough

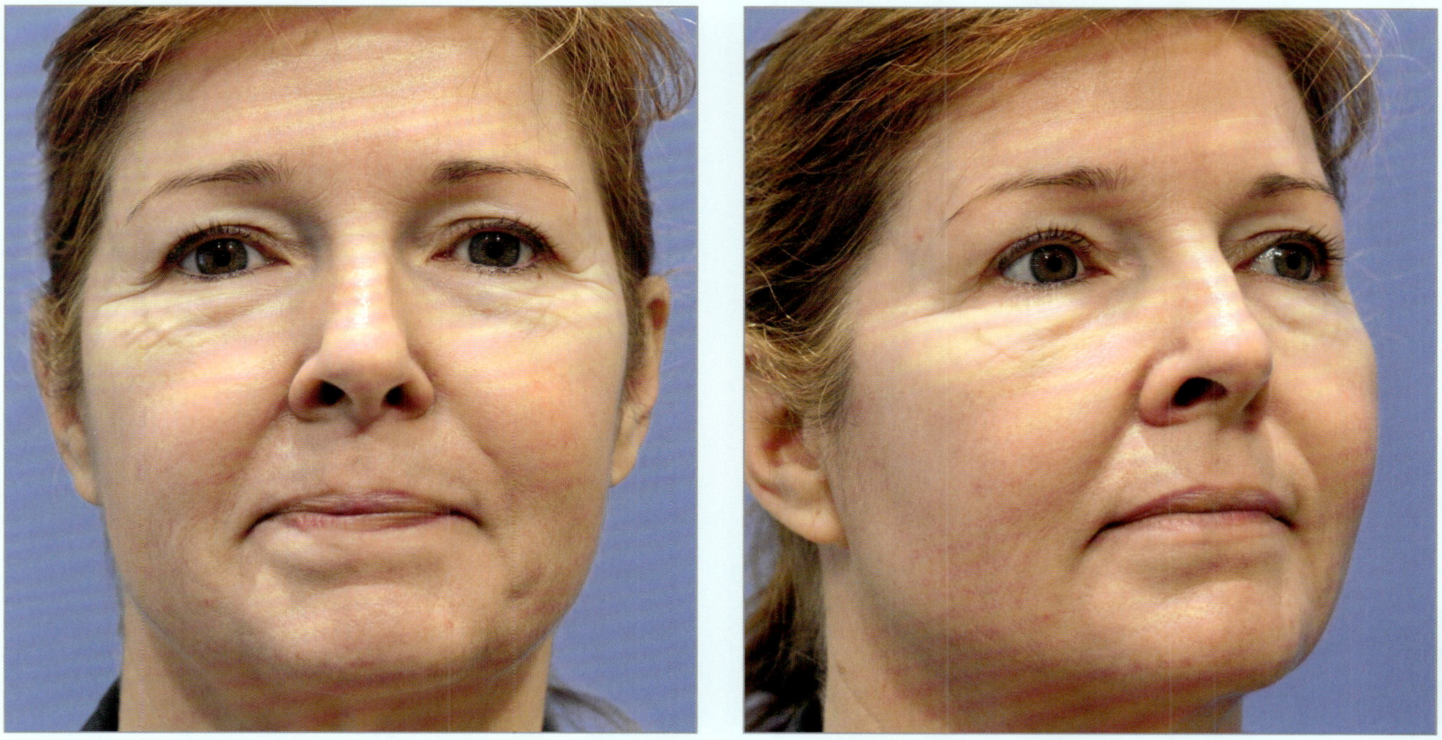

Baseline: 52-year-old female with incipient elastosis and volume loss around the eyes, mouth and cheeks. Furthermore, a marked asymmetry of the red lips is noted, particularly when assessed in dynamic repose.

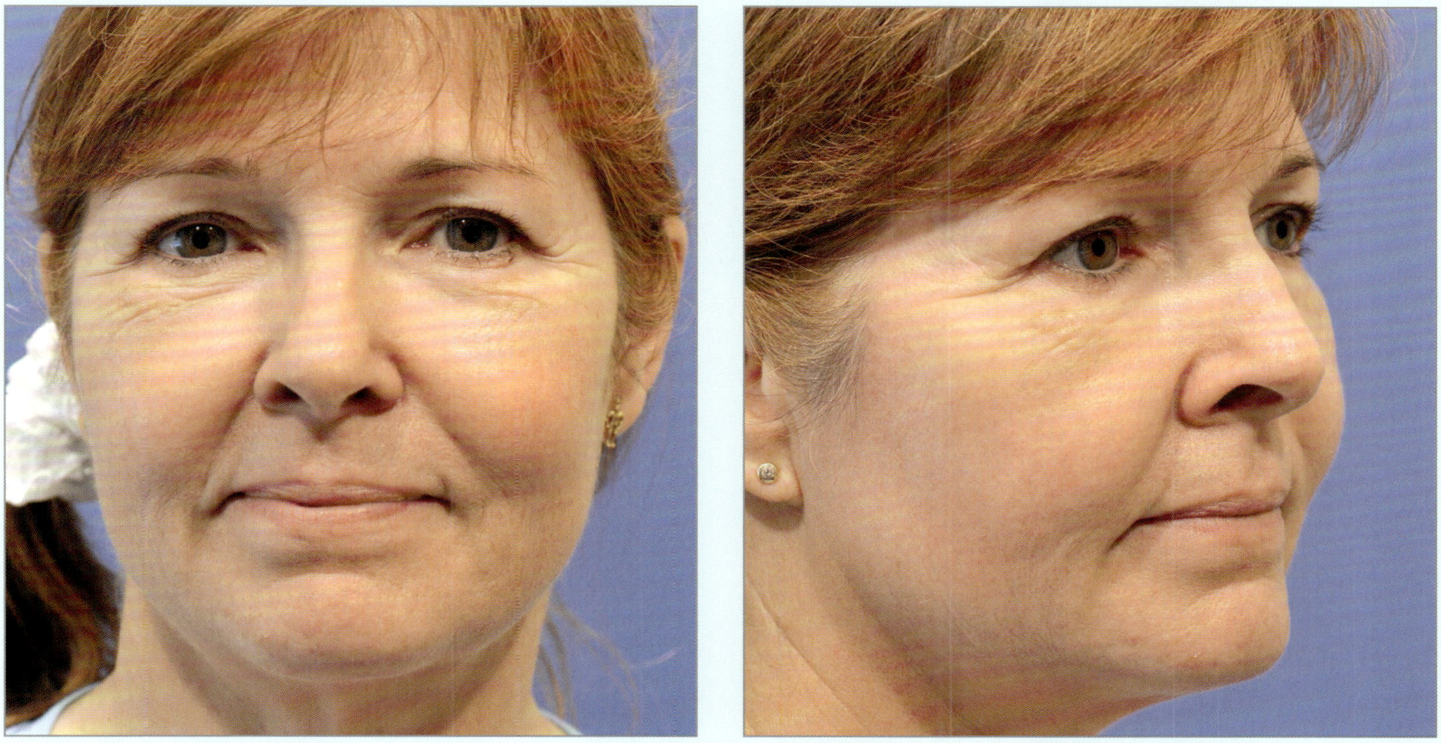

Result: 6 months after a single augmentation treatment with a hyaluronic acid filler using the vertical injection technique. A total volume of 3 ml was injected.

Case 16 – Advanced facial elastosis

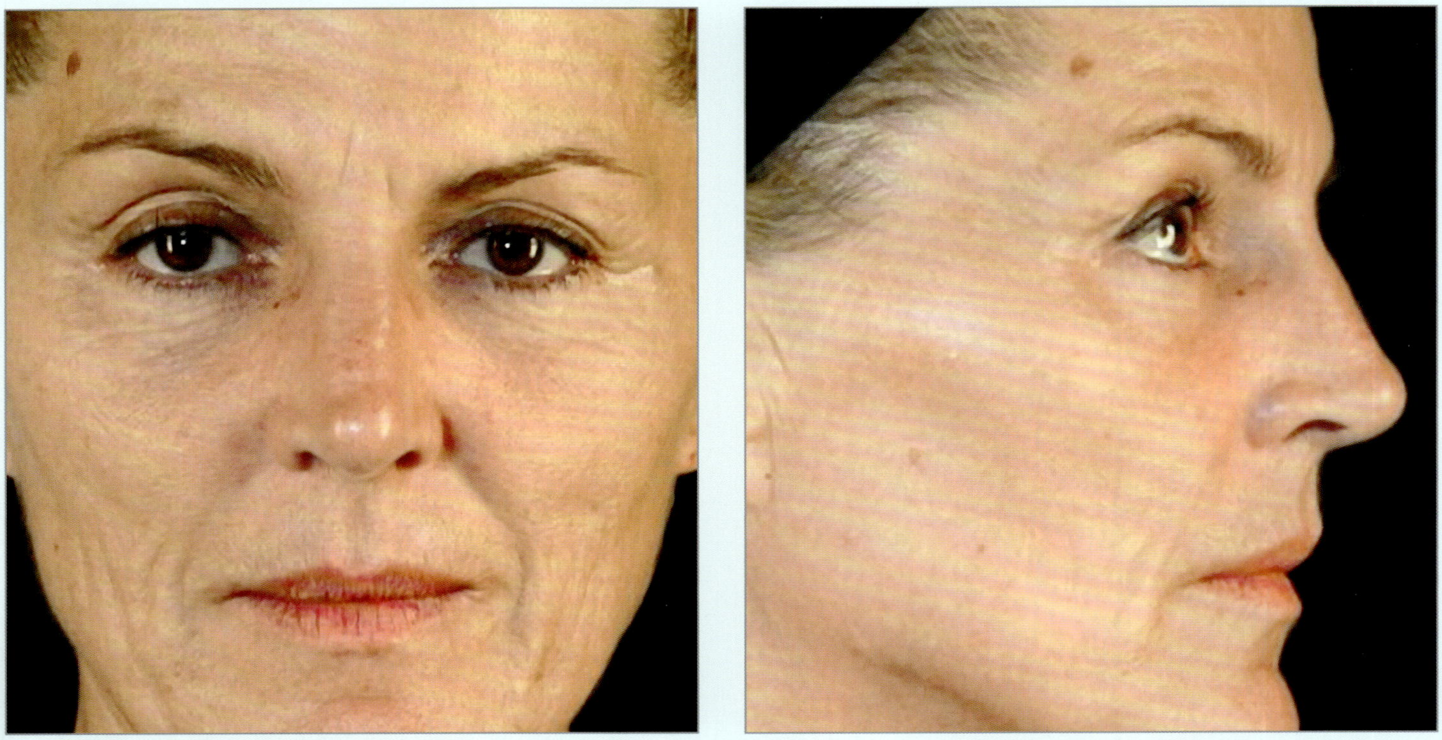

Baseline: 53-year-old female with global volume loss alongside senile elastosis.

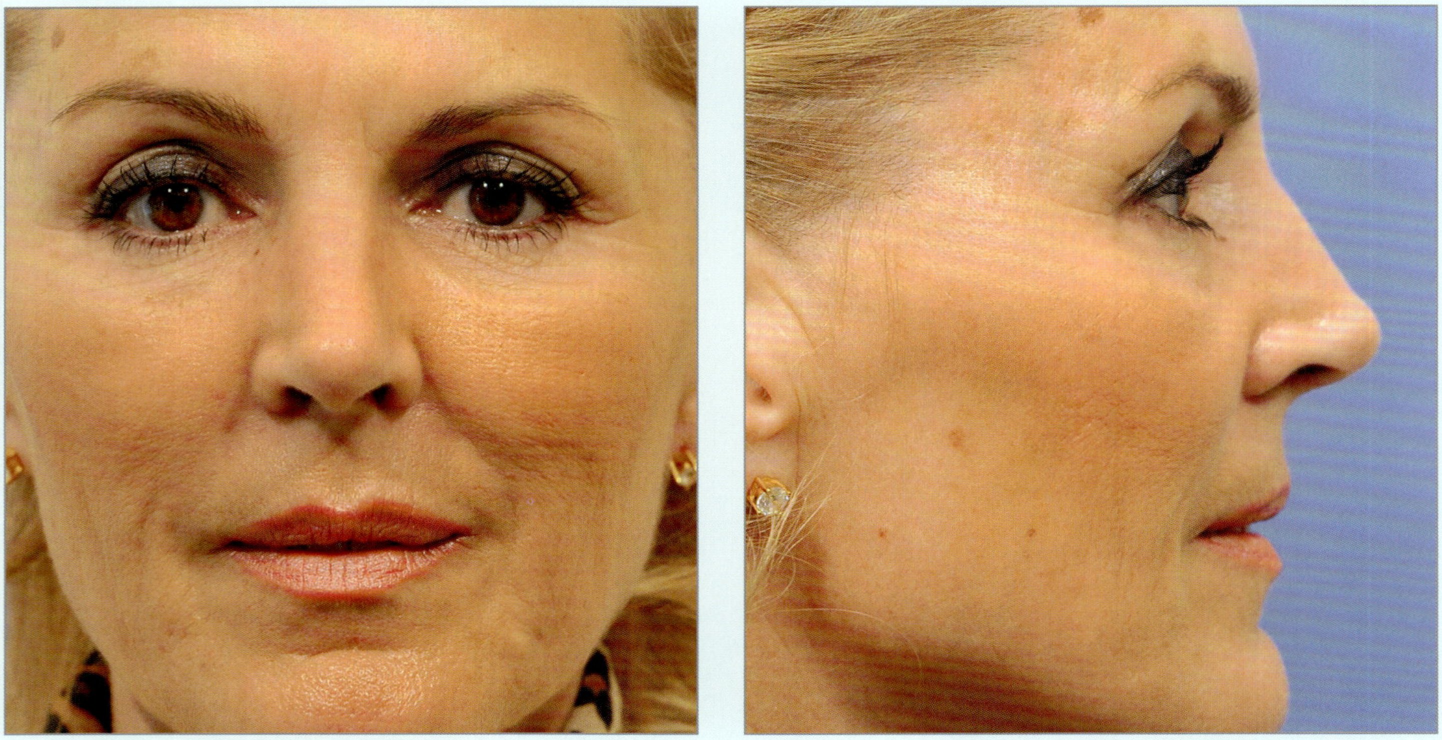

Result: 3 years after three augmentation treatments using hyaluronic acid fillers injected vertically into the infraorbital hollow and around the month. A total volume of 8 ml was injected. Additionally, four adjuvant treatments with botulinum toxin type-A in the forehead and glabellar region were performed.

Case 17 – Advanced elastosis and volume loss

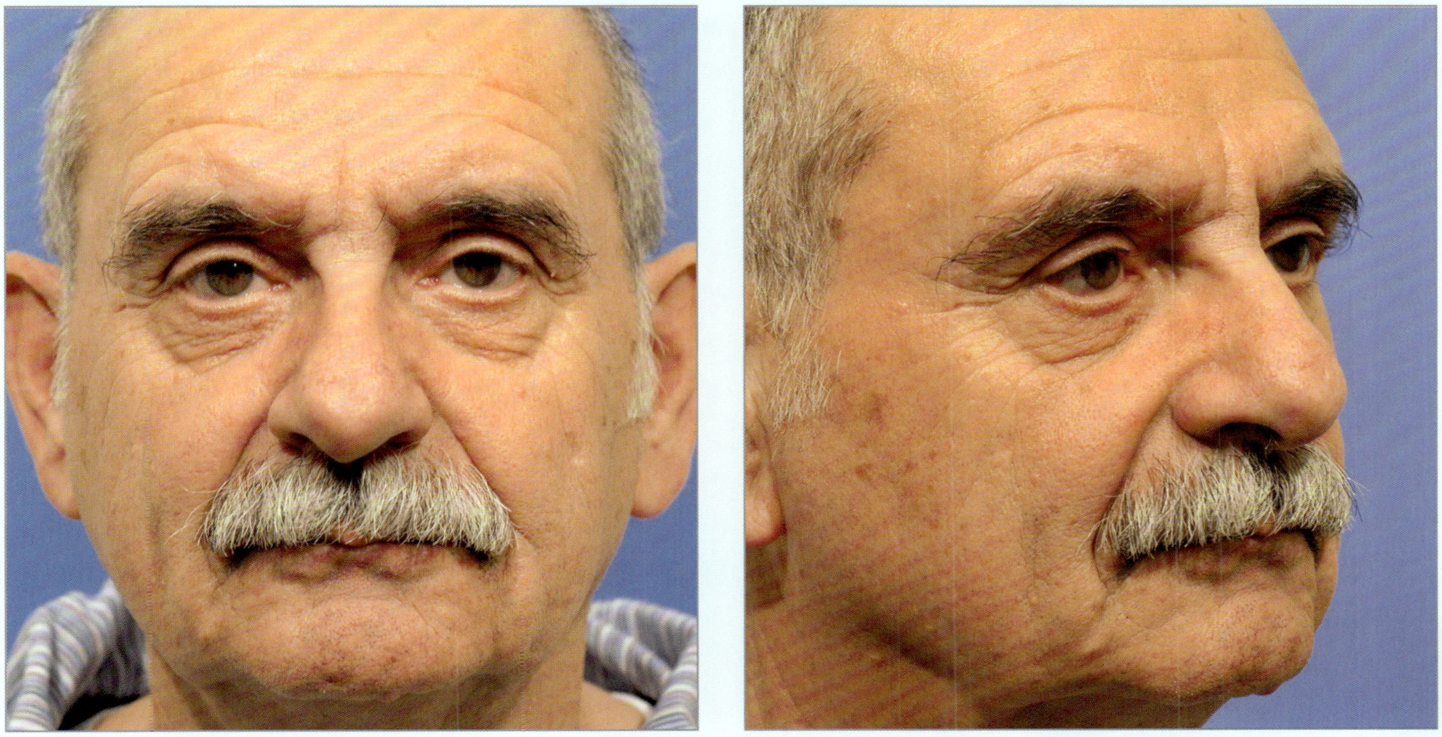

Baseline: 68-year-old male with advanced elastosis and volume loss around the eyes, mouth and cheeks. Furthermore, pronounced forehead and glabellar lines are also noted.

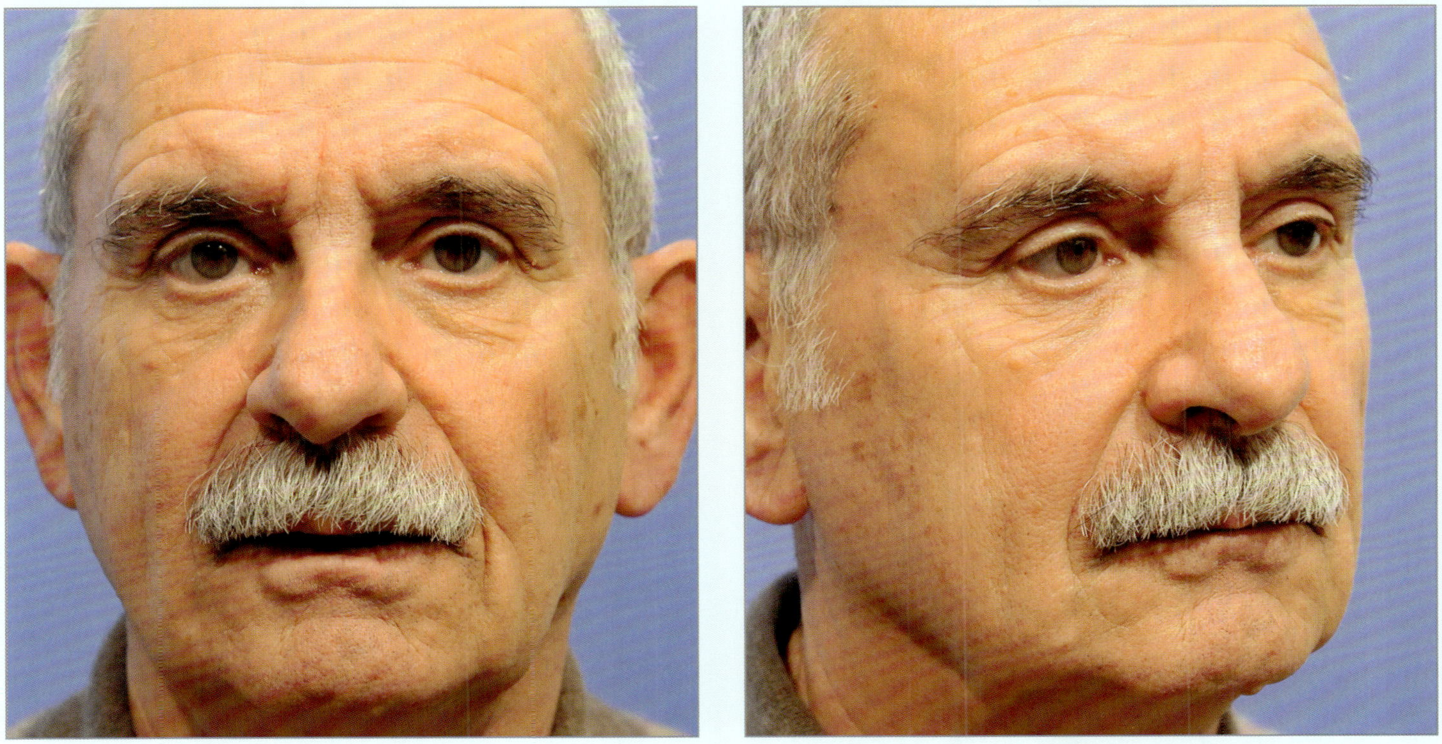

Result: 2 years after two augmentation treatments using a total volume of 6 ml of a hyaluronic acid filler injected vertically. Additionally, a further single botulinum toxin type-A treatment in the upper third of the face was performed.

Case 18 – Incipient elastosis and volume loss

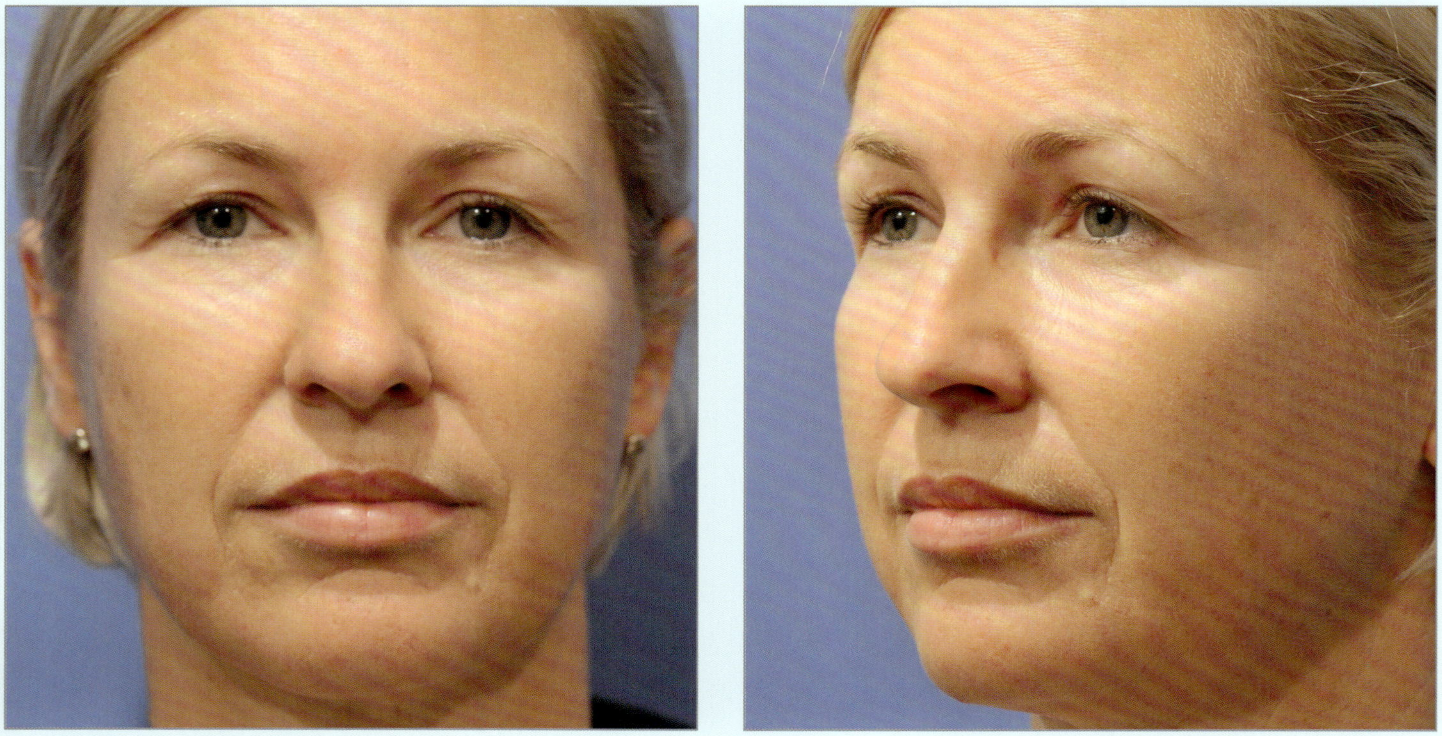

Baseline: 44-year-old female with incipient superficial elastosis and volume loss around the eyes, mouth and cheeks.

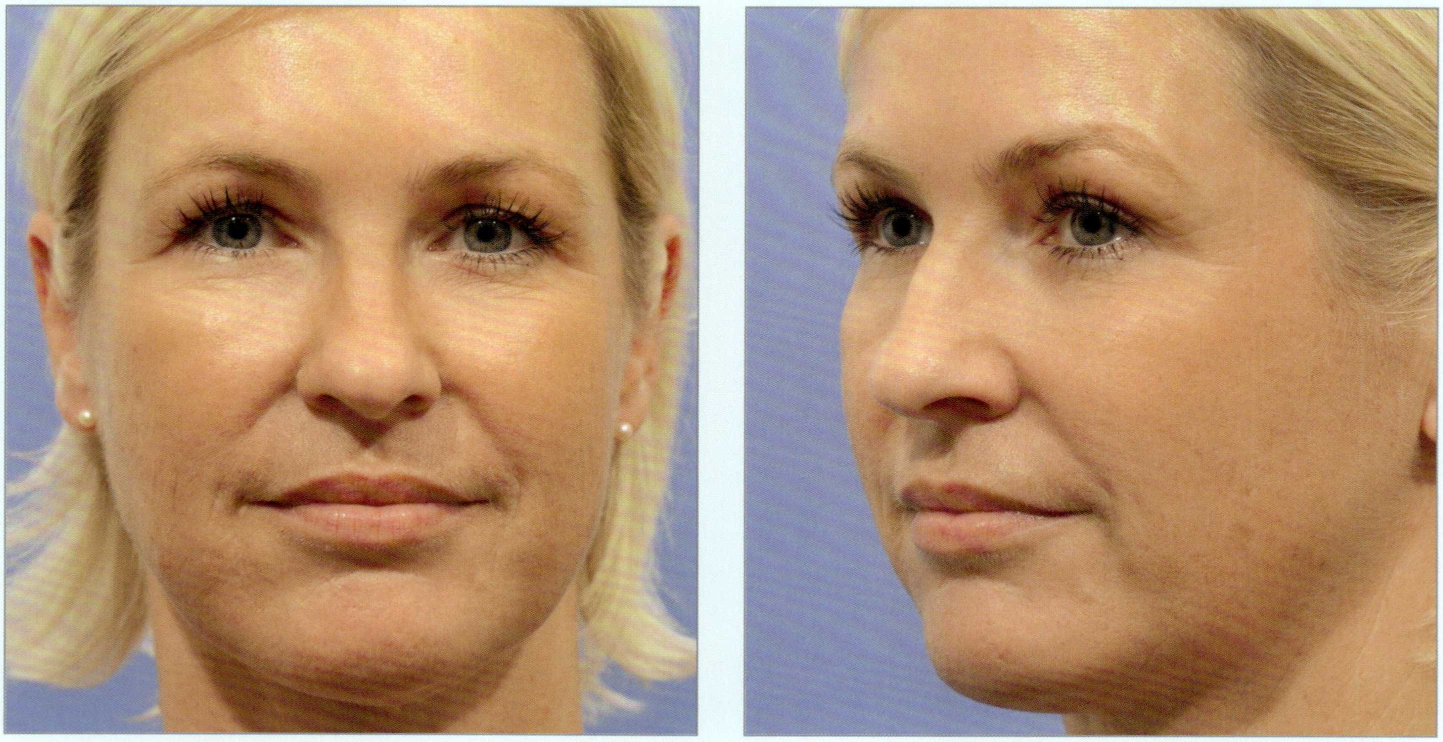

Result: 1 year after two augmentation treatments using a total of 6 ml of a hyaluronic acid filler injected vertically. A further two adjuvant treatments with botulinum toxin type-A were performed in the forehead and the glabellar region.

Case 19 – Advanced elastosis and volume loss

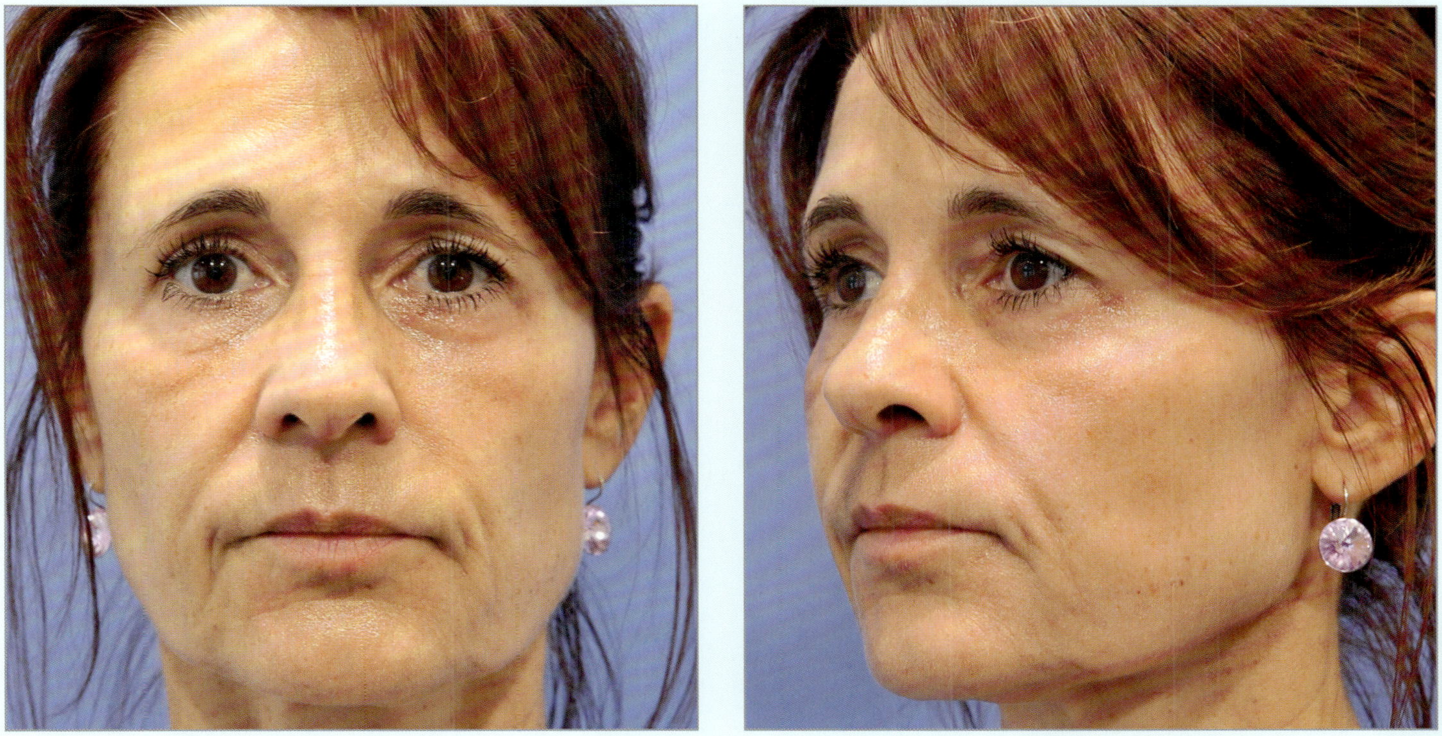

Baseline: 51-year-old female with pronounced superficial elastosis and volume loss around the eyes, mouth and cheeks.

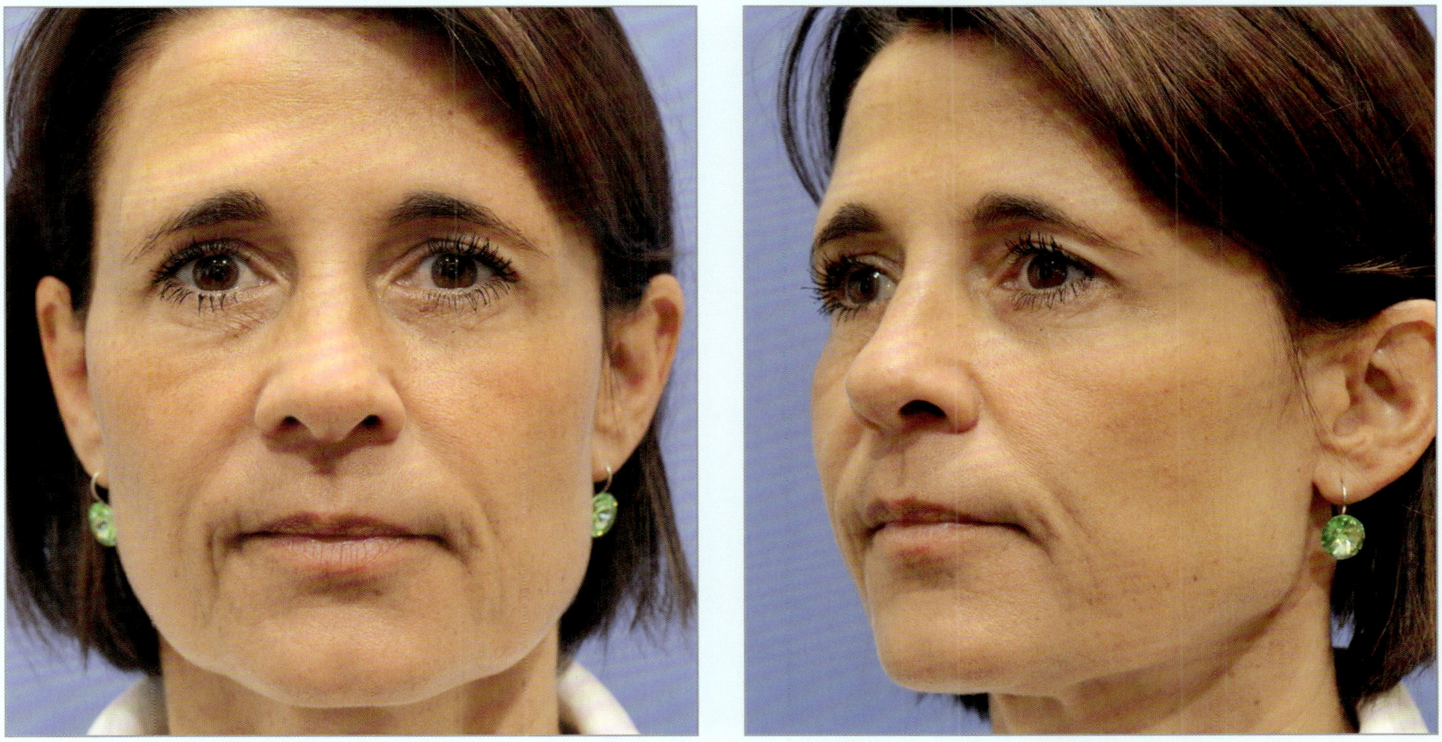

Result: 6 months after a single augmentation treatment with hyaluronic acid using the vertical injection technique. A total volume of 4 ml was injected. A single adjuvant treatment with botulinum toxin type-A in the forehead and the glabellar region was also performed.

Case 20 – Early perioral volume loss

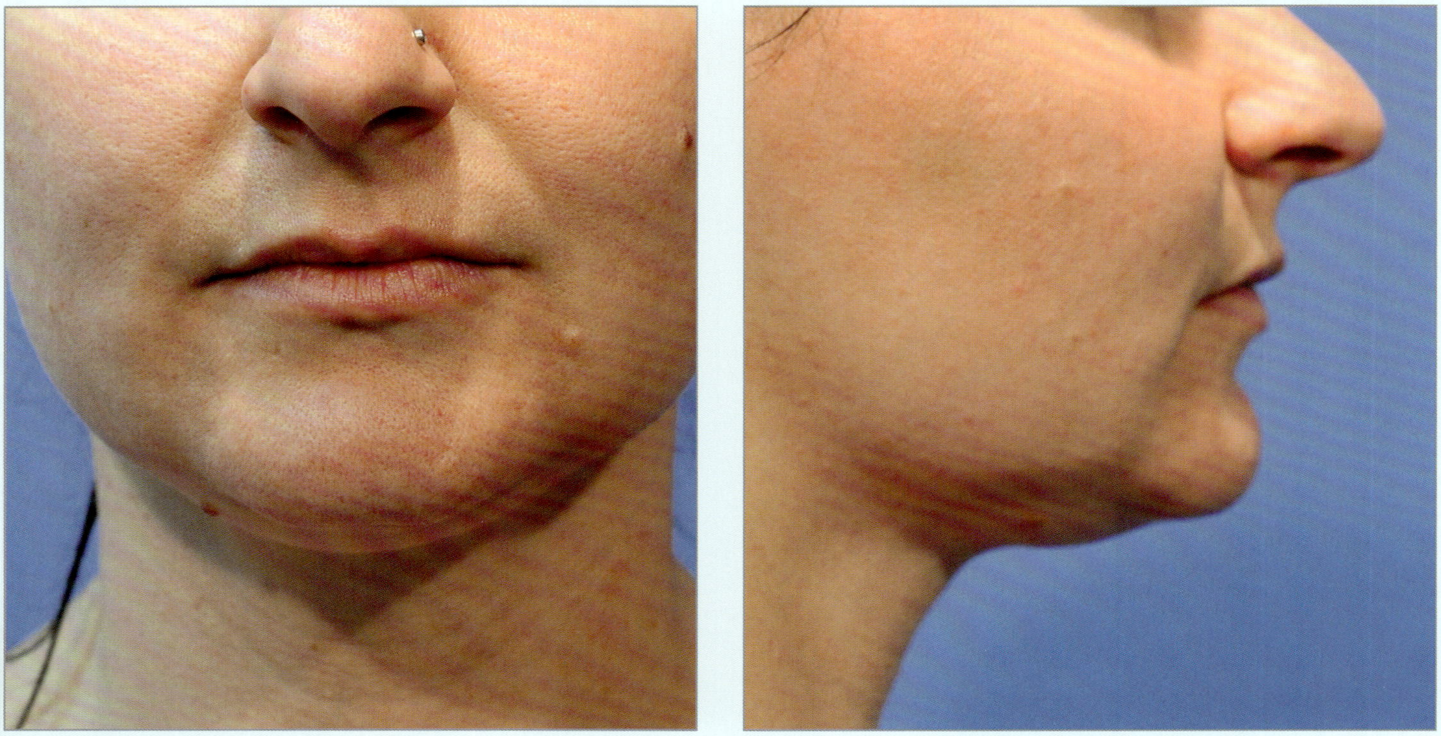

Baseline: 38-year-old female with advanced early volume loss around the mouth, particularly prominent at the marionette lines and in the region of the mandibular ligaments.

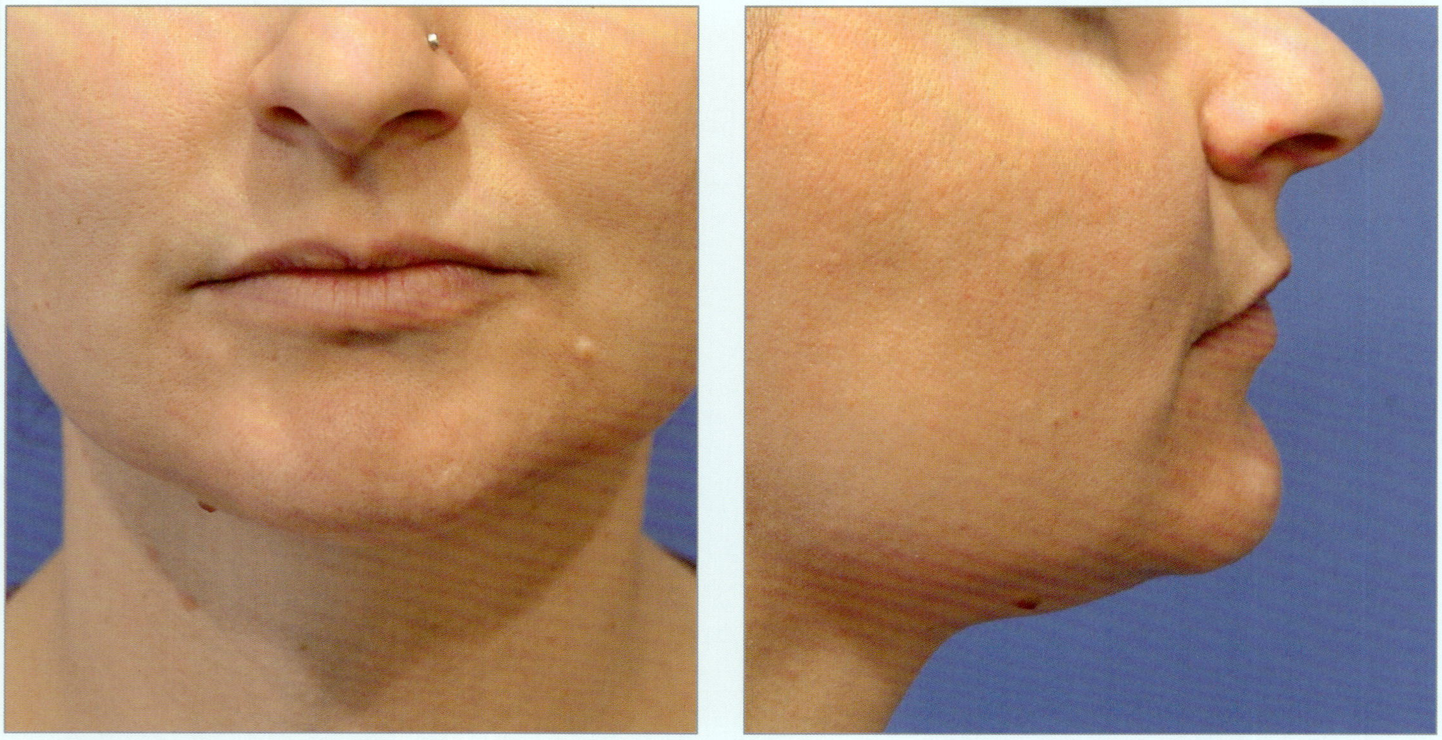

Result: 18 months after two augmentation treatments using a hyaluronic acid filler injected vertically into the ligaments, as well as horizontally at the marionette lines using a cannula. A total volume of 5 ml of a hyaluronic acid filler was injected.

Case 21 – Pronounced periorbital volume loss and elastosis

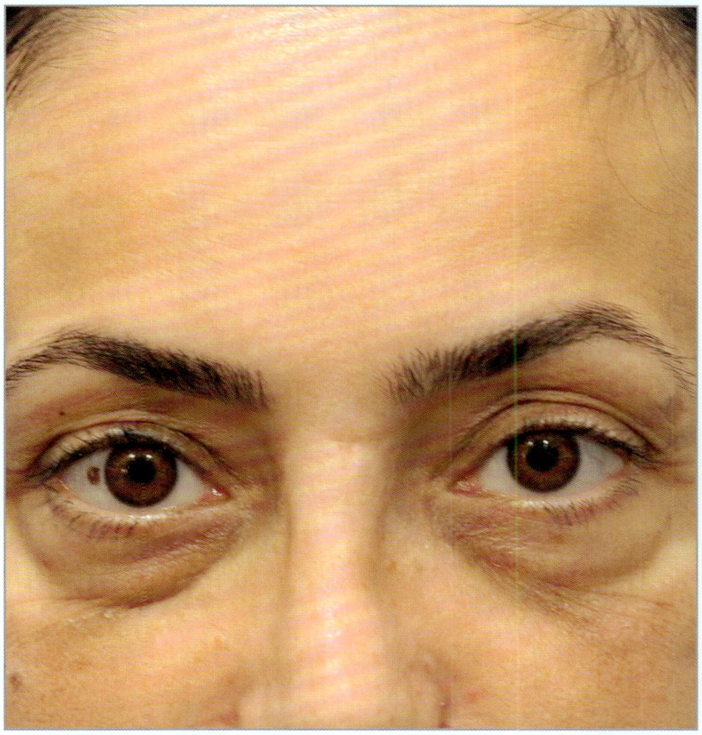

Baseline: 36-year-old female with advanced superficial elastosis and volume loss in the periorbital region.

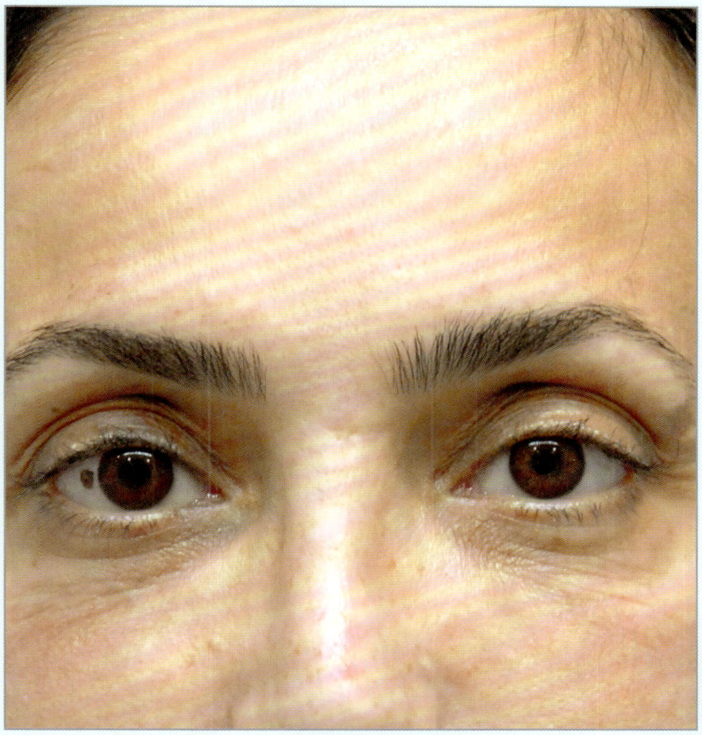

Result: 4 weeks after a single vertical injection into the infraorbital hollow using a total of 1 ml of a hyaluronic acid filler per side.

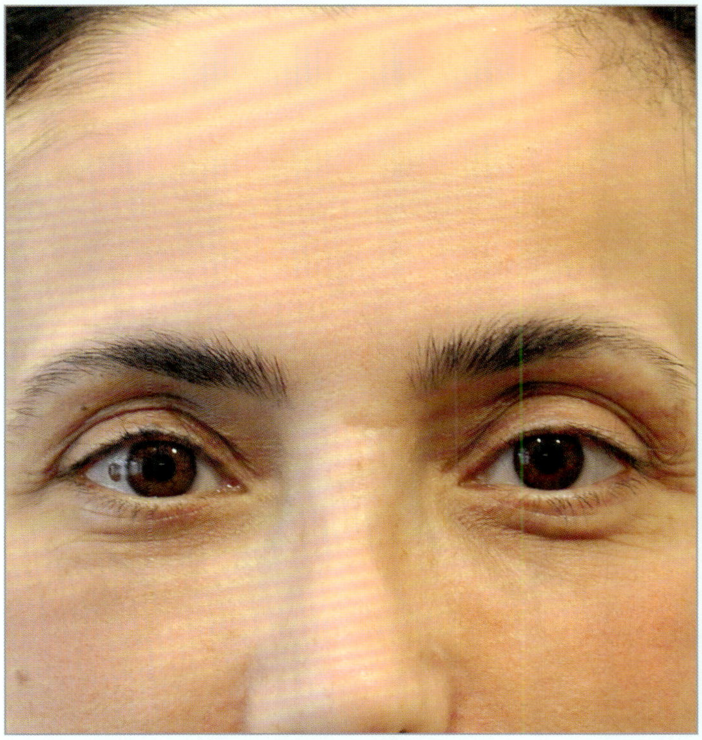

Result: 6 months after the treatment. No further injections were made.

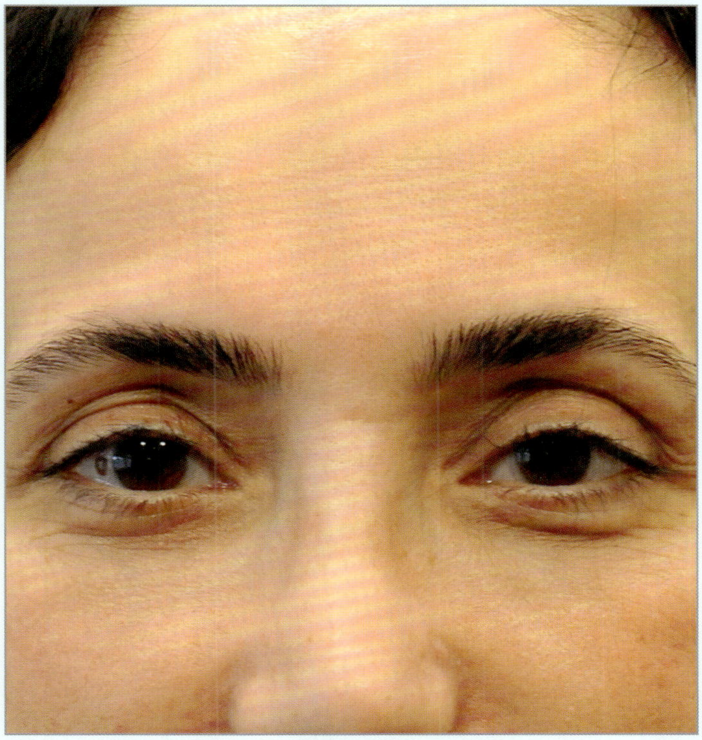

Result: 22 months after the treatment. No further injections were made with improvement still being noted.

Case 22 – Incipient periorbital volume loss and elastosis

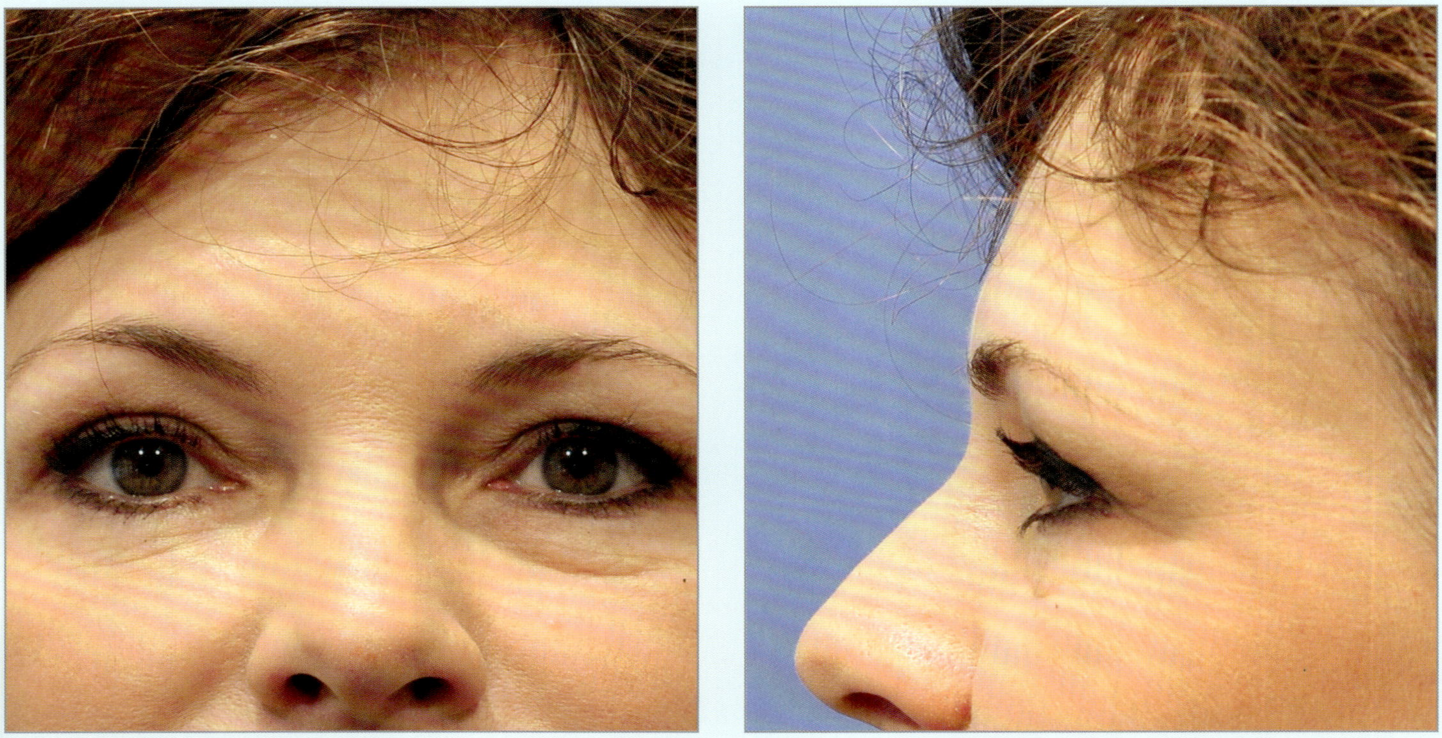

Baseline: 49-year-old female with superficial elastosis and incipient volume loss in the periorbital region.

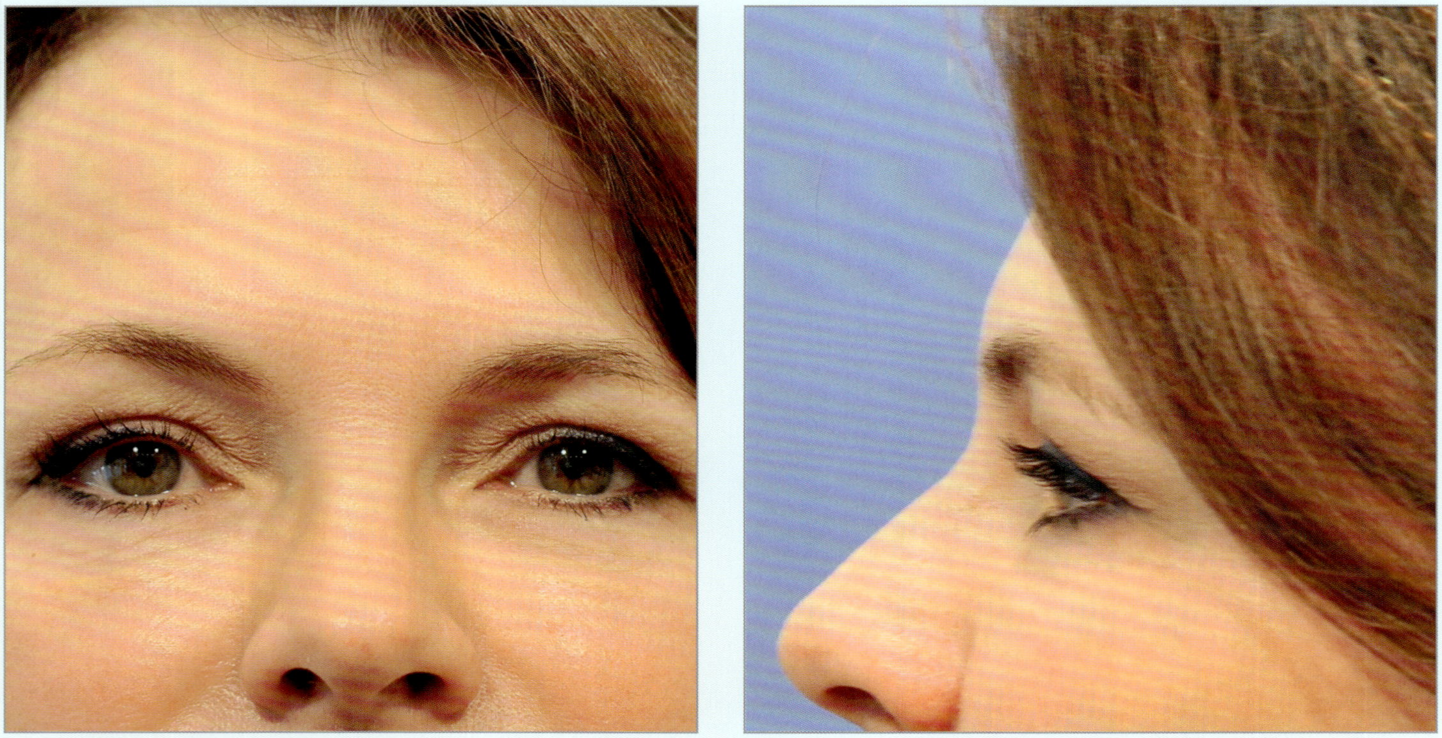

Result: 6 months after a single augmentation treatment with hyaluronic acid filler injected vertically into the infraorbital hollow. A total volume of 1.5 ml was injected.

Case 23 – Early volume loss

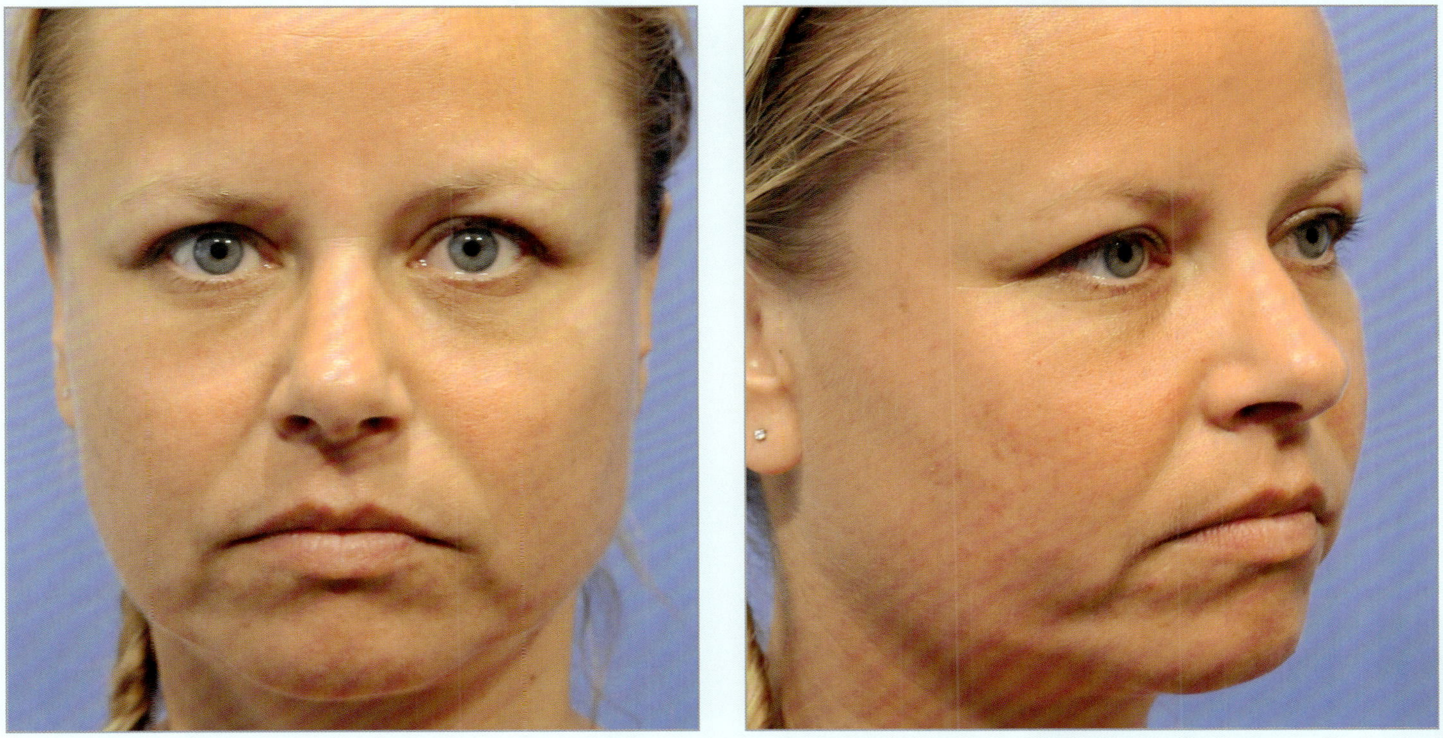

Baseline: 42-year-old, slim female with generalised volume deficits in the forehead, infraorbital region and cheeks, as well as in the lower third of the face. Additionally, marked brow ptosis, depressed corners of the mouth merging into marionette lines alongside chin atrophy is noted.

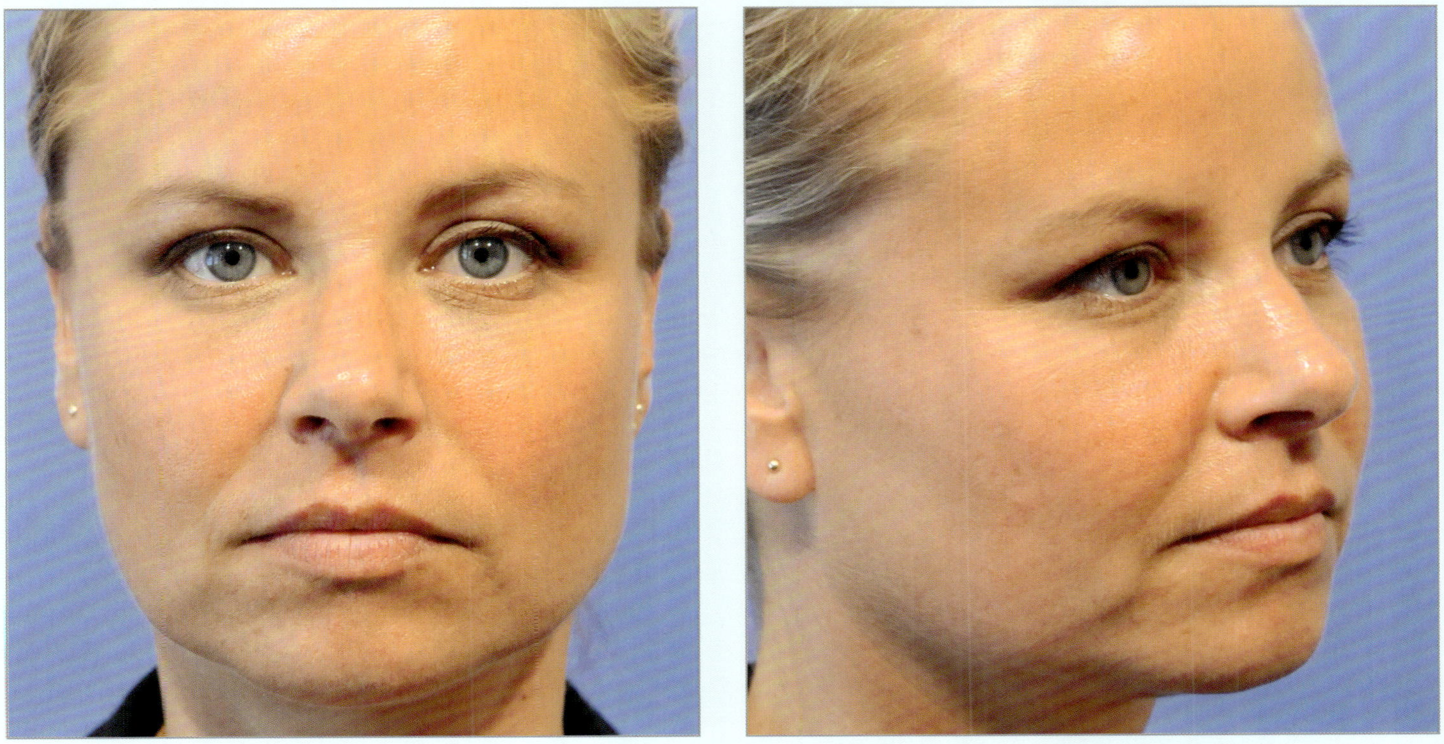

Result: 6 months after two augmentations treatments primarily using the vertical injection technique with hyaluronic acid fillers. A total volume of 6 ml was injected. A single adjuvant treatment with botulinum toxin type-A in the forehead and the glabellar region was also performed.

9 Aids for the Practitioner

9.1 Documentation Form

Documentation Form for Aesthetic Treatments

Name of patient ______ Date of birth ______ Medical Insurance ______

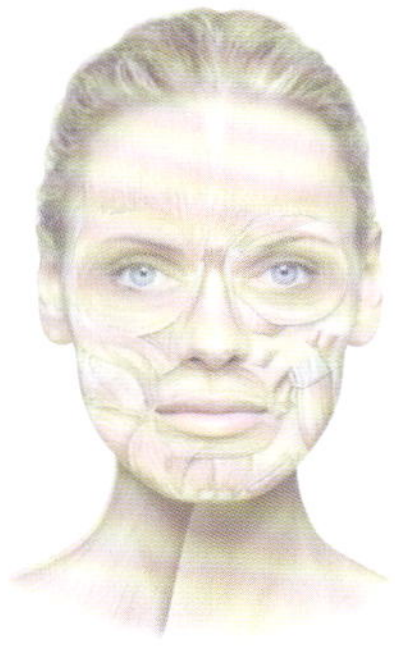

Treatment with: ☐ *Botulinum toxin* ☐ *Filler*

Products:

Batch numbers:

Units (ml):

Merz Scale:	*A*	*B*	*C*	*D*	*E*	*F*	*G*
Value:							
Merz Scale:	*H*	*I*	*J*	*K*	*L*	*M*	*N*
Value:							

Date:

Photo today: ☐ *Yes* ☐ *No*

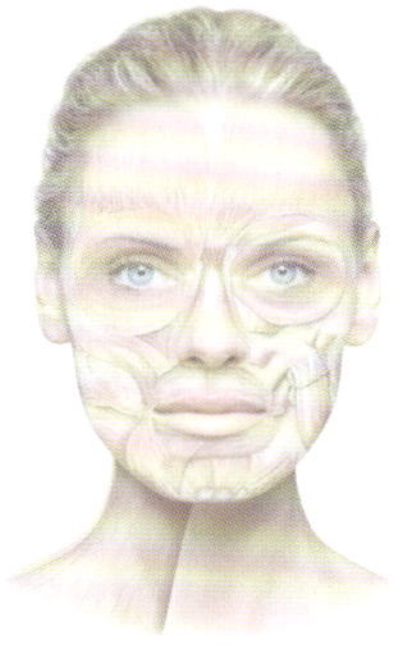

Treatment with: ☐ *Botulinum toxin* ☐ *Filler*

Products:

Batch numbers:

Units (ml):

Merz Scale:	*A*	*B*	*C*	*D*	*E*	*F*	*G*
Value:							
Merz Scale:	*H*	*I*	*J*	*K*	*L*	*M*	*N*
Value:							

Date:

Photo today: ☐ *Yes* ☐ *No*

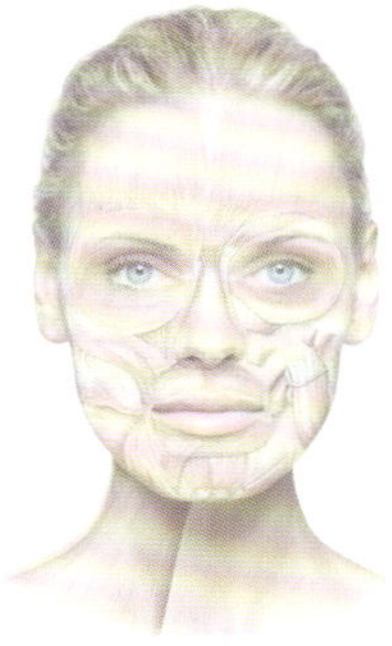

Treatment with: ☐ *Botulinum toxin* ☐ *Filler*

Products:

Batch numbers:

Units (ml):

Merz Scale:	*A*	*B*	*C*	*D*	*E*	*F*	*G*
Value:							
Merz Scale:	*H*	*I*	*J*	*K*	*L*	*M*	*N*
Value:							

Date:

Photo today: ☐ *Yes* ☐ *No*

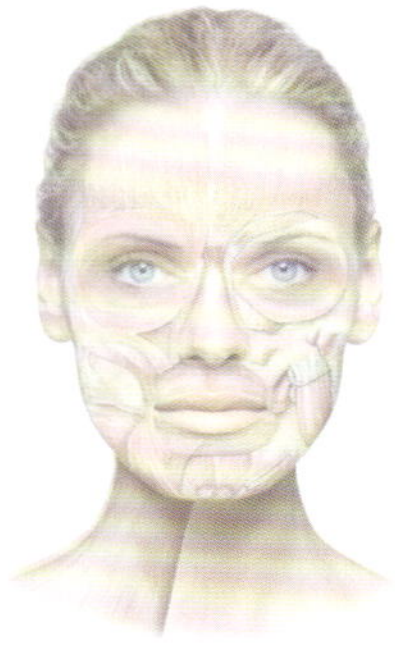

Treatment with: ☐ *Botulinum toxin* ☐ *Filler*

Products:

Batch numbers:

Units (ml):

Merz Scale:	*A*	*B*	*C*	*D*	*E*	*F*	*G*
Value:							
Merz Scale:	*H*	*I*	*J*	*K*	*L*	*M*	*N*
Value:							

Date:

Photo today: ☐ *Yes* ☐ *No*

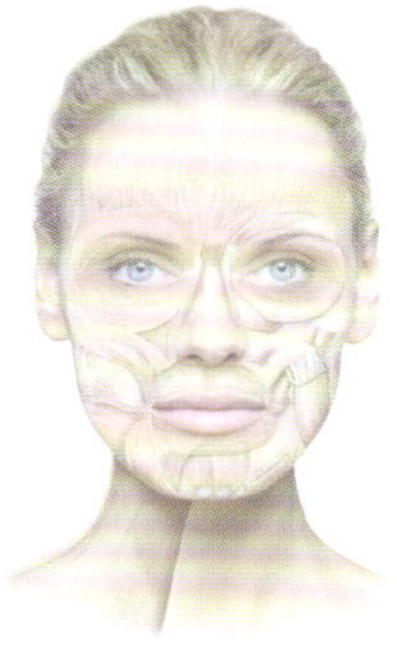

Treatment with: ☐ *Botulinum toxin* ☐ *Filler*

Products:

Batch numbers:

Units (ml):

Merz Scale:	*A*	*B*	*C*	*D*	*E*	*F*	*G*
Value:							
Merz Scale:	*H*	*I*	*J*	*K*	*L*	*M*	*N*
Value:							

Date:

Photo today: ☐ *Yes* ☐ *No*

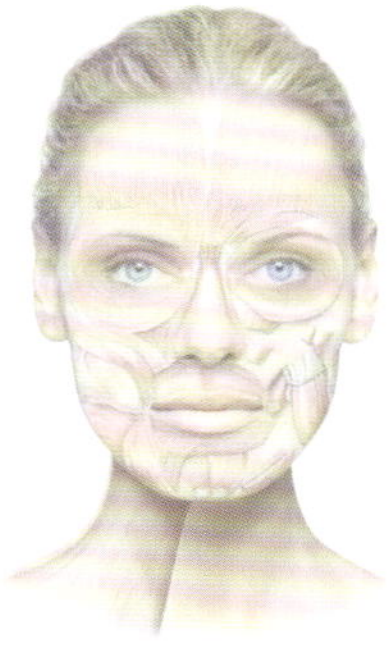

Treatment with: ☐ *Botulinum toxin* ☐ *Filler*

Products:

Batch numbers:

Units (ml):

Merz Scale:	*A*	*B*	*C*	*D*	*E*	*F*	*G*
Value:							
Merz Scale:	*H*	*I*	*J*	*K*	*L*	*M*	*N*
Value:							

Date:

Photo today: ☐ *Yes* ☐ *No*

9.2 Aesthetic Scales at Rest (by Merz)

A Forehead lines – at rest

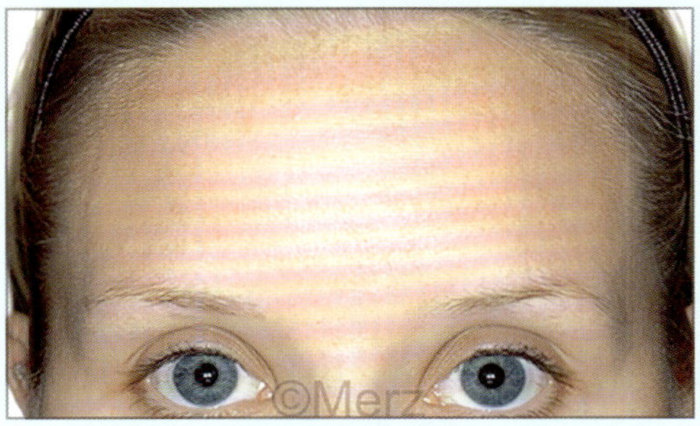

0
No wrinkles

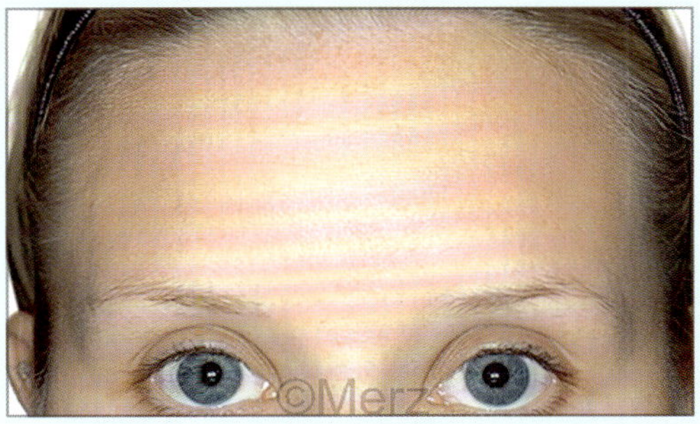

1
Mild wrinkles

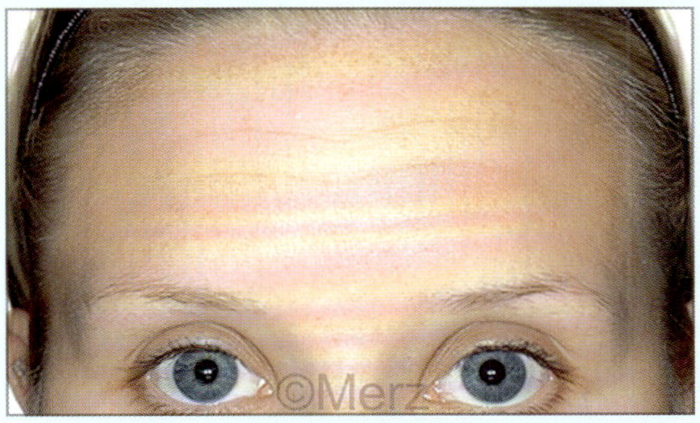

2
Moderate wrinkles

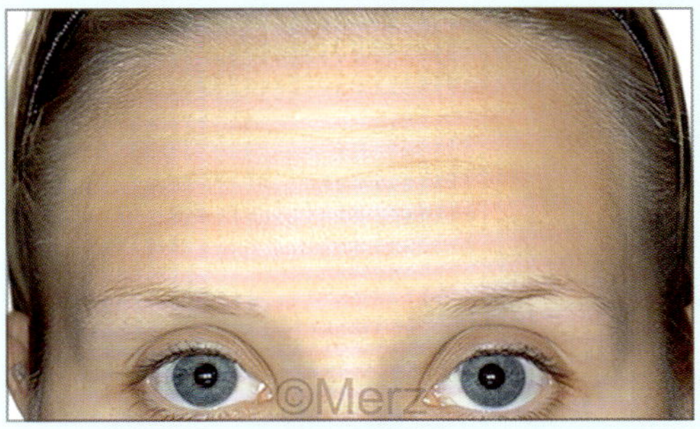

3
Severe wrinkles

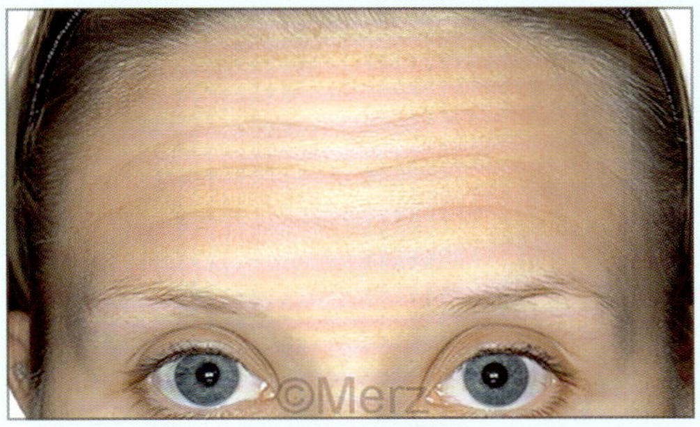

4
Very severe wrinkles

B Brow positioning

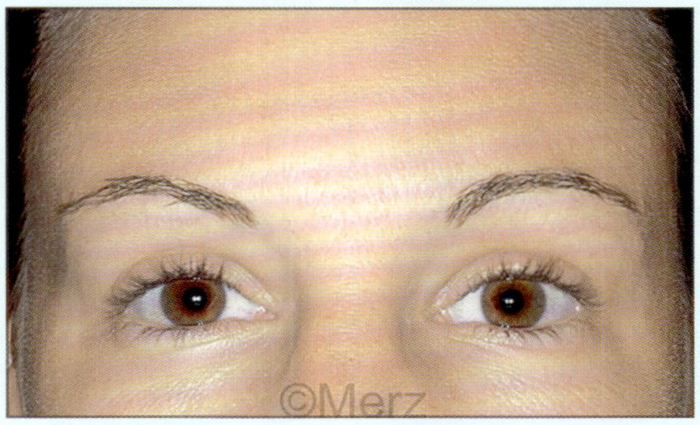

0
High arch of the eyebrow; youthful, refreshed look

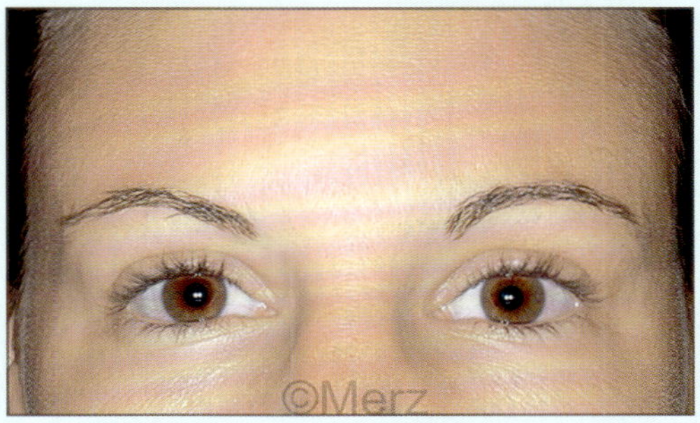

1
Medium high arch of the eyebrow

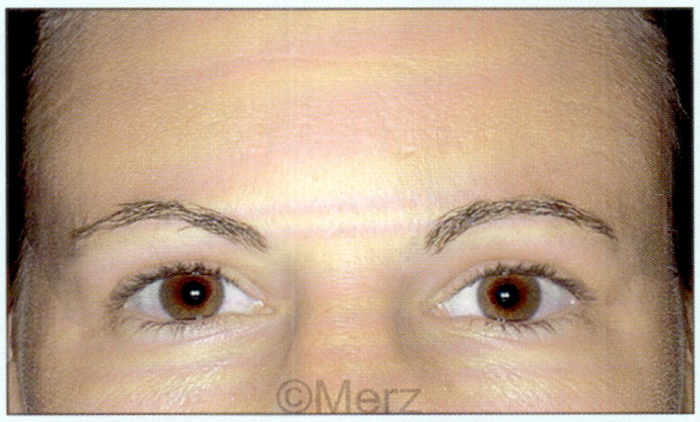

2
Slight arch of the eyebrow

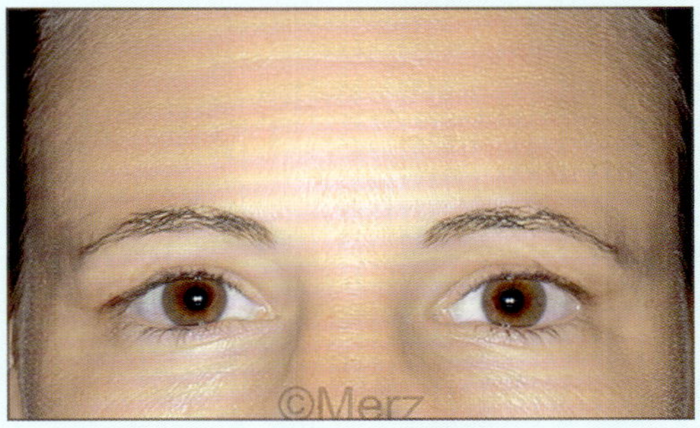

3
Flat arch of the eyebrow; mild ptosis, tired appearance

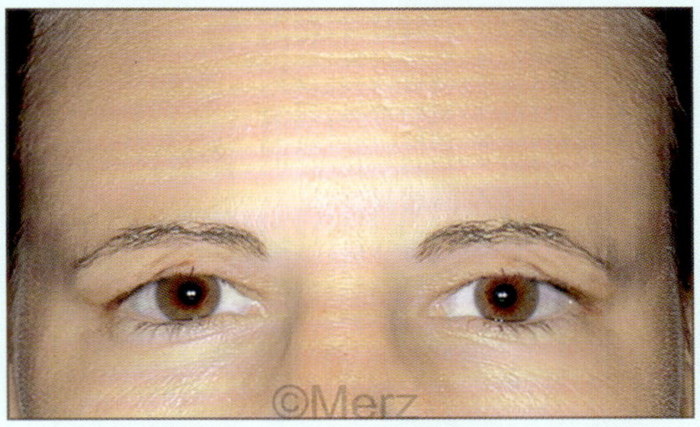

4
Sunken arch of the eyebrow; severe ptosis, very tired appearance

C Lateral canthal lines – at rest

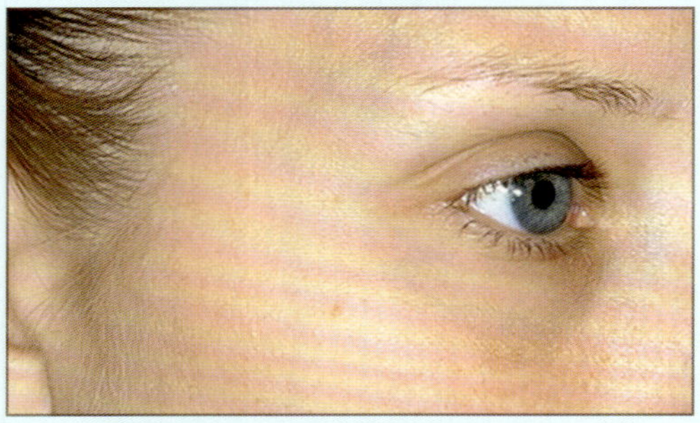

0
No wrinkles

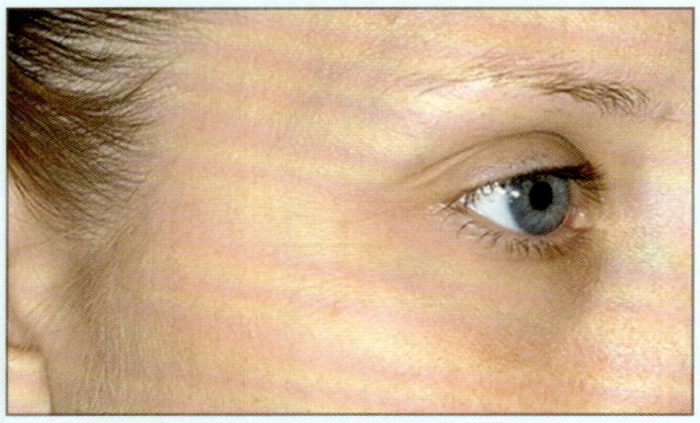

1
Mild wrinkles

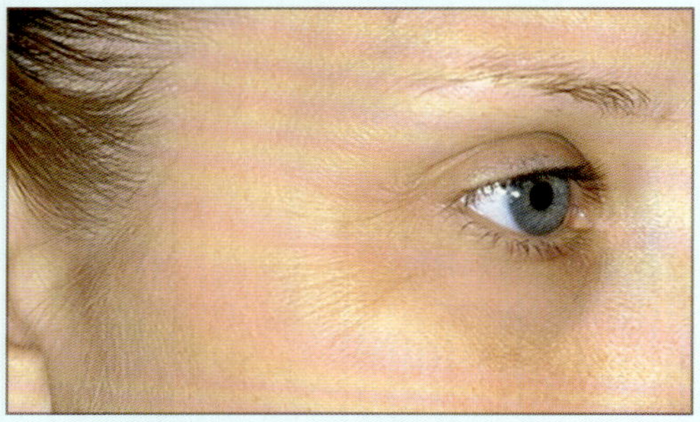

2
Moderate wrinkles

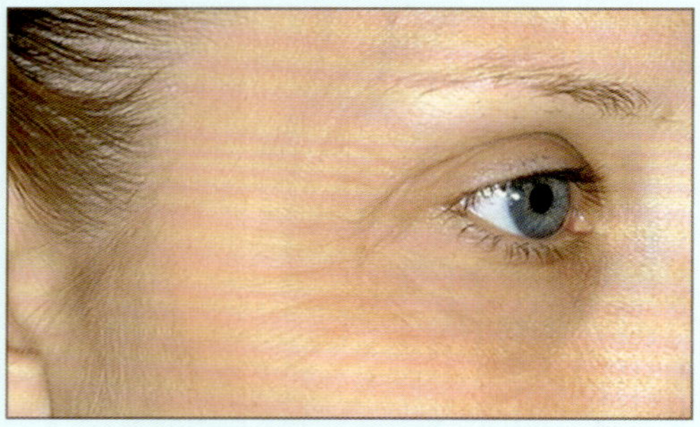

3
Severe wrinkles

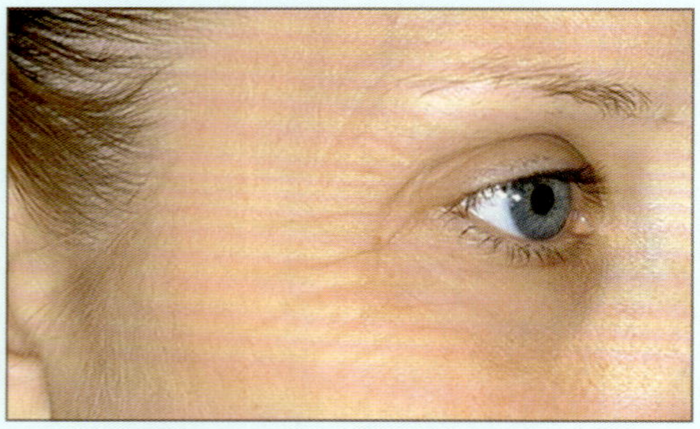

4
Very severe wrinkles

D Marionette lines

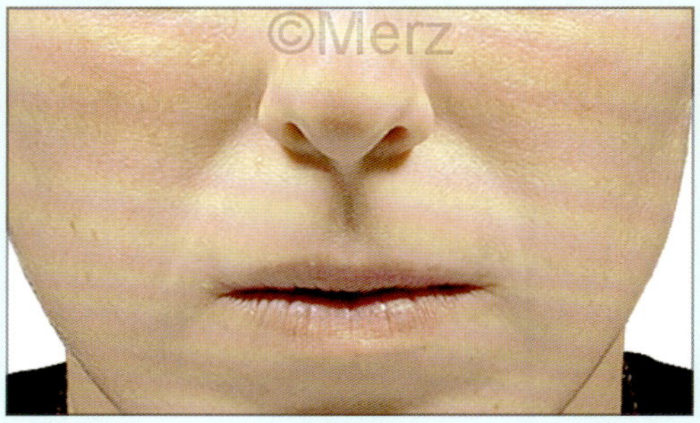

0
No lines

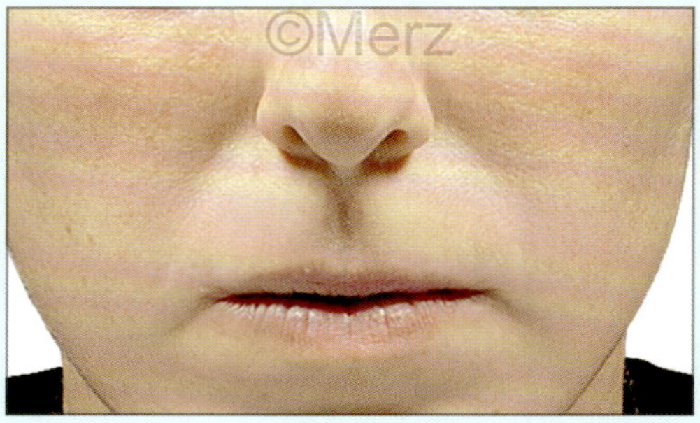

1
Mild lines

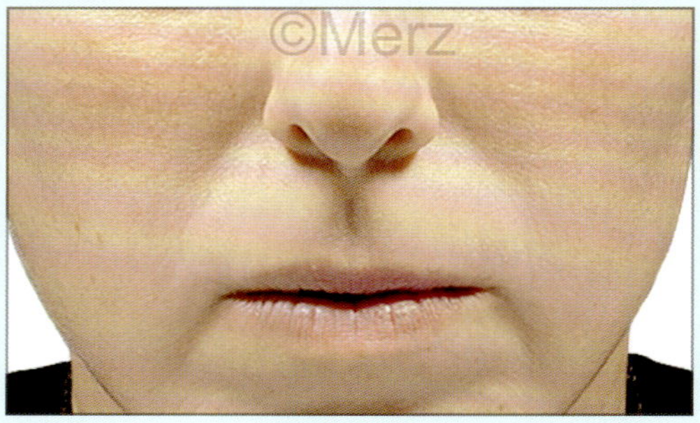

2
Moderate lines

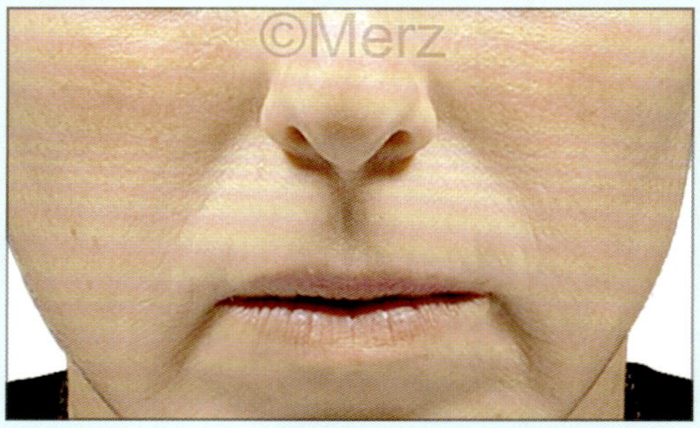

3
Severe lines

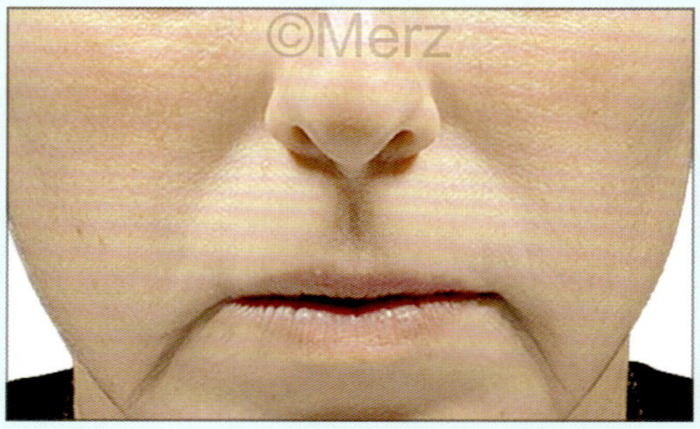

4
Very severe lines

E **Fullness of the upper lip**

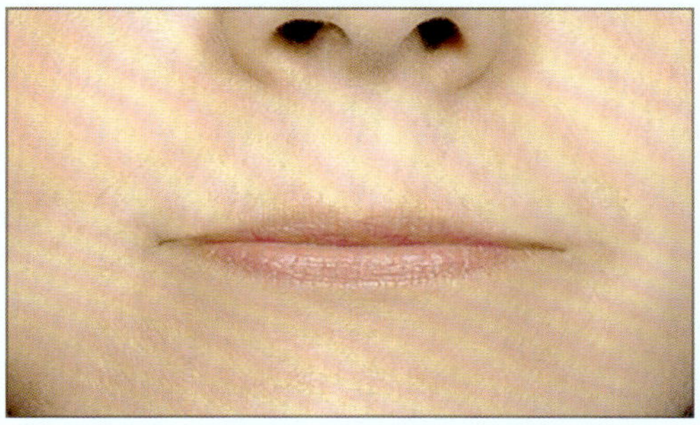

0
Very thin

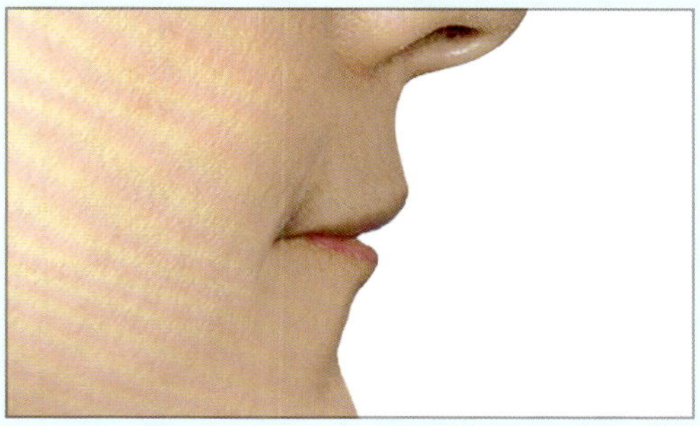

0
Very thin

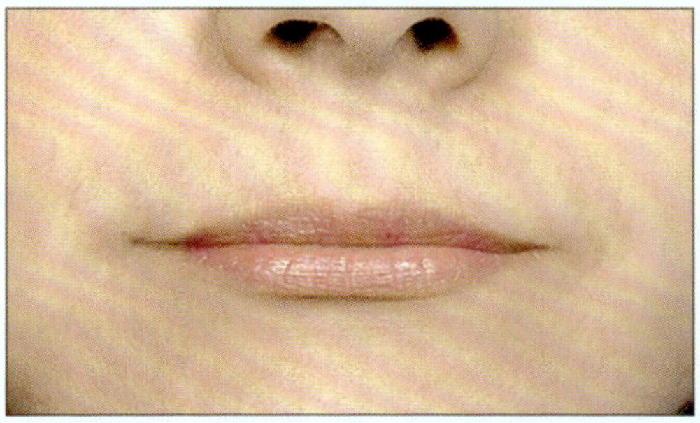

1
Thin

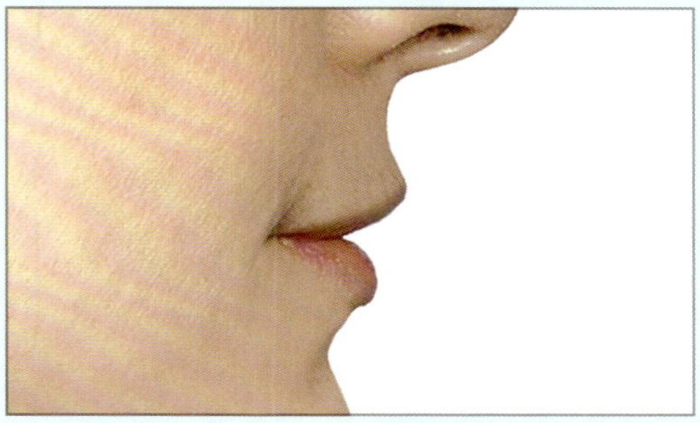

1
Thin

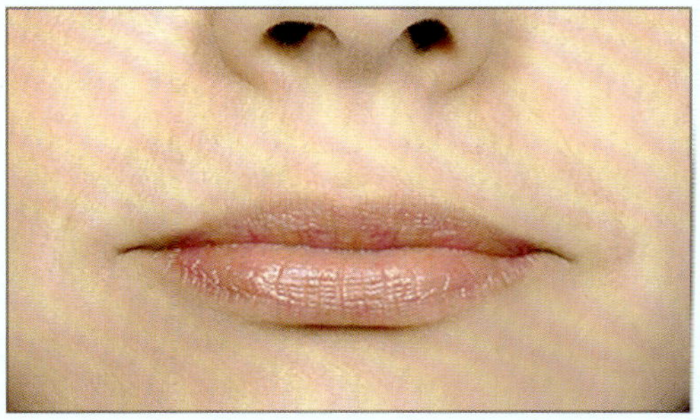

2
Normal fullness

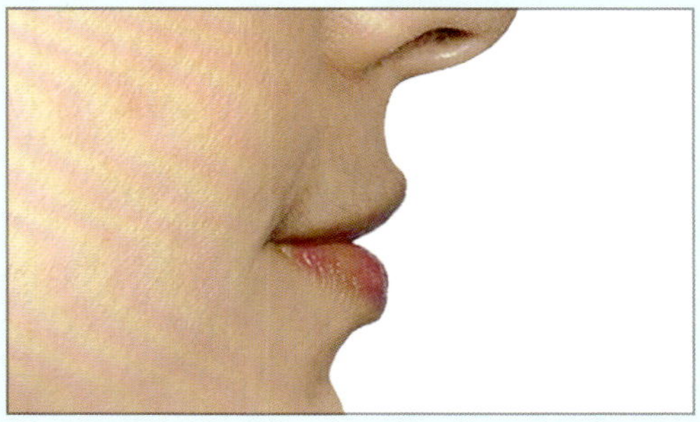

2
Normal fullness

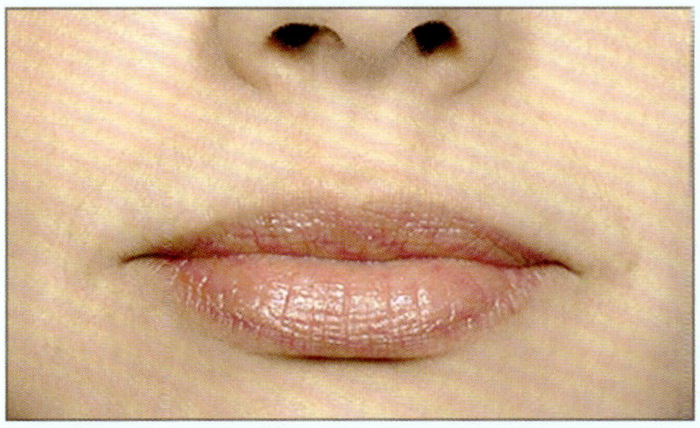

3
Full

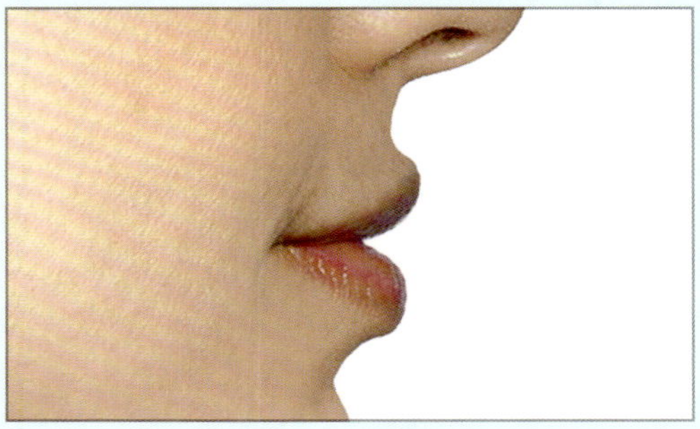

3
Full

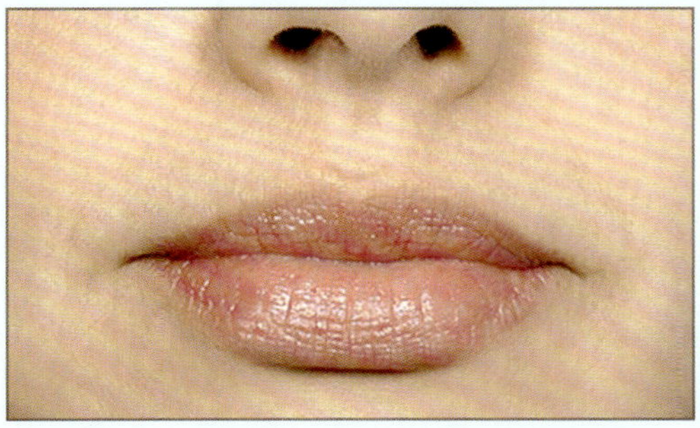

4
Very full

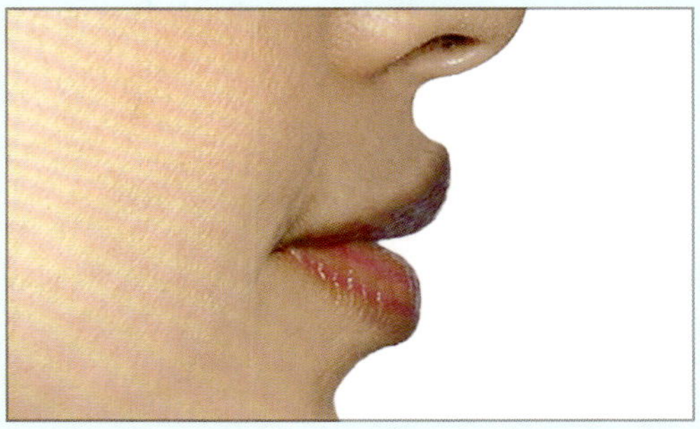

4
Very full

F **Fullness of the lower lip**

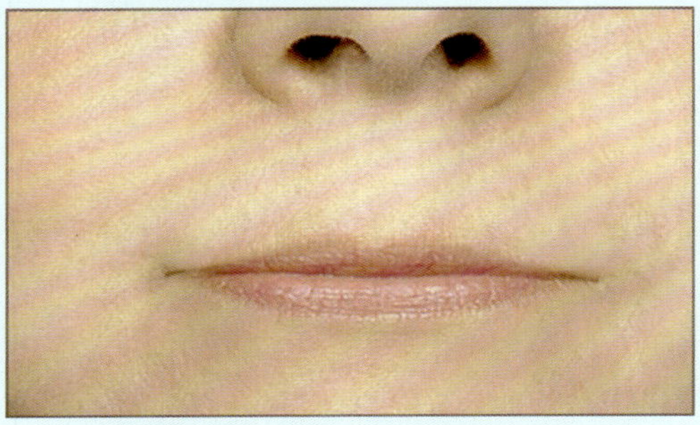

0
Very thin

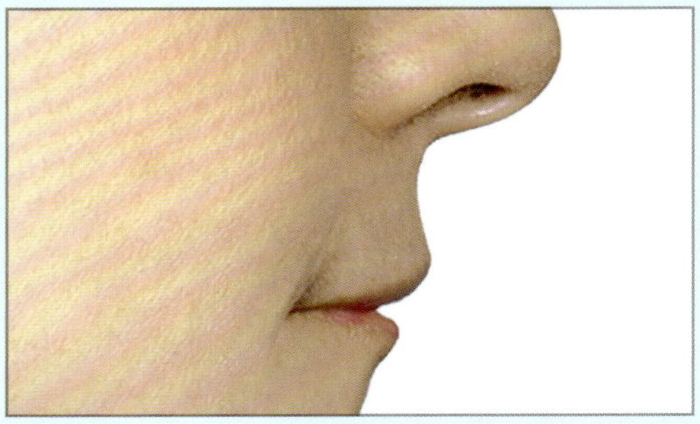

0
Very thin

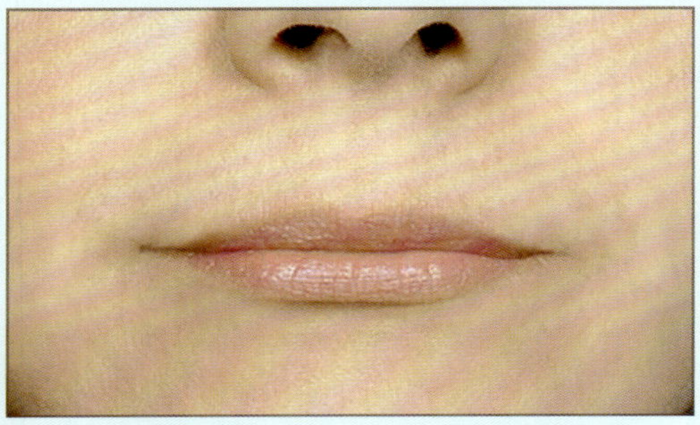

1
Thin

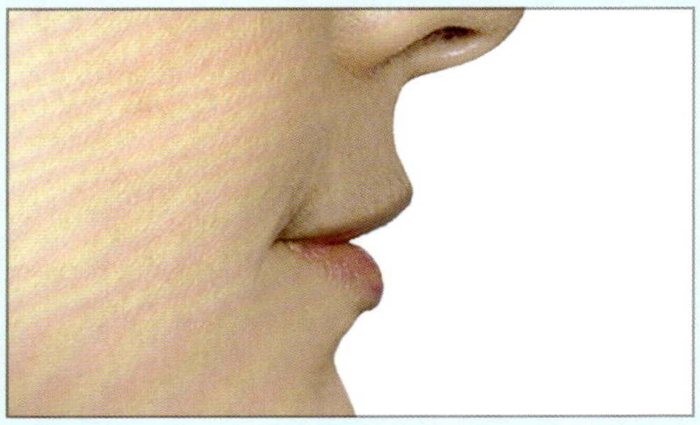

1
Thin

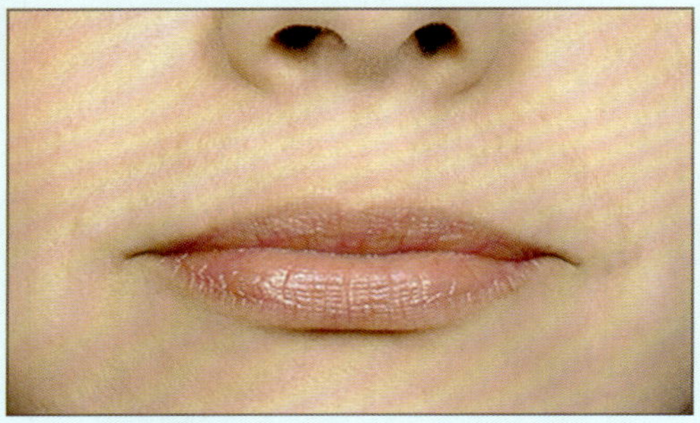

2
Normal fullness

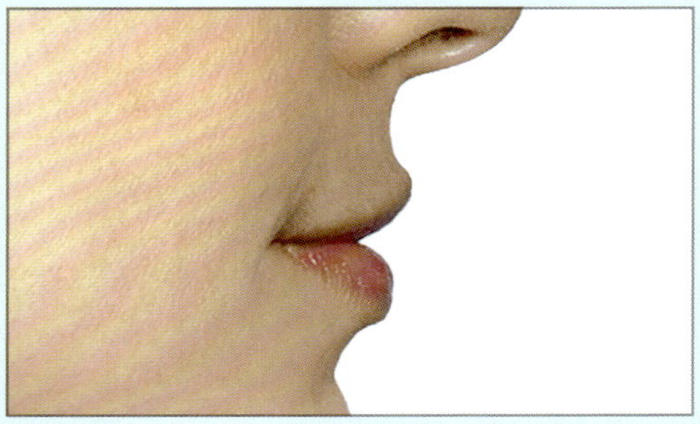

2
Normal fullness

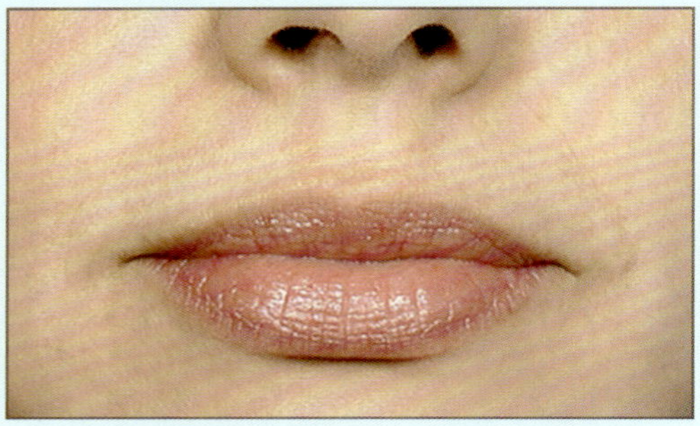

3
Full

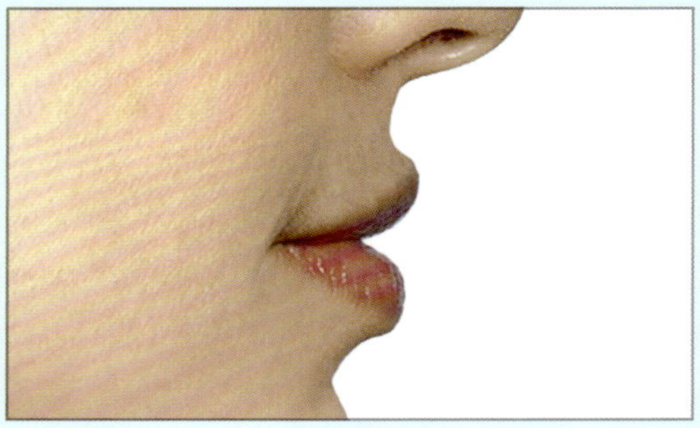

3
Full

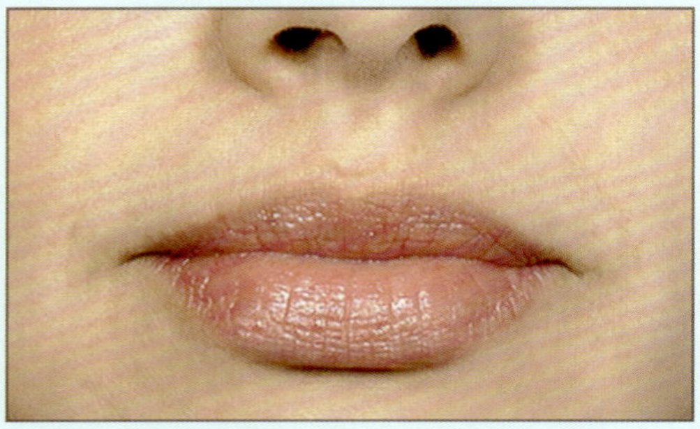

4
Very full

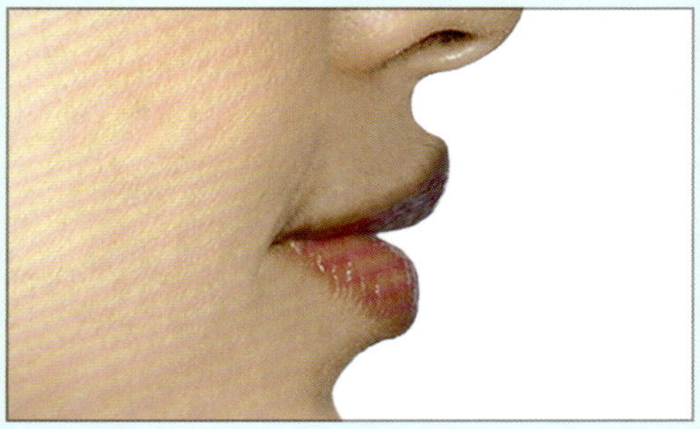

4
Very full

G Glabellar lines – at rest

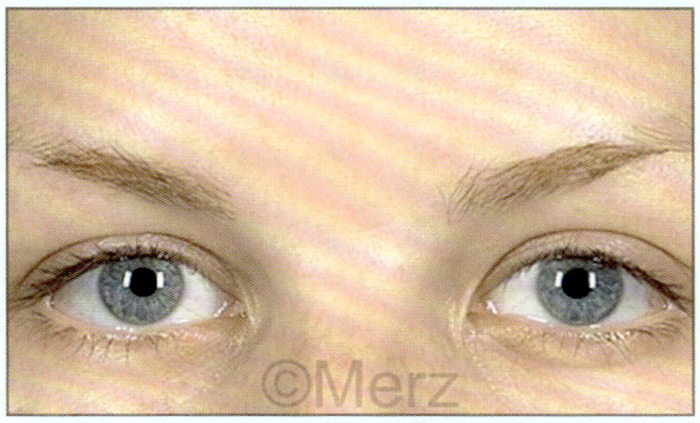

0
No wrinkles

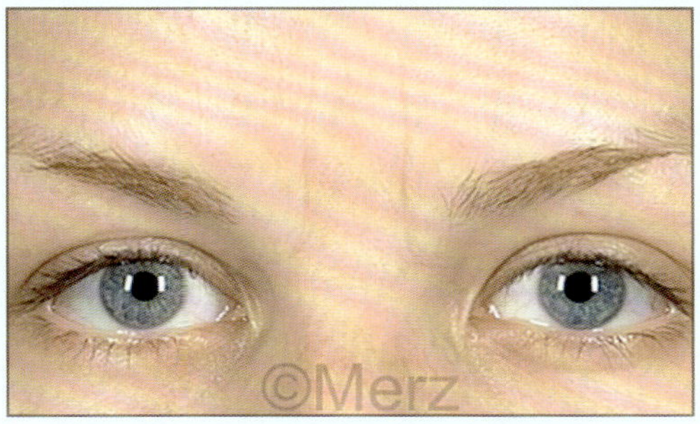

1
Mild wrinkles

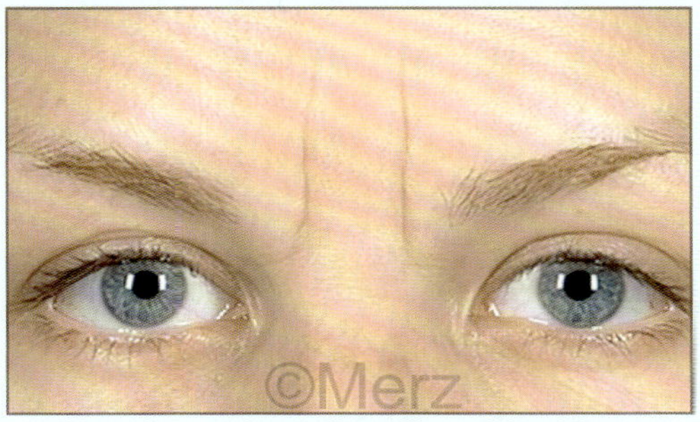

2
Moderate wrinkles

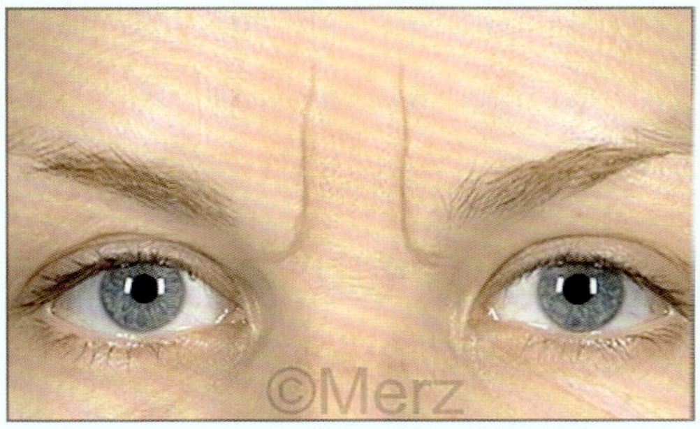

3
Severe wrinkles

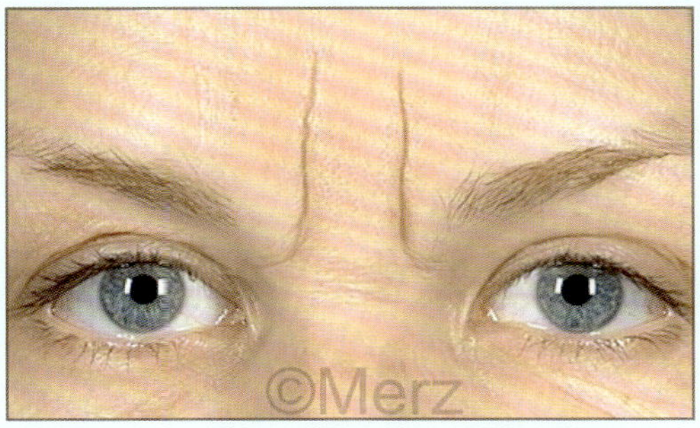

4
Very severe wrinkles

H Nasolabial lines – at rest

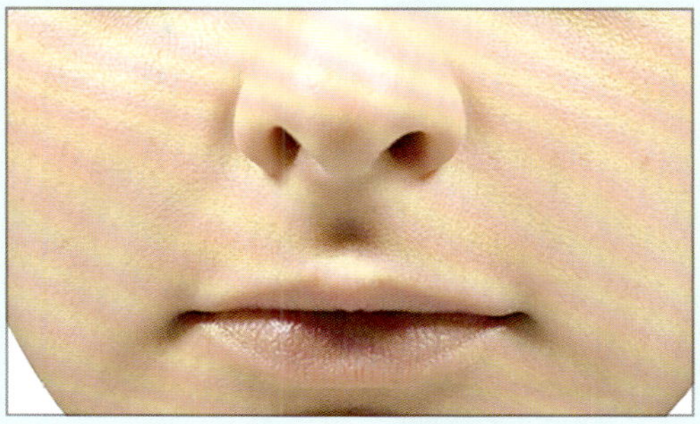

0
No lines

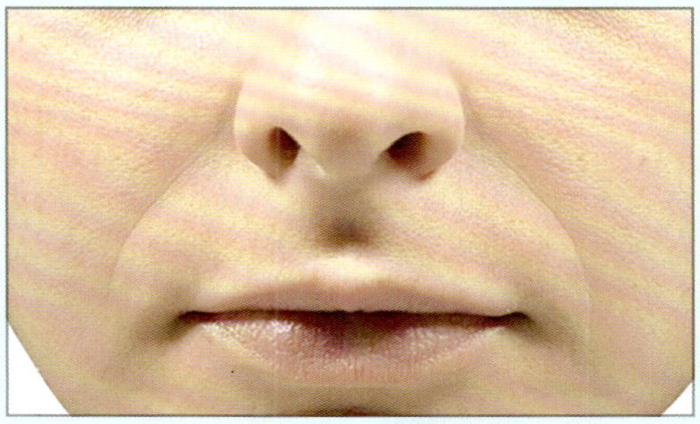

1
Mild lines

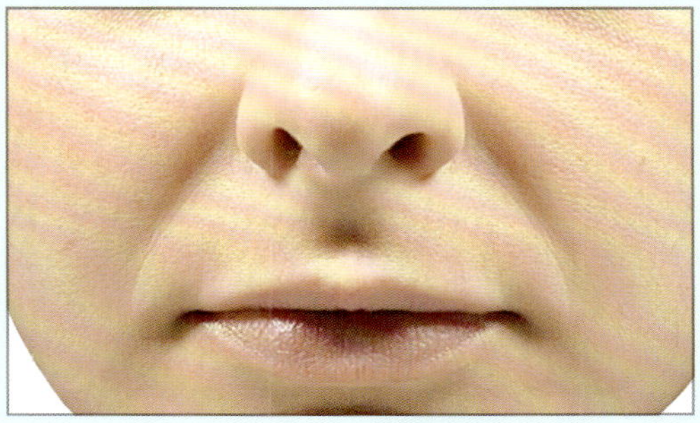

2
Moderate lines

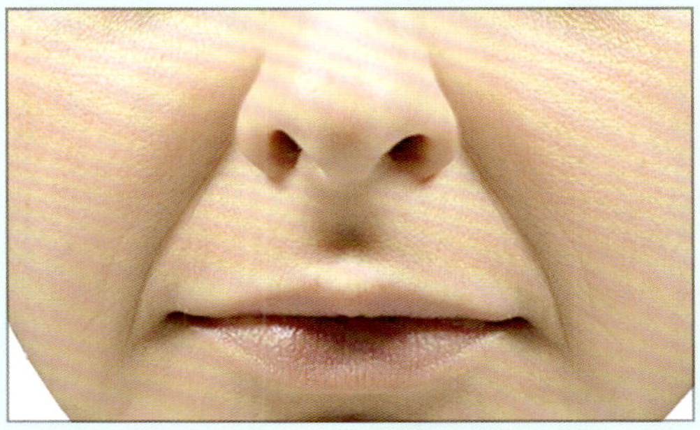

3
Severe lines

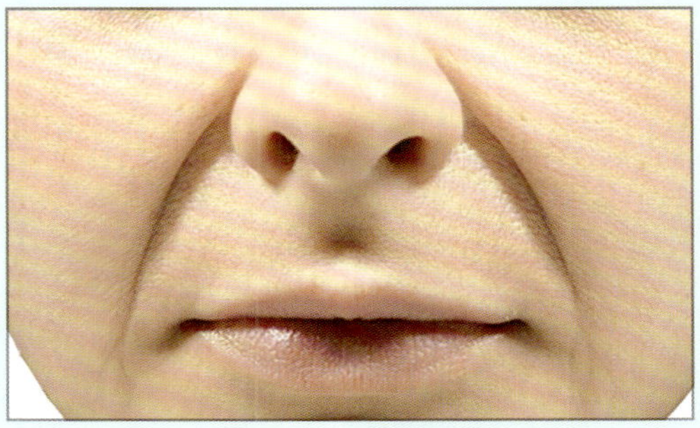

4
Very severe lines

I Lip wrinkles – at rest

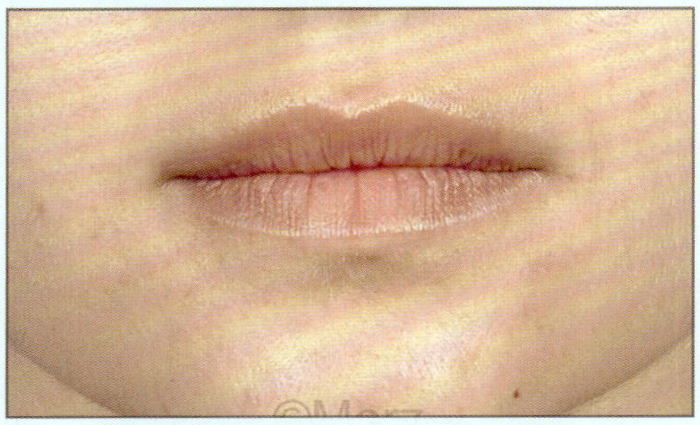

0
No wrinkles

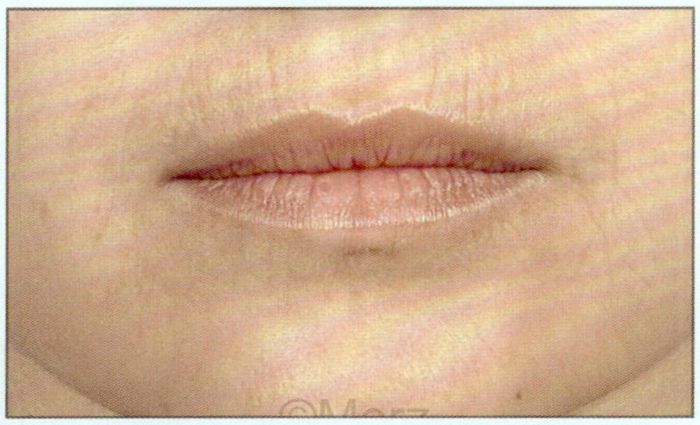

1
Mild wrinkles

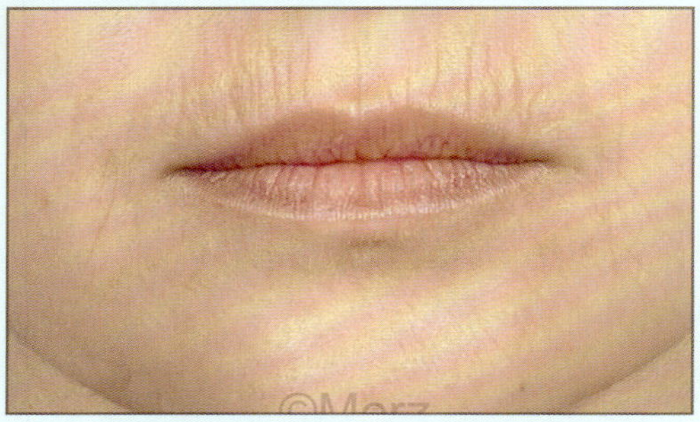

2
Moderate wrinkles

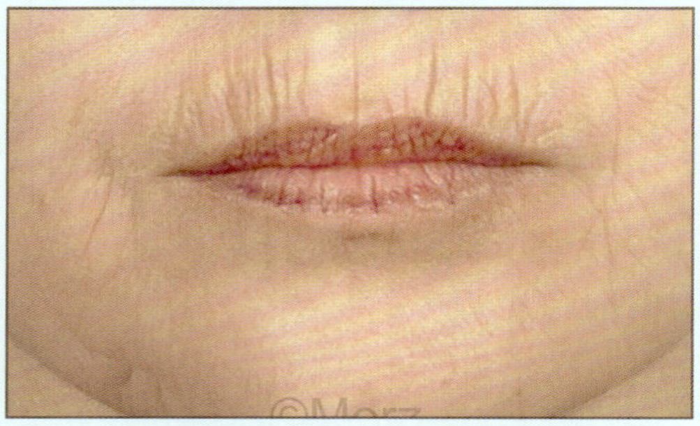

3
Severe wrinkles

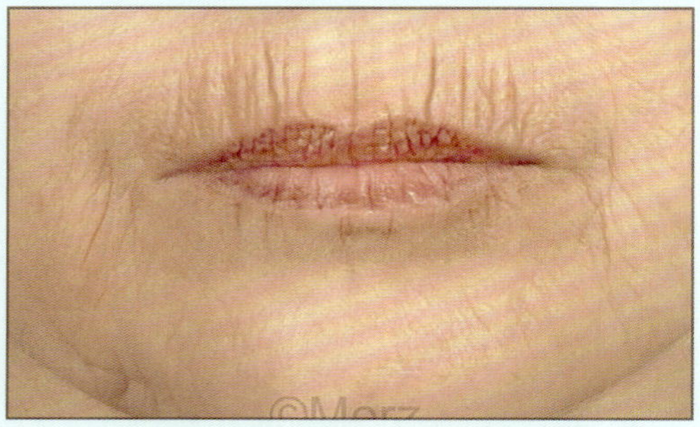

4
Very severe wrinkles

J Oral commissures

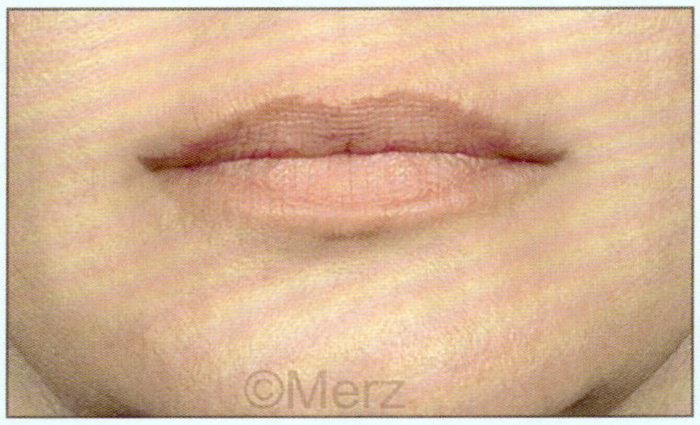

0
No sunken labial angles

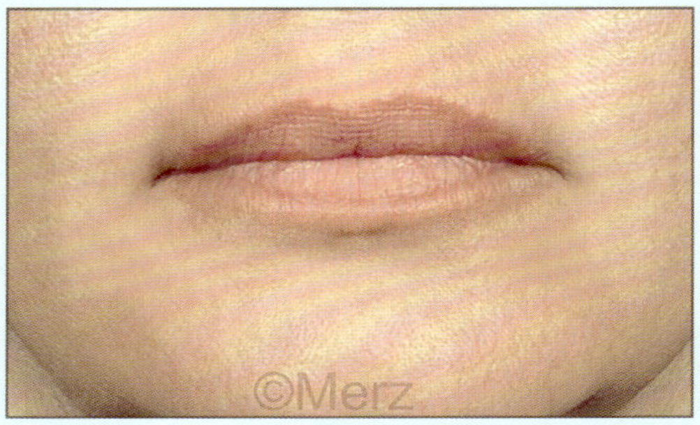

1
Mildly sunken labial angles

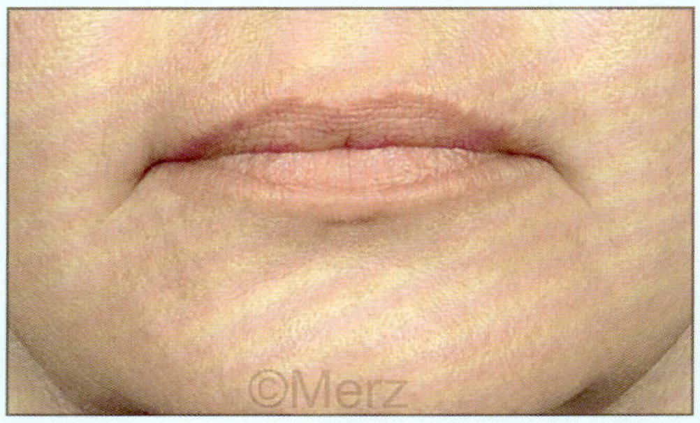

2
Moderately sunken labial angles

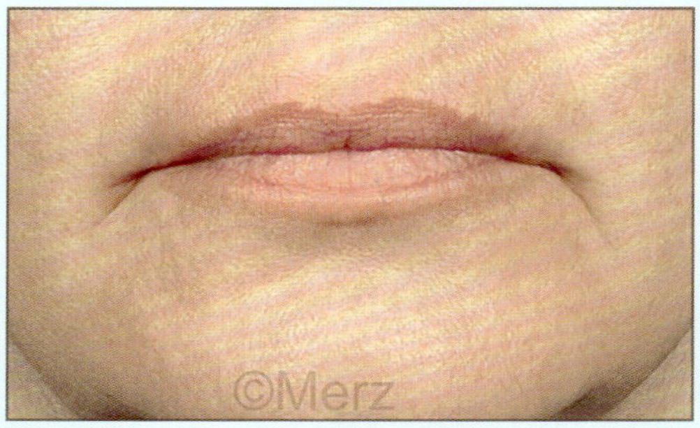

3
Heavily sunken labial angles

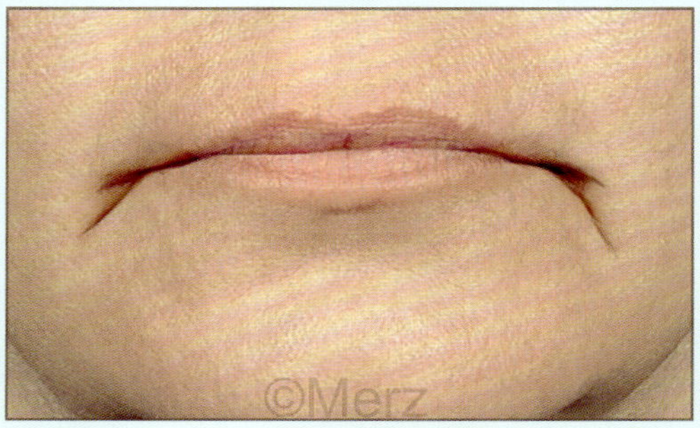

4
Very heavily sunken labial angles

9

K Jawline

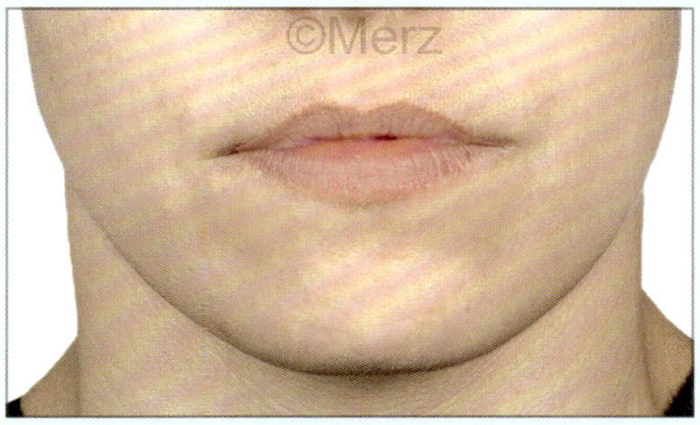

0
No relative sagging

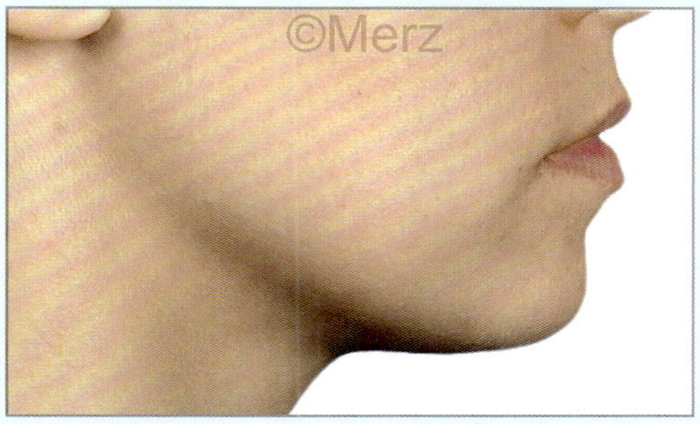

0
No relative sagging

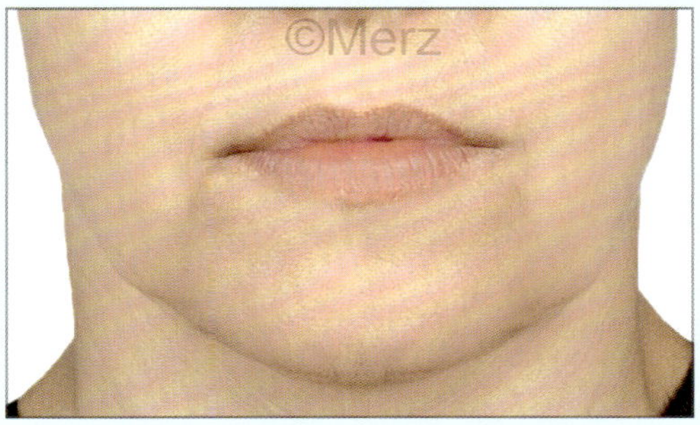

1
Mild relative sagging

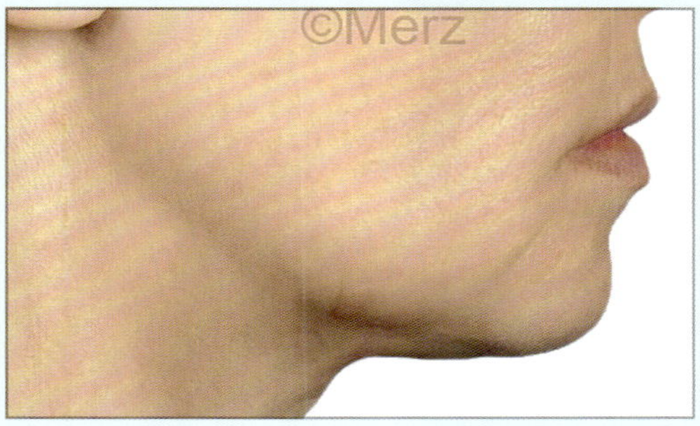

1
Mild relative sagging

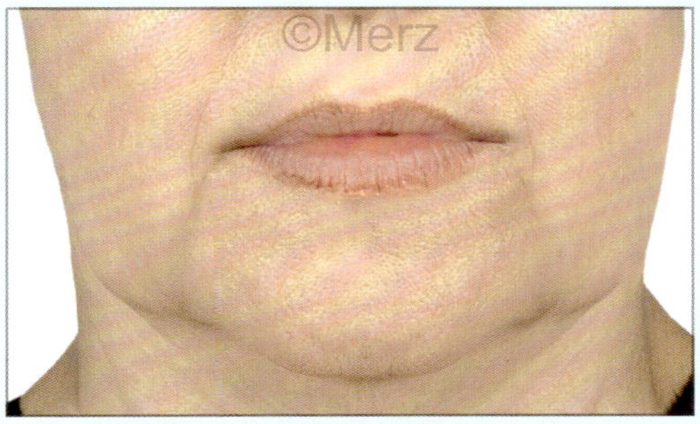

2
Moderate relative sagging

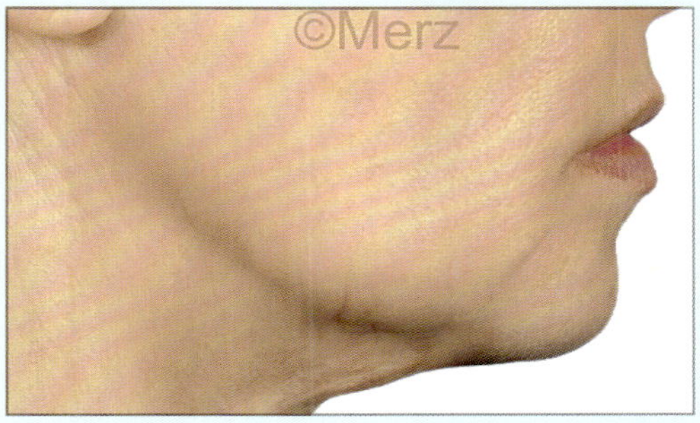

2
Moderate relative sagging

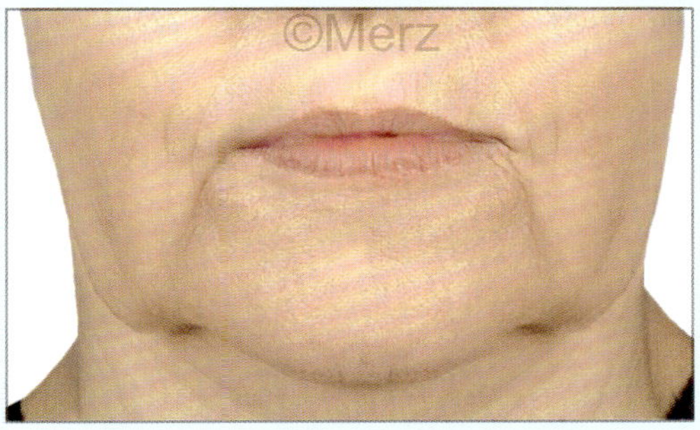

3
Severe relative sagging

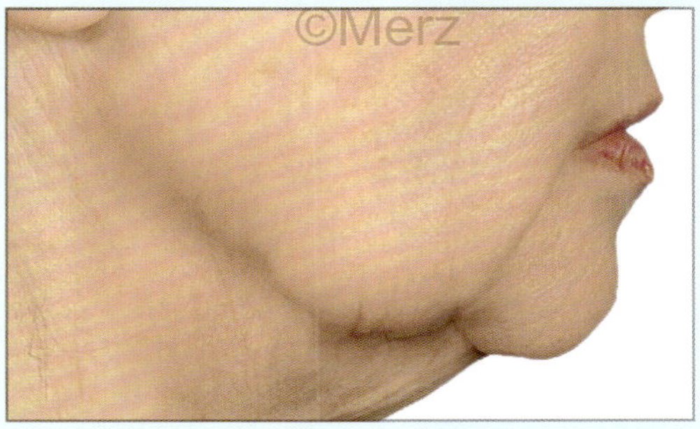

3
Severe relative sagging

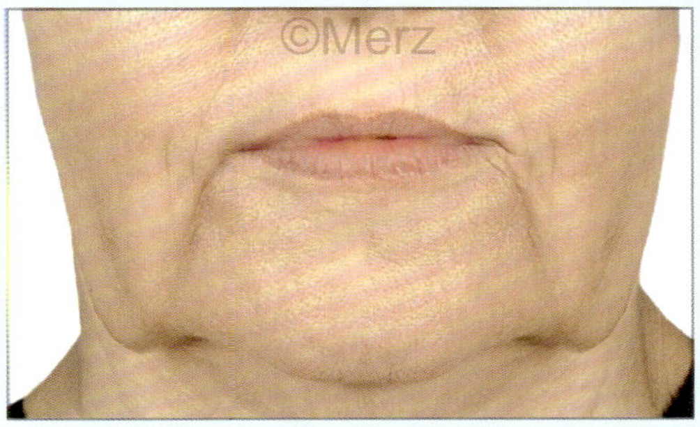

4
Very severe relative sagging

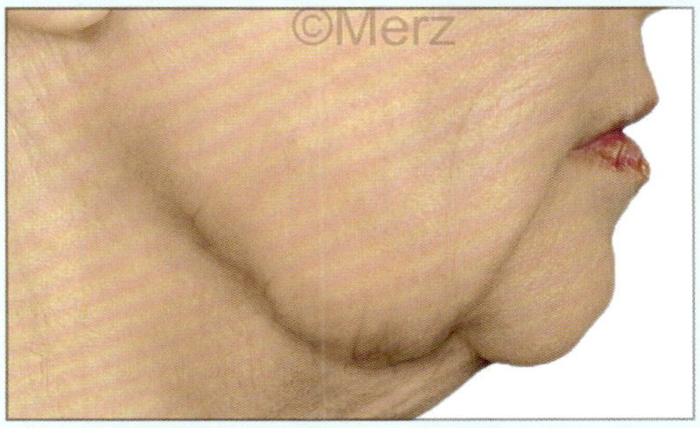

4
Very severe relative sagging

L Neck

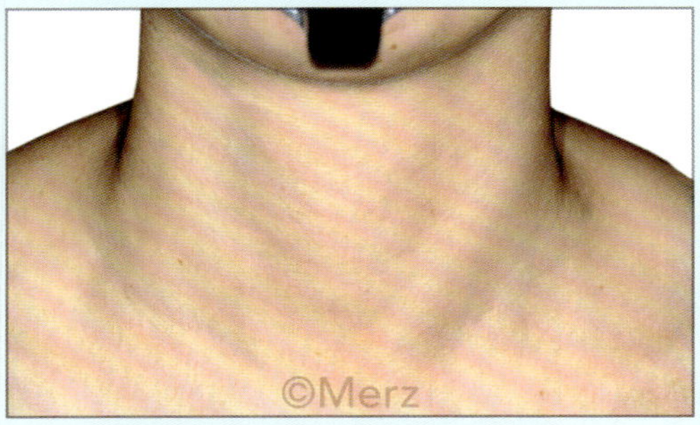

0

No horizontal lines and no elastosis

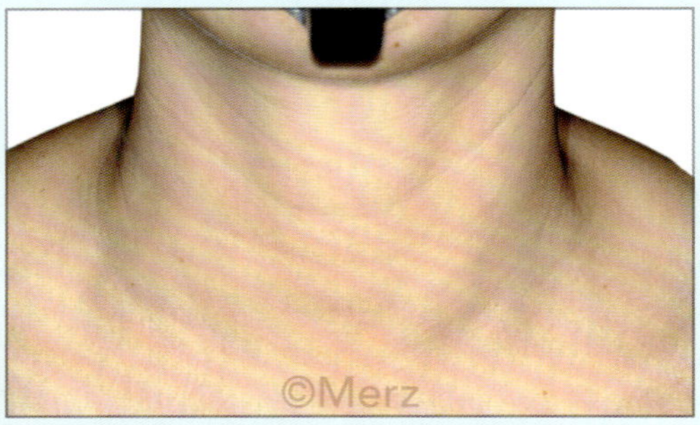

1

Mild horizontal lines and no elastosis

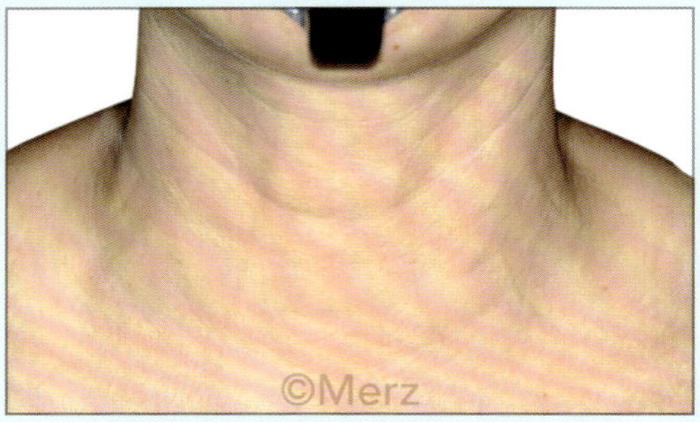

2

Moderate horizontal lines and initial elastosis

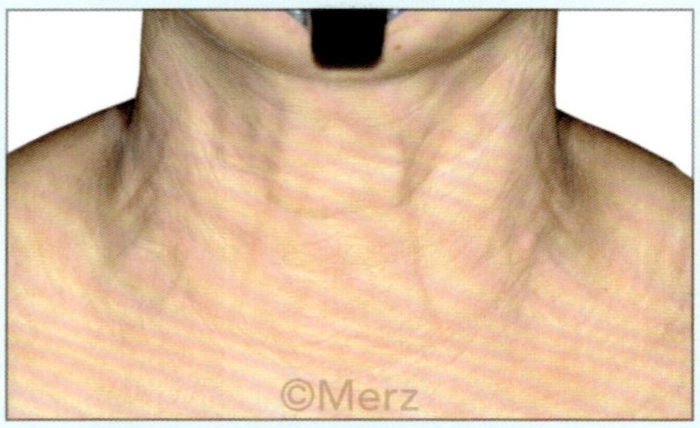

3

Severe horizontal lines and severe elastosis

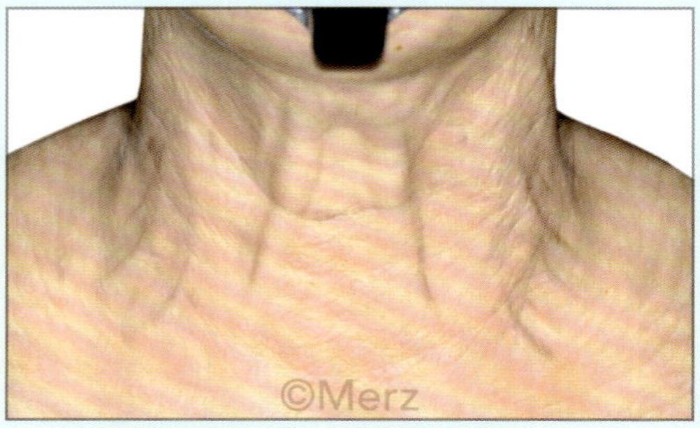

4

Very severe horizontal lines and very severe elastosis

M Back of the hands

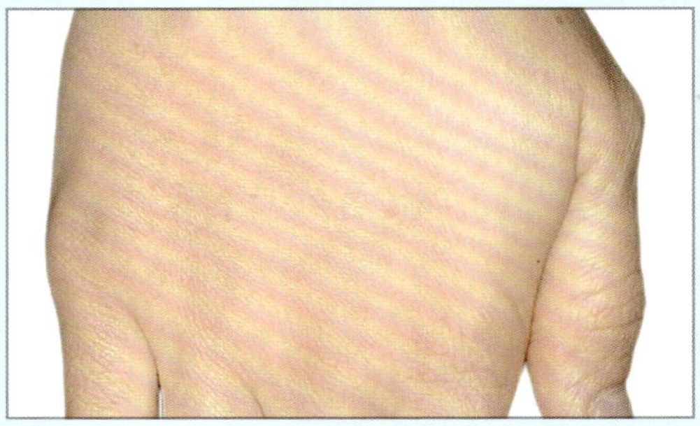

0

No volume loss, no skin ageing

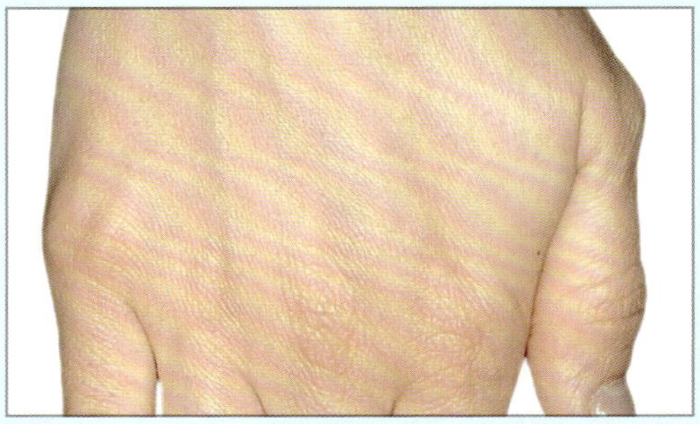

1

Mild volume loss, no skin ageing

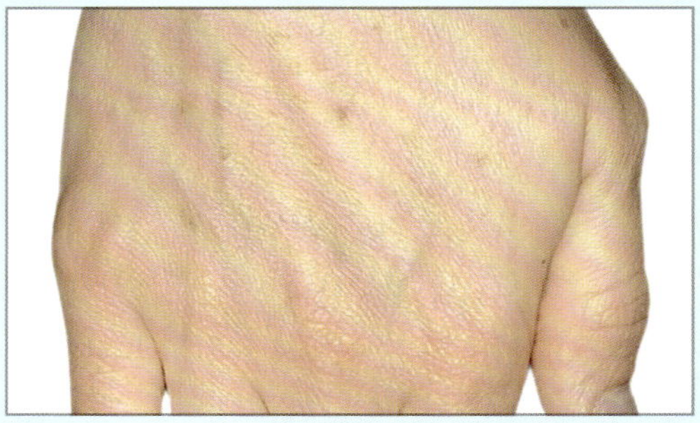

2

Moderate volume loss, initial skin ageing

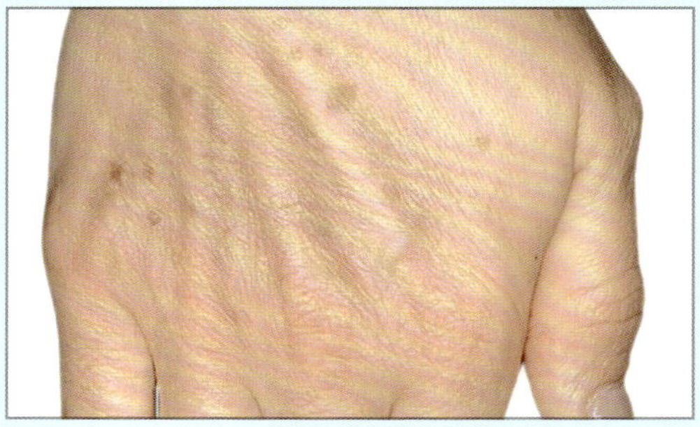

3

Severe volume loss, severe skin ageing

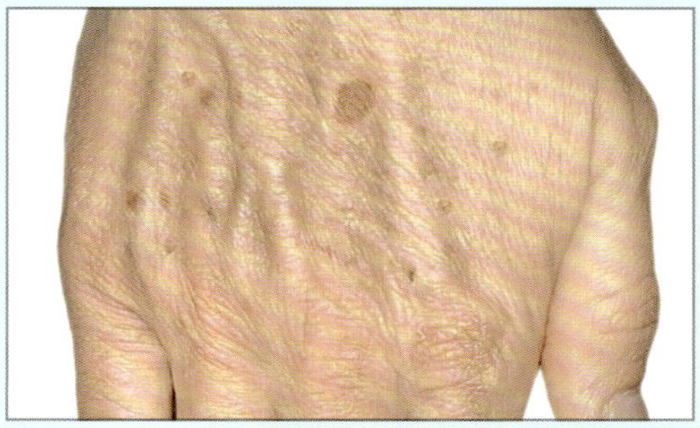

4

Very severe volume loss and very severe skin ageing

N **Infraorbital hollowness (IOH)**

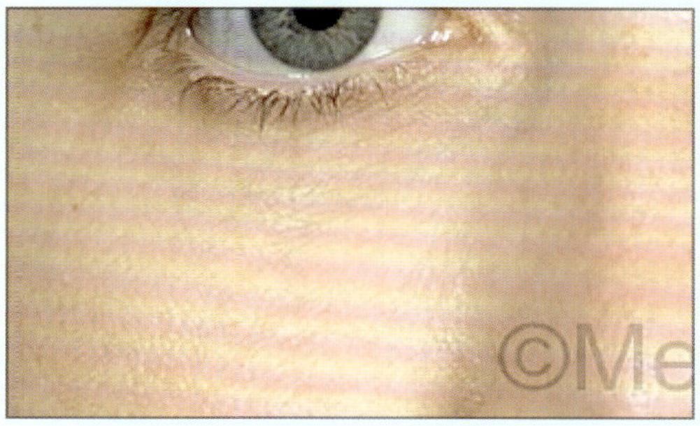

0
No hollowness

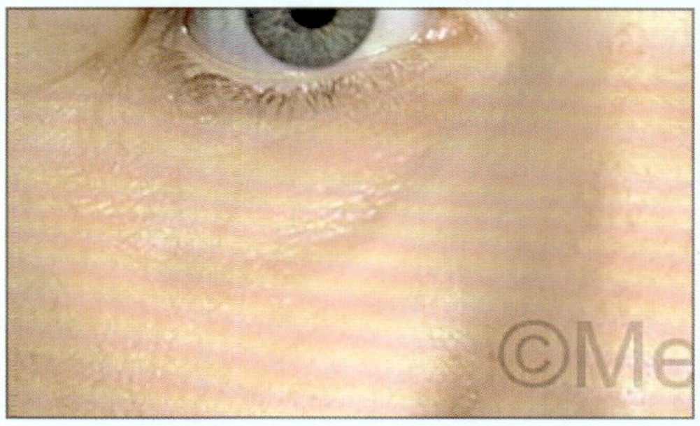

1
Mild hollowness

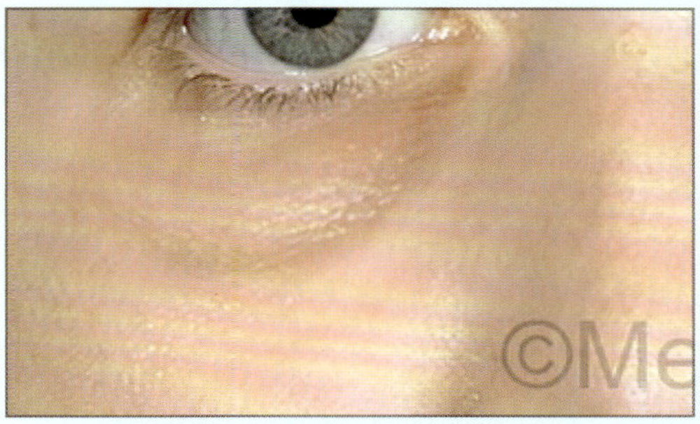

2
Moderate hollowness

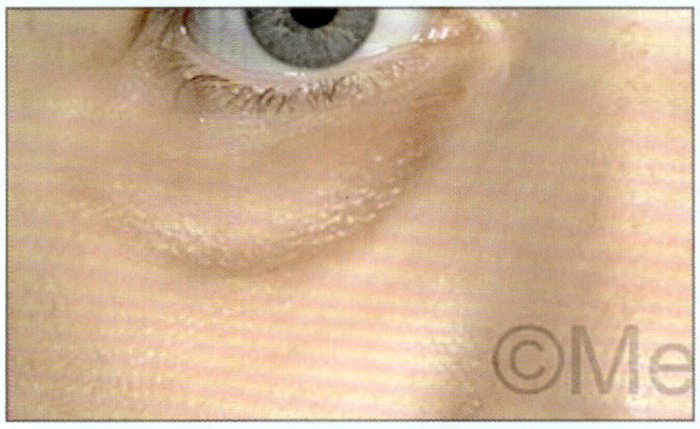

3
Severe hollowness

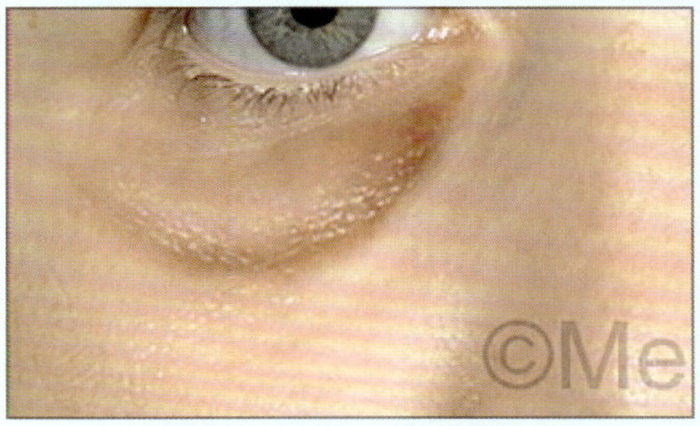

4
Very severe hollowness

10 Appendix

10 Appendix

10.1 Overview of Filler Products and Their Manufacturers

Allergan
Juvéderm® HYDRATE™
Juvéderm® ULTRA® 2
Juvéderm® ULTRA® 3
Juvéderm® ULTRA® 4
Juvéderm® ULTRA® SMILE
Juvéderm® VOLUMA
Juvéderm® VOLBELLA
Juvéderm® VOLIFT

Galderma
Emervel® Touch
Emervel® Classic
Emervel® Lips
Emervel® Deep
Emervel® Volume

Restylane® Skinboosters™ Vital
Restylane® Skinboosters™ Vital Light
Restylane®
Restylane® Perlane
Restylane® Lip Volume
Restylane® SubQ

Merz
BELOTERO® Hydro
BELOTERO® Soft Lidocaine
BELOTERO® Balance Lidocaine
BELOTERO® Intense Lidocaine
BELOTERO® Volume Lidocaine

Hyal® ACP

Radiesse®

Teoxane
TEOSYAL® First lines
TEOSYAL® Global Action
TEOSYAL® Deep Lines
TEOSYAL® Kiss
TEOSYAL® Redensity I
TEOSYAL® Redensity II
TEOSYAL® RHA1
TEOSYAL® RHA2
TEOSYAL® RHA3
TEOSYAL® RHA1
TEOSYAL® Ultimate
TEOSYAL® Ultra Deep
TEOSYAL® Meso

10.2 Addresses of the Manufacturers

Galderma S.A.
Avenue Gratta-Paille 2
CH – 1018 Lausanne
Switzerland

www.galderma.com

www.emervel.com

www.restylane.com

Merz Pharmaceuticals GmbH
Nibelungenplatz 3
60318 Frankfurt/Main
Germany

www.merz.com

www.merzaesthetics.eu

www.belotero.com

www.hyal-acp.de

www.radiesse.com

Pharm-Allergan GmbH
Pforzheimer Str. 160
76275 Ettlingen
Germany

www.allergan.com

www.juvederm.eu

Teoxane S.A.
105, Rue de Lyon
1203 Geneva
Switzerland

info@teoxane.com

www.teoxane.com

10.3 Manufacturer Directory

Omnican® 0.30 x 8 mm, single use insulin syringe with integrated needle: B Braun, Melsungen, Germany

1 ml Luer-Lok® Syringe, syringes: BD, Franklin Lakes, USA

Micro-Fine® 0.30 x 8 mm, insulin syringes: BD, Franklin Lakes, USA

Microlance® 0.30 x 13 mm, needles: BD, Franklin Lakes, USA

Steriject 0.25 x 13 mm, needles: TSK, Tochigi, Japan

Anteis Injection System: Anteis GmbH

VECTRA M3-System: Canfield Imaging Systems, 253 Passaic Ave., Fairfield, NJ 07004, USA

10.4 Image Sources

pp. 2–22:
Prof Dr Uwe Paasch, Leipzig, Germany

p. 58, p. 151, pp. 259–267:
Merz Pharmaceuticals GmbH, Frankfurt/Main, Germany

pp. 75–76:
Markus Karsten, Leipzig, Germany

p. 77:
Canon Deutschland GmbH, Krefeld, Germany

pp. 78–82:
Canfield Imaging Systems

pp. 232–255:
Dr Gerhard Sattler, Darmstadt, Germany

10.5 List of Videos

Title	Book page	QR-Code	URL
Tunneling Technique	102		http://www.kvm-tv.de/FIL/001.mp4
Stretching Technique	105		http://www.kvm-tv.de/FIL/002.mp4
Compression Technique	106		http://www.kvm-tv.de/FIL/003.mp4
VSDT	112		http://www.kvm-tv.de/FIL/004.mp4
Tower Technique	113		http://www.kvm-tv.de/FIL/005.mp4
HAC	115		http://www.kvm-tv.de/FIL/006.mp4
Forehead VSDT	138		http://www.kvm-tv.de/FIL/007.mp4
Glabella VSDT	144		http://www.kvm-tv.de/FIL/008.mp4
Temples DHAC	148		http://www.kvm-tv.de/FIL/009.mp4
Lat-can tunneling	160		http://www.kvm-tv.de/FIL/010mp4

Title	Book page	QR-Code	URL
IOH medially	168		http://www.kvm-tv.de/FIL/011.mp4
IOH laterally	168		http://www.kvm-tv.de/FIL/012.mp4
Bucco-maxillary ligament	180		http://www.kvm-tv.de/FIL/013.mp4
Malar fat pad	180		http://www.kvm-tv.de/FIL/014.mp4
Nasolabial fold DHAC	186		http://www.kvm-tv.de/FIL/015.mp4
Nasolabial fold TT	186		http://www.kvm-tv.de/FIL/016.mp4
Radial lines – stretching	192		http://www.kvm-tv.de/FIL/017.mp4
Mouth corners	204		http://www.kvm-tv.de/FIL/018.mp4
Marionette lines DHAC 2	210		http://www.kvm-tv.de/FIL/019.mp4
Marionette lines VSDT	210		http://www.kvm-tv.de/FIL/020.mp4
Chin superficial injections	214		http://www.kvm-tv.de/FIL/021.mp4

Title	Book page	QR-Code	URL
Chin VSDT	214		http://www.kvm-tv.de/FIL/022.mp4
Jawline VSDT	216		http://www.kvm-tv.de/FIL/023.mp4
Jawline and inferior cheek HAC	216		http://www.kvm-tv.de/FIL/024.mp4
Neck lines tunneling	220		http://www.kvm-tv.de/FIL/025.mp4
Neck lines deep	220		http://www.kvm-tv.de/FIL/026.mp4
Neck elastosis point	222		http://www.kvm-tv.de/FIL/027.mp4
Neck elastosis deep	222		http://www.kvm-tv.de/FIL/028.mp4
Hands point	228		http://www.kvm-tv.de/FIL/029.mp4
Hands DHAC	228		http://www.kvm-tv.de/FIL/030.mp4

10.6 References

Amar R.E., Fox D.M. (2011): The facial autologous muscular injection (FAMI) procedure: an anatomically targeted deep multiplane autologous fat-grafting technique using principles of facial fat injection. Aesthetic Plast Surg 35(4): 502–510.

Anderhuber F. et al. (2012): Anatomie des Menschen. DeGruyter Verlag.

Ascher B. (2008): Injection Treatments in Cosmetic Surgery. Informa Healthcare.

Beer K. R. (2007): Radiesse Nodule of the Lips from a Distant Injection Site. J Drugs Derm 6: 846–847.

Benninghoff A. (1994): Anatomie – Makroskopische Anatomie, Embryologie und Histologie des Menschen. Band 1, Urban & Schwarzenberg.

Berardesca E. et al. (1991): In vivo biophysical characterization of skin physiological differences in races. Dermatologica 182: 89–93.

Bergeret-Galley C. (2004): Comparison of Resorbable Soft Tissue Fillers. Aesthetic Surg J 24: 33–46.

Bergeret-Galley C. et al. (2001) :The value of New Filler Material in Cosmetic and Cosmetic Surgery: Dermalive®. Aesthetic Plast Surg 25: 2429–2255.

Braun C. (2001): Beautycheck – Ursachen und Folgen von Attraktivität. Report. Available from www.beautycheck.de.

Brody H. (2005): Hyaluronidase in the Treatment of Granulomatous Hyaluronic Acid Reactions or Unwanted Hyaluronic Misplacement. Dermatol Surg 31: 893–897.

Carruthers A. et al. (2008): A Validated Brow Positioning Grading Scale. Dermatol Surg 34: 150–154.

Carruthers A. et al. (2008): A Validated Hand Grading Scale. Dermatol Surg 34: 179–183.

Carruthers A. et al. (2008): A Validated Lip Fullness Grading Scale. Dermatol Surg 34: 161–166.

Carruthers A. et al. (2008): A Validated Grading Scale für Crow's Feet. Dermatol Surg 34: 173–178.

Carruthers A. et al. (2008): A Validated Grading Scale für Forehead Lines. Dermatol Surg 34: 155–160.

Carruthers A. et al. (2008): A Validated Grading Scale für Marionette Lines. Dermatol Surg 34: 167–172.

Christensen L. (2007): Normal and Pathologic Tissue reactions to Soft Tissue gel Fillers. Dermatol Surg 33: 168–176.

Donath A. S. et al. (2010): Quantitative Evaluation of Volume Augmentation in the Tear Trough with a Hyaluronic Acid-Based Filler: A Three-Dimensional Analysis. Plastic and Reconstructive Surgery 125, Issue 5: 1515–1522.

Duranti F. et al (1998): Injectable Hyaluronic gel für Soft Tissue Augmentation. Dermatol Surg 24: 1317–1325.

Fitzpatrick R. E. (1999):Treatment of inflamed hypertrophic scar using intralesional 5-FU. Dermatol Surg 25: 224–232.

Gelfer A. et al. (2007): The Natural History of Polymethylmethacrylate Microspheres Granulomas. Dermatol Surg 33: 614–6120.

Goldan O. et al. (2007): Early and Late Complications after a Nonabsorbable Hydrogel Polymer Injection: A Series of 14 Patients and Novel Management. Dermatol Surg 33: 199–206.

Glogau R. G. (1996): Aesthetic and anatomic analysis of the aging skin. Semin Cutan Med Surg 15(3): 134–138.

Halprin K. M. (1972): Epidermal "turnover time" – a re-examination. Br. J. Dermatol. 86: 14–19.

Klein A. W., Glogau R. G. (2006): Injectable Collagen. In: Klein A.W. (ed.): Tissue Augmentation in Clinical Practice. Taylor and Francis, 63–82.

Kligman A.M. (1959): The human hair cycle. J. Invest Dermatol. 33: 307–316.

Kollar E. J. (1970): The induction of hair follicles by embryonic dermal papillae. J. Invest Dermatol. 55: 374–378.

Kulick Michael I. (2010): Evaluation of a Noninvasive, Dual-Wavelength Laser-Suction and Massage Device für the Regional Treatment of Cellulite. Plastic and Reconstructive Surgery 125, Issue 6: 1788–1796.

Lefebvre-Vilardebo M. (2014): Anatomy and hand medical rejuvenation. Expert2expert Medical Publishing.

Lemperle G. et al. (2003): Soft tissue Augmentation with Artecoll®: 10 years History, Indications, Techniques and Complications. Dermatol Surg 29: 573–587.

Lowe N. J. et al. (2005): Adverse Reactions to dermal Fillers: Review. Dermatol Surg 31: 1616–1625.

De Lustro F. et al. (1998): Reaction to Injectable Collagen in Human Subjects. J Dermatol Surg Oncol 14, Suppl. 1: 49.

Monheit G. D. et al. (2009): Digital three-dimensional imaging für quantifiable measurement of lip augmentation with a 24 mg/mL hyaluronic acid gel implant. Journal of the American Academy of Dermatolgoy 60, Issue 3, Suppl. 1, AB187.

Montagna W. et al. (1989): Histology of sun-damaged human skin. J. Am. Acad. Dermatol. 21: 907–918.

Montagna W, Carlisle K. (1991): The architecture of black and white facial skin. J. Am. Acad. Dermatol. 24: 929–937.

Neuber G. A. (1893): Fetttransplantation. Bericht über die Verhandlungen der Deutschen Gesellschaft für Chirurgie. 22: 66.

Nouveau-Richard S. et al. (2005): Skin ageing: a comparison between Chinese and European populations. A pilot study. J. Dermatol. Sci. 40: 187–193.

Palastanga N. et al. (2002): Anatomy and human movement. 4. Auflage, Butterworth-Heinemann.

Pilsl U, et al. (2012): : Anatomy of the cheek: implications for soft tissue augmentation. Dermatologic Surgery 38 (7 Pt 2): 1254–1262.

Radlanski R. J., Wesker K. (2012): Das Gesicht. 2., überarbeitete Auflage. KVM-Verlag.

Reisberger E. M. et al. (2003): Foreign body granulomas caused by polymethylmethacrylate microspheres. Arch Dermatol 139: 17–20.

Rzany B. et al. (2009): Decrease of reported adverse events to injectable polylactic acid after recommending an increased dilution: 8-year results from the Injectable Filler Safety Study. J Cosmet Dermatol 8: 14–18.

Rzany B. et al. (2009): Risk of severe adverse reactions to an injectable filler based on a fixed combination of hydroxyethylmethacrylate and Ethylmethacrylate with hyaluronic acid. Dermatol Surg 35: 367–374.

Rzany B. et al. (2009): The spectrum of adverse reactions after treatment with injectable fillers in the glabellar region: results from the Injectable Filler Safety Study. Dermatol Surg 35, Suppl 2: 1629–1634.

Sasaki G. H. (2010): Quantification of Human Abdominal Tissue Tightening and Contraction After Component Treatments With 1064-nm/1320-nm Laser-Assisted Lipolysis. Clinical Implications. Aesthetic Surgery Journal 30(2): 239–245.

Sattler G. (2010): Bildatlas der ästhetischen Botulinumtoxin-Therapie. KVM-Verlag.

Sawyer R. et al. (2010): Quantitative analysis of normal smile with 3D stereophotogrammetry – an aid to facial reanimation. Journal of Plastic, Reconstructive and Aesthetic Surgery 63, Issue 1: 65–72.

Schünke M. et al. (2009): Prometheus – Kopf, Hals und Neuroanatomie. Thieme.

Sugiyama-Nakagiri Y. et al. (2009): Ethnic differences in the structural properties of facial skin. J. Dermatol. Sci. 53: 135–139.

Taylor A. et al. (2008): Prevalence of pigmentary disorders and their impact on quality of life: a prospective cohort study. J Cosmet. Dermatol. 7: 164–168.

Tepper O. M. et al. (2010): Mammometrics: The Standardization of Aesthetic and Reconstructive Breast Surgery. Plastic and Reconstructive Surgery 125, Issue 1: 393–400.

Wang F. et al. (2007): In vivo stimulation of de novo collagen production caused by cross-linked hyaluronic acid dermal filler injections in photodamaged human skin. Arch Dermatol Feb;143(2): 155–163.

Wiest L. G. et al. (2009): Electron Microscopic Documentation of Late Changes in Permanent Fillers and Clinical Management of Granulomas in Affected Patients. Dermatol Surg 35: 1681–1688.

Wiest L. G. (2009): Spektrum der Komplikationen nach Behandlung mit injizierbaren Füllmaterialien. Der MKG-Chirurg.

Yarbus A. L. (1967): Eye Movements and Vision. New York: Plenum Press.

Zielke H. et al. (2007): Risk Profiles of Different Ionjectable Fillers: Results from the Injectable Filler Safety Study (IFS Study). Dermatol Surg 34:1–10.

10.7 Index

1, 2, 3

A

B

10

10

10

10

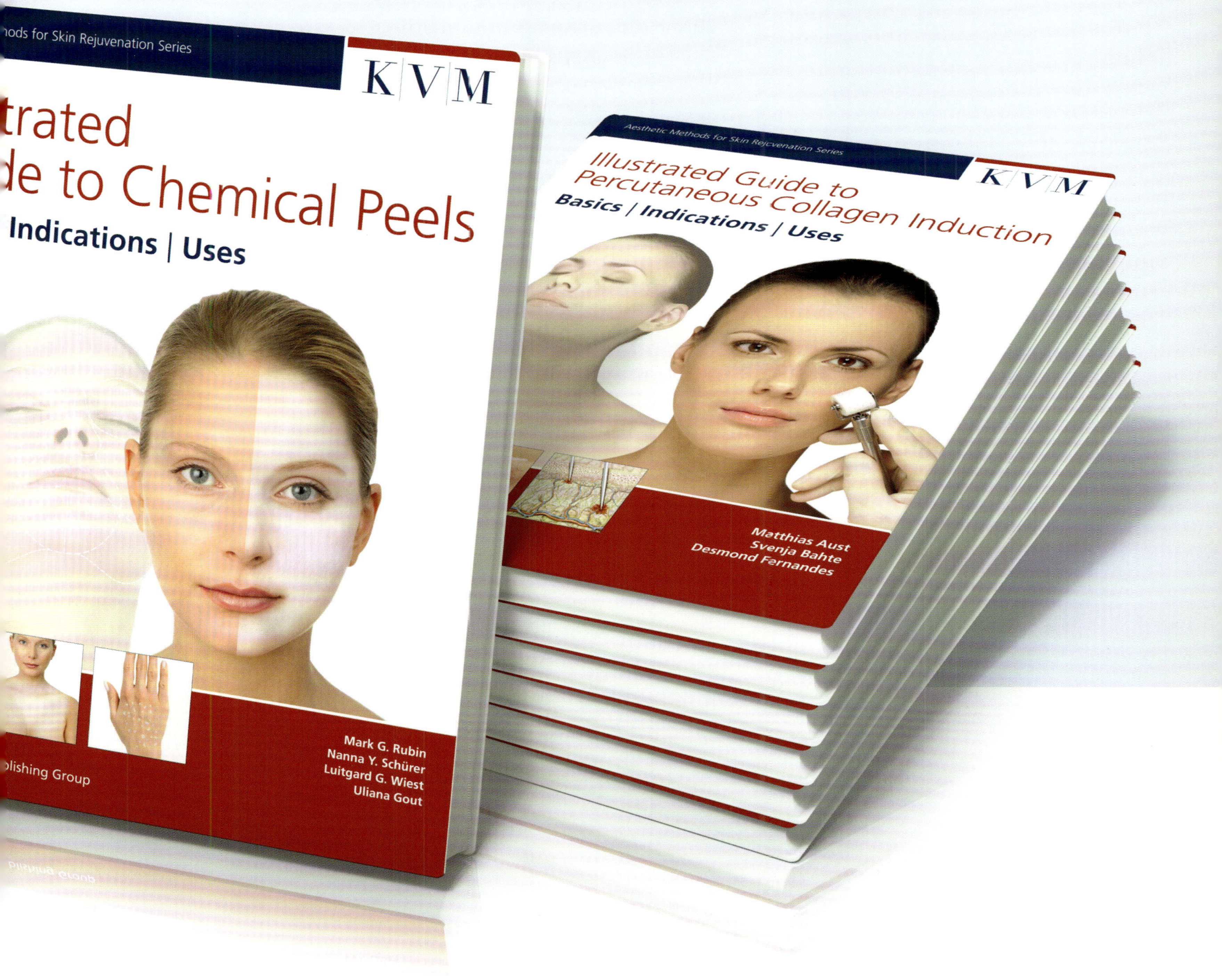

...hods for Skin Rejuvenation Series
KVM
...trated
...de to Chemical Peels
... Indications | Uses
Mark G. Rubin
Nanna Y. Schürer
Luitgard G. Wiest
Uliana Gout
...blishing Group
Aesthetic Methods for Skin Rejuvenation Series
Illustrated Guide to
Percutaneous Collagen Induction
Basics / Indications / Uses
Matthias Aust
Svenja Bahte
Desmond Fernandes